Clinical Education: An Anthology

American Physical Therapy Association
1111 North Fairfax Street
Alexandria, Virginia 22314-1488

ISBN # 0-912452-82-X

For more information about this and other APTA publications, contact the American Physical Therapy Association, 1111 North Fairfax Street, Alexandria, VA 22314-1488.
[Publication No. E-25]

FOREWORD

Growth in Clinical Education in Physical Therapy

This special collection of articles represents the current state of knowledge about clinical education in physical therapy in the following areas: clinical faculty; clinical environment and resources; design of clinical education, evaluation, and research; and academic resources. These clinical topics parallel the content areas addressed in both the American Physical Therapy Association's (APTA's) Plan for Clinical Education 1989-1991 and the Plan for Clinical Education 1992-1994; the articles provided some of the rich resources used in the development of these plans by APTA's Task Force on Clinical Education. The physical therapy literature has grown tremendously in these areas, demonstrating not only the importance of clinical education as a part of the curriculum, but also the extent to which the profession has seen fit to develop its theoretical and research basis in understanding diverse aspects of clinical education.

We wish we could have acknowledged all the individuals who have contributed to the body of literature in clinical education, but space does not permit reprinting of all the literature. A comprehensive bibliography of all related literature is available from APTA in a publication entitled "Clinical Education Resource Guide" (Publication No. P-71).

In reviewing this anthology, it is evident that many questions are posed routinely regarding the effectiveness and efficacy of clinical education. Yet it is also apparent that while we have begun to address some of these questions, we continue to raise new ones requiring further study. Many of the questions have sparked the need for innovative methods of study to expand our knowledge in both quantitative and qualitative measures to answer not only the "what," but also the "how" of what we provide in student clinical education. As we continue to develop our research skills and become more comfortable with alternative methods of exploring questions and developing theory, we will be able to respond to many of the complex questions that arise in the study of clinical education in physical therapy.

Physical therapy has made tremendous strides in the past ten years in developing a theoretical and research foundation in clinical education, and we anticipate that the next ten years will be equally fruitful as physical therapists with a vested interest in clinical education continue to contribute to the literature. We should take pride in the steps already taken, but not be satisfied to rest on our laurels. We anticipate that this anthology will enhance the accessibility and applicability of this knowledge to clinical educators, provide a comprehensive resource for use in clinical faculty development, provide the catalyst for future research in clinical education, and pique the interest of students — our future clinical educators.

We hope this anthology will serve as an inspiration for all involved with clinical education to continue to pose difficult questions and to be excited by the challenge of discovery in how we provide clinical education.

Jody Shapiro Gandy
Director of Clinical Education/Education Systems
American Physical Therapy Association

Table of Contents

Preface

Clinical Faculty

"If patients are to receive the physical therapy services they need now and in the foreseeable future, it will be necessary to utilize existing personnel more effectively and to find ways of preparing future personnel who will know how to spread their services without jeopardizing quality."

Catherine Worthingham, PhD, FAPTA

A Challenge to Clinical Educators: Compendium for Effective Clinical Education

Introduction

The future of the physical therapy profession is largely dependent on the quality of our educational system. Because clinical education is such a major component of this system, ensuring the continued development of clinicians who participate in this phase of curriculum is a high priority. The series of five articles that follows is intended to serve as a resource for physical therapists who wish to become clinical educators or who wish to enhance their existing skills in clinical teaching. The Compendium was designed to offer practical suggestions to address some of the most challenging issues in clinical education, and to stimulate discussion about additional strategies that can enhance the quality of our educational system.

The participating authors have drawn from their experience in the design, implementation, and evaluation of clinical education to prepare their articles. It is clear that an essential step in being a competent clinical educator is first to understand the concepts behind the practical challenges, and then to apply those concepts in individual settings. The articles in this series provide the clinical educator with both a conceptual understanding of issues relevant to professional education as well as a practical guide for improving clinical education in physical therapy. By synthesizing the literature and our experience, we hope to illustrate the complex nature of clinical education, demonstrate the dynamic character of teaching and learning in the clinic, and stimulate the reader's interest in participating in this essential and exciting phase of the professional curriculum.

Susan S Deusinger, PhD, PT
Acting Director
Program in Physical Therapy
Washington University School
of Medicine
St Louis, MO 63110

Resources for Clinical Education: Current Status and Future Challenges

Jan Gwyer, PhD, PT

ABSTRACT: *This article presents a brief overview of the resources available for clinical education in physical therapy. Resources for clinical education exist in the students, the clinical education centers, the clinical faculty, and the curriculum. This background information sets the stage for understanding the current status of physical therapy clinical education. Comparing our current status with objectives for improvement provides a framework for analyzing the strengths and weaknesses of the activities in clinical education and for developing strategies to foster growth in the profession.*

Dr Dwyer is Director of Graduate Studies, Department of Physical Therapy, Duke University, Durham, NC 27710.

RESOURCES IN CLINICAL EDUCATION: WHAT WE HAVE

Adequate resources are an essential component of any successful curriculum or program. Four major categories of resources should be considered in describing the current status of clinical education: the students, the clinical education centers, the clinical faculty, and the curriculum. Resources in each of these areas contribute to the overall quality of the educational experience in the clinic. Analyzing the resources in each of these categories and how these resources are changing will provide a description of the current status of clinical education.

The Students

Students, as the consumers of clinical education, are an essential resource.

Throughout the calendar year in this country there are approximately 11,700 physical therapist and physical therapist assistant students participating in clinical education activities. This pool includes 8,200 physical therapist students enrolled in 125 physical therapist education programs, and 3,500 physical therapist assistant students enrolled in the 90 physical therapist assistant programs (APTA Department of Education, personal communication, October 1989). These figures include all classes enrolled at any one point in time—for example, junior- and senior-year baccalaureate degree students or first-, second-, and third-year master's degree students enrolled in entry-level education programs for physical therapists.

Applicants to our education programs are

bright, capable, and experienced people who frequently pose pertinent questions about the education program's clinical education centers during the admissions process. The applicant pool for physical therapy education remains strong, with an average ratio of five applications to every available position. The 22,500 expected applications this year for approximately 4,100 positions overestimates the ratio of candidates to positions because of duplicate applications, but the actual ratio is probably not less than 3:1 (APTA Department of Education, personal communication, October 1989).

The Clinical Education Centers

A total of over 3,700 clinical education centers was identified by the APTA Department of Education in 1984.[1] This number is double the number of centers identified just 10 years earlier in a study of clinical education in physical therapy by Moore and Perry.[2] An average of 83 clinical education centers affiliate with each education program with a range from 21 to 180 centers.

The majority of education programs report that they choose a clinical education center based on specific criteria. These criteria include the qualifications of the clinical staff, adequate patient or client resources for teaching, the presence of an organized clinical education program, and the commitment of the clinical staff and administration to teaching.[1] Evaluation of these criteria is performed during site visits usually made by the academic coordinator of clinical education (ACCE) prior to beginning an affiliation with the center. The types of centers currently used for clinical education include public schools, pediatric and geriatric day-care centers, business- or industry-based clinics, and research laboratories.

Practice settings used for clinical education have changed in a manner similar to the changes in practice settings of physical therapists. In 1976, Moore and Perry reported that 58% of physical therapist education programs affiliated with home health agencies, 40% with sports physical therapy facilities, and only 3% with private practice physical therapists.[2] Needless to say, these percentages have changed over the years. In the mid-eighties, 77% of the education programs affiliated with home health agencies, 91% with sports physical therapy centers, and 100% with physical therapy private practices.[1] Data on the number and type of clinical education settings used by physical therapy education programs is currently being collected by the APTA.

Several education programs in the United States have clinical education agreements with clinical centers in Canada, Australia, and several countries in Western Europe. In addition, several physical therapy programs assist foreign physical therapy students who wish to complete their education by participating in clinical education in the United States. As no organization is known to be working to facilitate these types of international educational exchanges, these examples constitute purely individual cases. Possibly this is because these arrangements are made more difficult by educational requirements of the academic institutions and by government regulatory agencies. It would not be surprising to find, however, that the severe personnel shortage of physical therapists in the United States would lead health care corporations to pursue this international avenue of recruitment.

Clinical centers, therefore, represent an important resource in the context of physical therapy clinical education. Expansion of the variety and number of sites available to students in clinical education has been a significant product of growth over the last 20 years and continues to be a challenge for the future. This growth represents both an attempt to acquaint students with physical therapy practice in the growing variety of practice settings and an attempt to meet the clinical education needs of the increasing number of enrolled students.

The Clinical Faculty

Clinical faculty members are those persons employed by the clinical center who organize and/or teach in the clinical education center. Consistent with the demographics of physical therapists in practice, the majority of clinical faculty are young and female. A 1985 study of the physical therapy clinical faculty found 72% to be female with a mean age of 34 (range = 22–62).[3] It is customary for the education program to request that all clinical instructors (CIs) have at least one year of experience before teaching students in the clinic, a criterion that generally is feasible to meet and that is important for quality education. One third of our clinical faculty hold academic appointments from the education programs with which their center is affiliated, and some also serve as classroom instructors in an area of specialization. Forty percent of our clinical instructors also teach other types of students as part of their work responsibilities.[3]

Clinical faculty increasingly have been involved in organizing local support and resource groups (consortia) to promote the goals of clinical education. There are 30 or more clinical education consortia in the United States (APTA Department of Education, personal communication, July 1988). These consortia are composed of groups of clinical educators from both academic and clinical settings in a close geographical area. In some instances consortia are organized in a city (eg, in Chicago or Philadelphia), and in some instances consortia serve a state or region (eg, Texas or New England). These consortia allow persons interested in the clinical education of physical therapy students to meet and plan activities, conduct research, and sponsor education programs; all with the aim of improving the quality of clinical education. These consortia have been instrumental in improving the administrative aspects of clinical education (eg, scheduling clinical rotations and sharing information on site visits). They have also helped to improve the educational aspects of clinical education (eg, promoting a standardized method of student performance evaluation[4,5]).

From this author's perspective, the clinical faculty provide the most crucial resource for clinical education. Issues related to the continuing development of clinical faculty will command the majority of our efforts in the future.

The Curriculum

Several typical patterns of curriculum design exist for clinical education in physical therapist education programs. Using the term *clinical education rotation* to describe extended periods of full-time (eight hours per day, five days per week) clinical education, the average number of clinical rotations found in physical therapist education programs is three, with a range from two to five clinical rotations. These rotations are most commonly six weeks in length, although four- and eight-week rotations are also common. The average number of weeks a physical therapist student spends in full-time clinical education is 23, with a range from 15 to 72 weeks (APTA Department of Education, personal communication, October 1989). These clinical rotations occur throughout the calendar year; however, there is a much heavier pattern of usage between the months of January through August, and much lighter use from September through December.[1]

Integrated or part-time (less than eight hours per day and/or less than five days per week) clinical education experiences make up the other portion of clinical education. There appears to be less consensus on exactly what is occurring in this phase of clinical education, as is reflected in the variety of terms used to describe this part of the clinical education program. The terms clerkship, practicum, clinical laboratory, orientation, preceptorship, and pre-clinical have all been used to describe part-time experiences.

These experiences are usually interspersed throughout the curriculum, planned as half days or full days in the clinical setting. Taken together, the average number of days of part-time clinical education is 18, with a range from 3 to 40 days.[1] In the majority of education programs, the physical therapists in the clinical setting serve as the instructors, while in a very few, the academic faculty serve as clinical instructors for the students. The objectives for these part-time education experiences often are planned to allow the student to progress from observer to assistant in carrying out evaluation and treatment procedures with clients or patients. The student often is provided the opportunity to learn about physical therapy practice in a variety of specialty settings during this phase.

Even a passing glance such as this one reveals our clinical education system in physical therapy to be a remarkably large and complex system of communication and cooperation among many professionals. To create a successful learning experience, each student's affiliation depends on a sequence of numerous contacts in the planning stage, followed by many hours of preparation and implementation. When this is multiplied by the 10,000 students engaged in this process across the country, one understands the scope of this portion of our education system.

A closer look at what is current in clinical education would reveal a tremendous amount of creativity and sophistication in teaching and evaluation techniques. Examples of alternative teaching strategies include mock clinics, students teaching students, and individually planned and taught in-services. Some of the best educational research in physical therapy has taken advantage of the tremendous teaching resources and flexibility found in the clinical environment to design and evaluate new teaching techniques.[6-8] Investigators have studied the most effective theories of teaching and learning in the clinical setting, methods of giving feedback to the student, methods of evaluating student performance, and the characteristics of successful clinical teachers from the perspective of students and practitioners.[9-11] These advances in creative approaches to clinical teaching have resulted in a wealth of resources to foster the continued development of clinical education in physical therapy.

IMPROVING PHYSICAL THERAPY CLINICAL EDUCATION: WHAT WE WANT

Recognizing these numerous resources for clinical education does not eliminate the need to make projections about our future needs. The five goals in the areas of clinical faculty training and curriculum design presented below represent recognition of future resource concerns in physical therapy clinical education.

Clinical Faculty Training

1. Develop a credentialing process for clinical instructors. In addition to possessing clinical expertise, clinical faculty need to have a basic understanding of educational principles and demonstrated skill in teaching in the clinical setting. The responsibility for developing clinical instructors has been shared by the education program and the clinical center but has never been formalized to ensure consistent qualifications among clinical faculty.

Because physical therapists are geographically mobile, a national system to credential clinical instructors would balance the resources available for clinical faculty development at various education programs. Systems have been suggested that would credential persons for their respective roles as clinical instructor, center coordinator, and academic coordinator. Suggested methods of implementation range from on-site training courses to home-study or correspondence courses.[12]

2. Develop instructors with more clinical expertise. In the 1985 survey of clinical faculty, 41% of the clinical education faculty reported that they had less than one year's experience when they began to teach physical therapy students in the clinic.[3] With the shortage of personnel in some clinical settings, this percentage of inexperienced clinical instructors may increase. Montgomery has proposed a model for clinical education that would utilize experienced or master clinician/teachers as clinical instructors. These individuals would have "recognized proficiency in patient care" and would develop an expertise in clinical teaching prior to instructing a student in the clinic.[13(p7)] This model of clinical education would be characterized by a much smaller number of very prestigious clinical education centers and instructors. Although each center would teach a large number of students, it is doubtful that this model would meet the clinical education needs of an increasing number of students. Alternative models for increasing the clinical expertise of instructors should be considered.

Curriculum Design

1. Develop a national system of assigning clinical rotations. Given the numbers of students and clinical centers involved in physical therapy clinical education, some feel that a national system of clinical education rotation assignments is indicated. The system envisioned would model the medical residency matching program that employs a computerized system to match medical residents with approved clinical sites. To be feasible, two other goals may have to proceed this one: 1) developing a system of accrediting clinical education centers, and 2) (possibly) lengthening the clinical rotation period. Accrediting clinical education centers nationwide would require extensive resources to implement even the most simplistic paper-and-pencil evaluation process, not to mention the potentially prohibitive costs of incorporating site visits into the process. A rotation period longer than the typical six to eight weeks would be necessary to justify the resources needed to develop such a matching system.

2. Expand the length of time spent in clinical rotations. Our profession continues to consider whether it is appropriate to prescribe a minimum length of time for full-time clinical education experiences to be required in accredited education programs. This debate is fueled by the position that there now is insufficient full-time clinical education to accomplish the goals and objectives of the curriculum. It is argued that today's physical therapy student is not given sufficient experience in the administrative aspects of physical therapy practice during clinical rotations (eg, billing and scheduling procedures and supervision of support personnel).

More time is also needed for the complete professional socialization of the physical therapist student. There is a difference between a student who is technically competent and one who feels and acts with the moral commitments of a professional physical therapist. Achieving this goal requires a much more subtle and time-consuming process.

3. Improve methods of evaluating student performance in the clinic. Mechanisms to provide written and verbal feedback about a student's performance are abundant in physical therapy clinical education. We are constantly striving to improve our evaluation instruments and procedures, to make them more reliable and valid and easier to implement. The new trend in student performance evaluation is toward multiple methods of evaluation (eg, combining an objective written test on the topic of degenerative joint disease with an observation of a patient treatment session to evaluate the student's knowledge and skills in management of patients with this diagnosis). A more detailed discussion of the multimethod approach to evaluation of student performance will be found in a subsequent article in this journal.

CONCLUSION

The number of students involved in clinical education in physical therapy and the number and type of clinical centers participating in clinical education continues to increase. While this expansion adds resources to the clinical education program, it also accentuates the need for improving the clinical education program in two other areas: the quality of the clinical faculty and the patterns of curriculum design in clinical education. This article summarized the current status of clinical education resources and presented several goals for improving the quality of this important portion of the education program.

The external and internal forces affecting physical therapy clinical education may influence the achievement of some of our goals. In this period of shortages of physical therapy personnel in hospitals, more and more students may find themselves on clinical rotations in settings with reduced resources for patient care and education. One of the most critical characteristics of learning in the clinic—time with a patient—may not be available to the extent we would wish because of these staffing problems, an increased emphasis on productivity, and the reluctance of health insurance carriers to support the education of health care personnel.

Physical therapy educators must have accurate information regarding the profession's expectations of entry-level physical therapists and must design clinical and didactic education portions of the curriculum to produce a graduate with these skills and abilities. Working within the constraints of the health care system, academic and clinical faculty are challenged to develop clinical education programs that strengthen and promote the missions of our profession. Effective use of our current and future resources is essential for the development of clinical education programs that meet the expectations of the profession and the public. The following articles in this Compendium provide guidelines for using the resources described here.

REFERENCES

1. Current Patterns for Providing Clinical Education in Physical Therapy Education. Alexandria, VA, American Physical Therapy Association, 1985

2. Moore ML, Perry JF: Clinical Education in Physical Therapy: Present Status, Future Needs. Washington, DC, American Physical Therapy Association, 1976

3. Report on the Clinical Education Faculty in Physical Therapy Education, 1985. Alexandria, VA, American Physical Therapy Association, 1986

4. Kondela PM, Hatmaker T: Experience with a consortium for exploring and arranging clinical education programs. Phys Ther 58:156–158, 1978

5. Radtka S, Dragotta N, Needham S, et al: Texas consortium for physical therapy clinical education: A model for interinstitutional consortium arrangements. Phys Ther 63:971–974, 1983

6. Scully RM, Shepard KF: Clinical teaching in physical therapy education: An ethnographic study. Phys Ther 63:349–358, 1983

7. Sanders BR, Ruvolo JF: Mock clinic: An approach to clinical education. Phys Ther 61:1163–1167, 1981

8. Jacobson B: Role modeling in physical therapy. Phys Ther 54:244–250, 1974

9. Wightman ML, Wellock LM: Method of developing and evaluating a clinical performance program for physical therapy interns. Phys Ther 56:1125–1128, 1976

10. Emery MJ: Effectiveness of the clinical instructor: Student's perspective. Phys Ther 64:1079–1083, 1984

11. Henry JN: Using feedback and evaluation effectively in clinical supervision: Model for interaction characteristics and strategies. Phys Ther 65:354–357, 1985

12. Perry JF: Who is responsible for preparing clinical educators? In: Pivotal Issues in Clinical Education: Present Status/Future Needs. Alexandria, VA, American Physical Therapy Association, 1988

13. Montgomery J: Clinical faculty: Revitalization for 2001. In: Pivotal Issues in Clinical Education: Present Status/Future Needs. Alexandria, VA, American Physical Therapy Association, 1988

Establishing Clinical Education Programs: A Practical Guide

Susan S Deusinger, PhD, PT

ABSTRACT: This article evaluates the incentives that may attract physical therapists to participate in clinical education and the considerations needed to establish a program. Practical suggestions for creating an environment that promotes learning and fosters competence in clinical teaching are given. Self-assessment is emphasized as an appropriate process to determine readiness to start a clinical education program and to ascertain success in implementing quality clinical education.

Dr Deusinger is Acting Director, Program in Physical Therapy, Washington University School of Medicine, 660 S Euclid Ave, St. Louis, MO 63110.

INTRODUCTION

Participating in physical therapy clinical education is both an exceptional opportunity and a significant responsibility. This article offers suggestions about how to utilize our professional resources to design and implement quality clinical education programs. These suggestions are as relevent for clinical faculty who wish to alter or expand existing programs as they are for individuals interested in establishing new clinical education programs.

WHY BECOME INVOLVED?

Incentives to participate in clinical education have both tangible and intangible facets. From this author's perspective, intangible incentives are primarily responsible for a center's (or an individual's) decision to begin a clinical education program. Professional values for excellence in patient care and the desire to instill the same values in future colleagues motivates many clinicians to participate and to demonstrate a long-term commitment to quality clinical education in physical therapy. Both tangible and intangible incentives must be present, however, for a good clinical education program to be maintained.

The quality of patient care services offered by physical therapists can, in fact, be enhanced by incorporating students into the clinical environment.[1] By sharing record-keeping protocols, equipment designs, ideas for staffing patterns, and patient-evaluation schemas, the knowledge and experience bases of both faculty and students are enhanced. Students generally share these ideas with future colleagues in later clinical rotations and employment positions, a process that results in continual development for the profession.

The impact of role modeling by clinical faculty continues to be recognized as a powerful source of influence in professional education.[2] Students adopt both personal and professional characteristics of clinical faculty whom they perceive as competent clinicians, and incorporate these characteristics into behavioral repertoires that eventually lead to full professional status.[3] The cycle of influence that is created between students and clinical faculty not only serves the goals of professional education, but of practice as a whole.

In addition to being an effective educational process, role modeling also has been shown to yield significant personal and professional rewards for clinical faculty.[4] In addition to the satisfaction of seeing a student learn to be a competent practitioner, many clinical faculty find that the responsibility to model effective clinical behaviors actually serves as a stimulus for their own professional development. Through contact with students, clinical faculty have access to modern theories of practice and innovative approaches to patient care—a benefit often as valuable as other, more expensive forms of continuing education.

There is evidence that students often return as employees to facilities in which they have had positive clinical education experiences.[5] Thus, developing a clinical education program may have recruitment benefits to the facility. Although ideally not the primary reason for developing a program, facilitating recruitment is a professional concern of many physical therapists. A subsequent article in this Compendium will discuss the financial benefits in areas of recruitment and orientation when a site has a clinical education program—benefits of interest to administrators who are deciding whether to support development of a program.

Other incentives for a site to participate in a clinical education program include having access to educational materials, obtaining discounts for continuing education, and arranging consultation for the design of clinical research projects. The development of collegial relationships with academic faculty who offer additional professional perspectives may also occur as a result of establishing a clinical education program. These relationships inevitably enhance individual and collective growth.[1,4,6,7]

Additional benefits may ensue for practitioners interested in establishing a clinical education program if a site is located geographically close to a physical therapy education program. Many clinical faculty members receive library privileges, use of recreational facilities, tuition reimbursement for graduate studies, permission to audit new courses in the physical therapy curriculum, and the opportunity to serve as teaching assistants in the academic environment. Although they may be secondary incentives to participating in clinical education, these benefits do contribute to the resources a clinician has for professional development[1] and serve as rewards for maintaining a program over time.

Thus, developing a clinical education program has numerous benefits for the clinician who is interested in influencing the future status of the profession. The opportunity to serve as a role model and to become involved in collegial exchange with both students and academic faculty yields both tangible and intangible rewards. With the expansion of existing programs and development of new educational programs, ample opportunities exist for clinicians to participate in clinical education.

HOW DOES A SITE BECOME INVOLVED?

The potential exists in *all* physical therapy settings to provide quality clinical education. The basic ingredients for effective clinical education include an interest in promoting physical therapy through quality professional education, an efficient and ethical patient care service, a commitment to growth and development as a clinician and teacher, and a measure of administrative support. It is essential that the profession recognizes the value of developing clinical education programs in a wide variety of settings and geographic locations. This enables the responsibility for clinical education to be widely dispersed throughout the profession and to reflect the current trends in the health care system.

An effective clinical education program is grounded in clearly established philosophies of education and practice.[8] Both academic and clinical personnel must agree on a basic philosophy that will guide both patient care and education planning.[9] Ethical principles, standards of practice, institutional policies, expectations of the academic and clinical facilities, and individual preferences in teaching style should be examined honestly to determine whether a good "fit" can be achieved between the educational institution and the clinical site. To facilitate this, the academic coordinator of clinical education (ACCE) should provide information about the curriculum, the performance outcomes expected, and the benefits available to clinical faculty; in turn, the site should share procedures that affect students, evidence of administrative support, and expectations of the clinical institution.[10]

Establishing a clinical education program also requires negotiation of a legal agreement to protect the clinical site, the educational institution, and the individuals who teach and learn in the program.[8] Clinical sites already affiliated with educational institutions because of training programs in nursing or medicine may find that the legal framework for a clinical education program in physical therapy already exists. If not, this framework can generally be negotiated for any site willing to take the initiative to develop a program. Appropriate caution should be taken to determine the areas of protection necessary for each party (eg, malpractice coverage for students and faculty).

Because many educational programs are in urban regions, clinical sites in these areas may be overutilized and called on to take excessive numbers of students. As a result, rural or nontraditional settings may be underutilized.[8,10] An active effort to identify sites ready to establish or revitalize clinical education programs would assist the profession in serving all consumer groups. Although the ACCE often contacts potential clinical sites to determine interest in and feasibility of developing a clinical education relationship, this initial contact can be made just as legitimately by the site. Students also are a resource in making suggestions about sites that have specialized expertise, desirable geographical locations, or other attributes that contribute to quality education. Thus, an open attitude toward the types of sites that could be suitable for clinical education programs is essential.

Opportunities for quality clinical education abound in physical therapy because of the wide distribution of practice settings and the commitment to seeing the profession grow in the health care system. Developing an affiliation with an educational institution entails an initial period of discussion about goals, philosophy, and expected benefits of participating in clinical education. Legal agreements should not be negotiated until consensus has been reached about these issues. Once consensus is reached, planning can proceed for full development of the program.

HOW SHOULD A SITE PREPARE?

Self-assessment tools are useful in determining the specific strengths, limitations, and resources of a clinical site. Use of such tools is highly recommended before developing a clinical education program, and is very important for existing programs interested in modifying their design. A format for evaluating a clinical site's environment is provided in *Standards for Clinical Education in Physical Therapy: A Manual for Evaluation and Selection for Clinical Education Centers.*[11] This is an excellent resource for identifying specific criteria most academic institutions seek when developing a new clinical education site. These standards were developed with input received from both academic and clinical faculty throughout the nation[12] and are considered to be essential for providing quality clinical education. The Table lists characteristics that represent the 20 standards validated by Barr, Gwyer, and Talmor.[11]

Using these guidelines, a site can identify whether resources are sufficient to develop a clinical education program. Action should be taken to identify the impact each limitation in the learning environment may have on students and to modify the environment to make optimum use of current resources. Space, for example, is often a problem in clinical facilities. Increasing space allotments in the physical therapy department may not be in the purview of the clinical educator. Underutilized space elsewhere in the facility, however, may be identified as suitable for documentation, individual study, and instructor-student conferences. Clinical faculty should, therefore, look broadly for resources to meet the standards for quality learning environments.

Staffing is another resource of concern to many clinical sites when considering the development of a clinical education program. Innovative staffing patterns may be developed to address the needs of both patients and students. An effective learning environment can be created even in view of job sharing, split shifts, itinerant schedules, and other staffing idiosyncrasies. Recruitment and retention of clinical staff actually may be enhanced by the existence of a good clinical education program.[1] Sites where clinical education programs have been made a priority have access to applicant pools and sources of professional development not available to sites that do not serve students.

Developing a clinical education program may serve as an effective stimulus for change in the profession. Benefits accrue to the clinical facility as well as to the individual clinician who wants to develop expertise in

clinical teaching. Adding consultation from other clinicians and from academic faculty to the results of self-assessment may be important in preparing an environment that promotes student learning and in proceeding to set goals, establish objectives, and select specific learning experiences that would meet these objectives.

PROGRAM DESIGN: MODELS AND GUIDELINES

The design of clinical education programs should include systematic steps of planning, implementing, and evaluating learning experiences. Perry[13] outlined a useful eight-step process for designing learning experiences in clinical education. Her model of curriculum design applies principles from the literature to the specific case of clinical education. It prescribes collaboration between academic and clinical faculty in determining objectives for students, and recognition of differences in performance expectations for students in early, intermediate, and advanced phases of clinical education. It requires faculty to identify resource constraints at the clinical site before learning experiences are planned, and to have an organized sequence of activities that lead to achievement of terminal objectives. Finally, Perry specifies ongoing and frequent evaluation of the entire clinical education program to facilitate planning for improvements.[13]

The perspective of the clinician who wants to design a clinical education program has received attention because it is essentially the clinician's responsibility to implement the day-to-day operations of clinical education.[9,12] Accepting this responsibility has widespread implications for the site, the individual clinician, and the profession at large. Recognition of the pressures placed on clinicians for productivity, for professional development in areas other than clinical education, and for sharing in adminis-

tration of the department is essential for a clinical education program to be maintained over time. Adjustments in student and patient scheduling, in objectives for the program, and in lines of communication between the academic institution and the clinic may be necessary in view of these additional constraints.

Adoption of a model for planning and implementing a clinical education program is a wise decision for both academic and clinical institutions. Systematic design and evaluation of program elements is characteristic of quality clinical education. Input from all individuals involved is a necessary prerequisite for a program to serve the needs of academic and clinical institutions, students, clinicians, and ultimately the consumers who benefit from training of competent practitioners.

CONCLUSION

Clinical education is a key component in the preparation of competent physical therapists. Incentives for active involvement in clinical education are numerous, and the rewards are significant. Assessment of existing and potential resources that could enhance the learning environment of a clinical facility is an essential phase of developing a clinical education program and should precede contract negotiation. After a commitment to clinical education is made, full implementation of a quality clinical education program requires careful planning, coordination of resources at both academic and clinical institutions, and sufficient flexibility to enable appropriate responses to the dynamic, changing health care system in which clinical education occurs.

ACKNOWLEDGMENT

Appreciation is extended to Louise Huebusch, who contributed to the formulation

TABLE
Characteristics of Quality Clinical Education Sites[a]

An invigorating environment
Learning objectives targeted to specific needs
Ethical practices in the clinic
Congruent philosophy of site and school
Administrative support
Effective staff communications
Professional development and commitment
Sufficient support services
Adequate space and staff
Commitment to self-assessment

[a]Adapted from Barr JS, Gwyer J, Talmor Z: *Standards for Clinical Education in Physical Therapy: A Manual for Evaluation and Selection of Clinical Education Centers.*[11]

of these ideas while she was director of clinical education, Department of Physical Therapy and Exercise Science, State University of New York at Buffalo.

REFERENCES

1. Holder L: Paying for clinical education: Fact or fiction? J Allied Health 17(8):221–229, 1988
2. Jacobson B: Role modeling in physical therapy. Phys Ther 54:244–250, 1974
3. Emery MJ: Effectiveness of the clinical instructor: Students' perspectives. Phys Ther 64:1079–1083, 1984
4. Baker MA: Rewards and benefits for clinical faculty.

In: Pivotal Issues in Clinical Education: Present Status/Future Needs. Alexandria, VA, American Physical Therapy Association, 1988
5. Ciccone CD, Wolfner ML: Clinical affiliations and postgraduate job selection: A survey. Clinical Management in Physical Therapy 8:16–17, 1988
6. Hawken PL, Hillestad EA: Weighing the costs and the benefits of student education to service. Nursing and Health Care, April 1987, pp 223–227
7. Hillestad EA, Hawken PL: Weighing the costs and benefits of student education to service agencies: Part 2. Nursing and Health Care, May 1988, pp 277–281
8. Moore ML, Perry JF: Clinical Education in Physical Therapy: Present Status/Future Needs. Washington, DC, Section for Education, American Physical Therapy Association, 1976

9. Windom P: Developing a clinical education program from the clinician's perspective. Phys Ther 62:1604–1609, 1982
10. Sanders B: Implications for clinical centers. In: Planning for Clinical Education in 1990. Alexandria, VA, American Physical Therapy Association, 1984
11. Barr JS, Gwyer J, Talmor Z: Standards for Clinical Education in Physical Therapy: A Manual for Evaluation and Selection of Clinical Education Centers. Washington, DC, American Physical Therapy Association, 1981
12. Barr JS, Gwyer J, Talmor Z: Evaluation of clinical education centers in physical therapy. Phys Ther 62:850–861, 1982
13. Perry JF: A model for designing clinical education. Phys Ther 61:1427–1432, 1981

Teaching Students in the Clinical Setting: Managing the Problem Situation

Lynn Foord, MEd, MS, PT
Marilyn DeMont, MS, PT

ABSTRACT: Managing problem learning situations is a challenge for all clinical educators. This article presents a series of steps that can guide the clinical education team to identify and remediate student performance problems. Objective documentation, thorough analysis of the problem etiology, and comprehensive planning for a program of remediation are emphasized.

INTRODUCTION

The overall goal of clinical education is to produce a professional who will consistently provide quality patient care.[1] Clinical education becomes most challenging when the student has difficulty demonstrating expected levels of performance. Many difficult situations in clinical education can be effectively avoided or managed through a problem-solving team approach. This article describes a practical sequence of steps that clinical educators may use to address problem learning situations.

THE CLINICAL EDUCATION TEAM

Participation by all team members in this problem-solving process promotes a sup-

Ms Foord is Assistant Professor and Academic Coordinator of Clinical Education at Simmons College, 300 The Fenway, Boston, MA 02115. Ms DeMont is Assistant Professor and Academic Coordinator of Clinical Education at Boston University, Boston, MA 02115.

portive environment for the complete integrated learning of clinical practice.[2] The roles and responsibilities of the clinical education team are complex and interrelated; close coordination of all individuals is essential for a positive learning environment. The team should include the clinical instructor (CI), the student, the Center Coordinator of Clinical Education (CCCE), and the Academic Coordinator of Clinical Education (ACCE).

Effective clinical teaching, like clinical practice, involves facilitating behavioral change in the learner.[3] Although the CI and the student collaborate to plan the learning experiences, each individual has distinct responsibilities to ensure quality education. The student reviews all didactic material pertinent to that clinical setting, honestly and accurately self-assesses his or her level of skill and knowledge, actively participates in the experiences provided, asks questions that facilitate learning, and provides feedback to the clinical instructor as to what was attained from the experience. The clinical instructor is responsible first to his or her patients, but also carries significant responsibility for the student. A clinical instructor's responsibility to the student is to direct the student's learning with input from the student and to assess the student's ability to practice safely and effectively.[2,3]

The CCCE and the ACCE are responsible to both the CI and the student. Both the

CCCE and the ACCE are responsible for providing information and resources, for facilitating problem solving and communication among all team members, and for providing support to both the clinical instructor and the student. They function as ombudsmen, sounding boards, facilitators, and problem solvers. Finally, the ACCE, with the input of all the team members, is ultimately responsible for grading the student.

In addition to these responsibilities, each team member shares in three phases of problem solving in clinical education: 1) defining and analyzing the problem, 2) managing the problem, and 3) assessing outcomes. A sequential progression through these phases ensures a comprehensive approach to learning problems. Activities within each of these phases is illustrated below.

DEFINING AND ANALYZING THE PROBLEM

Initial assessment of a student requires sharp observation skills, a trust in one's intuitive senses, and a volume of nonjudgmental documentation. Documentation may take a variety of forms. A simple chronological diary of observations is usually a good start (Fig. 1). There are other formats that allow for a response from the student or organize the information in a manner similar to a flowsheet, thus placing the various incidents in perspective with one another.

Figure 1

The diary format for documentation

> **8/21/89**
>
> Followed all activities on the first day of orientation schedule. Daphne seems very easy to get along with and seems to feel comfortable with me. Plan to co-treat patients tomorrow. Daphne asked to be prepared for shoulder monitor, which she has done at past affil.
>
> **8/31/89**
>
> Daphne to re-eval Mr. "B," as I had told her on Friday. (Mr. "B" is returning with recurrent arthritic changes in his left shoulder after a motorcycle accident 16 months ago. He's been at his vacation house for a month). A straightforward upper quadrant eval.
>
> She took his history fairly well; although he "fed" her a lot of information. ROM done supine and some in sitting, but didn't eval either position completely; documentation was not accurate for which position. Forgot some MMT tests; most grades accurate.
>
> She put him on a HP, then came to find me to ask what treatments I wanted her to do. I told her I wanted her to do what *she* thought would be most appropriate and effective. She looked absolutely lost; "I've never seen this type of patient before. I don't know what he needs."

The Anecdotal Form (Fig. 2) and the Critical Incident Form (Fig. 3) are useful for these purposes.[4]

The student's level of performance must be identified accurately to provide appropriate learning experiences. Problem situations may first manifest themselves as apparently inconsequential or unrelated incidents. These incidents, when documented and later reviewed as a whole, often provide a clearer picture of the deficits in the student's safe and effective delivery of care. Careful documentation, initiated at the beginning of a student's experience, lays the framework for planning appropriate learning experiences and may effectively highlight a problematic behavior pattern that becomes apparent only when otherwise isolated incidents coalesce. Identifying these apparent deficits early can help to redirect the student's learning.

Analyzing a problem learning situation is a complex endeavor, which ultimately will challenge the skills and creativity of each member of the clinical education team. It is useful for all members to begin by diagnosing the stage at which the student is learning. The student's *stage of learning* refers to the maturity with which the student is able to learn in the clinical setting.[5,6]

In the earliest stage of clinical learning, *exposure*, the student functions as a novice, dependent on the CI for all aspects of instruction. As the student progresses in background knowledge and skill, he or she is able to participate in both the planning and the evaluation of a learning experience. In the second stage, *acquisition*, the student shares the responsibility for the learning experience with the CI. The most mature level of learning is *integration*, in which the student takes the primary responsibility for planning, implementing, and evaluating his

or her own learning experience. Knowing these stages assists the clinical education team in targeting expectations at appropriate levels.

The continued development of a professional depends on an ability to perform and interact in the three domains of learning. In the *cognitive* domain, the professional develops background information, as well as the ability to apply it in a variety of situations. Development of physical skill requires practitioners to perform in the *psychomotor* domain. Well-developed skills in interpersonal interactions involve a knowledge of self and one's values as described in the *affective* domain.[7]

Assessing the student's level of learning and the domain in which the problem resides are useful beginnings for the CI seeking to analyze a problem situation. There are additional analyses, familiar to the experienced clinician, which may also yield useful information. Questions that may further illuminate a learning problem include 1) Does the student have any secondary gain from the problem behaviors? 2) Under what circumstances does the problematic behavior occur? 3) Is there anything the CI is doing that supports the student's behavior? The example below illustrates how these different concepts can be applied by the clinical educator.

A PROBLEM SITUATION

Daphne is a physical therapy student in the second of three eight-week affiliations.

Figure 2

Anecdotal Record Form for documentation

> Date: 9/13/90
>
> Student: Daphne Rogers
> Evaluator: Jessica Williams
>
> **Setting:** M.C. is a 53 y.o. with L mastectomy 7/13/89, returned to clinic for review of exercises and treatment for decreased ROM and strength. She told Daphne that she couldn't do her exercises or treatment lying down because she had had a small (benign) skin cancer removed from her back and she was unable to lie on her back. Daphne's response was to show considerable creativity in thinking of ways to get M.C. to lie on her back; however, M.C. ultimately refused.
>
> **Student Action or Behavior:** Daphne was unable to modify M.C.'s tx program for positions other than supine. She hesitantly attempted several motions, stopped, changed positions, started again, and stopped. She continually looked to me to take over. I made several very specific suggestions and demonstrated some techniques for Daphne to follow. She then was able to complete only those exercises. Daphne did not adapt or change M.C.'s home program in any other way.
>
> **Evaluator Interpretation:** Daphne appears to be unable to adapt a treatment program. She appears apprehensive and gives up too easily without trying other options. When Daphne feels uncertain, she displays panic to her patient by stammering, physically withdrawing, and fumbling. Daphne needs to be prepared to adjust different treatments to meet the patient's needs, to learn not to panic when uncertain, and to be certain to elicit the patient's confidence at all times. Daphne's lack of confidence was conveyed to M.C., who seemed unnerved by the interaction and somewhat frustrated by Daphne's attempts at coercing her to lie on her back.
>
> _____   _____
> Student's signature   Evaluator's signature
>
> **Student's Comments:** I just didn't know what to do this time, because it was so unexpected. I do know how to adapt treatments; I just was caught by surprise this time. I would think that if a patient can't be treated, she shouldn't come in. I don't think she was aware that I wasn't sure what to do next. I think I would do better if the supervisor would just show me what to do when something happens that I haven't done before.

She has been working in a dynamic community hospital in the outpatient department. Within the first week, Daphne's CI, Jessica, notes that Daphne's performance in evaluation skills and treatment planning tends to be inconsistent. Jessica makes the following notes in her clinical education diary:

9-4 D. evaluated 35-yr-old police officer S/P medial meniscus repair. Eval was complete. Rx program safe and effective. Next patient was 53-yr-old housewife S/P L mastectomy returning to clinic for re-eval of ex program, also needs increased strength and ROM. Pt. was unable to perform exercises in supine. D. unable to adapt exercises, change Rx program. D. carried out specific "suggestions" I made for exercises.

9-8 D. continues to be effective with LE evals and Rx plans, but performance with UE involvement is problematic. ROM measurements are at least 10 degrees different from mine; her eval techniques are disorganized, time consuming; incomplete ROM and soft tissue assessment. Rx all pts with UE problems with HP, US, then she comes to me for help. When given accurate and complete eval findings, D. is unable to plan a treatment without significant help. She seems fairly independent in managing pts with LE problems.

This sort of inconsistent performance has continued throughout the first two to three weeks, and Jessica has tried a variety of techniques to help Daphne improve her performance. Daphne, however, continues to rely heavily on Jessica for input. During their weekly conference, Daphne listens carefully to Jessica's opening remarks about problem areas, and then asks her if she can have this Friday off to get ready for a party she is having on the weekend. The day Daphne has requested is the day on which her midterm evaluation has been scheduled. Jessica is perplexed by Daphne's response and tells Daphne that they will discuss these matters the next day.

However perplexed she might be, Jessica is now certain that a problem situation is brewing. She reviews her observation of Daphne up to this time and uses both an Anecdotal Form (Fig. 2) and a Critical Incident Form (Fig. 3) to more formally record the problem she has observed. She now is prepared to manage the problem situation.

MANAGING THE PROBLEM SITUATION
Seeking Information

Once a problem has been recognized, it is important for each member of the team to collaborate in its management. Jessica has begun by assessing the student's performance and documenting the behavior patterns that are interfering with Daphne's safe and effective delivery of care.

Jessica's next step might be to consult other individuals of the team. The CCCE generally has more experience in clinical teaching and is well-acquainted with the learning opportunities at the site. The CCCE can offer enormous support to the CI by assisting in further analysis of Daphne's problems. The CCCE might observe the student in her work with patients and then help Jessica develop her statements about the student's problems. The CCCE might also speak with Daphne to gather information about her opinion of the situation and to see that any issues concerning personality or supervisory style have been addressed and are not affecting the interpretation of Daphne's problems. Finally, the CCCE can work with the CI on her documentation to be sure that the documentation of the situation is as complete and objective as possible.

The ACCE can also assist in managing problem learning situations. The ACCE can encourage all members of the team to focus on changing the problem behaviors into desirable behaviors. By consulting with the CCCE, the CI, and the student, the ACCE can collate observations made by each team member and formulate a comprehensive picture of the problem situation. Based on the information collected, the ACCE can suggest the most realistic goals for Daphne, taking into consideration background information on both her academic and clinical experiences.

Implementing a program to correct performance in the clinic requires cooperation of all team members. The CCCE can support the CI to work with the student on a day-to-day basis. This support might take the form of a reduced caseload or regularly-scheduled meetings for assessing the progress made by the student. If possible, the CCCE might also observe the CI and the student working together to offer feedback to the CI as she creates an optimal learning environment for the student.

Throughout the remediation program, the ACCE must remain in close contact with the student, listening to the student's perspective on the problem, supporting the student's efforts, and facilitating the remediation process. The ACCE can present the problem situation to the student and assist the student in developing the most appropriate goals for behavior and performance. When there is a discrepancy between the student's report of the situation and the report given by the CCCE or the CI, it is the role of the ACCE to clarify the behaviors or skills at the heart of the problem. All planning should focus on these identified problems and how they can be resolved.

By working together, the ACCE and the CCCE can coordinate the program. To remedy Daphne's problem, each brings a different strength to the process. The CCCE is present, on the spot, and can observe the individuals in their daily interactions. The ACCE must be at a distance, but from that distance can offer an objective view of the progress made by all members of the clinical education team. The ACCE and the CCCE can be responsible for bringing all of the parties together through telephone or on-site dialogue. The ACCE and the CCCE make certain that all parties have the same information and are working toward the

Figure 3
Critical Incident Form for documentation

Student:		Evaluator:	
Date	Antecedents	Behaviors	Consequences
9/11	Student is on OP ortho rotation. Eval and treatment techniques are primary focus of affiliation. Has demonstrated repeated difficulties in eval and treatment situations, especially with the UE.	Student requests day off for mid-term evaluation in order to prepare for a party. This request followed CI's statement that midterm eval was coming up and that she felt there were some important issues for the student and the CI to discuss.	Leaves questions about the value this student holds for learning experiences and discussion with CI.

_____	_____
Student's signature	Evaluator's signature

same goals. The CI and the student—the other members of the clinical education team—interact with each coordinator, help to formulate the remediation program, and then carry it out on a daily basis.

Analyzing the Information

The program of remediation begins with the most accurate definition possible of the problem situation. Jessica has begun her role by not only completing her diary of Daphne's performance, but also by developing both a Critical Incident Form and an Anecdotal Form. By sharing this documentation with the CCCE, they will analyze it and begin to develop a program.

By reviewing the information that Daphne's school had sent to the facility prior to her affiliation, Jessica learned that Daphne's first affiliation had been in an inpatient orthopedics department at a large urban trauma center. Therefore, although Daphne was familiar with musculoskeletal evaluation and treatment techniques, her prior experience in applying them had been under significantly different circumstances. In view of the fact that Daphne's patients in her first affiliation were acutely ill, it was possible that her supervisor in that setting had encouraged Daphne to be quite dependent as a student. Daphne might, therefore, see her present behavior as "appropriate" instead of as "dependent." The fact that Daphne's prior clinical experience was exclusively with acutely ill patients might also explain her hesitance to do anything but familiar (and therefore safe and appropriate) treatments with patients with uncertain diagnoses.

Based on this analysis, Jessica concluded that Daphne was most comfortable in the exposure stage of learning and perhaps had not yet had the experience necessary to progress to the stage of acquisition. In considering the domains of learning, Jessica concluded that Daphne was functioning at a level on the cognitive domain in which she was able to understand information, instructions, and concepts but was unable to apply them independently. This is the level of *comprehension* in the cognitive domain. Jessica further concluded that Daphne was functioning at a similarly low level in the psychomotor domain. Daphne could perform a familiar treatment but could not adjust or initiate a new treatment without assistance. This is the level of *guided response*.

Jessica's CCCE suggested that the documentation indicated that Daphne also had problems in the affective domain. Her response, "If a patient can't be treated, she shouldn't come in" suggests an attitude toward patients that needs to be redirected. Her request for time off, particularly when her CI had expressed concern about her behavior, suggests that Daphne needs to examine her value system more closely to balance personal and professional concerns more appropriately. Thus analysis of the information collected can yield a comprehensive picture of the etiology of the problem, its severity, and options for remedy. Perspectives of all the team members are essential to consider in this phase of planning.

Selecting a Remedy

Once the documentation had been analyzed, it was necessary to formulate a plan for assessing Daphne's weaknesses and developing her strengths. Remediation plans can take a variety of forms, but there are a few elements that greatly improve the chances of success.

In developing the program of remediation, the CI should first clearly establish the minimal acceptable performance for this student at this facility. This is described in many student handbooks; however, all members of the team should have input into this pivotal component of the program. Once defined, it needs to be clearly stated so that there can be no misunderstandings about the minimal acceptable performance.[8]

Creating a flowsheet that chronicles the problem behaviors, goals, objectives, and learning experiences helps both student and CI focus on the goals of the program and sequence the learning experiences that are most likely to ensure success.

Even the most ideal remediation plan will not be successful, however, unless the CI and the student work together to develop an atmosphere conducive to learning. Communication between the two must be frank and assertive, and there must be a sense of mutual trust. The CI, as the one with the decision-making power, will need to show the student that he or she is trusted to participate in the plan for remediation. In fact, the more the student is trusted to bear responsibility for planning and implementation of the remediation program, the greater will be her commitment to its successful outcome.

It is likely that the CI will need to assist the student in taking mutual responsibility because most traditional students are accustomed to a more passive role in their learning. Students may need direction in identifying ways in which they can contribute to the plan. The CI can emphasize that the student needs to express his or her expectations about clinical learning in these goals, just as the CCCE at the facility has expressed his or her expectations.

Setting Goals

The student and the CI can then work together to describe the desired behaviors. The goals for each one should clearly state components of the desired behavior, the means by which the behavior will be measured, the conditions under which it will be measured, and the amount of time in which the student is expected to meet the goal.

It is not unusual for the CI and the student to establish a set of goals that, while comprehensive, is not realistic for the amount of time the student has to affiliate. The CCCE and the ACCE should work together with the student and the CI to focus on goals that meet the following conditions:

1. *Reasonable:* Are the goals at the appropriate level for the student's problems and educational level? Will the achievement of these goals result in a positive change in the student's performance?
2. *Necessary:* Will the goals lead the student to meeting the requirements of both the academic institution and the facility? Do any of the goals reflect a desire on the part of the CI to train the student to imitate the CI's behavior?
3. *Attainable:* Can the goals be achieved in the amount of time available to both the student and the CI?
4. *Sequenced for success:* Have the goals been written to "meet" the student at his or her present level of functioning and to help him or her progress in a stepwise fashion?

Selecting Learning Experiences

Once the appropriate set of goals has been established, the CI and the student can work together to design learning experiences available at the facility and to order these experiences into a stepwise formation that will gradually lead the student through a series of successful challenges to a higher level of safe and effective clinical practice. Planning these learning experiences requires an honest recognition of the resources a facility can offer. Patient availability and tolerance is a major consideration in effecting these experiences. The student's level of performance and rate of learning must also be considered for the plan to be successful.

In addition to her analysis of the stage at which Daphne was active in learning and the levels at which she was functioning within each domain, Jessica needed to include in her learning plan the communication skills she would focus on as the CI. For example, Jessica had noted that when she gave Daphne time to think through a treatment plan, Daphne was able to be more independent with patients with upper extremity problems. Based on these observations, Jessica decided to try to give Daphne time to think through unfamiliar situations whenever possible. The ACCE offered to speak to Daphne to see whether there were any issues in her personal life that were affecting her ability to perform at her highest possible level in the clinic.

When completed, the comprehensive remediation plan should contain the defined areas of deficits, desired behaviors that have been clearly defined, and a plan for attainment of each one. A series of ojectives written for each goal can serve to describe the strategy or approach that will be used to achieve the goal, while the various learning experiences will be the tactics that will be employed in the learning process. The final element necessary in an effective plan is to establish a calendar of weekly review of progress to assess the effectiveness of the plan and the progress of the student. These meetings not only keep both the CI and the student "on track" but also reinforce a sense of mutual responsibility throughout the course of the remediation process.

ASSESSING OUTCOMES
Identifying the Outcome
Everyone involved in the clinical education program should be involved in the development of this plan. While the primary responsibility may fall on the CI and the student, both the CCCE and the ACCE should be apprised of progress in the creation and implementation of the plan. In addition, both individuals can and should be relied on for consultation and support.

The remediation plan created by Daphne and Jessica was implemented beginning the week of the midterm of her affiliation.They met weekly to assess progress and were in frequent contact with both the CCCE and the ACCE. When the ACCE came to visit one week before the end of the affiliation, it was clear from the documentation that Daphne had made great progress in all areas of the remediation program. It was equally clear that Daphne was still functioning at a very low level in both the cognitive and psychomotor domains. Documentation of her interactions and performance with patients in a variety of situations supported this conclusion.

Success and Failure in Clinical Education
Daphne's clinical performance after seven weeks did not meet the university's requirements for successful completion of this second affiliation; the outcome was that Daphne did not successfully complete the affiliation. For some programs this would result in academic failure of the course; in others, it might simply delay the student's progress through the curriculum. Regardless of the individual academic outcome, in clinical terms "failure" is not the most pertinent concept by which to describe Daphne's experience.

Each affiliation offered through the professional curriculum is only a part of that student's clinical education. No one of the team members is responsible for that student either "passing" or "failing." The clinical educators are responsible only for doing the most they can for that student, in that facility, at that point in the student's education. To truly assess the outcome of their interventions, it is more useful to review the documentation of the problem behaviors, the remediation planning and implementation, and the feedback given to the student throughout the process. If the plan is complete and all the parties involved have fulfilled their responsibilities to the greatest possible degree, then where is the "failure"? Clinical educators should also be aware that the documentation and the remediation they have implemented can and often does serve as the basis for ongoing academic remediation. It also may be useful to the ACCE in planning additional clinical education experiences.

Unsuccessful completion of an affiliation is never a desirable outcome for any of the parties involved. It can, however, be the most valuable learning experience any one of them might have if it is handled in an open, mutually responsible manner.

Legal Implications
Unfortunately, even under the best of circumstances, there may be fear or even threats of litigation. There may be considerable financial consequences, as well as the emotional consequences associated with the final decision about a student's status. Although a relatively rare occurrence, it is a common concern and one best handled with participation by all team members.

Each member of the clinical education team has the responsibility to respect the legal rights of all the parties involved. The academic and clinical educators have a further responsibility to maintain a standard of competence for fellow practitioners and for patients.[9]

The history of decisions in cases of academic failure indicates that the courts support the ability of the faculty to make decisions about the student's technical, cognitive, and interpersonal skills. As the purveyor of education to the student (consumer), however, the CI is responsible for providing that:

1. The rules governing the student's performance have been clearly communicated to the student prior to the evaluation of that performance. In a well-managed clinical affiliation, this information is communicated to the student during the orientation.

2. The student has been treated fairly and given feedback regarding performance. Documentation of performance and records of meetings with the student become part of the legal record and, therefore, are essential. To the experienced clinician this will mean maintaining the same high standards for documentation of the clinical education process that are maintained in the process of patient care.

3. The instructors have not acted arbitrarily or capriciously. This is a professional responsibility in both clinical education and patient care. Documentation must include chronological accounts of all efforts in remediation that have been made by the parties involved.

4. The problem-solving process has been documented, as well as the student's behavior and response to feedback.

5. The ACCE, the CCCE, and the student have all been involved in any contract associations and decision making.[9]

CONCLUSION
Quality clinical education requires the mutual commitment of all members of the team: the CI, the student, the CCCE, and the ACCE. The CI bears a large part of the responsibility for planning the learning experiences for the student, observing and documenting the student's performance, and analyzing the student's progress. The student bears the responsibility for preparing to learn in the clinical setting and performing at his or her highest level of skill and judgment. The student shares the responsibility for analyzing his or her progress. Should a problem situation develop, the CI and the student should work together, with assistance and support from the CCCE and the ACCE, to develop a remediation plan that documents the problem behaviors and outlines specific strategies that assist the student in achieving clearly defined behavioral goals.

When all members of the clinical education team participate together to implement quality learning experiences in clinical education, the concept of failure becomes primarily an academic term. When the clinical education process is maintained effectively, the outcome is the development of committed, responsible professionals who will care for our patients and promote the growth of our field.

REFERENCES

1. Physical Therapy Education and Societal Needs: Guidelines for Physical Therapy Education. Alexandria, VA, American Physical Therapy Association, 1984

2. Shea ML, et al: Characteristics and Roles of the Clinical Instructor. Health Occupations Clinical Teacher Education Series for Secondary and Post-Secondary Educators. Urbana, IL, Illinois University Department of Vocational and Technical Education, 1985

3. Feldman E, Crook J: Personal characteristics of the health professional: Can they be changed by an education program? J Allied Health 13:163–168, 1984

4. Clinical Evaluation: The Use of Appropriate Evaluation Instruments. Illinois State Board of Education Health Occupations Clinical Teaching Education Series for Secondary and Post-Secondary Educators. Urbana, IL, University of Illinois at Urbana-Champaign, 1985

5. Stritter FT: Clinical instruction of students in the laboratory. Laboratory Medicine 14:795–798, 1983

6. Beck S, Youngblood P, Stritter F: Implementation and evaluation of a new approach to clinical instruction. J Allied Health 17:331–340, 1988

7. House JD, Burns EA: A study of the use of the adult learning theory. Family Practice Research Journal 5:241–246, 1986

8. Moeller P: Clinical supervision: Guidelines for managing the problem student. J Allied Health 13:205–211, 1984

9. Irby D: Legal guidelines for evaluating and dismissing medical students. N Engl J Med 304:180–184, 1981

Evaluating the Effectiveness of Clinical Education

Susan S Deusinger, PhD, PT

ABSTRACT: This article presents an overview of strategies that can be used to evaluate components of clinical education in physical therapy. The timing, targets, and methods of evaluation are examined for their strengths and limitations in today's challenging climate of professional education. Suggestions are made for improving the design of our evaluation systems and for enhancing the confidence placed in decisions made about the effectiveness of clinical education programs and the individuals who participate in them.

INTRODUCTION

Evaluation is an essential component of professional education. It is a process that involves collecting and interpreting information about people, facilities, and processes. It is integral to effective clinical teaching and necessary for growth and change in the learner. The purposes of this article are to examine the strategies currently used in evaluating physical therapy clinical education and to propose directions for change that can assist our profession in enhancing the quality of teaching and learning in the clinic.

THE RATIONALE OF EVALUATION

Evaluation is an integral process of professional education that informs decisions

Dr Deusinger is Acting Director, Program in Physical Therapy, Washington University School of Medicine, 660 S Euclid Ave, St. Louis, MO 63110.

about teaching and learning. It is a dynamic activity that can stimulate growth and change in the student, the faculty, and the educational system as a whole.[1,2] Data gathered from evaluation activities enable decisions to be made not only about the performance of students and the instructional effectiveness of clinical faculty, but about the quality of the clinical education program as a whole. Evaluation, therefore, is a process that affects the entire scheme of physical therapy education.

Evaluating student performance enables decisions to be made about whether learning has occurred in the classroom and in the clinical setting. Decisions about whether students are ready to be promoted to the next phase of clinical education and whether they are competent to graduate from the entry-level curriculum also are facilitated with evaluation. In addition, judgments about whether clinical teaching is effective, whether the curriculum is designed for optimal learning, and whether the clinical learning environment fosters appropriate socialization into the profession are made as a result of evaluation in clinical education. A comprehensive program of evaluation is required to ensure that the clinical education program is meeting the needs of students, faculty, and the profession.[3]

A broad and encompassing rationale for using a comprehensive system of evaluation in clinical education is evident. Decisions made as a result of evaluation in clinical education ultimately affect the health care system at large. Our commitment to quality professional education requires careful at-

tention to the strategies used to evaluate components of clinical education.

THE TARGETS OF EVALUATION

People, events, and facilities are all targets of evaluation in clinical education. The performance of people participating in clinical education is a central concern.[4] Effective clinical education relies on close coordination of the roles of many individuals; therefore, information should be collected on each person working to plan or implement the clinical learning experiences. Because the primary goal of entry-level education is to develop a competent practitioner, evaluation of student performance is a primary focus in clinical education. Student performance evaluation will receive the major emphasis later in this article. In addition to the student, however, the academic coordinator of clinical education (ACCE), the center coordinator of clinical education (CCCE), and the clinical instructor (CI) should be evaluated to determine whether working relationships are effective in achieving the missions of clinical education. Evaluation of these individuals can help to clarify the expectations inherent in each role and serve as a source of feedback to individuals seeking to improve their expertise in clinical education.

Although personnel may be the typical targets of evaluation in clinical education, other aspects of the clinical education program should also be addressed. Each of the following events requires thorough assessment to determine the contribution to the quality of the clinical education program:

1. Effectiveness of curriculum-planning sessions in establishing the goals of the clinical education program and in judging the congruence of the objectives set by clinical and academic faculty and by students.[4]

2. Adequacy of the orientation sessions provided to students before and after beginning a clinical rotation in clarifying the expectations set by the academic institution and clinical facility regarding personal and professional behavior.[4]

3. Effectiveness of faculty-development programs in preparing practitioners to function competently as clinical instructors.[5]

4. Usefulness of site visitation and consultation by academic faculty (the ACCE and others) in determining the progress of students and the needs of clinical faculty.

In addition to personnel and events, the characteristics and resources of the educational institution and clinical facility are also important targets of evaluation. Specific elements relevant to providing quality clinical education include the following:

1. Philosophies espoused by institutions and whether these are sufficiently congruent to form or maintain a relationship that will promote the goals of professional education.[6]

2. Financial resources allocated by both the academic institution and the clinical facility for clinical education and whether these resources yield sufficient benefit for the program to continue (or to begin).[7,8]

3. Space made available for the clinical education program and whether it is adequate for student-related activities (eg, patient care, independent study, conferences).[4]

Comprehensive systems of evaluation address the performance of people, the impact of policies and procedures, the fiscal outcomes, and the adequacy of educational planning. A variety of facets must be addressed to ensure informed decisions about students, faculty, and facilities in clinical education. Recognizing this, the profession can proceed to develop a consistent, comprehensive, and systematic approach to evaluating clinical education.

A SCHEDULE OF EVALUATION

Evaluation, regardless of the target, must be an ongoing phenomenon that is regular, frequent, and specifically timed to enable the various goals of education. In general, the evaluation process has three interrelated phases: needs assessment, formative check,

Figure
Phases of evaluation in clinical education

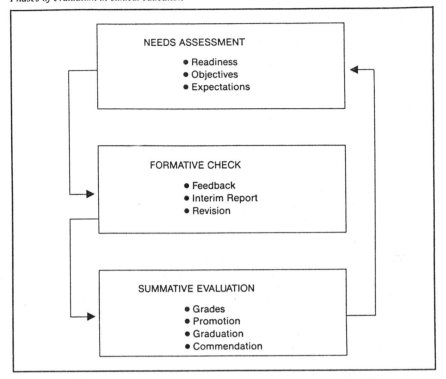

and summative evaluation. Although concerns about timing are relevant to other forms of assessment, the three phases of evaluation will be discussed using student performance evaluation as the target.

A *needs assessment* should be done initially to prescribe the level, intensity, and duration of clinical learning experiences appropriate for the student. This often occurs by reviewing a student's own objectives and expectations in conjunction with the performance goals of the educational institution. The effectiveness of clinical teaching is contingent on this phase of evaluation, which also includes determining whether 1) the site is ready to accept the student, 2) the caseload is appropriate for student learning, 3) the site and educational institution agree in their philosophy of professional practice, and 4) the clinician is ready to accept the responsibility for teaching.

The second phase of evaluation, the *formative check,* is performed periodically during the teaching process to determine the progress of the student's learning. The purpose of formative evaluation is to help *form* the ideas or skills of the person being evaluated. Formative checks rely heavily on regular documentation of situations in which performance and other outcomes are being judged. Critical incident reports and perfor-

mance logs often are used as formats for this documentation.[9] The results of formative checks may be communicated verbally in conversation with the student or in writing through reports of interim progress. These processes serve to guide subsequent teaching and learning.

Summative evaluation is intended to "sum up" the performance of a student. This type of evaluation occurs at the end of a specified period of learning and guides decisions about the next phase(s) of learning. Final course examinations, end-of-affiliation performance reports, and end-of-curriculum comprehensive tests are examples of summative evaluations. Results of these types of assessments are valued as meaningful measures of professional performance, growth, and development. The Figure illustrates the interrelationships of the three phases of evaluation in clinical education.

METHODS OF EVALUATION

Meaningful evaluation in clinical education relies on clearly specifying behaviors to be evaluated, reliable collection of data, and accurate interpretation of the data within the performance context.[1,10] Although these principles apply generally to the process of evaluation, this discussion will focus on assessment of students whose competent performance is regarded as a primary outcome of clinical education.

Direct observation of clinical behavior is the oldest and currently predominant system used for assessing student clinical competence. Use of this method entails specifying a set of observable behaviors, applying a standard (usually expressed with a rating scale) by which to judge the behaviors, and creating a format for recording ratings and supporting comments. Unfortunately, use of the direct-observation method has been cited for its poor reliability. The multiple distractions in the clinical setting, the considerable variability of human performance even under similar conditions, and the difficulty in maintaining a pool of trained observers all compromise the reliability of direct observations.[11] Thus, although it is common to almost all clinical education programs in physical therapy, use of the method may yield decisions that are suspect in their validity.

Careful training of clinical faculty is known to improve the reliability of performance assessments. Practice enables evaluators to focus on *observable* behaviors exhibited by students rather than on personal impressions. Training also assists the evaluator to remember and document *specific* examples of behavior that support achievement of required goals.[12] Objectivity and specificity are required characteristics of skilled evaluators. Keeping a log of comments about behaviors expected of a competent student enables the evaluator to make meaningful summative judgments at the completion of the learning period.

One of the most difficult aspects of evaluating performance in the clinic is interpreting the rating scales attached to lists of criterion behaviors.[13,14] These scales vary from dichotomous scales (allowing a choice of "yes" or "no") to multiple-level scales that offer many more choices. Rating scales contain a variety of dimensions that describe the standards we have for performance. These standards are reflected in the following questions:

1. *How often* is the student expected to perform a selected behavior?
2. *How much guidance* does the student require to perform correctly?
3. *What degree of accuracy* is the student expected to exhibit?

Multiple-level scales offer more freedom in describing the variations seen in behavior and may, therefore, be more meaningful in recognizing the range of behaviors students exhibit. Our interest is not just in whether a student is *able* to perform a behavior but in how habitually, how accurately, and how independently he or she performs. Percentage designations may be useful in communicating the degree to which students are expected to perform selected procedures correctly. Clinical faculty must thoroughly understand the rating scale applied to clinical performance instruments so that student behavior is accurately described. This understanding is gained through appropriate orientation to the evaluation system—an obligation of both the academic program and the clinical site.

A comprehensive evaluation system incorporates data collection from a variety of perspectives. Students benefit from feedback from academic faculty, clinical preceptors, supportive personnel, *and* patients. Input from all of these sources should be sought to form a complete picture of performance variables. Students also benefit from self-assessment. Incorporating self-assessment as a regular part of the scheme to evaluate student performance helps the student learn to make judgments about his or her own competence in professional practice,[2] a skill needed immediately by the entry-level physical therapist.

AN ALTERNATIVE SCHEME FOR SUMMATIVE EVALUATION

Clinical and academic educators share the responsibility to design and use evaluation schemes that are reliable, valid, and feasible for our educational system.[2,3,15] Because there is considerable turnover in clinical faculty, the profession is at a disadvantage in keeping the teaching and evaluation skills of preceptors current. In addition, the multiple distractions and work responsibilities present at clinical sites pose a serious practical threat to our current systems of evaluation. Clinicians often report that it is almost impossible to find sufficient time during the workday to evaluate students' needs, perform formative evaluations, and complete the summative assessments required by the educational institutions. One solution to this problem is to transfer the summative phase of evaluation to a setting where testing can occur in a controlled environment and at a time convenient to both students and faculty. The assessment-center methodology offers a useful format for accomplishing these purposes.

Assessment centers are characterized by the use of multiple forms of testing that are interpreted by multiple assessors in an environment simulating the actual workplace. The assessment-center method has been used in industry and the federal government to determine competence and potential for promotion of managers and other personnel. Although applying the method to summative evaluation in clinical education would be new for physical therapy, it has been used previously in our profession to promote postgraduate development of practicing clinicians.[16] Use of assessment centers to evaluate the competence of students participating in clinical education would be an innovative step toward addressing the psychometric and practical problems of evaluation noted above.

The complexity of performance required for quality patient care in the clinical setting limits the effectiveness of a single method (ie, direct observation) for evaluation of clinical competence. Multiple methods of testing are desirable to ensure that the numerous types of behaviors required of a competent clinician are evaluated thoroughly. The literature offers numerous options that could be incorporated in an assessment center to enhance our evaluation system. Role play and other simulations, review of medical records, and assessment of administrative acumen with methods such as in-basket tests can be used to complement the information obtained through direct observation when evaluating student performance.[2,3,16]

Development of an assessment center requires a considerable commitment of time and other resources.[15] Although it would be a major undertaking for the profession, use of assessment centers to evaluate student performance in clinical education may offer several benefits. Concerns are frequently voiced that our current system relies entirely on willing volunteers in the clinic who may have insufficient training to be consistent in their evaluations. Using the assessment-center methodology requires careful and consistent training of evaluators. Having a cadre of faculty (academic and clinical) who regularly participate in the centers might enhance our confidence in the promotion and graduation decisions currently being made about students.

Use of assessment centers might also increase collaboration between academic and clinical faculty in the summative phase of student-performance evaluation. Currently we rely almost exclusively on clinical faculty to conduct summative performance evaluations with students. Realistically, however, the decision to promote or to graduate a student remains with the academic institution. Participation by both academic and clinical faculty in the design and implementation of an assessment center would ensure that data collection and interpretation for decision-making were done collaboratively.

A comprehensive evaluation of clinical competence relies on systematically analyzing and understanding the domain of professional practice. Clinical educators voice concern about the generalizability of each clinical experience to the total repertoire of professional responsibility a physical therapist must assume. Assessment centers can be constructed to address a wide variety of practice issues and require competent performance across a significant variety of patient cases.[3,16] Successful completion of testing in a center designed with these characteristics shows the ability to adapt to the numerous challenges encountered by the physical therapy clinician.

The selection of tests appropriate for evaluation of student competence requires that we clearly describe the dimensions or aspects of performance required for quality patient care. Sufficient depth and breadth of knowledge, skill in interpersonal communication, the ability to prioritize and delegate tasks, psychomotor skills in handling patients, effectiveness in family teaching, and creativity in planning treatment programs are examples of performance dimensions expected in clinical education. Studies are needed in physical therapy to determine *essential* elements of practice and to clarify the optimal timing and method for assessment of each element. Tables 1, 2, and 3 illustrate how several types of tests could be incorporated into an assessment center at each of the three phases of assessment.

Table 1 depicts a blueprint of assessment systems that may be appropriate to test cognitive and affective aspects of practice. Assessment of these aspects is important in all evaluation phases, but is particularly essential in determining a student's readiness to participate in patient care activities. The blueprint proposed in Table 2 illustrates that a new set of assessment procedures may need to be adopted for the formative phase. Interest in the student's ability to accurately document patient care activities, effectively teach family members about

health regimens, and practice safely may be especially high in this phase. Similarly Table 3 suggests the testing of more complex skills in the summative phase by methods appropriate for each. These three blueprints represent proposed schema for designing an assessment center. In reality, the center must address many more performance dimensions and may include several more testing options to enable useful decisions about student performance.

Organizing assessment centers on a regional basis offers an additional benefit to clinical education programs. Because design and implementation of these centers may initially be expensive, several schools (or consortia) may wish to pool their resources to facilitate the process. Centers could be staffed by clinical and academic faculty trained in evaluation and responsible for implementing the standards set by the accreditation process of our profession and

by each educational institution. After initial costs are met, student examination fees eventually may be able to sustain the center's operations.

Finally, the opportunity to offer summative evaluation to students on an individually prescribed schedule may be an attractive benefit of using assessment centers. Currently most students progress through physical therapy education on a schedule defined more by the university calendar than by the learning needs of the student. Allowing students access to periodic evaluation sessions in the assessment center might enable them to anticipate learning needs and to be promoted to higher levels of clinical training (or to graduate) at individually appropriate times.

Developing an assessment center to serve the needs of physical therapy educators concerned with student performance evaluation should enhance the testing schemes already used by academic institutions, including written comprehensive examinations. This approach may also enhance our ability to recognize problems (as well as outstanding performance) in the clinic and enable students to progress through physical therapy education at a more individualized rate. At the very least, the method will increase collaboration among clinical and academic faculty concerned with the ultimate goal of producing clinically competent practitioners.

CONCLUSION

The rationale and process of evaluation in clinical education has been described as background for suggesting a method to improve

Table 1

Three-phase Evaluation System: Phase 1—Needs Assessment

Testing Method	Aspect of Competence		
	Knowledge	Communication	Professional Attitudes
Written test	X		
Role play		X	
Interview			X

Table 2

Three-phase Evaluation System: Phase 2—Formative Assessment

Testing Method	Aspect of Competence		
	Documentation	Family Teaching	Safety
Medical record review	X		
Case study		X	
Direct observation			X

Table 3

Three-phase Evaluation System: Phase 3—Summative Assessment

Testing Method	Aspect of Competence		
	Management Skills	Oral Presentation Skills	Patient Assessment Skills
In-basket	X		
Role play		X	
Simulated patient role play			X

this process. Although assessment of student performance is a primary concern of clinical educators, a comprehensive program of evaluation addresses a wide range of targets—people, procedures, philosophies, and other aspects of the educational program relevant to student learning. Clinical educators in the future will be challenged to be increasingly accountable for evaluation results. This will require designing and implementing evaluation systems that contribute useful information for deciding whether to graduate students and promote clinicians to faculty positions and for judging the overall quality of clinical education in physical therapy.

REFERENCES

1. Stritter FT, Flair MD: Effective Clinical Teaching. Bethesda, MD, US Department of Health Education and Welfare, National Medical Audiovisual Center/National Library of Medicine, 1980

2. Dinham S, Stritter FT: Research on professional education. In Wittrock MC: Handbook of Research on Teaching, ed 3. New York, NY, MacMillan Publishing Co, 1986

3. McGuire CH: Evaluation of student and practitioner competence. In McGuire CH, et al (eds): Handbook of Health Professions Education. San Francisco, CA, Jossey-Bass, Inc, Publishers, 1983

4. Barr JS, Gwyer J, Talmor Z: Standards for Clinical Education in Physical Therapy: A Manual for Evaluation and Selection of Clinical Education Centers. Washington, DC, American Physical Therapy Association, 1981

5. Perry JF: Handbook of Clinical Faculty Development. Chapel Hill, NC, University of North Carolina at Chapel Hill, 1971

6. Windom P: Developing a clinical education program for the clinician's perspective. Phys Ther 62:1604–1609, 1982

7. Lopopolo RB: Financial model to determine the effect of clinical education programs on physical therapy departments. Phys Ther 64:1396–1402, 1984

8. Gandy JS: Fiscal implications for clinical education. In: Pivotal Issues in Clinical Education: Present Status/Future Needs. Alexandria, VA, American Physical Therapy Association, 1988

9. Newble DI: The critical incident techniques: A new approach to the assessment of clinical performance. Med Educ 17:401–403, 1983

10. Michels E: Evaluation and research in physical therapy. Phys Ther 62:828–834, 1982

11. Wakefield J: Direct observation. In Neufeld VR, Normal G (eds): Assessing Clinical Competence. New York, NY, Springer Publishing Co, 1981

12. Wilson FR: Systematic rater training model: An aid to counselors in collecting observational data. Measurement and Evaluation in Guidance 14(4):187–194, 1982

13. Murphy KR, Garcia M, Kerker S, et al: Relationship between observational accuracy and accuracy in evaluating performance. J Appl Psychol 67(3):320–325, 1985

14. Wherry RJ, Bartlett CJ: The control of bias in ratings: A theory of rating. Personnel Psychology 35:521–551, 1982

15. Deusinger SS: Evaluation in clinical education. In: Pivotal Issues in Clinical Education: Present Status/Future Needs. Alexandria, VA, American Physical Therapy Association, 1988

16. Deusinger SS, Sindelar B, Stritter FT: Assessment center: A model for professional development and evaluation. Phys Ther 66:1119–1123, 1986

Costs and Benefits of Clinical Education

Jody Gandy, MS, PT
Barbara Sanders, MS, PT

ABSTRACT: *The purpose of this article is to discuss the costs and benefits of clinical education. The focus is on the three major components of the clinical education system: the clinical facility, the student, and the academic institution. Strategies to reduce costs are suggested, and current resources and available support systems are presented.*

INTRODUCTION

Today's rising health care costs are affected by cost-containment efforts that make institutional resources more scarce and competition for the health care dollar more prevalent.[1] As a result, health care professionals now are required to more thoroughly justify spending. Physical therapy is one of many health care professions under scrutiny for its cost effectiveness.[2] In addition to being concerned about the costs of patient

Ms Gandy is Assistant Professor and Academic Coordinator of Clinical Education at Temple University of the Commonwealth System of Higher Education, 3307 N Broad St, Philadelphia, PA 19141. Ms Sanders is Associate Professor and Director, Physical Therapy Program, School of Health Professions, Southwest Texas State University, San Marcos, Texas 78666.

care services, the profession also is concerned about the cost of training physical therapists in both academic institutions and clinical health care settings.

The purpose of this article is to address issues of cost in physical therapy clinical education. To achieve quality professional education, the clinical faculty, the student, and the academic institution must cooperate to ensure effective learning experiences. The costs and benefits affecting three components of the clinical education environment will be considered: the clinical site, the student, and the academic institution (Tabs. 1, 2). Strategies are offered to help minimize clinical education costs and to identify available resources and support systems to assist the individuals involved in clinical education.

THE CLINICAL FACILITY

The clinical site incurs both direct and indirect costs and benefits when sponsoring a clinical education program. Direct costs and benefits can be assessed in terms of tangible monetary losses or gains. Indirect costs and benefits are intangible yet critical to consider when evaluating the efficacy of clinical education in health care sites.

Direct Costs

Direct costs are represented by actual expenditures by the clinical facility to support the clinical education program. Direct costs are incurred by a facility when duties of departmental staff are specifically related to student clinical education, and when salary (and benefits) are accounted for in terms of time spent in clinical education.[3-5] In most cases individuals performing the role of clinical instructor (CI) are not compensated for their clinical education duties. In contrast, about 25% of the center coordinators of clinical education (CCCEs) are directly compensated through salary adjustments for their educational responsibilities.[6] In addition, some CCCEs carry a reduced patient caseload to provide time to adequately perform their responsibilities.

Direct costs for supporting students vary considerably among clinical facilities. These costs often are determined by a facility's budget, geographical accessibility, and desire to attract students. Possible student costs include room, board, parking, laundry, photocopying, uniforms, travel, telephone, malpractice insurance, or stipend. Clinical facilities operating on restricted budgets often limit many of these student benefits. Facilities may provide only parking and photocopying services, leaving the majority of the costs to be borne directly by the student.[3,6,7]

Other direct costs incurred by a facility that supports clinical education include postage, telephone, and written communication to the academic institution related to student programming.

Indirect Costs

In a physical therapy facility whose primary responsibility is patient care service, all costs associated with providing care can be allocated to chargeable procedures on the basis of direct labor by the physical therapist.[8] Mathematical models have been derived to assist clinical facilities in computing the costs and benefits of clinical education.[3,5,9] The physical therapist's time, therefore, is an economic commodity. Time taken to perform clinical education activities in lieu of patient care is considered an indirect cost (in terms of salary and benefits) to the facility. If therapists maintain their patient caseload in addition to supervising a student, however, it is not considered an indirect cost and in some cases may result in a direct benefit to the facility.

Cebulski and Sojkowski demonstrated that 72% of the CI-student teams they studied were more productive than just the CI alone. This team was most productive after the first week of student orientation and until the second-to-last week of the clinical affiliation.[10] Similarly, Carney and Keim reported that a clinical education program does not increase the hospital's cost and that the student-therapist team more than offsets any output loss.[11]

In examining different student affiliation levels, the early student affiliate has been shown not to generate sufficient revenue to cover costs, especially if the clinical experience is less than two weeks or is on a part-time basis.[3,6,7,10] Porter and Kincaid compared the cost/revenue generation of first- and second-year students at 35 diversified facilities and found that the second-year students generated more revenue than the first-year students using a one-to-one CI-student supervisory model.[12] Alternative supervisory models in selected clinical settings might provide more cost-effective methods of educating first-year students in the clinic.[13]

Clinical education activities performed by a CI that result in indirect costs to the facility include direct and indirect student supervision; evaluation and performance appraisal; documentation; and communication with the student, the CCCE, and at

Table 1
Costs of Clinical Education

Component	Direct Costs	Indirect Costs
Clinical facility	CCCE[a] salary and benefits Student support (room, board, parking, laundry, copying, travel, stipend) Program support (postage, telephone, scholarships) Scholarships for recruitment	CI[b] time (supervision, documentation, communication) Staff development Program development Secretarial support Staff burnout
Student	Tuition and fees Travel Room and board Uniforms Insurance	Loss of support system
Educational program	ACCE[c] salary and benefits Secretarial support Travel Clinical education workshops Liability insurance Tuition reduction	Adjunct faculty privileges (ID card, library access, recreational and entertainment access) Clinical faculty development

[a]Center coordinator of clinical education.
[b]Clinical instructor.
[c]Academic coordinator of clinical education.

times the academic coordinator of clinical education (ACCE). The time required for these activities varies based on both the student's and CI's level of experience, the difficulty of the clinical experience, the objectives of the affiliation, the student's academic preparation, and the time demands on the CI. Ideally as the CI gains more experience and the student progresses within the curriculum, the time commitment to perform these activities should progressively decrease as the student assumes greater patient care responsibilities and independence.

Activities performed by the CCCE that affect the cost of clinical education include supervision of both students and CIs; performance appraisal and documentation; CI training and development; development of clinical education materials and manuals; student scheduling; written and verbal communication with the ACCE; completion of contracts and forms, and meetings with students, the CI, and the ACCE. When analyzing the cost of the CCCE's participation in the clinical education program, consideration must be given to whether the CCCE has been given release time to perform these duties. Other indirect costs related to ancillary personnel in the physical therapy department are incurred when time is spent typing, photocopying, or performing other related activities.

Staff burnout may be considered another indirect cost of clinical education. Often CIs are asked to supervise students in addition to their patient care responsibilities when the facility may be understaffed. The therapist also may experience additional stress when there are limited numbers of experienced staff who are capable of providing student education. Because burnout may occur, facilities should be careful not to overextend their clinical education commitments to individual programs if appropriate staff resources are not available.

Direct Benefits

Direct benefits involve revenue-generating aspects of clinical education instead of expenditures. The direct benefits of clinical education may include the revenue generated by the student-therapist team, long-term staff recruitment and retention, and continuing education or tuition reduction at the academic institution.

As mentioned earlier, the later student affiliate-CI team is more productive and generates more patient revenue than the CI alone or the student in earlier affiliations. Page and MacKinnon determined that CI activities relating specifically to student teaching and learning occupied only 25% of their time. The majority of the

CI's time was devoted to patient care activities.[14] Perhaps the later student affiliate is more productive because CI teaching time is reduced while patient care activities substantially increase as the student becomes more independent. Likewise the student has prior clinical experiences that provide the foundation on which to build and refine clinical skills. This eliminates the need to teach the fundamentals of patient care and allows a focus on higher level clinical skills.

Another direct benefit of clinical education programs is staff recruitment.[4,15] Ciccone and Wolfner surveyed Ithaca College physical therapy graduates and found a strong symbiotic relationship between the student and the clinic. Fifty-one percent of the graduates actively sought employment at previous clinical affiliation sites, with 29% employed at a former clinical site at the time of the study.[16]

To assess the benefits of recruitment, a comparative cost analysis should be made between those facilities recruiting that have clinical education programs and those that do not have access to a student population. Items to consider when evaluating the direct cost or benefit of staff recruitment include the average number of staff vacancies per year, the length of time staff positions are vacant, advertising costs, the number of individuals interviewed to fill a staff vacancy, person(s) performing the interview, the length of time spent inter-

viewing the applicant; person(s) performing new staff orientation; the length of time to complete staff orientation, and the number of scholarships given to students. In some cases, clinical facilities offer scholarships to students at affiliating academic institutions to defray the costs of their education. In exchange, the student may be asked to work at the facility for a designated period of time if there is a vacancy or to pay back the scholarship with interest following graduation.

Direct benefits for recruitment from a clinical education program include 1) access to an applicant pool with minimal advertising; 2) fewer personnel required to interview because the applicant may already be personally known; and 3) a shorter staff orientation time, allowing the new staff to be more productive earlier.[6] In addition, facilities can advertise for staff and aide positions at the academic institution's health fair or career day or post recruitment announcements at the schools. Students also provide a rich resource by word of mouth to other students regarding the quality of a particular facility and potential staff vacancies.

In addition to recruitment benefits, clinical education programs also assist in staff retention. Two studies have reported that staff who were former student affiliates remain an average of 22 to 24 months at their first job—two to four months longer than those staff who were not student affiliates.[6,16]

Tuition reduction for university course work and continuing education are two additional direct benefits to the facility that supports clinical education. More specifically, continuing education programs related to clinical education may be provided free or at minimal cost. In a few cases, academic institutions may provide clinical facilities with a small stipend to be used toward the purchase of texts, equipment, or other resource materials.[4]

Indirect Benefits

Clinical education programs afford the facility indirect benefits that affect three general areas of concern: education, professional career growth, and prestige. Recognizing these indirect effects is critical when evaluating the benefits of clinical education.

Educational benefits ensue when academic faculty provide staff in-service workshops and consultations; when students do in-service workshops; when current didactic information is made available to staff; and when institutional resources such as the library, computer laboratories, and equipment are accessed.[4] Career growth and development occurs as a result of participation in clinical education. Assuming the position of the CI, the CCCE, or perhaps the ACCE entails additional responsibility that can lead to professional growth. Participation in clinical education also offers new opportunities for networking with other clinical educators, continuing education, and advanced graduate education. Students continue to stimulate physical therapists through the exchange of ideas and justification of treatment rationale.

Some facilities view having a clinical education program as prestigious. Academic institutions often acknowledge clinical educators through adjunct faculty appointments and certificates of appreciation. Clinical educators may have the opportunity to become teaching assistants because of their professional commitment and clinical skills. The clinic's association with an academic institution may augment and improve the facility's image within the community.[17] Because clinical education is such an integral component of physical therapy education, some physical therapists feel a professional obligation to return some of the benefits they have gained from the profession to produce future competent physical therapists. Nothing could be more prestigious (or satisfying) than to serve as professional role models for students aspiring to become physical therapists!

Table 2
Benefits of Clinical Education

Component	Direct Costs	Indirect Costs
Clinical facility	Revenue generated Staff recruitment Staff retention Continuing education Tuition reimbursement at the educational facility	Educational opportunities Professional career growth Prestige
Student	Skill development Stipends Housing, food, travel Preview of employment	Professional network development Role models Steps toward self-actualization
Educational program	Adjunct faculty, intructors Curriculum review and development Outside participation on committees (advisory, admissions) Variety of clinical settings and clinical specialists Opportunity for faculty practice Accessibility to equipment	Resources and input of a variety of clinicians

Participation in clinical education, therefore, entails numerous benefits—but not without some costs. Each clinical facility must evaluate whether the benefits outweigh the costs. All levels of personnel in the clinical education program must balance costs and benefits and determine whether the value of participation is equal to the effort.

THE STUDENT

As integral participants, students also incur both direct and indirect costs and benefits during the course of clinical education. This section addresses direct and indirect costs and benefits to students participating in clinical education.

Direct Costs

The primary and most tangible cost comes from tuition and fees paid to the educational institution. This cost varies and depends on the number of credit hours assigned to the course, the type of education facility (ie, public or private), and the residency status of the student.

As clinical facilities have tried to reduce their direct costs by eliminating such benefits to the student as stipends and room and board, the student has had to assume more of these costs.[6,7,18] In most instances the student is required to relocate and thus must bear the costs of temporary housing, food and incidentals, travel costs (public transportation, driving, parking), uniform or shoe expenses, and malpractice and health insurance. Many students in full-time clinical education must also give up outside employment because of relocation. This increases the impact of assuming other direct costs.

Indirect Costs

The temporary loss of a student's support system (ie, friends, family, and classmates) caused by relocation represents an important indirect cost of clinical education. The constant changes involved (eg, new housing arrangements, different cities, new supervisors, and new work environments) are emotionally stressful and may lead to transient losses in self-assurance and self-esteem.

Direct Benefits

The student, of course, benefits significantly from clinical education. The major benefit to the student is the opportunity to practice skills and implement classroom knowledge using real patients. Fewer clini-

cal facilities, however, are providing direct assistance to the student. When provided, the assistance may include stipends (rare), housing, food, travel stipends, laundry service, name tags, parking permits, and library privileges.

A valuable benefit to the student is the opportunity to investigate employment. During clinical education the student has had time to work with clinicians and the types of patients in the clinical environment that employment would provide. This saves many hours of consideration when seeking employment after graduation.

Indirect Benefits

There also are many indirect benefits that may not be recognized by the student or others involved in the clinical education process. The students have the opportunity to develop a network of professional associates and resources. Quite often, the relationship developed between a student and a CI endures much longer than when student-teacher contact is short-term. Clinical faculty serve as important role models in the process of professional socialization that occurs during clinical education. Clinical education provides the student with opportunities to enhance self-esteem and self-confidence, to improve interpersonal communication skills, and to develop and practice self-evaluation skills in patient care.

THE EDUCATIONAL PROGRAM

A physical therapy curriculum cannot exist without good clinical education facilities. The educational institution also incurs certain direct and indirect costs but reaps many benefits that are vital to the success of physical therapy education.

Direct Costs

The salary and benefits of the ACCE represent the primary cost to the educational program. Because of the comprehensive nature of the ACCE's responsibilities, this role may be filled by one or more full-time equivalents. The salaries and benefits of individuals providing administrative support to the ACCE also are included in the direct costs. One of the primary responsibilities of the ACCE is to schedule clinical education experiences. Although computerization has helped to facilitate this process, considerable time and effort are still put into scheduling. The development of new clinical education sites also requires a time (and financial) commitment, especially if site visits are required.

Other direct costs to the educational institution result from correspondence by phone and mail and the photocopying involved with major mailings, travel to clinical facilities during contract development or actual student placement, clinical education consortium meetings, continuing education workshops, and sponsored workshop programs.[7] Most education programs also sponsor some type of workshop for clinical faculty during the year. This type of program can be quite costly. In some states there are clinical education consortia that may require attendance by the ACCE at regular meetings as well as a membership fee. The education program also assumes costs for malpractice and liability insurance for its faculty (and students at some institutions).

Some universities also provide the CIs with a tuition-reduction program. This is a direct cost to the program. In a very few instances there is a payment to a clinical site for the cost of clinical education. Holder states that "cash payment for access to clinical education is the exception rather than the rule."[4] Hammersburg reported that stipends for students are quite rare and that more and more clinical facilities expect to be paid a share of the tuition by the educational institution for each student they teach.[18] This is attributed in part to accreditation agencies, third-party payers, and cost-containment efforts.

Indirect Costs

Examples of indirect costs to the educational institution include 1) privileges for adjunct academic appointments, 2) faculty identification cards, 3) library privileges, and 4) access to recreational, cultural, and sporting events. Clinical faculty development also is a cost carried by the educational institution and may include consultation by individual faculty members and/or applied courses in education, supervision, learning theory, counseling, and communication skills.

Direct Benefits

Clinical faculty members are a primary source from which adjunct faculty, laboratory instructors, course instructors, and lecturers may come. This pool of individuals represents a major resource—and thus a benefit—for the educational program. Other major benefits ensue from the opportunity for curriculum review and development, the participation of clinical specialists in academic curriculum, and the participation by clinical instructors on committees (eg, student selection, advisory, accreditation, and curriculum). According to Moore and Perry, "The educational institution also benefits by the participation of the clinical faculty in didactic courses, thus meshing the academic curriculum with the practical aspects of physical therapy services."[17]

The school also benefits from being able to place students in a variety of clinical settings. Attaining competence in many skills occurs more readily and more effectively in the clinical setting. Academicians can provide problem-solving sessions, simulations, and case studies, but the best place to truly develop problem-solving skills in patient care is the clinical setting. The clinic thus provides the final challenge in patient care.

Because maintaining clinical skills is an essential obligation of faculty, being in close proximity to a clinical site may offer academic faculty the opportunity to continue in practice. In addition, the clinics often can provide equipment that the educational program does not have. It is impractical to expect an educational institution to have more than one manufacturer's device for teaching; however, by working with local clinical facilities, the faculty and students may have access to major and current products needed in patient care.

Indirect Benefits

Clinical education demands a great commitment of time and effort from many people, and the rewards often are intangible. The staff of many clinical facilities volunteer this time, expecting no direct benefit. Moore and Perry stated:

> To reimburse the clinical facility and the clinical faculty for their support and time, the academic institution must recognize and accept its responsibility in providing both tangible and intangible rewards. Provision of these rewards serves many purposes in addition to thanking the clinical facility staff and the clinical faculty and recognizing their commitment.[17]

The more that people can be made to feel a part of the academic program, the more their commitment to the program. This commitment represents a primary indirect benefit to the educational institution. Ultimately all of these purposes serve the overall goal of improving physical therapy education and the profession of physical therapy.

MINIMIZING COSTS

There are many opportunities to minimize clinical education costs at all levels; as resources become more scarce, more creative approaches are being developed. Some possible alternatives to reduce the clinical facility's orientation costs include mailing policy and procedure manuals, expectations for students, and required readings prior to the student's arrival; orienting groups of students simultaneously; videotaping standard parts of the orientation; and utilizing one person to perform the orientation.

Direct supervisory costs may be minimized by the use of alternative models that allow one supervisor to work with more than one student, sharing supervisory responsibility with multiple staff members (instead of the traditional one staff to one student ratio), sending the same student to the two early consecutive affiliations, planning daily scheduled times to give student feedback during nonpatient treatment hours, and more effective use of the mock clinic within the academic curriculum. Emory and Nalette describe a model that uses a ratio of one CI to three students instead of a traditional one-to-one ratio.[13]

The use of regional consortia by academic programs can also provide collaborative efforts to reduce costs to the facility and academic programs while maximizing resources. The Texas Consortium for Physical Therapy Clinical Education has collaborated to develop a student and preceptor performance evaluation tool; the programs share a data bank for clinical facilities, work cooperatively to develop clinical schedules and site visits, and sponsor an annual clinical education workshop. Other consortia have been equally successful in maximizing similar resources.

Networks that are not formally developed as consortia can be equally effective in planning and implementing clinical education. Clinical facilities or CIs may form local study groups and meet on a regular basis. The educational institutions of a state or region may organize to provide one another with information about the clinical facilities within their immediate area.

Physical therapists who are participating in graduate education programs in areas that complement physical therapy (eg, education, psychology, or physical education) can be used to help defray the cost of clinical education. Employment by educational programs of these individuals as clinical instructors who accompany students to a clinical site, as teaching or laboratory assistants, as research assistants, or as part-time faculty is a productive use of community and professional resources.

Progressively more clinical facilities and organizations are providing student financial assistance programs in the form of scholarships or grants as a recruitment tool. As mentioned earlier, these programs generally assist the student with tuition and fees, books, and a monthly stipend in return for future employment that will forgive the grant or loan. This program also helps to minimize or even eliminate advertising costs for hiring new graduates because students are recruited prior to graduating. This is becoming a very popular program with students who do not meet the financial-need status required for traditional student financial aid.[19]

CONCLUSION

Clearly there are numerous costs and benefits associated with physical therapy clinical education. Recognition of these enables the individual educator and the program at large to develop creative cost-containment responses and to maximize the resources available to facilities, students, and educational institutions. Collaborative efforts to design effective responses to the challenges of planning and implementing quality clinical education in a complex health care system are essential.

REFERENCES

1. Del Polito CM: Future trends and opportunities: An assessment of enviromental factors affecting health professions education. In: Occupational Therapy Education: Target 2000 Proceedings. Promoting Excellence in Education, June 22–26, 1986, Nashville, TN. Rockville, MD, American Occupational Therapy Association, Inc, 1986

2. Davis K: Assessing physical therapy utilization in a prospective payment environment. Clinical Management in Physical Therapy 4:38–43, 1984

3. Lopopolo RB: Financial model to determine the effect of clinical education programs on physical therapy departments. Phys Ther 64:1396–1402, 1984

4. Holder L: Paying for clinical education: Fact or fiction? J Allied Health, August 1988, pp 221–229

5. Halonen RJ, Fitzgerald J, Simmon K: Measuring the costs and benefits of clinical education in departments utilizing allied health professionals. J Allied Health 5:5–12, 1976

6. Gandy JS: Financial Implications of Physical Therapy Clinical Education/PT Departments. Presented at the Combined Sections Meeting of the American Physical Therapy Association, Honolulu, HI, February 3, 1989

7. Meyers RS: The cost of clinical education in post-baccalaureate entry-level education. In: Leadership for Change in Physical Therapy Clinical Education. Proceedings from a Conference at Rock Eagle, GA, October 27–31, 1985. Alexandria, VA, American Physical Therapy Association, 1986

8. Ramsden EL, Fischir WT: Cost allocation for physical therapy in a teaching hospital. Phys Ther 50:660–664, 1970

9. Beaves RG, Joseph H, Rohrer JE, et al: Cost-effectiveness: How should it be determined? Evaluation and the Health Professions 11:213–230, 1988

10. Cebulski P, Sojkowski M: Clinical education and staff productivity. Clinical Management in Physical Therapy 8:26–29, 1988

11. Carney MK, Keim ST: Cost to the hospital of a clinical training program. J Allied Health 7:187–191, 1978

12. Porter RE, Kincaid CB: Financial aspects of clinical education to facilities. Phys Ther 57:905-909, 1977
13. Emery M, Nalette E: Student-staffed clinics: Creative clinical education during times of constraint. Clinical Mangement in Physical Therapy 6:6-10, 1986
14. Page GG, MacKinnon JR: Cost of clinical instructor's time in clinical education: Physical therapy students. Phys Ther 67:238–243, 1987
15. Hooper P: Recruitment: The art of being prepared. Clinical Management in Physical Therapy 5:36-37, 1985
16. Ciccone CD, Wolfner ML: Clinical affiliations and postgraduate job selection: A survey. Clinical Management in Physical Therapy 8:16-17, 1988
17. Moore ML, Perry JF: Clinical Education in Physical Therapy: Present Status/Future Needs, Washington, DC, American Physical Therapy Association, Section for Education, 1976
18. Hammersburg SS: A cost/benefit study of clinical education in selected allied health programs. J Allied Health, 1982, pp 35-41
19. Echternach JL, Sanders BS, Towne LL: Clinical Education in Physical Therapy: Consideration for Alternative Models. Alexandria, VA, American Physical Therapy Association, 1985

Summary and Future Initiatives

The responsibility for clinical education rests with the entire profession. Clinicians are challenged to accept their individual and collective obligation to contribute to the future of our profession by designing and implementing quality clinical learning experiences. The clinical educator is a significant source of influence in our profession and can serve as an effective change agent in today's health care system.

In the future lies a plethora of ideas, activities, and goals for clinical educators in the health professions. Included in each article of this Compendium were suggestions for change and initiatives for the future. As a summary, I would like to suggest the following as essential directions for change.

First, clinical educators are an important professional resource. Preparation as a clinical educator should begin as early as entry-level education and be reinforced through staff development, continuing education, and self-study. The knowledge and skills required to function competently as a clinical faculty member are quite similar to those required to provide effective patient education. Curricula, therefore, should consider incorporating study and practice of the methods by which one understands the needs of learners, the design of learning experiences, and the process of educational evaluation.

Second, although there are many intangible incentives to become and remain a clinical educator, development of some additional tangible incentives may be desirable. Rewards such as salary differentials, promotions, and other types of incentives should be developed to attract new clinical educators. These incentives also serve to recognize competence in clinical teaching and to ensure retention in the existing pool of clinical faculty. Certification of clinical instructors, accreditation of clinical sites, and association awards are appropriate initiatives to achieve this goal.

Third, consistency in the standards applied to all clinical learning experiences is an essential direction for the future. Adopting a common set of standards for clinical education is a most appropriate first step toward consistency throughout physical therapy. Such standards should address the characteristics of clinical centers that promote learning, the performance of students and faculty within the learning environment, and the methods that will best encourage leadership and professionalism in our new graduates. The goal of being consistent should not, however, overshadow the importance of recognizing individual differences in sites and students and legitimate variations in teaching methods.

Fourth, valid and reliable performance evaluation continues to be a challenging direction for the future. The literature in other health professions offers an important resource for determining what direction would be most productive to change our current system. Multi-method evaluation systems must be developed and used in physical therapy clinical education to ensure the competence of our future work force. Collaborative design of multi-method evaluation systems is essential if academic and clinical faculty are to place equal confidence in the outcomes of performance evaluation.

Lastly, focused research that addresses questions relevant to clinical education must be supported by institutions and funding agencies so that we develop a sound basis for planning and implementing clinical education. The study of costs in clinical education, for example, addresses long-standing concerns by administrators about the financial liabilities of student programs. Similar studies aimed at determining the most effective sequencing of clinical education in the curriculum, the impact of student participation on consumer satisfaction with physical therapy services, and other equally challenging issues will greatly enhance our effectiveness in working with an increasingly mature pool of students and sophisticated consumers.

Initiatives in other areas of concern to clinical educators must be taken also. The challenge of the twenty-first century is to see a parallel growth of practice, research, and education in physical therapy and to invite clinical educators to build on a dynamic past and to create an invigorating future.

Susan S Deusinger, PhD, PT
Acting Director
Program in Physical Therapy
Washington University School
of Medicine
St Louis, MO 63110

Academic Coordinator of Clinical Education

opinions and comments

The Dinosaur of Academic Physical Therapy

To the Editor:

The primary purpose of this letter is to suggest that—like the dinosaur—the position of Academic Coordinator of Clinical Education is no longer viable in the academic environment and is certain to become extinct in physical therapy education. We predict that future generations of academicians will look upon the ACCE with wonder, amazement, and great interest, but immediately will understand why this position vanished from the face of our academic earth. The viability of this position is threatened because of the present preoccupation with administrative logistics and student counseling, a preoccupation that prohibits full participation as an academic physical therapist. A restructuring of the ACCE's role is required if contributions to scholarly work, patient care, and teaching—all of which the academic environment demands—are to be made.

Administrative and counseling functions of clinical education should and must be performed as long as this phase of the curriculum remains within academic programs. Vesting these responsibilities exclusively in one faculty member, however, is a disservice to the individual and a waste of faculty resources. Performing these functions as a major work role is out of step with university expectations for academic productivity and hinders the faculty member from making important scholarly contributions to the profession. If mechanisms are not sought to allow the ACCE to establish a suitable distribution of functions that meet the expectations of the academic environment, then extinction is certain.

If administrative functions and counseling should not be the primary work roles of the ACCE, then what *are* the appropriate roles? The ACCE must be concerned with developing, substantiating, and communicating the practice implications of our knowledge base to students and colleagues. The changing mode of practice in physical therapy provides a fertile environment for determining the essential knowledge and skills that drive patient care in all specialty areas. Academic effort should be focused on developing a content expertise for the ACCE that is relevant both to practice and clinical education and that provides an academic focus for scholarship, teaching, and clinical practice. Establishing such a content expertise would allow the ACCE to be viewed in the same light as faculty members with expertise, for example, in anatomy, kinesiology, physical agents, or management of specific clinical entities. If this occurs, the ACCE would no longer be viewed as a faculty colleague whose major concerns are proposing the ideal duration or intensity of clinical learning experiences, mediating interpersonal conflicts between students and their clinical teachers, or negotiating legal agreements with clinical sites.

The real issue, then, is What *is* the knowledge base of this critical learning experience we call clinical education? Clinical education is focused on applying the basic and generic elements of clinical practice required across the profession, elements that have not yet been defined sufficiently in physical therapy. Defining these basic elements is an enormous undertaking. We propose that clinical decision making provides an essential focus for this definition and constitutes a generic base for both practice and education.

Educators in physical therapy must recognize and respond to the changes in practice that have increased the practitioner's responsibility to decide on management strategies for patients. The responsibility for developing skills and knowledge in clinical decision making in physical therapy students should be a major focus for the ACCE of the future. The science of clinical decision making is a recognized and respected area of research and scholarly activity, an area that has been given relatively little attention in physical therapy. The role of the ACCE is to adapt this science to the needs of students learning to practice physical therapy and to the needs of faculty who teach these students. This would require the ACCE to 1) participate in classroom and clinical teaching, 2) monitor students for progressive skill development in this area, 3) emphasize clinical decision making when structuring clinical education experiences, and 4) conduct research in this area.

To function effectively in clinical practice, physical therapists must be competent in psychosocial areas and in technical areas. Many ACCEs have associated themselves with the psychosocial area of interpersonal communications. In most cases, they seem to have emphasized the value of improving students as human beings functioning in society. Insufficient emphasis has been placed on the value of these skills in increasing the probability of obtaining the information required to make correct clinical decisions. The ACCE must provide students with learning experiences that emphasize that psychosocial knowledge and skills are essential for practice because they contribute directly to accurate patient assessment and not just to positive interpersonal relationships. The science of clinical decision making provides a mechanism for integrating these concerns.

We have suggested that the role of the ACCE needs to be redefined in order for this faculty member to survive the demands of academia and serve the needs of the profession. We have also suggested that a base of clinical decision making for teaching and scholarly activity would assist the ACCE in meeting the expectations of the academic environment. We propose that the ACCE serves an important and integral role in physical therapy education and hope that this letter stimulates further examination of the needs of clinical education.

SUSAN S. DEUSINGER, PHD, PT
Associate Director for Education
STEVEN J. ROSE, PHD, PT
Director
Program in Physical Therapy
Washington University
School of Medicine
Box 8083
660 S Euclid Ave
St. Louis, MO 63110

Role and Functions of the Academic Coordinator of Clinical Education in Physical Therapy Education: A Survey

BILLY U. PHILIPS, JR,
SUSAN McPHAIL,
and SHARON ROEMER

The Academic Coordinator of Clinical Education occupies a unique position in physical therapy education, often serving as the link between the didactic and the clinical domains of the program. A wealth of anecdotal information suggests the need for a more systematic study of the role and functions of the ACCE. A survey based on a self-administered questionnaire was sent to the ACCEs at 101 physical therapy education programs in the United States. A usable response rate of 79% was sufficient for the analysis. This study identifies some of the functions of the ACCEs, profiles their demographic characteristics, and describes the educational programs in which they work. The time ACCEs devote to participation in teaching, administrative, scholarly, and service activities is reported. In general, the ACCEs reported that the didactic and clinical curricula of their programs were well integrated.

Key Words: *Education, Physical therapy.*

The faculty member who serves as Academic Coordinator of Clinical Education in physical therapy serves as the liaison between the academic and the clinical faculties, often bridging the gap between what the clinical educators expect the student to know and what is possible to teach in an academic program. The ACCE also serves as the students' link to the academic faculty when participating in clinical assignments. Thus, the ACCE translates the multiple expectations of the academic faculty and of the clinical educators to the students in the program.

One of the specific responsibilities of the ACCE is to evaluate the learning experiences in the clinical portion of the curriculum to ensure that students progress in an orderly manner toward mastery of the competencies they will need.[1] The ACCE, thus, has the task of selecting an appropriate evaluation instrument and instructing the clinical faculty in its use.

Another function of the ACCE is to identify clinical facilities that would provide a good educational environment for students and then to negotiate and process affiliation agreements. The ACCE also is responsible for scheduling clinical assignments to match the resources of the facility, or of several facilities, to fulfill the educational needs of the students.

The travel that is required in the ACCE's role can be professionally isolating and may reduce the individual's full participation in regular teaching assignments, committee activities, and other routine functions shared with the academic faculty. This isolation may impair the integration of the didactic and the clinical portions of the curriculum.

Little information regarding the role of ACCEs or their demographic characteristics is currently available. Kondela-Cebulski reported on the role of the ACCE as a counselor,[2] but she did not mention the other functions of the ACCE, the requirements for the position, or the length of time ACCEs remain in their positions.

The purposes of this study were to describe the role of the ACCE in entry-level physical therapy education programs and to identify the demographic characteristics of the individuals serving as ACCEs. We also expected to describe the academic programs in which ACCEs serve, to document the range and distribution of activities of ACCEs (eg, teaching, administrative), to determine the extent of integration of the didactic and clinical curricula in each program, and to rate factors associated with the job satisfaction of ACCEs.

MATERIALS-METHOD

We developed a five-part questionnaire as the data collection instrument for our study. The five sections of the questionnaire were designed to elicit the following information:

1. Demographic characteristics of the ACCE (age, sex, educational level).
2. Characteristics of the ACCE's program (degree awarded, number of students).
3. The ACCE's duties and responsibilities (time utilization, administrative duties, student advising and evaluation).
4. Degree of integration of the didactic and clinical curricula.
5. The ACCE's opinions regarding various aspects of the program.

We conducted a pilot test of the questionnaire using a group of ACCEs. Based on their critique, some questions

Dr. Philips is Associate Dean and Associate Professor of Preventive Medicine and Community Health, The University of Texas School of Allied Health Sciences, Galveston, TX 77550 (USA).

Ms. McPhail is Assistant Professor and Academic Coordinator of Clinical Education, Department of Physical Therapy, The University of Texas School of Allied Health Sciences.

Ms. Roemer is a physical therapist with The Institute of Rehabilitation and Research, 1333 Moursund St, Houston, TX 77030.

This article was submitted January 16, 1985; was with the authors for revision 19 weeks; and was accepted November 1, 1985.

TABLE 1
Educational Level, Average Salary, and Years Experience as a Physical Therapist and as an ACCE

Educational Level	N (%)	Salary[a]	Years Experience as a Physical Therapist (Average)	Years Experience as an ACCE (Average)
Bachelor's	9 (11.2)	$24,374 (± $5,939)	13.0 (± 8.8)	3.3 (± 3.6)
Master's	66 (82.5)	$24,730 (± $4,841)	14.4 (± 7.2)	5.4 (± 5.0)
Doctorate	5 (6.2)	$31,499 (± $3,742)	22.8 (± 6.1)	8.2 (± 6.7)

[a] Respondents reported salary on a 12-month schedule in nine increments of $5,000 each, starting at less than $20,000. Average salary calculations were performed noting the midpoint of each interval as the amount for respondents selecting that category.

TABLE 2
Percentage Time by Categories of Activity

Category of Activity	Percentage of Time Spent in Activities by ACCEs[a]				
	0	1–10	11–25	26–50	51–100
Teaching[b]	0	0	0	7	73
Scholarly	21	46	11	2	0
Administrative	2	49	25	4	0
Service	12	55	13	0	0

[a] A total of 80 ACCEs responded to these questions.
[b] Clinical education is included in this category.

were clarified and a better response format was developed.

We mailed revised questionnaires and cover letters describing the purpose of the study and the process of informed consent to the ACCEs at all physical therapy programs in the October 1983 issue of PHYSICAL THERAPY. Four weeks after this initial mailing, a post card reminder was sent to those ACCEs who had not responded. No other follow-up was done. These two mailings resulted in the return of 83 of the questionnaires (82%). Three of the questionnaires (3%) were unusable (one was returned from a program that had closed, and two were completed by someone other than the ACCE of the program) and, therefore, the effective response rate was 79%.

The following terms are defined to permit an accurate comparison of the ACCEs:
1. Role—the attitudes, feelings, and expectations associated with the ACCE's position in the organization.
2. Functions—the duties and activities performed by the ACCEs in their position.
3. Integration—the amount of interaction between the clinical and academic faculties and the percentage of the total budget allocated for clinical education, as reported by the ACCEs. Responses to the portion of the analysis that related to role, functions, and integration were categorized according to these definitions.

The responses from all except 17 programs surveyed were included in our analysis. All entry-level master's degree programs were represented. We were unable to discern any differences between the programs that responded and those that did not respond. The survey had a sampling error of less than 2%. Analysis of the data from this survey was accomplished with descriptive statistical procedures.

RESULTS

Characteristics of Programs and Respondents

The physical therapy programs identified by respondents in our study included 69 baccalaureate programs, 21 master's degree programs, and 4 doctoral programs. The doctoral programs were represented because some respondents reported having more than one pro-

gram. The number of baccalaureate students in each program ranged from 14 to 479, with a median of 60 students. In the master's degree programs, the range was from 1 to 86 students, with a median of 30, and in the 4 doctoral programs the range was from 3 to 6 students, with a median of 3. The number of full-time academic faculty positions in the physical therapy programs ranged from 1 to 17, with a median of 6.

The compiled demographic information describes the average ACCE as a young, white woman without children (86% were women, and 91% had no dependents). The age range was 26 to 62 years, with a median age of 35 years and a mean age of 37 years. The respondents included 67 white women, 2 hispanic women, and 11 white men. Fifty percent of the survey group were single. The educational level, salary, and years of work experience of the respondents are shown in Table 1.

Eighteen ACCEs (22.5%) did not respond to the question regarding the ACCE's rank and position within a tenure track. Of the remaining 62 ACCEs, 48% reported being in a tenure track with the rank of assistant professor, 14% were instructors in a nontenure track, 14% were instructors in a tenure track, and 14% were associate professors in a tenure track.

Functions

In the third part of the survey, the ACCE indicated the percentage of time spent in teaching, scholarly, administrative, and service activities (to equal 100% of their time)—the same criterion that is used in annual faculty contract negotiations at The University of Texas School of Allied Health Sciences at Galveston and at many other institutions. Overall, 73 of the ACCEs (91%) spent over half of their time in teaching activities, including clinical education coordination. The majority of the ACCEs spent relatively little time on scholarly activities, and 21 (26%) reported that they devoted no time to this activity. All except 4 of the ACCEs (95%) devoted one quarter of their time or less to administrative activities. Twelve ACCEs (15%) allocated no time to service activities, and the remainder of respondents reported 25% of their time or less was used for service activities (Tab. 2).

The questionnaire divided teaching activity into six subcategories: basic science (anatomy, physiology, kinesiology), fundamental physical therapy courses (gait training, patient management, modalities), clinical education instruction (writing, problem solving, documentation), coordination of clinical education (site development, student assignments and visits), student advising, and other (eg, guest lectures, course coordination). The findings for each subcategory are summarized in Table 3.

The second general category, scholarly activity, was subdivided into research, writing for publication, instructional material development, grant writing, and other (eg, presentations to professional groups). Fifty-four percent of the ACCEs spent no time on research, 73% spent no time writing for publication, 56% devoted no time to instructional materials development, 88% devoted no time to grant writing, and 95% devoted no time to giving presentations at professional meetings. Overall, the ACCEs were able to devote a median of only 5% of their time to scholarly activities.

The administrative activity category was subdivided into departmental committees, school committees, university committees, faculty or university senates, and other (eg, clinical forums, consortia). Most of the ACCEs did not serve on university committees (63%) or in a faculty or university senate (90%). Thirty-two ACCEs (41%) did not serve on school committees, and 40 of the other 47 respondents reported that they spent less than 5% of their time on school committees. The majority of the ACCEs did serve on departmental committees. Sixteen ACCEs (20%) spent less than 5% of their time on departmental committees, 48 (60%) devoted between 6% and 10% of their time, and 9 (11%) devoted between 11% and 25% of their time.

The category of service activity was subdivided into activities involving the American Physical Therapy Association at the national, chapter, district-area, and community levels, and activities involving other organizations. Twelve of the ACCEs (15%) engaged in no service activities, and another 35 (44%) spent less than 5% of their time in service activities. The largest percentage of time devoted to service activity was spent in district and chapter activities of the APTA.

TABLE 3
Number of Respondents Reporting Percentage of Time Spent in Subcategories of Teaching Activity

Subcategory of Teaching Activity	Percentage of Time							
	0	1–5	6–10	11–25	26–50	51–75	76–100	TOTAL
Basic science	59	7	3	7	0	0	0	76[a]
Fundamental physical therapy	16	8	14	21	20	1	0	80
Clinical education instruction	25	34	12	8	1	0	0	80
Clinical coordination	0	0	1	16	45	9	4	75[a]
Student advisement	13	38	19	6	1	0	0	77[a]
Other	70	3	4	2	1	0	0	80

[a] Total less than 80 because some respondents did not answer all components of the question.

Clinical Coordination

The next section of the questionnaire concerned the interactions between the ACCEs and the clinical and academic faculties, which included negotiating and updating contracts and maintaining relationships with clinical faculty members. The total number of clinical sites visited by the ACCEs varied each year, ranging from 20 to 180, with a median of 80. In the academic year 1982–1983, the number of clinical sites visited by the ACCEs ranged from 0 (a new program) to 140, with a median of 64 visits. The individual ACCEs reported having visited from 0 to 103 facilities, with a median of 35 site visits. They reported that other faculty members visited from 0 to 67 facilities; 25 ACCEs reported that no other faculty members made site visits, and 27 reported that 1 to 10 visits were made by other faculty members.

The ACCE also is responsible for evaluating the students' performance in the clinic. Sixty-six of the ACCEs who responded to this section of the questionnaire (83%) had the authority to choose the evaluation instrument, and all had the responsibility to instruct the students and the clinical faculty in the use of the evaluation tool. The majority of the ACCEs who answered this part of the questionnaire (89%) reported that they alone had the final responsibility for assigning students' grades. The programs used different types of evaluation instruments: 60% were competency-based questionnaires, 25% were rating scales, and 15% were check lists or narratives. The extent of the integration of the didactic and clinical curricula was evaluated using various criteria, especially budgetary support and the amount of interaction between the academic and clinical faculties. Informa-

tion concerning the annual budget for clinical education, including communication costs, educational expenses, reimbursement for facilities, and emoluments to clinicians, was requested on the questionnaire. Of the 71 respondents who answered this question, 55 (77%) reported having budgets of less than $5,000. The median budget was within the range of $2,000 to $2,999, and the quartiles below and above the median were in the $1,000 to $1,999 and $4,000 to $4,999 ranges, respectively.

Clinical faculty input into the educational program was accomplished by various means, including participation on academic committees. Sixty-four ACCEs reported that clinical faculty members serve on at least one school committee (eg, curriculum, grading and promotion, admissions, awards), and half of the ACCEs responded that clinical faculty members serve on more than one committee. Sixty-two ACCEs reported that clinical faculty members had direct teaching responsibilities, and 26 ACCEs reported that clinical faculty members participated in research activities with academic faculty members.

The ACCEs also were asked to enumerate the number of meetings held by their school during the 1982–1983 academic year that included clinical faculty members, such as meetings for clinical education orientation, continuing education, curriculum redesign, and course design. The 80 respondents reported that a total of 219 meetings included clinical faculty members, with a range in each program from 0 to 15 meetings (median, 2).

To determine the amount of academic faculty input into clinical education curricula, participation in specific

TABLE 4
Perceptions of ACCEs Regarding Their Role in Clinical Education

Statement	Agree	Disagree	No Opinion	TOTAL
1. Clinical education is well integrated into the didactic curriculum at your program.	70	9	1	80
2. The clinical faculty have an appropriate amount of input into your curriculum.	59	19	2	80
3. The academic faculty who are physical therapists at your program are aware of current clinical practices.	75	5	0	80
4. All academic faculty who are physical therapists should be required to deliver direct patient care.	52	27	1	80
5. The rest of the academic faculty view the ACCE as essential to the program's success as any other academic faculty position.	75	4	1	80
6. The academic faculty are aware of the ACCE's responsibilities.	65	14	1	80
7. The final decision in resolving student problems during the clinical sequence should rest with the academic faculty (or faculty committee) even if this is contrary to the recommendation(s) of the ACCE.	36	41	3	80
8. If cuts must be made in the budget for the program, the clinical education budget should be given priority for retention.	71	3	6	80

activities was evaluated. Sixteen ACCEs reported that other academic faculty members participated in the selection of the evaluation tool. The ACCEs reported that 14 academic faculty members assisted in the assignment of students to facilities, 49 visited clinical facilities for student conferences with other faculty members, and 34 assisted in student telephone conferences. Forty-seven ACCEs reported academic faculty input in determining policies for clinical education, such as deciding the length of affiliations or identifying clinical competencies.

The ACCEs reported a wide range (0% to 100%) in the percentage of full-time academic faculty members involved in clinical practice. Thirty-two of the ACCEs (40%) reported that less than half of their academic faculty members were practicing clinically. Fifty-five ACCEs reported that academic faculty members provided in-service or continuing education to clinics; 41 indicated that academic faculty members provided direct patient care in clinical facilities; 50 reported that academic faculty members consulted clinical faculty members concerning patient problems;

25 reported that academic faculty members consulted clinical faculty members about administrative issues, such as new program development or quality assurance; and 39 reported that academic faculty members offer their research expertise to clinical facilities.

The final part of the survey included eight questions, designed for measurement on the Likert scale, to elicit the ACCEs' perceptions about the integration of academic and clinical curricula and their role in the program. The scale items were assigned numerical values of 1 (strongly agree) to 4 (strongly disagree) and, therefore, the theoretical range of the scale was 8 to 32. The distribution of scores ranged from 9 to 28, with a median of 14, a mean of 14.73, and a standard deviation of ± 3.04. The distribution of responses to the eight questions is shown in Table 4. This information will be discussed in a future article.

DISCUSSION

This study provides a contemporary view of the role and functions of the ACCE in physical therapy education

that confirms much of the anecdotal information about the position. Several of our findings have positive implications for job satisfaction and the stability of the ACCE position in the academic environment. Although the ACCEs' responses to questions concerning the didactic and clinical aspects of their programs suggest that the programs are well integrated, our study raises several fundamental issues in clinical education.

The typical ACCE profile is that of a 37-year-old white woman, without dependents, holding a master's degree, and having 15 years' experience in physical therapy. The typical ACCE, however, earns only $25,000 a year, with the rank of assistant professor within a tenure track. From the point of view of the academic institution, the ACCE is a junior faculty member who is subject to meeting the standards for tenure at the institution.

The ACCE, therefore, is in a position that may jeopardize the traditional path to tenure. Ninety-one percent of ACCEs spend over half of their time in teaching activities, a substantial portion of which is devoted to the coordination of clinical education, and they spend a very small amount of time in scholarly activities. The ACCEs also tend to serve primarily on committees within their departments and rarely on school- or university-wide committees. Consequently, they have little opportunity to communicate their unique concerns or to advocate changes in promotion and tenure policies.

Professionals involved in physical therapy education must look for ways to enhance the job satisfaction of ACCEs and to promote the continued integration of the didactic and clinical aspects of their programs. Several strategies have been recommended, including encouraging other faculty members to assist ACCEs with some of their duties, lobbying for changes in promotion and tenure policies, and supporting ACCEs in their attempts to meet the traditional standards for promotion and tenure.[3]

This study demonstrates that many of these strategies are already being used. Travel, for example, appears to be a significant part of the ACCE's job, with about 35 facilities to visit each year, despite an average annual budget of less than $5,000. This relatively small budget may burden the ACCE financially, especially if the sites are very far apart. Our survey did not investigate the

ACCEs' perceptions regarding whether the budget was sufficient, but it did show that 61% of the ACCEs are assisted in site visits by other faculty members.

Another area in which the ACCE may be supported is to enhance their image of authority among clinical educators by assigning them the responsibilities of choosing the evaluation tool and assigning students' grades. Fifty-nine percent of the ACCEs received input from their academic and clinical faculties regarding clinical education policies, although 64% believed that their faculty members should not override their recommendations for resolving student problems in the clinic. It is encouraging that 82% of the ACCEs perceived other faculty members to be aware of their responsibilities and that 93% believed that they were considered to be essential to their programs.

One area of concern that emerged during our study was that academic faculty members appeared to be less involved with the activities of the clinical faculties than the clinical faculty members were with the activities of the academic faculties. This discrepancy may be a result of the fact that an average of less than half of the academic faculty members in the 80 programs surveyed participated in direct patient care. Ninety-four percent of the ACCEs agreed that their academic faculty members were aware of current clinical practices, although 65% believed that academic faculty members should be required to deliver direct patient care. This finding emphasizes the ACCEs' strong commitment to clinical practice. Interestingly, despite their minimal contact with clinical practitioners, 87% of the ACCEs agreed that their didactic and clinical curricula were well integrated.

The problems of functioning as an ACCE that have been identified in this study are related primarily to integrating didactic and clinical components of education. These problems are not common in most academic programs and, thus, may not be familiar to other faculty members in the university. The best way to deal with these problems is based on a general strategy of education and involvement. Physical therapy faculties must do a better job of informing others in the university community about the unique nature of physical therapy education and the contributions it makes to the total climate of learning and scholarship at their institution. The ACCEs must advocate increased involvement of the clinical and didactic faculties in the operational phases of the program. This involvement is one way of illustrating to other faculty members what is required for a successful program. Physical therapy program directors must be sensitive to the economic, physical, and social demands of the ACCE position to find effective mechanisms to support the people in these positions. Finally, physical therapy as a profession must continue to encourage clinicians to become active in the didactic aspects of their programs and academic faculty members to remain active clinically.

REFERENCES

1. Scully RM: The role of the coordinator of clinical education. Section for Education Newsletter, American Physical Therapy Association, Spring, 1966
2. Kondela-Cebulski PM: Counseling function of academic coordinators of clinical education from select entry-level physical therapy educational programs. Phys Ther 62:470–476, 1982
3. Mettler P, Bork CE: Tenure and the allied health professions: Issues and alternatives. J Allied Health 14:119–127, 1985

The Academic Coordinator of Clinical Education: Current Status, Questions, and Challenges for the 1990s and Beyond

Elizabeth Mostrom Strickler, MS, PT

ABSTRACT: The academic coordinator of clinical education (ACCE) has a unique role and multiple responsibilities in physical therapy education. The singularity of the ACCE position in physical therapy, allied health, and higher education, however, produces special problems in the academic environment: this is the dilemma of the ACCE in academe. This article presents the results of a national survey of ACCEs conducted in 1989. The survey was designed to collect information on the current characteristics, status, and activities of ACCEs and to identify how the ACCE position is presently defined and structured in various institutions. The physical therapy programs and ACCEs that responded are characterized, and the ways that the dilemma of the ACCE position is being approached in different institutions are described and discussed. Questions regarding the ACCE role and position are posed for consideration by physical therapy educators, and some challenges related to this issue for physical therapy programs and ACCEs for the 1990s and beyond are identified.

INTRODUCTION

The role and position of the academic coordinator of clinical education (ACCE) is unique: it is often singular within physical therapy departments, and it is uncommon in higher education. Over the last decade, several authors have attempted to examine and clarify the role and functions of the ACCE.[1–6] All of these authors described the varied and extensive responsibilities of the ACCE and the unique and multidimensional characteristics of the ACCE role and position. Within

Ms Strickler is Assistant Professor, Department of Physical Therapy, Grand Valley State University, Allendale, MI 49401. She is a doctoral student; School of Health Education, Human Performance, and Counseling Psychology; Michigan State University; East Lansing, MI 48823. She was Academic Coordinator of Clinical Education at Grand Valley State University at the time this study was conducted.

physical therapy programs or departments, it is often the ACCE who serves most visibly as the critical link between the academic and clinical components of the program, helping to create and maintain the bridge that permits students to successfully complete the journey from the classroom to the profession.

Anecdotal evidence suggests that frequently it is the multidimensionality and unique challenges of the ACCE role and the opportunity to bridge the gap between the didactic and clinical components of the curriculum that attract individuals to the ACCE position and into the academy. Yet it may be precisely these same characteristics that force individuals to leave the position and the academic environment. Although this hypothesis requires further investigation, it is clear that "the position and role of the ACCE presents a dilemma in academe because of its singularity, and this dilemma becomes an issue most often at the time of faculty evaluation for promotion and tenure."[4]

The challenge of achieving a "fit" in academia and providing avenues for promotion and tenure of allied health and physical therapy faculty members, including ACCEs, has been a topic of discussion in the literature in fields where expansion of professional practice, concomitant educational change, and faculty shortages demand systematic and effective approaches toward faculty recruitment and retention.[7–12] In physical therapy, the frequency and intensity of these discussions has increased substantially over the past decade, and in particular over the past five years, as movement toward the entry-level master's degree in physical therapy has gained momentum. Specifically, the discussion has often focused on evolving methods to increase the number of doctorally prepared physical therapy faculty and methods to foster increased scholarly activity and productivity of faculty members. In turn, doctoral preparation and expanded scholarly activity among faculty members is expected to ensure survival and longevity in the aca-

demic environment, to ultimately permit greater contribution to our body of knowledge, and to advance the profession.

One of the greatest challenges, however, to achieving a "fit" in academia for allied health faculty is the qualitative difference between the socialization of clinicians to a primarily professional service role and the preparation and socialization of faculty members for a professional academic role. Because the great majority of physical therapists enter academia as clinicians socialized to a service role, their integration into the academic environment can be problematic. Patrick Ford described this problem in his 1989 address at an American Physical Therapy Association conference entitled "Expectations for Higher Education" and stated that physical therapists "bring to the academy an ethos and a set of values and expectations that are frequently quite at odds with the prevailing value structure within higher education."[11] Jane Mathews, in her 1989 Presidential Address to members of the APTA, highlighted the problem posed by such divergent socialization paths and suggested that we reexamine our methods of recruitment and retention of faculty, recognize this critical difference, and encourage a more proactive rather than reactive response to the problem.[8]

Perhaps there is no position within physical therapy education that creates greater challenges in achieving a "fit" in academia (or socializing to the academy) than the ACCE position and role. ACCEs are, by nature of their position, asked to fulfill a faculty role and to meet all of the demands and requirements of that professional academic role while also maintaining, modeling, and supporting a professional service role as they constantly traverse the bridge between the academic and clinical environments. The dilemma is this: the faculty role and the ACCE role are not inherently compatible as currently defined, although the great majority of ACCEs have regular faculty appointments.[3–6] This is a dilemma for the individual, the physical therapy department, and the

Table 1

Distribution of Survey Responses by Accrediting Regions

Accrediting Region	Frequency	Percentage
New England	6	8.3
Middle states	10	13.9
Southern	17	23.6
North Central	32	44.4
Northwest	5	6.9
Western	2	2.8
TOTAL	72	

university. If physical therapy educators agree that the ACCE is a valuable member of the faculty team and that this is a role and position that we should retain in physical therapy education, then the challenge is to find a balance or to create a congruity between these two roles. Another option is to redefine what the ACCE is and does to legitimize the role and functions of the ACCE so that not only survival, but respect, is possible in academia.

In 1986, at a national ACCE conference that explored the roles and image of the ACCE in physical therapy education, Steve Rose[13] and Sam Feitelberg[14] debated this question: Is the ACCE a "dinosaur" in physical therapy education or a "rising phoenix"? Although these appear to be opposite perspectives, the speakers really were articulating the same message. Both saw the ACCE position as a potentially threatened position and suggested that to prevent the ACCE from becoming a "dinosaur" and to permit the ACCE to be a "phoenix," ACCEs must do the following: 1) be flexible and responsive to the needs and demands of the profession and the academy, 2) be responsive to demographic and health care changes that drive clinical education, and 3) establish a valid and valued domain for research in clinical education and become researchers in this domain.[13,14] ACCEs were encouraged to continue or expand their roles as administrators, counselors, communicators, teachers, mentors, scholars and researchers, problem solvers, and change agents and to do this visibly both within and outside of the academic environment. ACCEs were challenged to socialize into the academy, to develop research capabilities, and to be innovative and creative in addressing the clinical education problems or questions of the future. Although these were monumental challenges, most ACCEs, including myself, left the meeting inspired and happy to accept such challenges.

Unfortunately, many ACCEs who accept and meet these challenges and make significant contributions to their students, departments, institutions, and the profession are still at risk in the tenure and promotion process in higher education because of their unusual role and multiple responsibilities (which often are poorly understood outside of their own departments). Anecdotal evidence and my own experience suggest that many ACCEs 1) leave the position prior to tenure or promotion decisions, 2) assume nontenure-track positions, 3) are provided with mixed faculty and administrative appointments that may or may not be tenure-track appointments, or 4) encounter some difficulty in the tenure and promotion process because of the distinctive nature of their position. As the latter occurred at my own institution, the need for additional information on the ACCE role and position in physical therapy departments around the country was recognized.

In 1989, a survey was conducted to gather new information to answer questions at our institution (and potentially others) regarding the ACCE. The purpose of the survey was to add to findings from surveys of ACCEs conducted four to five years earlier[3–5] and to document the current faculty status, role, and activities of ACCEs. We also hoped to gather supplemental information on physical therapy education programs and to identify the ways that the dilemma of the ACCE position described earlier was being addressed in colleges and universities around the country. This article presents the results of this survey and attempts to explore and discuss the implications of the results in light of the past history and future directions of physical therapy education and the physical therapy profession.

METHOD

Subjects

The study population included ACCEs from all accredited entry-level education programs for physical therapists identified in a listing published by the APTA in April of 1989.[15]

Procedure

The data collection instrument was a five-part survey questionnaire that sought the following information:

1. *General information*—respondent name (optional), title, and work address.
2. *Respondent information*—type of entry-level degree earned, highest earned degree, whether currently enrolled in a degree program.
3. *Program information*—size (students, faculty, and support staff) and length of professional program, number of active affiliating clinical sites.
4. *Position information*—position title and faculty rank, type of appointment (full-time versus part-time, administrative, length, tenure track or nontenure track), job description, division of time in specific activities during contractual year, and staff assistance provided for clinical education administrative duties.
5. *University faculty load calculation information*—use of contact hours, values of contact hours for lecture and laboratory time, methods for calculating clinical education contact hours.

The survey was mailed in the fall of 1989 to the ACCEs at the 114 identified programs with a cover letter describing the purpose of the study.

Data Analysis

Descriptive statistics, frequency distributions, and percentages were generated for data as appropriate. For subjective or narrative data, responses were reviewed and classified for summary purposes.

RESULTS

Seventy-two of the questionnaires were returned for a response rate of 63%.

Program Information

Responses were received from ACCEs representing programs in all six of the institutional accrediting regions as shown in Table 1. The highest number of surveys was received from the North Central region, which also has the highest percentage of entry-level programs of all the accrediting regions.[16,17] The number of students admitted into the professional program each year ranged from 18 to 130, with a mean of 43.51. The programs were then divided into five groups according to the number of students admitted each year: 29 or fewer students, 30 to 50, 51 to 75, 76 to 100, or more than 100 students. The frequency and percentage of programs by number of students admitted each year is shown in Table 2. The majority of programs (55.6%) admitted 30 to 50 students per year into the professional program. Table 2 also shows the number of faculty and support staff for programs by the admitting class size. For the modal category of programs (30 to 50 students admitted per year) the mean, median, and mode of full-time equivalent (FTE) faculty was seven, and the majority of these programs had two support staff ($\bar{X}$=1.84 ± .78, median=2, mode=2, range=1–4). Respondents also were asked to provide the titles of their support staff. Most often, support staff consisted of a combination of secretaries and administrative assistants.

There were 71 usable responses regarding the length of the professional program. The mean length (in years) of the programs was 2.38 ± .83, with a median and mode of 2 years and a range from 1.3 to 5 years. Forty-six of the programs (64.8%) had professional programs of two years or less, and 25 (35.2%) had professional programs of more than two years.

Seventy respondents provided information on the number of active clinical affiliation sites. For all programs, the minimum number of sites was 50 (a program admitting 30 students per year), and the maximum number of sites was 315 (a program admitting 100 students per year), with a mean of 137.67 sites and a median of 122.5. A frequency distribution of the number of affiliation sites (Figure) shows that the greatest number of programs (N=14; 20%) had between 140 and 169 active clinical affiliation sites and 13 (18.57%) programs each had 80 to 109 or 110 to 139 active affiliation sites. Overall, 57% of the programs had between 80 and 169 affiliated clinical sites.

Respondent Information

All respondents were physical therapists. Forty-nine (68.1%) of the respondents had a baccalaureate entry-level degree, 18 (25.0%) had a certificate in physical therapy, and 5 (6.9%) had an entry-level master's degree. Seven (9.7%) of the respondents had a baccalaureate degree as their highest earned degree; five of these seven individuals were enrolled in a master's-degree program. One (1.4%) individual had a certificate as the highest earned degree, 58 (80.6%) respondents had a master's degree, and 6 (8.3%) had a doctoral degree (PhD or EdD) as the highest earned degree. Twenty-one (29%) respondents were enrolled in a degree program at the time of the survey. Of these 21 respondents, 8 (38%) were seeking a master's degree, and 13 (62%) were seeking a doctoral degree (PhD=9, EdD=4).

Position Information

Seventy of the respondents had the title of ACCE, and two respondents had the title of

director of clinical education or associate director of clinical education. Some individuals had other titles in addition to the ACCE title, such as assistant director or assistant chair of the department. Faculty rank of the respondents is shown in Table 3. The individual who reported no faculty rank had an exclusively administrative appointment. Those individuals reporting "other" rank typically had a faculty title such as clinical assistant professor, adjunct assistant professor, clinical associate, or lecturer. Of the individuals reporting a rank of instructor, 7 (33.3%) held a baccalaureate degree, 1 (4.8%) held a certificate, and 13 (61.9%) held a master's degree. At the assistant professor level, 28 (90.3%) individuals held a master's degree and 3 (9.7%) held a doctoral degree. The nine individuals who reported a faculty rank of associate professor all held a master's degree, and the two respondents who reported a faculty rank of professor both held a doctoral degree.

The great majority of respondents (N=67; 93%) held full-time positions at the university (Tab. 3). The five respondents that had part-time appointments reported their FTEs as .3, .5, .5, .75, and .75. Twenty-two respondents (30%) reported that they had some type of administrative appointment (Tab. 3). Twenty of these individuals had administrative appointments in addition to or with their faculty appointments; for example, an individual might have a nine-month faculty appointment and a three-month administrative appointment. The percentage of administrative appointment for individuals with such appointments ranged from 25% to 60%, and there was great variability among respondents with administrative appointments in regard to tenure status. For example, some respondents with a 50% administrative appointment were on tenure tracks, while others were not. The one individual that reported an administrative appointment of 60% was not on a tenure track. Two respondents reported that they held exclusively administrative appointments, and both of these individuals did not have tenure-track appointments.

Table 2

Number of Students Admitted into Professional Program Each Year and Number of Faculty and Support Staff by Class Size

Number of Students Admitted per Year	Frequency	%	FTE Faculty[a]			Support Staff[b]		
			$\bar{X}$	Median	Mode	$\bar{X}$	Median	Mode
≤ 29	17	23.6	5.82	5	4	1.93	1.5	1
30–50	40	55.6	7.04	7	7	1.84	2	2
51–75	8	11.1	9.28	8.5	12	2.63	2	2
76–100	5	6.9	13.20	14	16	4.17	4	
> 100	2	2.8	22.5	12.25	15	4.0	3	

[a]FTE = full-time equivalent; based on 72 responses.
[b]Based on 62 responses.

Table 3

Faculty Rank and Appointment Characteristics for Academic Coordinators of Clinical Education

Position Information	N	%
Faculty rank		
None	1	1.4
Instructor	21	29.2
Assistant professor	31	43.1
Associate professor	9	12.5
Professor	2	2.8
Other	8	11.1
Type of appointment		
Full-time	67	93.1
Part-time	5	6.9
Administrative		
Yes	22	30
No	50	70
Tenure-track[a]	34	49
Nontenure-track	33	47
Tenure not awarded	3	4

[a]Two respondents did not indicate their tenure status.

Table 4
Percentage of Time Spent in Activities by Academic Coordinators of Clinical Education

Activity	Number of Usable Responses	Percentage of Time		
		$\bar{X}$	Median	Mode
Clinical education[a]	68	51.8	53	60
Classroom teaching[b]	68	24.1	20	10
Professional/Community service[c]	66	10.67	10	10
Program/University service	66	7.27	5	5
Scholarly activity	66	6.17	5	5

[a]Includes clinical education teaching/counseling and administration.
[b]Includes nonclinical education teaching.
[c]Some respondents included clinical practice in this category.

Overall, 34 (49%) of the respondents had tenure-track appointments, 33 (47%) had nontenure-track appointments, and 3 (4%) institutions did not award tenure (Tab. 3). Two respondents did not indicate their tenure status. For 15 of the 33 individuals who reported that they had nontenure-track appointments, tenure-track appointments were available to them if desired. Therefore, if tenure was awarded at an institution, 49 (70%) of the ACCEs responding to this question had tenure-track appointments or had the option to have a tenure-track appointment.

The survey asked respondents to provide information on the length of their appointment per year. If individuals reported that they had permanent summer appointments (usually of two- or three-month lengths) in addition to their regular 9- or 10-month appointments, these individuals were classified as having 11- or 12-month appointments. Using this definition, 12.5% of the respondents had 9- or 10-month appointments, and 87.5% of the respondents had 11- or 12-month appointments.

In an attempt to clarify how ACCEs are fulfilling their role, respondents were asked to approximate how their time was spent during a contractual year in the following areas (to equal 100% of their time): 1) clinical education teaching and counseling (one-to-one or group interaction with students, instructors, and clinical coordinators) and clinical education coordination and administration (correspondence, phone calls, contract negotiations, site development and evaluation, and student assignments), 2) nonclinical education classroom teaching (lecture and laboratory), 3) professional and community activity and service, 4) program and university service (program, department and university committees, faculty senates, clinical forums, and consortia) and 5) scholarly activity (research, writing for publication, grant writing, professional presentations). Results are shown in Table 4.

The respondents spent the majority of their time in clinical education activities (as defined in this survey), with the remainder of their time divided between classroom teaching, professional and community service, program and university service, and scholarly activity. Sixty-five percent of the ACCEs responding to this question spent more than 50% of their time on clinical education activities. Although this distribution of time is clearly unusual when compared with that of most faculty members, 64% of the respondents reported that they did not have a written job description or listing of the role and functions of the ACCE for their program or university.

Lastly, because it was recognized that administrative responsibilities consume a considerable amount of time for most ACCEs, the survey asked whether the ACCEs had support staff to assist with or assume responsibilities for some of the administrative aspects of clinical coordination. Seventy-four percent of the respondents reported that they do have some assistance from support staff primarily in the form of secretarial support. This included assistance with tasks like typing, filing, photocopying, generation of routine correspondence, updating of information, and record keeping. A few ACCEs reported that other faculty assisted them in completing student clinical education assignments and student visitations.

The final part of the survey requested information on how faculty loads were determined at the ACCE's institution. Of 70 institutions reporting, 48 (68.6%) use contact hours for determining faculty teaching loads. All (100%) of these institutions reported that one lecture hour was equal to one contact hour in their formulas, but there were extremely variable formulas for calculating laboratory contact hours. Most institutions did not count one laboratory hour as one contact hour; rather, a laboratory hour usually counted as some percentage of a contact hour.

If a university used contact hours in determining faculty loads, ACCEs at those institutions were asked to describe how their nonclassroom clinical education responsibilities (eg, clinical site and student visits, travel time, phone interviews, student scheduling, correspondence, and individual counseling with students) were counted. The most frequent types of responses to this question were "they aren't," "no one knows," or "negotiated informally within the department." Virtually all respondents suggested that this was a problematic and difficult issue at their institution. A few institutions had devised formulas or methods for calculating contact hours for clinical education activities. Some ACCEs received one contact hour for each credit hour of clinical education courses taught, some received one contact hour for a specific number of students that they were supervising at any given time, and others received a certain number of hours of release time each semester to enable them to fulfill their clinical education responsibilities. For those individuals with administrative appointments, clinical education activities outside of the classroom were counted as their administrative duties.

ACCEs were then asked to provide their average contact hours per week in the classroom. Forty-five usable responses to this question were obtained. The mean number of classroom contact hours reported by the ACCEs was 7.06 hours, with a median of 6.5. In this subsample of 45 respondents, 16 (35.6%) individuals reported less than 5 average contact hours per week, 8 (17.8%) reported between 5 and 7 contact hours per week, 12 (26.7%) reported between 7.1 and 10 contact hours per week, and 9 (20%) reported more than 10 contact hours in the classroom per week.

DISCUSSION

The past five years represent a time of significant change in physical therapy practice and education. This study updates and extends the findings of investigations conducted four to five years ago on the ACCE role and responsibilities.[3-5] Comparison of the results of this survey with previous studies sheds light on some of the questions posed by earlier investigators and helps to identify the direction of change, if any, that has occurred over the past five years. When viewed in the contemporary practice and educational milieu, the results of this study help to identify current issues that surround the ACCE position in physical therapy education and may foster further consideration of and action on these issues.

The sample for this study, although not inclusive of all entry-level physical therapy education programs, seems to represent enough of a diversity of programs to make the results useful and applicable to faculty in a variety of programs and institutions. Institutions from all six accrediting regions were represented, and programs of varying size in terms of number of students admitted, faculty, and support staff are represented. The length of the professional programs in this sample is slightly longer than that of the programs surveyed recently by the APTA.[16,17]

Because the ACCE serves as a liaison between the university and affiliated clinical facilities and between students, academic faculty, and clinical faculty, the number of active affiliation sites for the programs is of interest. The ACCE must routinely interact with clinical sites; whether it is to initiate affiliation agreements, to assist the development of clinical education programs or clinical faculty at the site, to evaluate the educational experiences provided at the site, or to monitor student performance during clinical affiliations. Given such responsibility and the fact that, in this sample, the majority of programs have over 100 active clinical affiliation sites, it is not surprising that ACCEs are spending a large percentage of their time in clinical education activities rather than in the classroom. In fact, 65% of ACCEs spent the majority of their time in clinical education activities (as defined in this survey), with the remainder of their time divided between, in descending order, classroom teaching, professional and community service, program and university service, and scholarly activity (Tab. 4).

The categorization of activities selected for use in this survey is similar, in some respects, to that used by Philips et al[3] but is different insofar as nonclinical education classroom teaching and clinical education activities are treated as two distinct categories. This division was chosen based on an impression, developed through discussions with other ACCEs and from experience, that clinical coordination, student counseling, and clinical education instruction are not often considered teaching activities as such at many institutions. This impression appears to be supported by the results of this survey for institutions that use contact hours in calculating faculty load. ACCEs reported low values for average classroom contact hours, with a mean of 7.06 per week; this value is similar to recent data reporting a mean of 7.1 for ACCEs teaching in entry-level master's degree programs and 7.8 for ACCEs teaching in baccalaureate degree programs in 1989 to 1990.[17] The majority of ACCEs also described a lack of systematic methods for calculating contact hours for clinical education activities in many institutions.

Despite the difference in categorization of ACCE activities, the pattern of distribution of time in various activities shown in this survey is very similar to that seen by Philips et al[3] and Myers[4] in 1985. It is clear that most ACCEs have had, and continue to have, an unusual division of their time compared with regular academic faculty. This fact, paired with the unusual and often poorly understood role and functions of the ACCE, places the ACCE in jeopardy at the time of promotion and tenure determinations.

Although this problem has been identified previously,[3–5] it is worth reiterating. This study shows that the majority of ACCEs have full-time faculty appointments, and many are on tenure tracks or have the option to have tenure-track appointments. Tenure criteria for most institutions include evidence of 1) effective teaching performance, 2) scholarly activity and productivity, 3) service to the university, and 4) service to the profession and community.[9,12,18] Although the relative importance of each of these areas in tenure or promotion determinations is decided by the university, most institutions give greatest attention to either teaching or scholarly activity, depending on their institutional mission. The distribution of time in activities for ACCEs shown in this survey demonstrates why the ACCE is at such great risk in the tenure and promotion process. On average, the respondents spend less than half of their time in activities that are considered in tenure and promotion determinations. Yet, despite their unusual role and responsibilities, many ACCEs do not have formal job descriptions that delineate their responsibilities or outline how their time might be spent fulfilling their role. The ACCE's risk in the tenure process is further heightened by the fact that most ACCEs have a master's degree as their highest earned degree. This study found that 80.6% of the ACCEs presently have a master's degree, and other studies (APTA; unpublished data; 1990)[3,5] have found a similar percentage of ACCEs with a master's degree as their highest earned degree.

In the face of significant faculty shortages in physical therapy[16,17,19] and the difficulty in recruitment and retention of faculty, we must address the problems posed by the ACCE position in physical therapy education and the question of whether the ACCE can survive in academia. The answer to this question requires the recognition that the ACCE dilemma is not a simple or overriding problem and that there are multiple factors working against the ACCE in terms of survival. Serious examination of some philosophic, professional, and practical issues will be necessary. Physical therapy educators must ask themselves these questions: 1) Do we believe in and value the role of the ACCE? 2) What do we need and want this role to be

Figure

Frequency distribution: Number of active clinical affiliation sites.

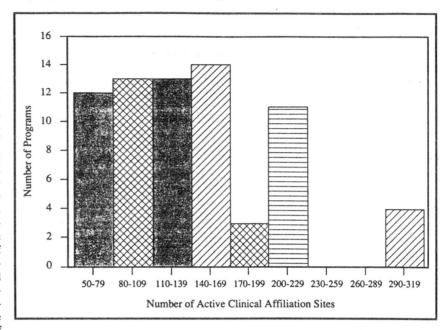

for the 1990s and beyond? 3) Should we redefine the role and functions of the ACCE? 4) If we believe in this role, how can we make this an attractive and stable position within our programs, considering the context and boundaries of higher education within which this individual and our programs must function? The answers to these questions should form the underpinnings of any attempts to ensure survival of the ACCE.

A general solution, applicable to all institutions, to the dilemma of the ACCE position is unlikely or impossible. Several approaches that are being taken to the ACCE dilemma are suggested by this survey and warrant examination. Each approach or potential solution raises specific questions and issues of its own and has advantages and disadvantages that must be carefully weighed.

One approach used at a few of the institutions surveyed is to devise a formula that allows clinical education coordination and administration activities to count as classroom contact hours or to be used in determining faculty load. The potential advantage of this method is that it allows for equity in loads across faculty and places academic value on the coordinating, counseling, and mentoring activities of the ACCE, occurring in a variety of settings, by equating clinical coordination with classroom teaching. While this approach may be readily accepted within physical therapy departments, it may be viewed with skepticism by other faculty, departments, and administrators, particularly those that are not familiar with allied health and professional education. Because faculty and administrators outside of the physical therapy departments often will be involved in peer reviews and personnel decisions, it would be extremely important to educate these individuals and to obtain their understanding and support for this method of determining faculty loads for the ACCE.

Another approach to managing the unusual and time-consuming responsibilities of the ACCE is to shift some of the routine administrative duties to an administrative assistant or secretary and to have other physical therapy faculty assist with site and student visitation. Although 74% of the respondents to this survey reported that they did have support staff assisting with routine secretarial and some administrative tasks, they still reported that a large percentage of their time is devoted to this aspect of their work. Perhaps support staff are being underutilized for routine clinical education tasks or support staff are already burdened with work for other department faculty members and are unable to take on additional responsibility for clinical education activities. The amount

of assistance provided by faculty for ACCE activities was not investigated formally in this survey.

Twenty of the institutions represented in this sample have provided ACCEs with administrative appointments in addition to or as part of their faculty appointment. The tenure status of ACCEs with such administrative appointments was variable and apparently depends on institutional requirements. Informal interviews with several ACCEs with this type of arrangement suggest that some institutions require that individuals move out of tenure-track appointments if they have administrative appointments of 20% to 25% or more. So, while this approach addresses the diminished faculty load problem for the ACCE, it may, in some cases, also diminish or eliminate their chances for promotion or tenure. More importantly, it may jeopardize their status within the institution or, as Ford suggests, place them in some kind of "limbo . . . lacking the privileges of academic citizenship, the protection of tenured status, and the prequisites and prestige that full-fledged faculty status confers."[11] When ACCEs move off of tenure tracks and out of standard faculty positions, they may not retain all the rights and privileges of regular faculty in academic governance although they may continue to participate as faculty members in their own department. This may not be true in all institutions, but it is certainly the case in some. The way that this type of appointment is used and managed apparently varies greatly among universities and deserves further examination.

While there has been much debate over the value and validity of the tenure system in academia,[20] it is the issue of academic citizenry that is probably the most important issue to consider as we address the ACCE dilemma. This is brought into even sharper focus by the fact that there are some ACCEs who have full-time administrative appointments. Although only two of the respondents had such an appointment, this type of approach to the ACCE position deserves attention because of some of the philosophic questions it raises. Both of these appointments were nontenure-track appointments and would typically be classified as professional staff positions. In most institutions of higher education, such positions do not carry all of the attendant rights and privileges of faculty positions (eg, involvement in academic governance and decision making). More information is needed on how these positions are working and why they were instituted, but the existence of such administrative positions and the variable types of ACCE positions described earlier raise several cen-

tral questions: Is the ACCE primarily an administrator or an educator? Is this a legitimate faculty role? Should ACCEs be on the tenure track? Can they achieve promotion, tenure, longevity, and respect in academia while fulfilling the ACCE role as currently defined? If so, how?

Only the profession and physical therapy educators can answer these questions, but careful examination of the current status of the ACCE and a consideration of future challenges for ACCEs and physical therapy clinical education in general is essential. A recent Delphi study conducted by Elder[21] found consensus among administrators in schools of allied health on 16 objectives rated as important for their schools for the year 2000. Among these 16 objectives were seven that were directly related to clinical instruction.[21] This underscores the importance of engaging in dialogue about the role and position of the ACCE, because it is these individuals who are most intimately involved with the clinical education components of physical therapy curricula.

In their "educator" and "scholar" roles, ACCEs have the potential to become experts and researchers in the process of professional education, particularly as it relates to the realm of integration into the clinical environment and the acceptance of professional behaviors versus technical skills. Our growth as a profession and our continuing transition to the entry-level master's degree demands this. Mathews[8] and Shepard and Jensen[22] have encouraged us to reexamine physical therapy curricula in the 1990s and to attempt to educate reflective practitioners. ACCEs could play a major role in researching and identifying the attitudes and behaviors of the reflective practitioners we seek to develop and could be instrumental in revamping or designing curricula to help physical therapy education achieve such a goal. There is a plethora of ideas and questions relating to the domain of clinical education that requires investigation. ACCEs, collaboratively and individually, can engage in such scholarly activity to legitimize their existence and to ensure their viability in academia. This may require, however, a redefinition or reorganization of the administrative responsibilities of the ACCE to permit the extension of the faculty role of the ACCE.

To enable and encourage expanded scholarly pursuit in the realm of clinical education, we need to increase our numbers of doctorally prepared ACCEs. A recent study on scholarly productivity of physical therapy faculty found that the majority of respondents reported that their own academic preparation for research was the factor that most assisted them in scholarly activities, followed by the availability of promotion opportunities and disciplinary prestige.[10] Doctoral preparation should not only enable more ACCEs to engage in research activities but should enhance promotion opportunities and disciplinary prestige within the academic and professional environment. Eighteen percent of the ACCEs responding to this survey were seeking doctoral degrees. We should, however, be very concerned about Harris's finding that doctorally prepared ACCEs had high levels of dissatisfaction with their jobs as compared with other ACCEs.[5] Although this finding requires further investigation, anecdotal evidence suggests that, for all ACCEs, some of the day-to-day administrative demands of the position are wearing and frustrating at the least, and this frustration may be accentuated for doctorally prepared ACCEs.

If the ACCE role is defined as largely administrative, however, a different spectrum of ACCE characteristics, activities, and responsibilities is likely. Further discussion of the specific nature of such an administrative role for the ACCE and the position within the department and university would be imperative. Furthermore, the philosophic issues that emanate from such a position for the ACCE must be carefully considered.

The ACCE role can be exciting and rewarding and critical to the success of students and to the achievement of the goals of physical therapy education programs. It is important, however, that ACCEs, physical therapy faculty and departments, and institutions that house physical therapy programs carefully consider some of the questions and issues raised here. The outcome of such consideration and future discussion may be a vision of the ACCE as a "rising phoenix"; an identification of a "fit" for the ACCE in academe that best serves our students, departments, the university, and our profession; and a dedication of all involved to work toward achieving that fit.

REFERENCES

1. Barr JS, Gwyer J, Talmor Z: Standards for Clinical Education in Physical Therapy: A Manual for Evaluation and Selection of Clinical Education Centers. Washington, DC, American Physical Therapy Association, 1981

2. Kondela-Cebulski PM: Counseling function of academic coordinators of clinical education from select entry-level physical therapy educational programs. Phys Ther 62:470–476, 1982

3. Philips BU Jr, McPhail S, Roemer S: Role and functions of the academic coordinator for clinical education in physical therapy education: A survey. Phys Ther 66:981–985, 1986

4. Myers RS: Current Patterns for Providing Clinical Education in Physical Therapy Education. Alexandria, VA, Department of Education, American Physical Therapy Association, 1985

5. Harris MJ, Fogel M, Blacconiere M: Job satisfaction among academic coordinators of clinical education in physical therapy. Phys Ther 67:958–963, 1987

6. Strickler EM: The role of the academic coordinator of clinical education: A dilemma in academe. J Allied Health 19:95–101, 1990

7. Conine TA: Prevention instead of remediation: Changing the nature of faculty development. J Allied Health 18:157–165, 1989

8. Mathews JS: Preparation for the twenty-first century: The educational challenge. Phys Ther 69:981–986, 1989

9. Rothman J, Rinehart ME: A profile of faculty development in physical therapy education programs. Phys Ther 70:310–313, 1990

10. Holcomb JD, Selker LG, Roush RE: Scholarly productivity: A regional study of physical therapy faculty in schools of allied health. Phys Ther 70:118–124, 1990

11. Ford PJ: The nature of graduate professional education: Some implications for raising the entry level. Journal of Physical Therapy Education 4:3–6, 1990

12. Mettler P, Bork CE: Tenure and the allied health professions: Issues and alternatives. J Allied Health 14:119–127, 1985

13. Rose SJ: The ACCE: The Dinosaur of the Physical Therapy Education Program. Presented at the Second National ACCE Conference, Chicago, IL, September 26–28, 1986

14. Feitelberg SB: Clinical Education: Dinosaur or Phoenix? Presented at the Second National ACCE Conference, Chicago, IL, September 26–28, 1986

15. Careers in Physical Therapy. Alexandria, VA, American Physical Therapy Association, 1989

16. Physical Therapy Education. Alexandria, VA, Department of Education, American Physical Therapy Association, 1988

17. Physical Therapy Education. Alexandria, VA, Department of Education, American Physical Therapy Association, 1990

18. Lewis LS: Getting tenure: Change and continuity. Academe 66:373–381, 1980

19. The Plan to Address the Faculty Shortage in Physical Therapy Education. Alexandria, VA, American Physical Therapy Association, 1985

20. Smith BL (ed): The Tenure Debate. San Francisco, CA, Jossey-Bass, Publishers Inc, 1973

21. Elder OC: Looking for the 21st century in schools of allied health. J Allied Health 19:237–244, 1990

22. Shepard KF, Jensen GM: Physical therapist curricula for the 1990s: Educating the reflective practitioner. Phys Ther 70:566–573, 1990

Job Satisfaction Among Academic Coordinators of Clinical Education in Physical Therapy

MARY JANE HARRIS,
MARVIN FOGEL,
and MICHAEL BLACCONIERE

The Academic Coordinator of Clinical Education is the physical therapy faculty member who is responsible for the clinical component of the curriculum. The responsibilities involved in the ACCE's job are such that ACCEs seem to be at risk for job dissatisfaction and burnout. The purpose of this descriptive study was to investigate the levels and patterns of job satisfaction among ACCEs in physical therapy. A questionnaire, including a 32-item job satisfaction inventory, was sent to the ACCE at each accredited entry-level education program for physical therapists and physical therapist assistants (N = 169). One hundred twelve (66.3%) responses were received and analyzed. Demographic characteristics of the respondents are reported. The results of the study showed that ACCEs, in general, expressed low levels of occupational dissatisfaction and burnout. Satisfaction with the aspects of the job involving self-esteem, achievement, and creativity seems to outweigh dissatisfaction with the time available, the work load, and organizational efficiency. Those ACCEs with doctoral degrees expressed the highest levels of dissatisfaction and burnout. Those ACCEs working in entry-level master's degree programs expressed the lowest level of dissatisfaction; those in tenure-track positions expressed the lowest level of burnout. Factors contributing to job satisfaction and dissatisfaction are discussed.

Key Words: *Education, Faculty, Job satisfaction, Physical therapy.*

The Academic Coordinator of Clinical Education has multiple responsibilities as a physical therapy education program faculty member. They are involved, to varying degrees, in activities common to physical therapy faculty: classroom teaching, nonclinical education administration, committee work, counseling, scholarly activity, and patient care.[1-3] In addition, the ACCE is responsible for the management of the clinical component of the curriculum, which involves selection and development of clinical facilities, negotiation and update of contracts with clinical facilities, maintenance of relationships with clinical faculty members, scheduling of clinical assignments, clinical site visits, evaluation of student clinical performance, and clinical faculty development. The importance of the clinical education component of the curriculum is such that the ACCE often devotes more time and effort to it than to other activities.

Consequently, as ACCEs face the daily pressures of their many responsibilities, they would seem to be at some risk for job frustration.[2] Additionally, the extent of the ACCE's involvement in clinical education activities appears to limit the ACCE's involvement in service and scholarly activity and, thus, puts the ACCE at risk in the traditional tenure process.[4]

The variety of duties required of ACCEs suggests that they have greater potential for dissatisfaction and burnout than other faculty members. The stress associated with the job and the potential difficulty in achieving tenure might contribute to ACCE dissatisfaction, burnout, and attrition. Identification of the factors that influence ACCE job satisfaction is an important first step in efforts to foster ACCE retention, which is particularly relevant in this time of recognized faculty shortages.

A review of the literature on occupational stress revealed a wealth of information related to job satisfaction and professional burnout.[5-9] Relatively little information, however, was found that directly relates these concepts to allied health care personnel or to allied health care educators.[10-16] No information was found that specifically applies these concepts to physical therapy faculty members or to ACCEs.

The purpose of this study was to identify the levels of job satisfaction among ACCEs in entry-level physical therapy education programs. Specifically, the study was designed to 1) identify the demographic characteristics of ACCEs, 2) measure the levels of self-expressed occupational burnout among ACCEs, 3) identify the levels of ACCE job satisfaction, and 4) identify the factors that contribute to job satisfaction and dissatisfaction among ACCEs.

METHOD

Procedure

The study population included the ACCEs from all accredited programs offering entry-level education for physical

Ms. Harris is Assistant Professor and Academic Coordinator of Clinical Education, Physical Therapy Program, School of Allied Health Professions, Northern Illinois University, DeKalb, IL 60115-2854 (USA).

Dr. Fogel is Professor, Community Health Program, School of Allied Health Professions, Northern Illinois University.

Mr. Blacconiere is a doctoral candidate, Department of Psychology, Northern Illinois University.

This article was submitted October 28, 1985; was with the authors for revision 22 weeks; and was accepted September 5, 1986. Potential Conflict of Interest: 4.

therapists and physical therapist assistants. The programs were identified from a list published by the American Physical Therapy Association.[17]

We assembled a two-page, three-part questionnaire entitled "Occupational Needs Survey: Academic Coordinators of Clinical Education" for this study. The first section was designed to collect demographic data that we thought might be related to job satisfaction: age, sex, number of years as an ACCE, highest degree held, tenure status, terminal degree offered by the program in which employed, amount of time allotted to various activities, and class size.

The second section asked the respondent to indicate, on a subjective scale of 5% to 95%, their degree of occupational burnout. We used the following operational definition of occupational burnout: "Feeling that in your job, you are constantly being drained of more energy through stressful experiences than is being replenished through positive experiences and rewards."

The third section was a 32-item inventory entitled "Occupational Needs Questionnaire" (ON-Q). The ON-Q is a research instrument designed to measure levels and patterns of job satisfaction and frustration and is based on contemporary theories of job satisfaction, including those of Herzberg et al,[5] French et al,[6] and Vroom.[8] The ON-Q items are designed to measure job factors in eight areas: 1) pay and benefits, 2) organization, 3) supervision, 4) time and work load, 5) work, 6) self-esteem, 7) achievement, and 8) creativity (Appendix). Doctoral research provides support for the item groupings and indicates acceptable levels of reliability and validity: Test-retest and internal consistency studies yielded acceptable reliability coefficients; concurrent validity studies with the Job Descriptive Index and the Minnesota Satisfaction Questionnaire yielded moderate correlations on general scores and moderate to high correlations on selected subscores.[18] Research populations have included samples from the university faculty, health care professionals, and private-sector industrial managers and hourly employees.

In completing the ON-Q, subjects are asked to respond twice to each of the 32 job satisfaction need statements. They first are asked to indicate, on a nine-point scale, how important each need is for them to be happy in their work. They then are asked to indicate, again on a nine-point scale, the degree to which that need is being met through their current job. Each item then is scored, taking into consideration the difference between what they "need" and what they "get." A weighted scoring system yields a range of 0 to 72 for each item and a composite mean. Scores are interpreted as follows: 0 to 10 indicates satisfaction, 11 to 20 indicates mild dissatisfaction, 21 to 30 indicates moderate dissatisfaction, and 31–72 indicates intense dissatisfaction.

The questionnaire was sent to the ACCE at each of the identified programs, along with a cover letter explaining the purpose of the study and a postage-paid return envelope. Each questionnaire was coded for statistical purposes. Six weeks after the questionnaires were mailed, we began our data analysis. Responses received after that time were not used.

Data Analysis

Descriptive statistics were calculated for the demographic data. Mean percentages of self-assessed burnout were calculated for all respondents and for several subgroups. Job satisfaction scores and profiles were generated for the entire group and for the subgroups.

RESULTS

One hundred twelve (66.3%) of the total of 169 questionnaires were returned and analyzed.

Demographic Data

The mean age of the respondents was 37.9 ± 8.7 years with a range of 25 to 64 years. Eighty-eight (78.6%) of the respondents were female; 24 (21.4%) were male. Seventy (62.5%) of the respondents held advanced master's degrees, 20 (17.8%) held bachelor's degrees, 16 (14.3%) held entry-level master's degrees, and 6 (5.4%) held doctoral degrees. The mean length of time as an ACCE was 5.2 ± 5.0 years, with a range of 1 to 30 years. Sixty-two (55.3%) of the respondents held positions in baccalaureate degree programs, 38 (33.9%) in associate's degree programs, 6 (5.4%) in entry-level master's degree programs, and 6 (5.4%) in certificate and combined academic level programs. Thirty-two (28.6%) of the respondents were tenured, 35 (31.2%) were on a tenure track, and 42 (37.5%) were not on a tenure track. Three respondents (2.7%) did not indicate their tenure status. The greatest mean percentage of work time

a year was allotted to ACCE activities ($\overline{X}$ = 46.9% ± 19.8%, range = 15%–100%) with classroom teaching ($\overline{X}$ = 32.9% ± 19.3%, range = 0%-75%) ranking second. Considerably less time was allotted to other activities: committee-service activities ($\overline{X}$ = 9.8% ± 10.2%, range = 0%-50%), professional practice ($\overline{X}$ = 7.2% ± 10.1%, range = 0%-50%), and research ($\overline{X}$ = 2.8% ± 4.6%, range = 0%-25%). The mean class size was 32.1 ± 18.1 students, with a range of 7 to 100 students. These demographic characteristics were comparable to those reported by other authors.[1-4]

Self-perceived Burnout

The mean percentage of self-perceived burnout for all respondents was 39.2% ± 26.4%, with a range of 0% to 95%. Those ACCEs holding doctoral degrees expressed the highest mean percentage of burnout, and tenure-track faculty members expressed the lowest mean percentage. The mean percentages of self-perceived burnout for all subgroups are presented in the Table.

Job Satisfaction

The mean job satisfaction score for all respondents on the ON-Q ($\overline{X}$ = 13) indicated only mild dissatisfaction. The mean job satisfaction scores for all subgroups are shown in the Table. The job satisfaction profiles generated for all respondents, for the most satisfied subgroup (ACCEs in entry-level master's degree programs), and for the least satisfied group (ACCEs holding doctoral degrees) are shown in Figure 1.

Comparisons of job satisfaction profiles of the subgroups are presented in Figures 2 through 5. In Figure 2, the ACCEs are compared by sex; in Figure 3, they are compared by the highest degree held; in Figure 4, they are compared by tenure status; and in Figure 5, they are compared by the type of educational program in which they work.

Because the profiles represent composite scores for four items within each area, variations among the individual item ratings are not evident in the figures. Noteworthy single-item responses that are clouded by the composite scores include the following: 1) ACCEs in associate's degree programs, ACCEs with bachelor's degrees, and tenured ACCEs expressed high levels of dissatisfaction with the time available to accomplish tasks (ON-Q scores of 35, 35, and 36, respectively) and 2) ACCEs with doctoral degrees expressed high levels of

TABLE
Mean Percentages of Self-perceived Burnout and Job Satisfaction Scores for Academic Coordinators of Clinical Education by Subgroups

Subgroup	n	Self-perceived Burnout (%)		Job Satisfaction Score
		X̄	s	
Sex				
Male	24	38.0	29.1	15
Female	88	39.5	25.7	13
Degree				
Bachelor's	20	35.2	23.2	16
Entry-level master's	16	40.9	25.5	12
Advanced master's	70	39.2	27.5	13
Doctorate	6	52.5	13.7	18
Type of program				
Associate's degree	38	43.6	27.7	16
Bachelor's degree	62	37.7	25.0	12
Entry-level master's degree	6	32.5	29.4	8
Certificate-combined degrees	6	44.0	23.3	14
Tenure status*				
Tenured	32	45.5	28.8	15
On tenure track	35	29.8	21.6	12
Not on tenure track	42	43.6	23.8	13

ª Three respondents did not indicate their tenure status.

dissatisfaction with the need to feel that their capabilities are not wasted and to earn a comfortable living (ON-Q scores of 38 and 31, respectively).

DISCUSSION

Analysis of the self-perceived burnout levels reveals some surprising results. Given the variety and extent of ACCE responsibilities, we expected the level of self-perceived burnout to be higher than reported. Although a wide range of levels of burnout was reported by individuals, the mean is relatively low. The low mean level of burnout is supported, however, by the ON-Q scores indicating relatively high levels of job satisfaction.

We also expected that ACCEs on a tenure track would express higher levels of burnout than tenured or nontenure-track ACCEs because of the increased pressures often inherent in the tenure process. Those ACCEs on a tenure track, however, expressed the lowest burnout level of all groups. Because the data obtained from this study do not provide information about why this response was expressed, future research on this finding is warranted.

Analysis of the job satisfaction inventory results indicates that, overall, ACCEs are dissatisfied only mildly with their jobs. Given the nature and extent of the ACCE's responsibilities, it is not surprising that ACCEs expressed dissat-

isfaction with their work load, the time available to accomplish tasks, and organizational efficiency. These responses, however, must be considered in light of previous ON-Q research indicating that many occupational groups tend to express high levels of dissatisfaction in these areas.[18] When viewed in the con-

text of Maslow's hierarchy of needs theory,[9] the ACCEs expressed satisfaction with those aspects of their jobs that allow them to meet their higher order motivational needs (ie, being able to help others through their work, having the responsibility to implement important activities, having freedom in their job activities, having opportunities for creativity, and experiencing friendship among co-workers). Satisfaction with these areas would appear to outweigh the dissatisfactions expressed.

When grouped according to sex, the female ACCEs expressed greater overall satisfaction than the male ACCEs. Except for the area of pay and benefits, women expressed greater satisfaction than men in each of the areas identified in the profile, although the pattern of satisfaction is similar for both sexes (Fig. 2), indicating that both groups find satisfaction and dissatisfaction in similar aspects of the job.

When grouped according to the highest degree held, ACCEs with entry-level master's degrees expressed the greatest overall level of satisfaction, followed by those with advanced master's degrees, those with bachelor's degrees, and those with doctoral degrees. This relationship generally is maintained throughout the subgroup profiles (Fig. 3). The master's degree groups show considerable consistency in their profile patterns indica-

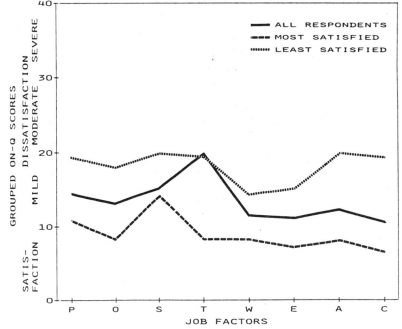

Fig. 1. Job satisfaction profiles of all Academic Coordinators of Clinical Education, the most satisfied group (ACCEs in entry-level master's degree programs) and the least satisfied group (ACCEs with doctoral degrees). (P = pay and benefits, O = organization, S = supervision, T = time and work load, W = work, E = self-esteem, A = achievement, C = creativity.)

ting that they find similar aspects of the job satisfactory and dissatisfactory. The profile patterns of the bachelor's and doctoral degree groups is less consistent. Though both groups generally show high levels of dissatisfaction throughout the profiles, time is a greater source of dissatisfaction for the bachelor's degree group than for the doctoral degree group, whereas the work itself is a source of some dissatisfaction for the doctoral degree group. The levels of dissatisfaction in the area of achievement expressed by the bachelor's and doctoral degree groups are the highest expressed by any of the subgroups. The doctoral degree group also expressed the highest level of dissatisfaction relative to creativity.

The extent of dissatisfaction expressed by ACCEs holding doctoral degrees is only partially evident in the profile. The grouping of items into categorical areas obscures this group's high level of dissatisfaction with the need to feel that their capabilities are not being wasted (ON-Q score = 38), because also included in the self-esteem area is the item related to friendship, which this group reported to be highly satisfactory (ON-Q score = 1). The high ON-Q score for the item related to use of capabilities, together with the overall level and pattern of dissatisfaction, suggests that ACCEs with doctoral degrees may not

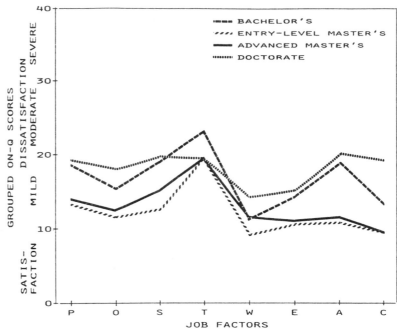

Fig. 3. Job satisfaction profiles of Academic Coordinators of Clinical Education grouped according to highest degree obtained. (P = pay and benefits, O = organization, S = supervision, T = time and work load, W = work, E = self-esteem, A = achievement, C = creativity.)

be realizing their full potential within the current academic structure. Further study of this group appears to be warranted.

When grouped according to tenure status, ACCEs on a tenure track expressed the greatest overall level of sat-

isfaction, followed by those who are not on a tenure track and those who are tenured. The overall pattern of satisfaction remains generally the same throughout the profiles (Fig. 4). The relationship between the groups, however, does not remain consistent. This finding indicates that, with the exception of the pay and benefit area, these groups find satisfaction and dissatisfaction in the same job factors, but to differing degrees. The high level of dissatisfaction expressed by ACCEs with tenure is an interesting finding and warrants further investigation.

When grouped according to the type of educational program in which they work, ACCEs in entry-level master's degree programs expressed the greatest overall level of satisfaction, followed by those in bachelor's degree programs, those in certificate-combined degree level programs, and those in associate's degree programs. This relationship is maintained throughout three of the subgroup profiles (Fig. 5); the certificate-combined degree level program profile is atypical. The profile patterns lack the same degree of consistency seen in previous groupings. The profile of ACCEs in bachelor's degree programs is typical of most subgroup curves with one notable exception: expressed satisfaction with the area related to achievement. The atypical nature of the certificate-combined degree level program profile

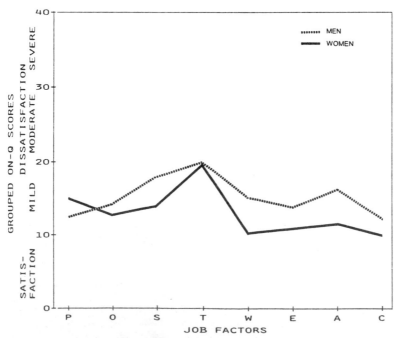

Fig. 2. Job satisfaction profiles of Academic Coordinators of Clinical Education grouped according to sex. (P = pay and benefits, O = organization, S = supervision, T = time and work load, W = work, E = self-esteem, A = achievement, C = creativity.)

may be related to the diversity of such programs.

Of particular interest is the level and pattern of satisfaction expressed by ACCEs in entry-level master's degree programs. Only the supervision area is a source of major dissatisfaction for this group. This finding is noteworthy only because it deviates substantially from the satisfaction level expressed in the other areas. This group also is the only subgroup to express relative satisfaction with time and work load.

The profile of ACCEs in associate's degree programs is also of interest because this group clearly is more dissatisfied than the others. The level of dissatisfaction expressed in the area related to the organization is the highest of all the subgroups. That most of these programs are located in community colleges may be a significant factor influencing this group's level of dissatisfaction, although other factors may be important as well. Further study of this group is warranted, especially because the problems of ACCEs in associate's degree programs may be considerably different from those of ACCEs in entry-level programs for the physical therapist.

Considered together, the job satisfaction scores and profiles for all subgroups suggest that the most satisfied ACCE would be a woman, have a master's degree, and be on a tenure track in an entry-level master's degree program, whereas the least satisfied ACCE would be a man, have a doctoral degree, and be tenured in an associate's degree program. The trend toward postbaccalaureate entry-level education for the physical therapist, therefore, would bode well for the job satisfaction of ACCEs in educational programs for the physical therapist, provided that doctoral degree level preparation is not mandatory.

CONCLUSIONS

The results of this descriptive study indicate that the overall level of job satisfaction among ACCEs is relatively high, and the overall level of burnout is relatively low. Academic Coordinators of Clinical Education appear to find satisfaction in those areas of the job that allow them to meet their needs for self-esteem, achievement, and creativity. The level of satisfaction in these areas appears to outweigh the dissatisfaction that they express with the work load, time constraints, and organizational efficiency. The levels of overall satisfaction and the areas of expressed satisfac-

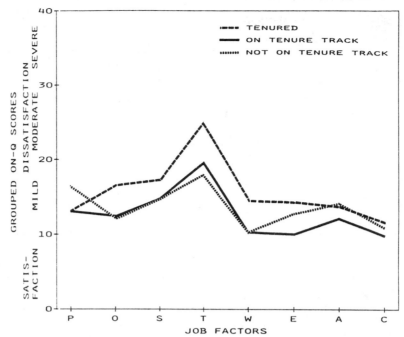

Fig. 4. Job satisfaction profiles of Academic Coordinators of Clinical Education grouped according to tenure status. (P = pay and benefits, O = organization, S = supervision, T = time and work load, W = work, E = self-esteem, A = achievement, C = creativity.)

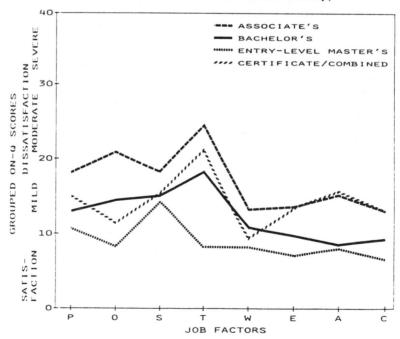

Fig. 5. Job satisfaction profiles of Academic Coordinators of Clinical Education grouped according to the type of program in which they work. (P = pay and benefits, O = organization, S = supervision, T = time and work load, W = work, E = self-esteem, A = achievement, C = creativity.)

tion and dissatisfaction vary among subgroups: ACCEs in entry-level master's degree programs expressed the highest level of satisfaction, whereas ACCEs with doctoral degrees expressed the lowest level of satisfaction.

Insofar as the job expectations of ACCEs are similar to those of other allied health care professionals, the results of this study provide a basic description of job satisfaction among ACCEs. Other factors unique to the

ACCE's job may exist, however, that were not addressed in the inventory used for this study. Further investigation is needed to determine whether such factors exist and, if so, to what extent they might affect job satisfaction levels. Additionally, a replication of this study after 1990 might be warranted to determine whether the shift to postbaccalaureate entry-level education for the physical therapist affects the job satisfaction of ACCEs.

REFERENCES

1. Moore ML, Perry JF: Clinical Education in Physical Therapy: Present Status/Future Needs. Washington, DC, Section for Education, American Physical Therapy Association, 1976
2. McPhail S: Role of the Academic Coordinator of Clinical Education. Read at the First National Academic Coordinators of Clinical Education Workshop, St. Louis, MO, November 8-9, 1984
3. Kondela-Cebulski PM: Counseling function of academic coordinators of clinical education from select entry-level physical therapy educational programs. Phys Ther 62:470–476, 1982
4. Philips BU Jr, McPhail S, Roemer S: Role and functions of the academic coordinator of clinical education in physical therapy education: A survey. Phys Ther 66:981–985, 1986
5. Herzberg F, Mausner B, Snyderman BB: The Motivation to Work. New York, NY, John Wiley & Sons Inc, 1959
6. French JRP, Rogers W, Cobb S: A model of person-environment fit. In Coelho GV, et al (eds): Coping and Adaptation. New York, NY, Basic Books Inc, Publishers, 1974
7. Maslach C, Jackson D: The measurement of experienced burnout. Journal of Occupational Behavior 2:99–113, 1981
8. Vroom VH: Work and Motivation. New York, NY, John Wiley & Sons Inc, 1964
9. Maslow AH (ed): Motivation and Personality, ed 2. New York, NY, Harper & Row, Publishers Inc, 1970
10. Broski D, Cook S: The job satisfaction of allied health professionals. J Allied Health 7:281–287, 1978
11. French RM, Renzler AG: Personality and job satisfaction of medical technologists. Am J Med Technol 42:92–103, 1976
12. Rogers DA: Stress and job satisfaction of clinical laboratory scientists. Am J Med Technol 49:183–188, 1983
13. Wolfe GA: Burnout of therapists: Inevitable or preventable? Phys Ther 61:1046–1050, 1981
14. Schuster ND, Nelson DL, Quisling C: Burnout among physical therapists. Phys Ther 64:299–303, 1984
15. Atwood CA, Woolf DA: Job satisfaction of physical therapists. Health Care Manage Rev 7(1):81–86, 1982
16. Selker LG, Rozier CK, Vogt MT: Locus of decision-making and job satisfaction of department chairpersons in schools of allied health. J Allied Health 12:21–29, 1983
17. Careers in Physical Therapy. Washington, DC, American Physical Therapy Association, 1984
18. Berger P: Occupational Needs Questionnaire. Doctoral Dissertation. DeKalb, IL, Northern Illinois University, 1983

APPENDIX
Occupational Needs Questionnaire Items

PAY AND BENEFITS
5. To earn a comfortable living.
12. To get training to develop new work skills.
13. To have job security.
15. To make significant financial gains from my wages.

THE ORGANIZATION
8. To have clearly defined organizational policies.
17. To be a part of an organization of which I can feel proud.
25. To have adequate equipment and supplies to do the job.
29. To have a pleasant physical work environment.

THE SUPERVISION
10. To know clearly what my employer expects of me.
18. To have a supervisor I can respect.
22. To be treated fairly by my employer.
30. To receive recognition from my supervisors for my good work.

THE TIME
7. To have enough time to do the work required.
9. To have a manageable work load.
24. To feel that my organization gets things done efficiently.
28. To be satisfied with the work hours and schedules.

THE WORK
1. To be free from boring tasks.
4. To be engaged in work that is in and of itself enjoyable.
21. To have responsibility for carrying out important activities.
26. To be doing things that agree with my conscience.

SELF-ESTEEM
2. To help others through my work.
3. To feel that my job is considered important by people meaningful to me.
16. To experience friendship among my co-workers.
31. To feel that my capabilities are not being wasted.

ACHIEVEMENT
14. To feel that I have achieved importance in life through my work.
19. To experience personal growth through my work.
27. To advance up the ladder of career success.
32. To have enough authority to take action without clearance through superiors.

CREATIVITY
6. To feel a sense of adventure in my work.
11. To feel a sense of excitement in my work.
20. To have opportunities to be creative on the job.
23. To have freedom in what I do rather than having to follow set rules.

Role Modeling Behaviors and the Clinical Instructor

Characteristics of Physical Therapy Role Models

BARBARA F. JACOBSON, MS

This study examined the personal and technical characteristics used in an investigation of role modeling in physical therapy. Recently graduated physical therapists performed a forced-choice Q sort composed of 49 physical therapist characteristics to describe 1) themselves, 2) their model academic instructor, and 3) their model clinical instructor. A significant difference between the frequency of personal and technical characteristics placed in the Most Descriptive section resulted for the self sort. The 10 characteristics ranked by highest mean values were all personal for self sorts, the majority were personal for the clinical model and combined sorts, and were equally divided between personal and technical for the academic model sorts.

This study focused on the professional characteristics which provide a basis for the identification, modeling, and role-taking processes students may go through in becoming physical therapists. The investigation addressed the general question of whether recently graduated physical therapists would describe themselves, their clinical role models, and their academic role models primarily with personal or technical characteristics.

In a previous investigation, these recent graduates' self-descriptions correlated significantly with descriptions of their model clinical instructors, but not with descriptions of their model academic instructors.[1]

REVIEW OF LITERATURE

Just as society defines or describes a person by his or her behavior or by assigning abstract psychological characteristics on the basis of behavior, members of different professions also identify themselves by certain behaviors and qualities. These characteristics may be held informally in a mental image or they may be specifically listed by a professional group or organization. Studies of professional socialization of doctors,[2,3] nurses,[4-6] and educators[7] present various concepts and models of people in different roles. Professional characteristics vary among members of the medical profession, depending on their positions or specialty areas. Various lists of characteristics considered essential for being a physical therapist have been developed primarily for screening and evaluation purposes. Bergman writes about certain personality characteristics of physical therapy students entering a university program.[8] Extending these characteristics, she describes a practicing therapist. Brollier's study also focuses on cognitive and personality traits of physical therapy students.[9] More recently, questionnaires were used to obtain descriptions of the clinical physical therapists who supervise students.[10,11]

As in most professional education, the study of physical therapy includes learning in the cognitive, psychomotor, and affective realms. During much of the profession's educational history, however, most emphasis has been on the acquisition of medical facts, therapeutic procedures, and clinical skills. One assumption may have been that students enter training already possessing certain basic personal qualities. The affective realm has received more attention in recent years as an area in which to plan learning experiences and in which students should be evaluated. Nevertheless, evaluating personal qualities remains more difficult than testing knowledge and skill. While intellectual or cognitive development is the main focus in the classroom,[9,12] the development of professional attitudes and behaviors seems to receive more emphasis during clinical practice. Most clinical evaluation forms are designed to assess the student's skills, knowledge, and personal characteristics. According to Watts, learning in the affective domain is strongly related to the process of becoming a professional.[13] She likens "the process of initiating (physical therapy) students into their professional role" to the development for physicians, as described in *Boys in White*.[2]

Ms. Jacobson conducted this study in partial fulfillment of requirements for a graduate program at Sargent College, Boston University, 1971. She is currently a physical therapist with the Durham County Health Department. She resides at 96 Hamilton Rd, Chapel Hill, NC 27514.

THE SPECIFIC PROBLEM

Assuming that the process of becoming a professional is closely related to the development of the affective domain, much of this process must occur in the clinic where personal qualities are stressed. Models must be present in the clinic who possess the positive characteristics with which the students can identify or which they can emulate. Are students cognizant of the personal qualities of the physical therapists who supervise them? Would personal quality characteristics be chosen more frequently by the students to describe their model clinical instructor or their model academic instructor? This study attempts to answer these specific questions: In a forced-choice Q sort would personal characteristics be placed more frequently than technical (knowledge-skill) characteristics in the *Most Descriptive* section of the Q sort by new graduate physical therapists when describing themselves, their model academic instructor, and their model clinical instructor? What are the characteristics which rank highest and lowest in being most and least descriptive, respectively, of these three types of physical therapists?

METHOD

Instrument

To measure the amount of identification or similarity between students and their role models, the method of measurement of trait-by-trait comparison seemed the most reliable and valid of the methods reviewed.[14] The Q sort is an appropriate measurement technique consisting of descriptive statements placed on a continuum to describe a person, subject, or feeling. A Q sort of 49 favorable professional characteristics was derived from physical therapy educational objectives and evaluation forms, nursing studies, a teacher Q sort, personality trait lists, and interviews with therapists. The items represented overt and inferred characteristics, either of a personal-social (affective) or technical (cognitive-psychomotor) nature, and were applicable to clinical staff therapists, clinical supervisors, and academic instructors. The validity of the Q-sort items was tested before data collection began. Six judges who were physical therapy graduate students with clinical experience determined, by five/sixths or total agreement, whether items were technical or personal characteristics, and whether they would validly describe a clinical staff member, a clinical supervisor, and an academic instructor. Of the original 86 items, 49 were acceptable—26 personal and 23

technical characteristics. To determine reliability of the Q sort, six female physical therapists (two teachers and four clinical therapists—all graduate students) sorted the items to describe a physical therapist. After 48 hours they resorted the items. The Pearson product moment correlation was .804.

Subjects

Two-hundred and sixty women, recent graduates, were randomly selected from the American Physical Therapy Association membership list and contacted for participation in the study. The subjects were the 95 respondents who correctly completed all three Q sorts. The women contacted were 1970 graduates of 49 approved physical therapy schools and were currently employed. Their ages ranged from 21 through 25 years.

The following descriptive data on the subjects and their model therapists are taken from the previously mentioned study.[1] The recent graduates' modal age was 23 years. Their modal clinical affiliation time was 12 weeks. They were employed at their first job (82%) in a hospital department (70%), working between nine and eleven months (53%). The majority of subjects described the academic models as between the ages of 30 and 60 years with daily contact between nine and 14 months. The clinical models were between the ages of 20 and 30 years and had daily contact with the students for a period of from four to six weeks.

The data collection materials with the Q sorts were mailed to each subject, requesting her to describe 1) herself as a practicing physical therapist, 2) her model classroom instructor (female physical therapist), and 3) her model clinical supervisor (female physical therapist). The model therapists to be described were to be "therapists whom the participants admired most and wanted to be like."

The subjects were instructed to sort the 49 items into nine piles of varying predetermined sizes, ranging from *Least Descriptive* through *Somewhat Descriptive* to *Most Descriptive* (Tab. 1). An item could be placed in any pile thought appropriate and would be ranked according to the pile number, nine being the highest value. For this analysis the last three piles numbered 7, 8, and 9 were designated the *Most Descriptive* section and piles 1, 2, and 3, the *Least Descriptive* section, with each containing 12 items.

Analysis

Three forms of analysis were performed:
1. The frequency with which personal and technical

TABLE 1

Q-sorting Pattern

Pile #	(1)	(2)	(3)	(4)	(5)	(6)	(7)	(8)	(9)
# of items to be placed in each pile	2	4	6	8	9	8	6	4	2
Descriptive range		Least Describes			Somewhat Describes			Most Describes	

characteristics were placed in the *Most Descriptive* section for the three different sorts was obtained. The chi square test of significance at the .01 level was calculated to test the differences between expected and observed frequencies of the two types of characteristics.

2. The mean or average rank of each characteristic for each group sort was derived and the characteristics with the 10 highest means were ranked for each group sort and combined sorts.

3. The six characteristics with the lowest means for the model sorts and all sorts combined were also identified.

RESULTS

A total of 1,140 items were placed in the *Most Descriptive* sections of each group of Q sorts. The frequency with which technical and personal items were placed in the *Most Descriptive* sections varied significantly for each sort as revealed by the chi square test (Tab. 2). Both the self and clinical model sorts contained a larger number of personal than technical items, whereas the academic model sort contained a higher number of technical than personal items.

The mean or average rank of each characteristic for each group sort was derived by giving the item the value number or rank of the column, combining the values for the subjects (95) and obtaining the average. Table 3 depicts the items ranked according to the 10 highest means for the three sorts and the combined sorts for each characteristic. All high-

ranking characteristics were personal for the self sort. The majority of the characteristics were personal for the clinical model, models combined, and total sorts. Personal and technical characteristics were equally divided for the academic sort.

A sample of the Q sort items are listed in Table 4 with the mean rankings shown in Tables 3 and 5. The following characteristics, all personal, ranked in the top ten for all three sorts and combined sorts:

Item 31. The physical therapist appears to have care and concern for the individual with whom she is working.

Item 23. The physical therapist has good rapport with people she instructs.

Item 26. The physical therapist always tries to do the best job that she can in the time that is available.

The self and clinical model sorts had these items, all personal, in common in the top 10 rankings:

Item 1. The physical therapist is industrious and hard-working.

Item 30. The physical therapist has an optimistic and positive attitude toward people with whom she comes in contact.

Item 37. The physical therapist seems to have good common sense which she uses in her work situation.

The role models had only item 8 in common: The physical therapist is generally well-informed in most areas involving physical therapy theory and treatment techniques and skills.

Items selected in the top 10 for self only were numbers 4, 5, 29, and 36, for clinical models only—numbers 10, 3, and 43, and for academic models only—numbers 9, 24, 27, 35, 46, and 49. By

TABLE 2

Chi Square Table for Type of Item Frequency in the Most Descriptive Section of the Q Sort

Model	Type	Expected	Observed	Chi Square[a]
Self	Personal	604.9	855	21.92
	Technical	535.1	285	
Academic	Personal	604.9	501	3.75
	Technical	535.1	639	
Clinical	Personal	604.9	682	2.07
	Technical	535.1	458	

[a] at .01 level with 1 df, $x^2 = 6.64$ for one-tailed test

combining academic and clinical Q sorts as role models, some otherwise lower-ranked items for each model (numbers 1, 3, 9, and 49) received a higher ranking, giving the impression that they could be considered important characteristics for an overall physical therapy role model.

Table 5 depicts the items ranked according to the six lowest means for the model sorts and all sorts combined for each characteristic. The majority of these six characteristics were technical. Item 39 ranked lowest for almost all group and combined sorts:

> The physical therapist presents an idealistic view of the practice of physical therapy to the students.

Other items ranking lowest, and therefore least descriptive of physical therapist models, were numbers 2, 14, 15, 18, and 40 (Tabs. 4, 5).

DISCUSSION

The 10 items with the highest means are referred to by the author as *most descriptive* because of their placement at the *most descriptive* end of the Q sort. To the recent graduates, these items must have seemed important and of intrinsic value, because they were assigning characteristics to their role models—persons whom they admired or wanted to be like. Whether the graduates projected these characteristics onto the models or the models, in fact, displayed the characteristics is beyond the scope of this study. Forced-choice sorting builds in a limitation in choosing most descriptive items but causes the subjects to be discriminating in their choices.

Personal items were chosen as *most descriptive* of self and clinical models by the recent graduates (Tabs. 2, 3). Therapists working in the clinic were identified by the same six personal items. Why were these personal items chosen more frequently by the recent graduates than technical items for the clinical models and the self? One influencing factor may have been related to most students' primary objective of clinical work prior to and throughout the formal training period. Another factor may have been that at the sorting time the majority of subjects were working in clinical settings, thus identifying more readily with the clinical models. Closeness in age and continuous contact between the subjects and the clinical models could have been a contributing factor. Because students are used to being evaluated by others in terms of technical abilities, identifying themselves with personal items may have been easier. Also, the subjects may still have be-

lieved themselves to be weak in the cognitive-skills area because they lacked experience. Due to contact with a variety of people and situations present in the hospital, the daily interactions of the clinical model may define her personal qualities in an obvious and identifiable manner for the students. Recent graduates associated more technical characteristics with the classroom model than with the clinical model. The academic models had daily contact over a long period, at least nine months, but I assume that this contact was in a fairly formal setting with limited personal interaction. The academic models were older than the clinical models.

According to this study, some technical attributes, considered necessary for being a competent physical therapist by the "profession,"[15] appear more descriptive of the academic therapist than the clinical therapist. Items 27, 35, and 46 ranked in the top 10 for the academic model (Tabs. 3, 4). The previously mentioned study concluded that the primary model for the novice was the clinical model.[1] Perhaps, if the academic models were in situations where the students would identify more with them, the students would also incorporate some of the important technical characteristics. For the most effective modeling, classroom instructors might work directly with patients either by treating their own limited patient loads while students are in the clinic or by supervising students who are treating patients. McMillan[16] and Borden[17] have suggested that academic models work primarily with patients of their speciality areas in the clinic, as a carry-over from their major teaching subjects in the classroom. Faculty members, however, may not have easy access to the clinic. Classroom demonstrations of treatments with patients or students or filmed treatment incidents may have to serve as second best, but the students would at least see the academic model acting as a clinician. The clinical therapist could also increase didactic teaching in the classroom or clinic to more obviously display possession of the technical-skills characteristic to the role-taker.

I base the above discussion on the assumption that some common characteristics are desired and promoted for all therapists. Not only do admission committees of physical therapy schools emphasize certain characteristics in their selection of students, but, as stated by Bartlett, our complex society demands "a clear identification of our professional role."[18] On the other hand, specialty areas continue to proliferate in the profession. According to medical specialization studies[4, 6, 19] and the distribution of characteristics for the two models in this study (Tabs. 3, 5), specialization may promote diversity of characteristics in professional membership. Literature written on specialists versus generalists in schools or on the job emphasizes the existence of, and necessity for, both to exist concurrently.[20] Members with a wide variety of professional characteristics may become the norm, but some common professional identity is necessary to separate physical therapists from other health professionals. As this study indicated, the profession may thrive best in a "paradoxical state," as many professions are doing, with some important characteristics remaining common to all physical therapists and other prominent characteristics describing only the specializing therapists.

CONCLUSIONS AND SUGGESTIONS

Looking at the frequency of personal and technical items placed in the *Most Descriptive* section of

the Q sort for the groups of sorts, personal items were chosen significantly more than technical items for the self and slightly more for clinical model sorts, whereas technical items were chosen slightly more often for the academic model sorts.

This investigation points up the strong emphasis on certain personal characteristics considered important for physical therapists to possess, particularly the qualities of "care and concern for the individual with whom she is working" and "has good rapport with the people she instructs." A technical characteristic that also must be considered important for the physical therapy role model is that she "is generally well-informed in most areas involving physical therapy theory and treatment techniques and skill."

Because personal quality characteristics were selected more frequently as most descriptive of the clinical models, the study indicates that the personal

TABLE 3
Characteristics with the Ten Highest Means Ranked for the Sorts

Item #	Individual Sorts						Combined Sorts			
	Self[a]	R[b]	Clin.[a]	R[b]	Acad.[a]	R[b]	Mods.[a]	R[b]	Tots.[a]	R[b]
31 – P	7.75	1	6.81	1	6.04	7	6.43	2	6.81	1
23 – P	6.52	3	6.27	4	6.33	4	6.30	3	6.37	2
26 – P	6.40	5.5	6.11	5	6.11	5.5	6.07	4	6.18	3
8 – T	5.30		6.52	2	6.55	2	6.54	1	6.12	4
1 – P	6.25	8.5	5.81	8	5.57		5.69	7	5.88	5
10 – T	5.51		6.35	3	5.77		6.06	5	5.87	6
37 – P	6.25	8.5	5.97	6	5.26		5.67	8	5.83	7
36 – P	6.40	5.5	5.47		5.28		5.38		5.72	8
5 – P	6.50	4	5.36		5.22		5.29		5.69	9
30 – P	6.20	10	5.72	10	4.96		5.34		5.63	10
9 – T	3.36		5.13		6.60	1	5.87	6	5.03	
49 – P	5.60		5.33		5.92	9	5.63	9	5.61	
3 – P	5.32		5.92	7	5.28		5.60	10	5.51	
4 – P	6.85	2	5.57		4.40		4.88		5.61	
29 – P	6.36	7	4.91		5.37		5.14		5.27	
43 – P	5.78		5.75	9	4.55		5.15		5.36	
35 – T	3.90		4.37		6.34	3	5.36		4.87	
27 – P	4.72		5.04		5.96	8	5.50		5.24	
24 – T	4.01		5.04		6.11	5.5	5.58		5.25	
46 – T	3.26		4.39		5.87	10	5.13		4.52	

[a] Means.   P Personal.
[b] Rank.   T Technical.

TABLE 4

Sample of Physical Therapist Characteristics on Q Sort[a] Items

Item #	Type[b] Characteristics	The physical therapist . . .
1	(P)	. . . is industrious and hard-working.
2	(P)	. . . prefers clearly defined work situations where each person is responsible for her job and her job alone.
3	(P)	. . . motivates people to work to their capacity while helping them to realize limitations.
4	(P)	. . . is responsive to the moods and needs of others.
5	(P)	. . . has a good sense of humor which uplifts the others' moods or situation.
8	(T)	. . . is generally well-informed in most areas involving physical therapy theory and treatment techniques and skills.
9	(T)	. . . knows how to teach physical therapy material in an interesting manner.
10	(T)	. . . applies her knowledge and skills of the latest techniques in patient treatment planning.
14	(T)	. . . demonstrates abnormal body movements for teaching purposes in the use of aids.
15	(P)	. . . prefers to work independently.
18	(T)	. . . participates in research projects which may contribute to the professional body of knowledge.
23	(P)	. . . has good rapport with the people she instructs.
24	(T)	. . . presents information to the learner in a clear and concise manner.
26	(P)	. . . always tries to do the best job that she can in the time that is available.
27	(T)	. . . gives a comprehensive explanation of the rationale behind a treatment program.
29	(P)	. . . recognizes her own abilities and short-comings.
30	(P)	. . . has an optimistic and positive attitude toward people with whom she comes in contact.
31	(P)	. . . appears to have care and concern for the individual with whom she is working.
35	(T)	. . . is interested in the current problems and trends in the establishment and development of physical therapy as a profession.
36	(P)	. . . is willing to help out where needed, even if the work extends beyond her expected duties.
37	(P)	. . . seems to have good common sense which she uses in her work situation.
39	(T)	. . . presents an idealistic view of the practice of physical therapy to the student.
40	(T)	. . . displays interest in research by reading research articles and discussing problem areas in physical therapy.
43	(P)	. . . is flexible, adapting readily to a variety of situations or crises.
46	(T)	. . . has special knowledge and skills in one or two areas in which she concentrates.
49	(P)	. . . is observant and aware of things going on in the department or classroom.

[a] Q sort limited to the items mentioned in this text
[b] (P) = Personal. (T) = Technical

attributes of the clinical therapists are of noted importance. The personal characteristics they possess may help to determine the amount of influence they exert or the degree to which they serve as positive models for the students. The recent graduates, also, described themselves primarily with personal qualities. Many of these qualities are the same as for the clinical models. This pattern is congruent with the current emphasis on the affective realm in the clinical physical therapy professional program.

Limitations existed in this study and some questions are raised. Because this study was performed in retrospect with the subjects already practicing in the clinic, the recent graduates might be expected to identify more with the clinical instructor model than with the academic instructor model. A more exacting study might have the students perform the Q sorts at the end of the formal didactic study period and again at the end of the clinical education period. The characteristics themselves, because they may have been neither inclusive enough nor labeled accurately as personal or technical, and because selection was by new members of the profession, may have affected the results of this study. The members of the profession set the tone for characteristics which are projected and promote those they think important. As an interesting and timely study, experienced physical therapists could sort their description of a physical therapist model or models. Would their descriptions of academic and clinical therapists differ? With more therapists specializing within the profession, will more therapists with diverse characteristics be found? As in medicine, do certain characteristics accompany particular specialties? Or should the emphasis continue to be on

TABLE 5
Characteristics with the Lowest Means Ranked for the Sorts

Item #	Individual Sorts						Combined Sorts			
	Self[a]	R[b]	Clin.[a]	R[b]	Acad.[a]	R[b]	Mods.[a]	R[b]	Tots.[a]	R[b]
40−T	2.8	47	3.6	44	5.0		3.8	44	3.8	44
14−T	3.1	46	2.8	47	3.6	46	3.2	46	3.4	45.5
18−T	2.3	49	3.1		4.8		3.4	45	3.4	45.5
15−P	3.8		2.9	46	2.7	48	2.8	47	3.1	47
2−P	3.5		2.6	48	2.7	47	2.7	48	3.0	48
39−T	2.5	48	2.5	49	2.6	49	2.6	49	2.54	49

[a] Means.
[b] Rank.
T Technical.
P Personal.

many characteristics which are held in common by all physical therapists? How are the profession and its educational institutions approaching the dichotomy of similarity and diversity of personal qualities and abilities among its present and potential members?

Acknowledgment. The author wishes to acknowledge with appreciation the assistance of Irma Wilhelm, Research Associate, Division of Physical Therapy, University of North Carolina School of Medicine, Chapel Hill, NC, in the preparation of this paper.

REFERENCES

1. Jacobson B: Role modeling in physical therapy. Phys Ther 54:244-250, 1974
2. Becker H, Greer B, Hughes E, et al: Boys in White. Chicago, The University Press, 1961
3. Merton R: Some preliminaries to a sociology of medical education. In Merton R, Kendall P (eds): The Student Physician. Cambridge, Harvard University Press, 1957, pp 3-79
4. Corwin R, Taves M: Some concomitants of bureaucratic and professional conceptions of the nurse role. Nurs Res 2:223-227, 1962
5. Heidgerken L: Preference for a teaching or clinical nursing career: Influence of significant others. Nurs Res 19:292-302, 1970
6. Kramer M: Role models, role conceptions, and role deprivation. Nurs Res 17:115-120, 1968
7. Becker H, Carper J: The development of identification with an occupation. Am J Soc 61:289, 1956
8. Bergman J: A Comparative Study of Certain Personality Characteristics of Students Enrolled in Selected Health Programs at the University of Alabama in Birmingham. Dissertation. Birmingham, AL, University of Alabama, 1974
9. Brollier C: Personality and Cognitive Style Characteristics of Physical Therapists, Physical Dysfunction Occupational Therapists, Psychiatric Occupational Therapists, and Social Workers. Thesis. Boston, MA, Boston University, 1969
10. Woodard K: The Characteristics of Effective Clinical Instructors, A Pilot Study. Senior Paper, Chapel Hill, NC, University of North Carolina, 1976
11. Project on Clinical Education in Physical Therapy. Washington, DC, American Physical Therapy Association, 1974
12. Dewton R: Correlative Findings of Student Performance in a Physical Therapy Professional Curriculum. Thesis. Boston, MA, Boston University, 1969
13. Watts N: The affective domain in learning. In MacQueen S (ed): Learning in Physical Therapy Education, APTA-VRA Institute Papers. New York, American Physical Therapy Association, 1966, p 50
14. McAllister L, Neuringer C: A comparative investigation of commonly used methods of measuring the identification process. J Gen Psychol 80:229-242, 1969
15. May B: Evaluation of a competency-based educational system. Phys Ther 57:28-33, 1977
16. McMillan J: Should physical therapy faculty engage in clinical practice? Phys Ther 54:187, 1974
17. Borden R: Should physical therapy faculty engage in clinical practice? Phys Ther 54:188, 1974
18. Bartlett R: A conversation with the president. Progress Report, APTA Membership Newsletter 6 (5):2, 1977
19. Kendall P, Selvin H: Tendencies toward specialization in medical training. In Merton R, Kendall P (eds): The Student Physician. Cambridge, Harvard University Press, 1957, pp 158-174
20. Commach J, Johnson G, Hogue R, et al: What's the answer? Phys Ther 52:447-451, 1972

Role Modeling in Physical Therapy

BARBARA JACOBSON, M.S.

The influence of the instructor in the clinical affiliation period on the professional development of physical therapy students was investigated. Recent graduates' concepts of their academic instructors were compared to those of their clinical instructors as role models for the students by use of a professional characteristics Q sort. A significant difference was found in the amount of agreement between the two relationships. The importance of the supervising clinical therapists in the professional socialization of physical therapy students is emphasized.

The increased amount of theory and the new technical skills of the past decade have necessitated taking a new look at physical therapy education. Should more emphasis be placed on the academic-classroom period or on the clinical education segment? In making this determination, one must consider the influence on the student of both the clinical therapist and the classroom instructor. Which type of therapist has the most influence on the novice?

REVIEW OF LITERATURE

Socialization and Professionalization

The student and teacher both have their own concepts of the physical therapy educational process. To the student, becoming a physical therapist may mean one or two years of physical therapy school with classes, reading, dissecting, practicing on other students, and finally working with patients in the clinic. To the teacher, becoming a physical therapist may

mean that the student attends classes, learns, and applies his new knowledge in patient treatment. All of these activities and more are part of professional socialization. In addition to acquiring an adult role and self-identity through *developmental socialization,* the student is moving from layman to professional man through *professional socialization.*[1] Greenwood defines professional socialization as the acquisition of the body of knowledge and technical skills along with the acculturation process of internalizing the social values, the behavior norms, and the symbols of an occupational group.[2]

Professional socialization or professionalization involves processes which are also common to human development in general. Processes used in a person's general socialization such as identification, modeling, and role-taking are used in his professional development, as well. The various concepts of these processes proposed by theorists of different disciplines overlap; nevertheless, all these processes affect the development of a person's self-concept (or professional concept).

Identification is defined in this study as the modeling of one's self in thought, feeling, or actions after another person,[3] consciously or unconsciously, with the result of assuming abstract psychological characteristics of a

Miss Jacobson is a Clinical Associate and Staff Physical Therapist, Department of Physical Therapy, North Carolina Memorial Hospital, Chapel Hill, NC 27514.

This study was conducted in 1971 while Miss Jacobson was in the graduate program in physical therapy at Boston University.

model such as those termed motives, attitudes, values, ideals, roles, or affective states,[4] as well as behavioral activity.[5,6] Schafer's concept of identification as a secondary-process (the other person is viewed as a model and a basis for comparison) may apply more to some subjects in this investigation than the primary process theory (a positive relationship, with love or respect, and *modeling after someone with qualities they aspire to have*).[3]

Modeling incorporates identification. First, parents are the prime models for the child; then, as the child expands his environment, other significant figures become his models. The teacher may be one of these "significant others." Mager summarizes Bandura's modeling experiments by stating that "if we would maximize subject matter approach tendencies in our students, we must behave the way we want our students to behave."[7]

The model has taken a role, but the learner is in the process of "taking the role of the other" from the role model. Role-taking, an active state, not a one-way process, may be direct or indirect. The person who is enacting the role of a model is continually in a relationship with the model. Not only is the model's role performance observed and acted, but the model's reactions to the observer's role performance are taken into account. Each continually identifies with the other's role and gives identity to his own. Role-taking, a variant of identification, cannot be made without identifying the model. Appearance facilitates identification.[8]

Affected by modeling, identification, and role-taking processes, the self-concept is a learned constellation of perceptions and values which develops largely from observing the reactions one gets from other persons. The parents are the most consistent and earliest influence.[9] Rubin believes that identification is part of the process which enters into the formation of the self-concept; however, self-concept is broader than identity. He states that self-conceptualization and identity formation may occur together and throughout life with one more predominant than the other at a particular time. A person who matures normally will undergo the psychological process of assimilating self-concepts through his experiences and the reactions of others to form his particular identities.[10,11] Identity includes all previous experiences and personal qualities,

while aspects or parts of the self-concept may be modified, given up, or replaced. As a result of growth patterns, various external circumstances, and changing identifications, the self-concept may change throughout life.[11] This alteration in self-concept, resulting from imitation and identification in socially (or professionally) determined situations, provides another basis for this study.

Medical Professionalization

The socialization process of physical therapists has not been studied significantly. Perhaps,. Merton's reference to socialization of doctors would be similar to that of physical therapy students. The medical student develops his professional self with its characteristic values, attitudes, knowledge, and skills, fusing these in such a way as to govern his behavior in a wide variety of professional (and extraprofessional) situations.[2]

Studies have been done in nursing, as well as in medicine, about the person from whom the role is taken—the professional role model. These studies relate to the concepts that nurses develop about their profession and themselves because of the type of nursing model they worked with—instructor versus practitioner or professional versus practical nurse.[13-15] The most relevant article, written by Heidgerken,[16] considered the influence of significant others on a preference for a teaching or clinical nursing practice career. She wanted to know if either the nurse teacher or professional nurse practitioner influenced the neophyte. Teachers were identified 131 times and nurse practitioners 23 times as a major role model influence. Heidgerken believed that the teachers' strong influence might have resulted from the increasing localization of control of nursing education within educational institutions. Because of such control, the opportunity for student nurses to learn the nurse role through imitation or modeling of the nurse practitioner decreases.

In physical therapy, investigations of the most influential role model have not been conducted. Although the clinical therapist is believed to be the most influential, no research by the profession supports this belief. From various studies, research, and theories written on socialization, however, one can presume that role models are important for the professionalization of the physical therapy aspirant. Through role-taking from the physical therapy model, the student's professional identifications are internalized and the role concept of self is formed and stabilized. Identification of the student with the therapist is a result of the modeling process.

THE SPECIFIC PROBLEM

In determining identification between subject and model in the physical therapy educational realm, characteristics of both persons must be evident. For this study, the professional self-concept or image was sought in terms of Rubin's definition of self-concept: "a sum of descriptive attributes of self."[11] A set of professional characteristics was used to show identification of the student with the role models. These characteristics were developed on the theoretical basis of qualities in the role behavior area of actions, skills, and knowledge and in the psychological processes area of traits, attitudes, values, motives, beliefs, interests, ideals, and other affective states.[4,5] With these specific characteristics, I sought to answer the investigative question: What is the degree of agreement or amount of similarity between the perceived professional charactertistics of the recent graduate and the two types of physical therapy role models?

METHOD

In seeking a means of measuring the amount of identification between the student and her physical therapy role model, primary consideration was given to an article by McAllister and Neuringer.[3] The method of measurement in terms of similarity and absolute, trait-by-trait comparison by which students rated themselves and their supervisors seemed the most reliable and valid of the methods tested. Since the testing was to be ex post facto, concurrent testing was not practical.

Instrument

The Q sort, a measurement technique developed by Stephenson,[17] which consists of descriptive statements that can be placed on a continuum to represent a particular subject or person, was used as the method of measurement. Suinn has used Q sorts to measure correlations of both perceived self-sort and ideal self-sort with perceived father-sort for self-father similarity.[18] The latter means of measurement was followed with the assumption that similarity represents identification. Since a physical therapy Q sort did not exist, one consisting of forty-nine favorable professional characteristics was derived from educational objectives and evaluation forms, nursing studies, a teacher Q sort, personality trait lists, and interviews with therapists. The items represented overt and inferred characteristics, either of a personal-social (affective) or technical (cognitive-psychomotor) nature, and were applicable to clinical, supervising, and classroom instructor physical therapists. The items were tested for reliability (.804) and validity.

Subjects and Data Collection

The sample came from 260 randomly selected female physical therapists on the American Physical Therapy Association membership list who were twenty-one through twenty-five years of age, who were 1970 graduates of forty-nine approved physical therapy schools, and who were currently employed.

The data collection materials and Q sorts were mailed to each subject, requesting her to describe 1) herself as a practicing therapist, 2) her model classroom instructor (female physical therapist), and 3) her model clinical affiliation supervisor (female physical therapist). The model therapists were identified as therapists whom the participants most admired and wanted to be like because they had certain qualities which the subject wanted to make her own.

Analysis

The amount of similarity or assumed identification between the subject and each of the model therapists was compared by correlation of the Q sorts of each recent graduate to each chosen role model. The significance of differences was determined by the t test for correlated pairs.

TABLE 1
*Significance of Differences in Correlations
between Subjects and Models*

Sort-Corr.	Mean	S.D.	S.E.	Max.	Min.	t test
Self-Acad.	.140	.217	.022	.678	−.472	$t = 5.88$[a]
Self-Clin.	.338	.277	.028	.929	−.662	

[a] Significant at .001 level, $t_{.001} = 3.46$ (94 d.f., one-tailed).

TABLE 2
Critical Values of the Pearson r

Sort-Corr.	Mean	df
Self-Acad.	.140	93
Self-Clin.	.338[a]	

[a] Significant at the .05 level, $t_{.05} = .1702$ (93 d.f., one-tailed).

TABLE 3
*Role of Physical Therapist Who Was
Considered Most Like the Graduate's Ideal
Therapist (N = 85)*

Role of Therapist	Percent
Classroom instructor	27.0
Therapist who supervised daily during a clinical affiliation	37.6
Staff therapist during clinical affiliations (did not supervise)	11.8
Therapist at first or second place of employment	21.2
Other	2.4

RESULTS

Descriptive Data

Subjects. Of 260 subjects contacted, 53 percent (138) responded. Thrity-seven percent (N = 95) of the total had usable returns. The following information was reported by the subjects about themselves. The recent graduates' model age was twenty-three years. The majority of the subjects were from baccalaureate degree programs (82%) and from classes of over twenty students (79%). All subjects finished their physical therapy programs in 1970. Although schools were attended throughout the United States, the eastern part of the country had the model value of 33 percent attendance. The majority of the subjects reported having full-time clinical affiliations lasting between twelve (22%) and eighteen (21%) weeks. They were currently employed at their first job (82%) in a hospital department (70%) where they had worked between nine and eleven months (53%).

Academic model. As generally described by the majority of the subjects, the academic model was between the ages of thirty and sixty, single, and had had daily contact with the student for a period between nine and fourteen months. The model was most admired as a teacher and then as a person.

Clinical model. The clinical model was between the ages of twenty and thirty, single, and had had daily contact with the students for a period of four to six weeks. This model was admired first as a practitioner, then as a person, and third as a teacher.

Analytical Data

After deriving the Pearson product-moment coefficients of correlation for each subject's Q sorts between self and her academic model and between self and her clinical model and using z transformations for each correlation, the means from each group were subjected to the t test (Tab. 1). The perceived professional characteristics of the physical therapist graduate correlated significantly higher with the assigned characteristics of a clinical instructor than with the assigned characteristics of a classroom instructor.

When similarity in chosen characteristics is equated to identification, then the recent graduate identified more with her clinical model than her academic model (Tab. 2). Correlation of the recent graduate's self-description with the clinical model was high enough to be significant at the .05 level; the correlation with the academic model was not enough to be significant.

Additional descriptive data from the information sheet that each recent graduate completed appear in Table 3. When asked if they had encountered an ideal physical therapist,

89.5 percent of the graduates indicated they had; 10.5 percent said they had not. The supervising therapist was selected as the ideal physical therapist 37.6 percent of the time. When supervising therapists and staff therapists during clinical affiliations were combined into one category, that category included the ideal therapist of 49 percent of the responders. When all clinical therapists were combined (including those in the first or second place of employment), this group represented the ideal therapist of 71.8 percent of the responders.

DISCUSSION

Clinical Education

Clinical education has always been considered an important aspect of physical therapy education. Early in the development of the physical therapy profession, the clinical education period was a time to practice the skills learned, interact with patients in a realistic setting, and treat patients under supervision. Now, all of these aspects plus developing attitudes, values, and manners of the physical therapy profession are considered a part of the professional socialization process. The results of this study lend support to the hypothesis that much emphasis should continue to be placed on the clinical setting and the practicing therapists as a critical part of physical therapy socialization.

Identification with the Role Models

Even more important than the setting are the therapists in the setting, especially those with whom the students work most closely. Contacts with therapists have been recognized in this study in terms of identification through role-taking and modeling. As Merton observed in his study of medical students,[12] physical therapists also directly and indirectly engage in role-taking. Identification with the physical therapy profession as a whole is promoted through the members working in the profession. For the novice, the classroom teachers and clinical instructors are the members who function as the primary models. The results of this investigation indicate that the beginning therapist identifies more with the therapist instructor in the clinic than in the classroom. Eighty-three percent of the self-clinical correlations were higher than their corresponding self-academic correlations. Even among those subjects who commented that they had not encountered their ideal therapist but who completed the Q sorts, only 27 percent had a higher correlation with their academic models.

Two reasons may support the general assumption held by therapists and educators that a student therapist and a practicing therapist identify more with a clinical therapist. The student aspires to be a clinical therapist—to work with the patients directly. Newly practicing therapists consider themselves as having characteristics of the clinical therapist that they are.

The results of this study appear to conflict with those of Heidgerken.[16] Her findings portrayed that undergraduate students preferring teaching careers (21.4%) and those preferring practicing careers (18.2%) selected a teacher role model over a practitioner role model. The difference in the results of the two studies may relate to the fact that the nurse teacher role model is more continuously visible than the physical therapy academic role model. Also, as stated earlier, nursing education has had increasing localization of control within the educational institutions, thus providing less opportunity for the student to learn the practicing nurse role through modeling.

Although the majority of ideal therapists were found in the clinical setting, if therapists similar to the students' ideal model are considered, the educational therapists encountered during physical therapy education were selected over three times as frequently as the therapist encountered after graduating from physical therapy school. Since the graduate is still undergoing professional socialization as she enters and works on the first job, the importance of role model therapists at this time must be recognized. Many students may find relatively inexperienced therapists or therapists who practice in a traditional and inflexible manner at their first place of employment. Lack of a progressive role model for the beginning therapist may promote imitation and identification with the more traditional practices of physical therapy. Instead of maintaining a progressive professional self-concept as a physical therapist and taking an active role in a developing profession, she may lose interest and become dissatisfied.

Of eighty-five subjects, 17.8 percent chose a therapist at their first place of employment as the ideal therapist. A few therapists (4) who were at their second job indicated that during this time they encountered their most ideal physical therapist.

Description of the Clinical Model

A look at some of the descriptive information indicated by the recent graduates about their academic and clinical models suggests some of the characteristics which may promote identification with the clinical model more than the academic model. Bandura's research, as reported by Mager, has pointed out that stimulus properties of the model such as age, sex, status, and the model's similarity to the subject increase identification.[7] As mentioned earlier, the majority of physical therapy students aspire to be clinical practitioners. Students who want to be clinical practitioners may already have more characteristics in common with clinical therapists because of general interests. The age range from twenty to twenty-nine years was most predominant (65%) among the clinical therapists and was closer to that of the students. When choosing whether they admired the models as a person, woman, or friend, as a person was most frequently chosen for both models (average 81.5%). The recent graduates admired their clinical models more (12%) as a woman than their academic models. Perhaps this is a minor influencing aspect for identification. Admiration as a friend was almost equal to that of admiration as a woman. The graduates also appeared to admire the clinical models as teachers more than they admired the academic therapists as practitioners. Perhaps, finding more of the teacher qualities in the practitioner added another dimension for identification with the clinical model. Both aspects which a student would seek in a professional educational model seemed to be more obviously displayed in the clinical model.

The length of contact with the two models did not seem to influence the amount of identification since the student had longer contact with the less-identified-with academic model. The frequency of daily contact with the clinical model, however, may have affected this process. Consideration must be given to the fact that, throughout the day, a student will usually have more personal, direct contact on an individual basis with her supervising therapist and more time for observation of this therapist. The intensity and closeness in contact, the involvement of the student, and the observation time and situation in which the student and model function seemed to have more effect on modeling than the length of time in professional socialization.

Description of the Academic Model

Twenty-two of the Q sorts averaged a higher correlation of self with the academic model than with the clinical model. Identification of the recent graduate with the academic model was not significant. Since personal qualities were more closely associated with the clinical models, identification could have been facilitated more readily with the clinical instructor. Perhaps the cognitive aspects of learning about physical therapy can be learned more easily from the academic model without as much identification, whereas the affective learning of physical therapy which is emphasized during clinical practice requires more identification and modeling.

Three of Mager's conclusions for student learning from Bandura's modeling experiments are applied to this study.[7] One would think that the academic teacher model would have more prestige, and thus influence, for modeling on the student. The physical therapy student may be so interested in treating the patient, however, that, contrary to some other professions, the actual worker has more prestige in the eyes of the student. A physical therapy student may imitate a clinical model more because he observes this model receiving greater reinforcement than the academic model receives. The patient may be the prime reinforcer of the physical therapy role behavior. If the student sees a therapist classroom teacher being pressured by external or internal forces, fewer other models are around to present a rewarding model picture. In the clinical situation, more people are present who may reward the practitioner—patient, staff, doctors, family, and students.

Modeling involves identifying with certain characteristics of the model who, in physical therapy, is usually the clinical therapist. If the academic or teacher model in physical therapy is to become a more prominent model, perhaps the specific characteristics applied to the two types of therapists need to be considered. The secondary aspect of this study focused on certain characteristics of the therapist, since they were used as the basis for identification or similarity. More thought and planning needs to be given to the functioning of the academic physical therapist in the clinic as a practitioner when students are present, especially if the profession is to develop in a scientific manner.

CONCLUSIONS

Self-perceived professional characteristics of the recent physical therapy graduate showed more positive correlations with the assigned characteristics of a clinical instructor than with the assigned characteristics of a classroom instructor. If we assume that assignment of similar characteristics to self and model represents identification, the recent graduate identified more with the therapist who supervised her during clinical affiliations than with a classroom instructor. Thus, this study indicates that the clinical therapist has a greater influence than the academic instructor in the socialization process. In conclusion, the clinical practice period and the clinical therapist, the most important model, do remain a vital segment of physical therapy education.

REFERENCES

1. Olesen V, Whittaker E: The Silent Dialogue. San Francisco, Jossey-Bass, Inc., Publishers, 1968, p 9
2. Greenwood E: Attributes of a profession. In Professionalization, edited by Howard Vollmer and Donald Mills. Englewood Cliffs, New Jersey, Prentice-Hall, Inc., 1966, p 18
3. McAllister L, Neuringer C: A comparative investigation of commonly used methods of measuring the identification process. J Gen Psychol 80:229, 1969
4. Gewirtz J, Stingle K: Learning of generalized imitation as the basis for identification. Psychol Rev 75:375, 1968
5. Maier H: Three Theories of Child Development. New York, Harper & Row, Publishers, 1965, p 196
6. Mussen P, Conger J, Kagen J: Child Development and Personality. New York, Harper & Row, Publishers, 1969, p 356
7. Mager R: Developing Attitude Toward Learning. Palo Alto, Fearson Publishers, 1968, p 63
8. Turner R: Role-taking: Process Versus Conformity. In Human Behavior and Social Processes, edited by Rose Arnold. Boston, Houghton Mifflin Company, 1962, p 23
9. Wylie R: The Self Concept. Lincoln, University of Nebraska Press, 1961, p 7
10. Foote N: Identification as the basis for a theory of motivation. Am Sociol Rev 16:16, 1951
11. Rubin J: Self-awareness and body image, self-concept and identity. In The Ego, edited by Jules Masserman. New York, Grune & Stratton, Inc., 1967, p 62
12. Merton R, Reader G, Kendall P: The Student-Physician. Cambridge, Harvard University Press, 1957, p 287
13. Corwin R: Role conception and career aspiration: A study of identity in nursing. Sociol Q 2:119, 1961
14. Corwin R, Taves M: Concomitants of bureaucratic and professional conceptions of the nurse role. Nurs Res 11:223-227, 1962
15. Kramer M: Role models, role conceptions, and role deprivation. Nurs Res 17:115, 1968
16. Heidgerken L: Preference for a teaching or clinical nursing practice career: Influence of significant others. Nurs Res 19:292-302, 1970
17. Stephenson W: The Study of Behavior: Q Technique and Its Methodology. Chicago, University of Chicago Press, 1953
18. Suinn R: The relationship between self-acceptance and acceptance of others: a learning theory analysis. In Theories of Personality, edited by Hall C and Lindzey G. New York, John Wiley & Sons, Inc., 1957, pp 499-504

THE AUTHOR

Barbara Jacobson received a bachelor's degree from Texas Christian University, a certificate in physical therapy from the University of Texas, and a master's degree in physical therapy from Boston University. She is currently employed at North Carolina Memorial Hospital as a staff physical therapist.

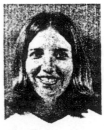

Effectiveness of the Clinical Instructor

Students' Perspective

MICHAEL J. EMERY

I conducted a survey of 102 senior physical therapy students to identify, from the students' perspective, training needs for clinical instructors. The literature identified 43 clinical instructor behaviors in four categories (communication, interpersonal relations, professional skills, and teaching behaviors). Students scored these behaviors for their importance and frequency. Results demonstrated all behaviors were perceived as somewhat significant and frequent. The students scored communication as most important followed by interpersonal relations, teaching, and professional skills behaviors. Frequency of the 43 behaviors was evenly distributed among the four categories. Correlational analysis of the perceived importance with the frequency of each behavior yielded 9 statistically significant positive correlations, no negative correlations, and 16 near random correlations. Positive correlations were 56 percent professional skills and 44 percent teaching behaviors. Near random correlations were 38 percent communication, 6 percent interpersonal relations, 6 percent professional skills behaviors, and 50 percent teaching. These 16 behaviors are identified as the target for clinical instructor training programs. This method in individual clinical settings is discussed briefly.

Key Words: *Education, Physical therapy.*

Clinical education is important in preparing physical therapists for working with patients.[1,2] Clinical education in physical therapy is learning by doing in the presence of a clinical model. Internship is a vital extension of the academic program because students practice and refine their newly-learned psychomotor skills and assume a role that incorporates the attitudes, values, and beliefs of the physical therapy profession. Despite the importance of clinical education, the education of clinical instructors remains very inconsistent. One possible reason for this is the lack of understanding of what content is most needed by clinical instructors. Good teaching is the degree to which the teacher moves the student toward an outcome.[3] The questions that arise are, 1) How can good teaching be measured? 2) What objectives are appropriate? 3) Who should set them? and 4) How can progress be measured?[3] Beyond these is

the unique problem of how well the practitioner functions as a teacher and how this can be assessed. Little work has been done in the evaluation of the teacher when the teacher is also a full-time clinician. The research has been introductory in nature and often too broad in its description to be useful as an evaluative tool.[4] Herein lies the problem this paper will address: With little known about the characteristics or qualities of clinical teaching, it is very difficult to prepare the clinician with any sense of certainty for this significant role as clinical instructor.

Clinical education incorporates both affective and psychomotor learning objectives. The clinical instructor's education often consists only of on-the-job training with undefined and inconsistent outcomes.[5] Such haphazard training does not imply that the physical therapy practitioner lacks respect for his role as clinical instructor. On the contrary, the physical therapist is sensitive, even apprehensive of, this responsibility. Realizing the importance of the clinical education experience, however, does not mean that the physical therapist is prepared to assume the role of clinical instructor.[6]

Researchers have done studies to clarify the educational needs of clinical instructors in physical therapy and several other health and medical professions. These studies have identified broad cat-

egories of performance but, for the most part, have not defined observable behaviors.[7]

Preparation of the clinical instructor requires both the educator and the clinical instructor to have a clear understanding of what competencies that role requires, those the clinical instructor brings to that role, and those that remain deficient. If deficiencies are identified, a relevant plan for training can be developed and appropriate methodologies selected. The purpose of this study was to identify, by student opinion, the perceived importance and frequency of some 43 previously identified clinical instructor behaviors. I designed the study to correlate these opinions of behavior importance and behavior frequency. The results offer insight into the educational needs of clinical instructors through a new perspective: the student consumer.

I expected the students to assess all behaviors as highly or moderately important in facilitating their learning because physical therapy educators had identified all 43 behaviors previously as significant. I collected this descriptive data because the frequency that students perceive these behaviors to occur appropriately could not be predicted. I postulated that if a behavior was important, it should also be observed frequently.

I expected positive correlation to exist between the perceived importance and

Mr. Emery is an Advanced Clinician, Department of Physical Therapy, Medical Center Hospital of Vermont, and Clinical Assistant Professor, University of Vermont, Burlington, VT 05401 (USA). At the time of this study, he was an Educational Specialist, Department of Rehabilitation Medicine, Mary Hitchcock Memorial Hospital, Hanover, NH 03755. This article was adapted from his master's thesis, completed at the University of Vermont, May 1981.

This article was submitted May 7, 1982; was with the author for revision 71 weeks; and was accepted January 24, 1984.

TABLE 1
Interval Scales Used to Score Each Clinical Instructor Behavior

Behavior	
Importance	Frequency
1. Significant	1. Frequent (75–100% of time)
2. Moderately significant	2. More than not (50–75% of time)
3. Somewhat significant	3. Occasional (25–50% of time)
4. Not at all significant	4. Seldom (0–25% of time)

TABLE 2
Ranking by Importance of Behavior

Behavior	Ranking (%)			
	1–10	11–20	21–30	31–43
Communication	60	20	10	10
Interpersonal relations	17	33	50	0
Professional skills	11	0	22	66
Teaching behaviors	11	33	22	33

the appropriate frequency of each behavior. A lack of correlation or negative correlation suggested clinical instructor behaviors that students believed needed further development. Identification of behaviors would be valuable in designing clinical instructor training programs.

METHOD

Subjects

The subjects for this study were 102 senior physical therapy students who had completed their clinical education. Approximately one-third of the sample came from each of three undergraduate physical therapy schools. Students were selected randomly from each school to participate in this study. In two of the school curricula, three full-time clinical affiliations were required. In one school curriculum, two full-time clinical affiliations were required.

A general profile of the clinical education program at each of the three schools suggested that the programs were basically similar in size and format. The only major variation was that one school used a formal co-op program in which students, during the first three years of the professional education, worked in physical therapy clinics during their semesters away from the academic program. The other schools had less intensive early exposure programs to physical therapy clinics for students in the first three years. Formal clinical

education experiences for the last year were organized similarly in all programs.

Design

Review of the clinical education literature in physical therapy revealed numerous characteristics and broad areas of competence necessary to be an effective clinical instructor.[1,5,8] I identified 43 observable behaviors from these characteristics and assigned them to one of four categories of behavior: communication, interpersonal relations, professional skills, and teaching behaviors (Appendix). I constructed a questionnaire using these behaviors and asked students to score each behavior twice, corresponding to 1) how important the clinical instructor behavior was in achieving effective clinical education and 2) how frequently the student had observed clinical instructors exhibit the behavior. In both cases, the behaviors

were scored using a four-point interval scale (Tab. 1).

Before I administered the student sample, the questionnaire was reviewed by three physical therapists considered to be experts in the field of clinical education and an undergraduate class of senior physical therapy students in another region of the country. I made corrections in terminology and editorial changes in the behavioral statements because of this review.

Questionnaires were administered in person to all students in the study about two months before they completed their undergraduate studies and after they completed all clinical education assignments. Response to the questionnaire was 100 percent.

Data Analysis

I compiled scores for importance and frequency of each behavior and calculated means and standard deviations for both. Using these means, I ranked behaviors for both importance and frequency, and where means were equal, I used the standard deviation to determine rank. I cross-tabulated the importance with the frequency of each behavior and calculated correlational analysis using a Pearson correlation coefficient (r) from the cross-tabulation of each behavior to assess the relationship between importance and frequency of each.

Statistical analysis of this data was computer-assisted using the Statistical Package for Social Sciences (SPSS) system. Specific analysis was done on subprograms: frequencies and cross-tabulations.[9,10]

RESULTS

Importance of Behaviors

Mean scores for the 43 behaviors ranged from 1.1 to 2.6 on the possible scale of 1.0 to 4.0, or roughly within the

TABLE 3
Ranking by Frequency of Behavior

Behavior	Ranking (%)			
	1–10	11–20	21–30	31–43
Communication	30	30	20	20
Interpersonal relations	17	17	67	0
Professional skills	33	11	33	22
Teaching behaviors	17	28	6	50

upper one-half of the available scale. Standard deviations ranged from 0.4 to 0.9 and averaged 0.6 for the 43 behaviors. Only 1 behavior's mean score fell below 2.0 (Demonstrates leadership among peers, 2.6). Ranking behaviors using the mean scores described above allows a comparison of behavioral categories. The majority (60%) of communication behaviors ranked in the top 10, but interpersonal relations were more central in the ranking (33% ranked 11–20, 50% ranked 21–30). Professional skills behaviors ranked lowest with 66 percent ranking 31–43. Teaching behaviors were more evenly distributed (Tab. 2).

Frequency of Behaviors

Mean scores of the 43 behaviors ranged from 1.2 to 2.2 on a possible scale of 1.0 to 4.0. Standard deviations ranged from 0.5 to 0.9 and averaged 0.7 for the 43 behaviors. Seventy-four percent of all behaviors demonstrated greater variability in scoring of frequency compared with importance of the behavior as evidenced by the standard deviation. All but 4 behaviors demonstrated a score less than 2.0 (Observed performance in a discreet manner, 2.1; Plans learning experience before the student arrives, 2.2; Helps student define specific objectives for the clinical education experience, 2.2; and Schedules regular meetings with the student, 2.2). Communication and professional skills behaviors were more evenly distributed through the ranking. Interpersonal relations ranked low with the majority (67%) in the 21–30 ranking. Teaching behaviors ranked lowest with 50 percent ranking 31–43 and 28 percent ranking 11–20 (Tab. 3).

Correlation of Importance with Frequency

Correlational analysis of the importance and frequency of each behavior produced four behaviors that demonstrated statistically significant ($p < .01$) positive correlations. Three of the four behaviors were in the category of professional skills behaviors. An additional five behaviors demonstrated a weaker positive correlation ($p < .05$). No negative correlations demonstrated significance (Tab. 4).

Behaviors demonstrating significant positive correlation ($p < .01$) repre-

TABLE 4
Behaviors Demonstrating Positive Correlation

Behavior	r
Professional skills behaviors	
Demonstrates leadership among peers	.46[a]
Clearly explains physiological basis of physical therapy evaluation	.38[a]
Clearly explains physiological basis of physical therapy treatment	.27[a]
Demonstrates systematic approach to problem-solving	.20[b]
Demonstrates professional behaviors as a member of the health-care team	.20[b]
Teaching	
Is timely in documenting student evaluation	.29[a]
Observes performance in a discreet manner	.19[b]
Schedules regular meeting with student	.20[b]
Is accurate in documenting student evaluation	.20[b]

[a] Significant at $p < .01$.
[b] Significant at $p < .05$.

TABLE 5
Behaviors Demonstrating Near Random Correlation

Behavior	r
Communication	
Is an active listener	.017
Communicates in a nonthreatening manner	.070
Provides useful feedback	.014
Provides positive feedback on performance	.031
Is open in discussing issues between student and self	.017
Provides feedback in private	.047
Interpersonal relations	
Demonstrates positive regard for the student separate from the student's performance	.088
Professional skills behaviors	
Manages own time well	.021
Teaching	
Makes relation between academic knowledge and clinical practice	.082
Plans effective learning experience	.018
Allows student progressive, appropriate independence	.064
Questions/coaches in a way to facilitate student's learning	.062
Manages student's time well	.046
Is available to the student	.094
Provides a variety of patients	.070
Provides unique learning experiences available at the facility	.085

sented 22 percent of the teaching behaviors category and 56 percent of the professional skills behaviors category. I found no significant correlations in the behavior categories of communication or interpersonal relations.

Sixteen behaviors demonstrated almost random correlation between importance and frequency as defined by a correlation coefficient ranging between .10 and −.10 (Tab. 5). These behaviors represent 60 percent of the communication category, 17 percent of the interpersonal relations category, 11 percent of the professional skills behaviors category, and 44 percent of the teaching category.

DISCUSSION

All behaviors appeared to be important to students. I expected this finding because all behaviors were taken from previous works devoted to the identification of pertinent clinical instructor behaviors in clinical education. No insignificant items were added to this compilation of clinical instructor behaviors.

From the ranking of behaviors, students clearly recognized the categories of communication, interpersonal relations, and teaching behaviors as the most valuable instructor behaviors in the clinical education process. These results are consistent with those of Irby who found the largest differences between "best" and "worst" teachers as rated by students to be the following characteristics: "enthusiastic, clear and well-organized, and adept at interacting with students."[1] Irby also found, as I did in this study, the smallest differences between "best" and "worst" teachers in areas of professional skills and knowledge.

Ranking behaviors by frequency showed all behaviors occurred relatively the same. In ranking, students did not select one category of behavior over another for greatest frequency. I noted considerable variation among individuals and schools in the scoring of frequency of behaviors. All these factors support the notion that the process of clinical instruction remains inconsistent as evidenced by the disparity in these students' experiences. Each student's experience or perception of importance also could have caused him or her to be more sensitive to the frequency of one behavior or another.

Correlational analysis of each of the 43 behaviors allowed greater scrutiny of the behaviors categorically and on an individual basis. Behaviors that demonstrated positive correlation between importance and frequency were those behaviors that were less important to students, that is, professional skills behaviors and teaching behaviors. Although significant, these correlations were admittedly low. Behaviors that demonstrated almost random correlation between importance and frequency were ironically those that were more important, primarily, communication and secondarily, interpersonal relations and teaching. I found two-thirds of these behaviors with near random correlations in the top half of the ranking of behaviors by importance.

From these students' perspectives, I found that many behaviors of the clinical instructor identified as necessary for effective teaching were the same behaviors that the students ranked as weak in their instructors. The clinician does not disagree with this. As a component of a comprehensive study of clinical education in physical therapy, Moore and Perry surveyed clinicians who ranked selected behaviors of communication and interpersonal relations to be the most important traits of an effective clinical instructor.[8] Moore and Perry pointed out that the selection process for clinical instructors is based primarily on patient-care performance and other professional skills behaviors. The discrepancy between selection criteria and traits perceived as important suggests a lack of adequate preparation rather than lack of appreciation on the part of the clinical instructor. Moore and Perry's data support this finding and demonstrate that only 25 percent of the clinical instructors surveyed had attended any kind of teacher's training.

Training programs for clinical instructors can be developed with behavioral objectives that incorporate the specific deficient behaviors identified in this study. This approach offers both efficiency and effectiveness by targeting the program at these perceived needs. Student input, gathered routinely, may be useful to identify changing clinical instructor training needs.

Individual use of the students' assessment of clinical instructor behaviors by clinical centers would allow custom designing of instructor training programs to meet that center's particular needs.

This study provided one perspective, that of the student, in helping to identify the training needs of clinical instructors

---

APPENDIX
Clinical Instructor Behaviors

Communication Behaviors
1. Makes himself/herself understood
2. Provides useful feedback
3. Is an active listener
4. Provides positive feedback on performance
5. Communicates in a nonthreatening manner
6. Openly and honestly reveals perceptions that the clinical instructor has of the student
7. Provides timely feedback
8. Is open in discussing issues with the student
9. Teaches in an interactive way; encourages dialogue
10. Provides feedback in private

Interpersonal Relations Behaviors
1. Establishes an environment in which the student feels comfortable
2. Provides appropriate support for student concerns, frustrations, anxieties
3. Empathic
4. Demonstrates a genuine concern for patients
5. Presents student as a professional to others
6. Demonstrates positive regard for student as a person

Professional Skills Behaviors
1. Employs physical therapy practice with competence
2. Demonstrates professional behavior as a member of the health-care team
3. Demonstrates systematic approach to problem-solving
4. Explains physiological basis of physical therapy treatment
5. Explains physiological basis of physical therapy evaluation
6. Demonstrates appropriate role of physical therapy as part of total health care
7. Serves as an appropriate role model
8. Manages own time well
9. Demonstrates leadership among peers

Teaching Behaviors
1. Allows the student progressive, appropriate independence
2. Is available to the student
3. Makes the formal evaluation a constructive process
4. Makes effective learning experience out of situations as they arise
5. Plans effective learning experiences
6. Provides a variety of patients
7. Questions/coaches in a way to facilitate student learning
8. Points out discrepancies in student's performance
9. Provides unique learning experiences
10. Makes relationship between academic knowledge and clinical practice
11. Is accurate in documenting student evaluation
12. Helps student define specific objectives for the clinical education experience
13. Observes performance in a discreet manner
14. Schedules regular meetings with the student
15. Plans learning experiences before the student arrives
16. Manages student's time well
17. Is timely in documenting the student's evaluation
18. Is perceived as a consistent extension of the academic program

in physical therapy. Further study is needed, also using specific behavioral statements, to ascertain other key perspectives such as those of the clinical instructor, the academic clinical coordinator, and the clinical site coordinator to complete the process of identifying the specific training needs of the clinical instructor. From this variety of perspectives, a clinical instructor training institute with a standardized format could be developed. This format would allow a more objective evaluation of clinical education, clinical instructors, and their impact on students.

CONCLUSION

The results demonstrated that effective communication, interpersonal relations, and teaching behaviors were the most important, yet the least apparent, clinical instructor behaviors from the students' perspective. Professional skills behaviors appeared more frequently but concerned students less. These findings were not new or contrary to the opinion of clinical instructors and seemed to reflect a lack of adequate preparation for the role of clinical instructor. Suggestions were made on how this assessment of clinical instructor behaviors can be used in the development of a clinical instructor training program and the further evaluation of clinical instruction.

Acknowledgments. I thank the students and Academic Coordinators of Clinical Education from the following physical therapy programs for their interest and participation in this study: University of Vermont, Burlington, VT; Northeastern University, Boston, MA; and Boston University, Boston, MA.

REFERENCES

1. Dickinson R, Dervitz HL, Meida HM: Handbook for Physical Therapy Teachers. New York, NY, American Physical Therapy Association, 1967, pp ix–x
2. Jacobson B: Role modeling in physical therapy. Phys Ther 54:244–250, 1974
3. Hildebrandt M: Evaluating University Teaching. Berkeley, CA, University of California Press, 1971, p 39
4. Stritter F: Clinical teaching re-examined. J Med Educ 50:876–882, 1975
5. Scully R: Clinical Teaching of Physical Therapy Students in Clinical Education. Doctoral dissertation. New York, NY, Columbia University, 1976
6. Ramsden E, Dervitz HL: Clinical education: Interpersonal foundations. Phys Ther 52:1060–1066, 1972
7. Irby D: Clinical teacher effectiveness in medicine. J Med Educ 53:808–815, 1978
8. Moore ML, Perry JF: Clinical Education in Physical Therapy: Present Status/Future Needs. Washington, DC, Section for Education, American Physical Therapy Association, 1976, p 4.45
9. Nie N, Hull CH, Jenkins JG, et al: Statistical Package for the Social Sciences, ed 2. New York, NY, McGraw-Hill Inc, 1975, p 223
10. Hull CH, Nie N: SPSS Update 7–9, New York, NY, McGraw-Hill Inc, 1981, pp 301–304

Clinical Teaching in Physical Therapy

Clinical Teaching in Physical Therapy Education

An Ethnographic Study

ROSEMARY M. SCULLY
and KATHERINE F. SHEPARD

The purpose of this ethnographic study was to examine the process of clinical education from the viewpoint of clinical teachers. A three-month field study based on a grounded theory approach and involving simultaneous collection and codification of data led to the discovery and explication of two major components of the clinical education process. One component, the clinical teaching situation, identified the organizational and human factors that influence the type, quality, and quantity of the student learning. The second component, teaching tools used by the clinical teachers, identified the strategies used to pace the student to professional competence. The authors view the findings as a beginning understanding of how and why clinical education is fundamentally different from academic education.

Key Words: *Affiliations, clinical; Education, clinical; Teaching.*

Much of the literature in physical therapy clinical education is based on personal experience and opinion rather than on systematic investigation. With little systematically obtained data on the process of clinical education, it is difficult for physical therapy educators to plan for clinical education or to train clinical teachers (CTs) from a rational basis. This paper describes a field research method used to explore the clinical education process and to identify and explain some of its components. Clinical education may be studied from several perspectives; this study focuses on CTs—what they do, why they do it, and factors that facilitate or constrain their activities.

RESEARCH DESIGN

Field research methods have often been used to study the social and psychological environments of various organizational settings. One method called participant observation has been found to be particularly effective where environments are complex and essential data cannot be retrieved by pen and paper methods.[1] In participant observation, the researcher becomes part of the social milieu to be studied and performs on-site recording of all incidents related to the theme being studied. As McCall and Simmons suggest, "If one seeks to know and understand what exists or what is happening, the commonsense impulse is to go and look at it, closely and repeatedly."[2]

The theoretical framework for data gathering and analysis in this study was grounded theory as described by Glaser and Strauss.[3,4] This method involves generating theory rather than verifying it.[5-7] The investigator's approach is to enter the field without predetermined theoretical guidelines. Analytical categories are constructed out of similarities and differences that emerge from the study of the situation and are analyzed using a method of comparative analysis.

The research tools of the grounded theory include theoretical sampling and the constant comparative method:

> Theoretical sampling is the process of data collecting for generating theory whereby the analyst jointly collects, codes and analyzes his data and decides what data to collect next and where to find them, in order to develop his theory as it emerges. This process of data collection is controlled by the emerging theory, whether substantive or formal. The initial decision for theoretical collection of data is based only on a general sociological perspective and on the general subject or problem area.... The researcher will choose any groups that will help generate, to the fullest extent, as many properties of the categories as possible.[3(pp45-47)]

Dr. Scully is Associate Professor and Director, Program in Physical Therapy, School of Health Related Professions, University of Pittsburgh, Pittsburgh, PA 15261 (USA).

Dr. Shepard is Assistant Professor, Division of Physical Therapy, School of Medicine, Stanford University, Stanford, CA 94305.

This article was submitted November 30, 1981, and accepted November 8, 1982.

The analysis of data proceeding concurrently with the collection of the data calls for a continuous testing of the validity of emerging categories against comparable situations. This is referred to as the constant comparative method.

METHOD

Five hospitals in New York City were selected as the setting for this study for several reasons: they were available to the investigator, they had clinical education programs in progress during the three summer months the investigator collected data, they had students from a number of different academic programs, and they represented a variety of clinical settings in which clinical teaching was conducted. The five facilities selected were a large private voluntary teaching hospital, a rehabilitation hospital, a Veterans Administration hospital, a large city hospital, and a smaller private hospital. All of these hospitals had been conducting clinical education programs for over 10 years and all of them had students from more than two academic programs. In four facilities the students were junior, senior, and certificate students affiliating both part-time and full time; the rehabilitation center accepted the same categories of students but only on full-time affiliations.

The selection of the CTs to participate in this study was limited to those individuals assigned as CTs in the programs during the period of the study. In all, 31 CTs responsible for clinical education experiences on neurological, orthopedic, pulmonary, intensive care, and rehabilitation services and on general medical and surgical wards were observed. The male and female CTs ranged in age from 23 to 57 years. They were graduates of 10 different physical therapy educational programs, and six had master's degrees in physical therapy.

Data were collected solely by the primary author by observing the CTs work, that is, in the clinical education setting, seeing what they did, when, with whom, and under what circumstances. Informal interviewing was used to query them about the reasons for their actions. Before being observed, the CTs were reassured that their teaching techniques and physical therapy skills were not being evaluated. The investigator was there only to observe what they did and possibly to ask them why they did it.

After a day in the field, the investigator spent the next day transcribing rough field notes to typewritten, close-to-verbatim accounts of what was seen and heard. After several days had been spent in the field, these verbatim field notes were organized into categories as shown in the Figure.

During the first month of the study, as an increasing number of categories emerged from field notes, the categories were cross-checked with all the field data. This was done to ensure that the categories were typical of clinical teaching situations and CT actions and to determine how various categories interrelated.

After observing and recording the activities of the CT, the investigator discussed with CTs the reasons for their actions. This explanatory data and its analysis led to the re-coding of categories into two major components—the clinical teaching situation and teaching tools used by CTs. These two components provided the theoretical framework for explaining and understanding the process of clinical teaching.

RESULTS: THE CLINICAL TEACHING SITUATION

The clinical teaching situation has organizational and human factors that influence the type, quality, and quantity of the student learning. Organizational factors are primarily givens or ground rules that

Field Notes		Categories
Clinical Teacher—	"Do you see anything particular happening when he moves his hip?"	Questioning
Student—	"He moves his pelvis."	
Clinical Teacher—	"Why do you think he is doing that?"	Questioning
Clinical Teacher—	"I lost my cool back there." (Referring to her confusion in directing aides to position the patient for his treatment.) She also went on to admit, "and my sterile technique was not the greatest. I wasn't prepared."	Candor
Clinical Teacher—	"It's patients that need a break from students . . . They need to be treated by their physical therapist . . ."	Concern for the Patient

Figure. Example of how field notes were organized into categories.

emanate from academic programs, health care institutions, and the physical therapy departments within those institutions. The human factors are the perspectives CTs hold and the level of professional maturity students bring to the clinical setting.

Academic Ground Rules

The number of students, the level and quality of their training, their part-time or full-time assignments to clinical settings, and the time of year and length of these assignments are ground rules that emanate primarily from academic programs. These ground rules from academic programs tend to be fairly inflexible given academic admission policies, budget constraints, the quarter or semester curriculum design, faculty hiring policies, teaching schedules, and research assignments. Also, CTs are requested by those in academic programs to submit written formal evaluations of student performance during each full-time clinical education experience. These evaluation forms have traditionally been designed by those in academic programs, sometimes with the assistance of clinical advisory committees.

Health Care Institution Ground Rules

Factors inherent in the structure or functioning of any health care organization affects the clinical teaching situation. The following factors appear to influence the degree of immediate supervision provided to the students during their performance of patient care activities.

Physical structure. This includes the distance between clinical treatment areas and the size and the degree of privacy of the treatment area. For example, bedside treatment in a private room seems to yield greater immediate supervision than treatment in a large open gymnasium.

Patient factors. These include the total number of patients, fluctuation of patient load, availability of patients during scheduled treatment times, and the complexity of evaluation and treatment programs. For example, in a setting such as an in-patient rehabilitation center where the CTs' loads remain relatively constant, the students may have less opportunity to perform patient treatments independently. In this situation, CTs may have less patient care responsibility and more time that may be used to check and observe the students during their performance.

Temporal factors. These include the length of time students are assigned to a particular facility or treatment area, the length of time of the patients' hospitalization, and the length of the treatment programs. For example, the more time students spend in a facility, the more they are taken out of a student's role and placed in a temporary staff therapist's role

in which they assume greater responsibility for patient treatments.

Circumstantial factors. Sudden illness of the CT or a "spontaneous happening" may defer or enhance the achievement of patient treatment and the amount of student independence allowed. For example,

> I threw you into ice water yesterday having you help me treat that patient. But I wanted you to work with the athetoid patient yesterday and get some idea of the problems they present. We don't get too many of them and if we didn't do it yesterday when the opportunity presented itself at clinic I wasn't sure if you would have another chance to work with a patient like this. (Field Note)

House rules. Clinical teachers as employees of an institution pass on to students in-house policies and procedures ranging from dress codes to standardized treatment protocols. For example,

> The clinical teacher and the student were going over ways to wrap a below knee stump; the student had previous experience doing this in another facility, but the clinical teacher said, 'Let me show you how we do it here. It's kind of standardized. All the therapists and other personnel here use this method . . . there is less confusion this way. While you are in our facility, we will want you to use the method adopted by this center.' (Field Note)

Along with constraints resulting from overt policies there is a more unobtrusive but equally powerful ground rule falling under House Rules called "guest-in-the-house."[8] These rules include those expected of all good guests, such as arriving on time and being properly attired for the situation. Although some of the guest rules are explained to students, they are often thought of as better guests when "they know to help without being asked."

Professional image. Clinical teachers have a concern for their profession and how physical therapy is seen by patients and other health care professionals. For example,

> I don't like to carry on a discussion of the values of one technique or another . . . with a student in front of the patient. I have seen doctors do this on rounds. . . . This kind of discussion raises questions in the patient's mind like, 'they really don't know how to treat me.' In addition to my concern for the patient's feelings in this kind of situation, this kind of discussion is not good for physical therapy. (Field Note)

Physical Therapy Department Ground Rules

Several ground rules in the clinical teaching situation that originate within physical therapy departments appeared to be commonly shared among the clinical settings studied. One of these ground rules was rotating the responsibility of clinical teaching among the staff therapists. With few exceptions, every staff member in the facility was expected to assume responsibility for clinical teaching. This responsibility was assigned on a rotating basis by the clinical coordinator or departmental supervisor to give the staff as well as the patients of that staff member a "break" from students. Another common finding reported by CTs was their perceived lack of preparation for roles as CTs.

Clinical teachers in this study received no extra compensation for their involvement in student education. Without this compensation, CTs felt more like "free agents" and exhibited little reluctance to state their own guidelines for their behavior. If they demonstrated allegiance at all, it was to rules that were formulated within the institution paying their salaries.

One additional common ground rule that can originate from the academic institution, the physical therapy department, or both is the convention of "limited knowledge" of the student. Often clinical preceptors know little more about the students than what schools they are from, length of time in the clinical setting, course work covered to date, and lists of prior clinical affiliations. Faculty, clinicians, and students are all reluctant to share additional information about the students, using the rationale that the CTs do not want to be prejudiced or biased toward the students.

Clinical Teachers' Perspectives

The delivery of theoretical knowledge and clinical skill elements to students is constantly shaped by three forces influencing the CTs: their concern for patient primacy and their perception of the rewards and hardships of the clinical education experience.

Patient primacy. Physical therapy CTs have a deep concern for the welfare of their patients. This concern has personal, ethical, and legal bases and is related to a clinician's primary role, that of being responsible for patient treatment. The concern for patient primacy exerts omnipresent influence on all clinical education activities, from assignment of CTs, to patient selection, to on-the-spot feedback given to students. As one clinician stated:

> I assign the student to patients when I know he is capable of giving the treatment and that the patient will be getting a proper treatment and hopefully one that will allow the patient to make progress toward his recovery. (Field Note)

Because patient primacy may run contrary to student educational goals, the teaching tools used in a clinical teaching situation are uniquely shaped and often vastly different from teaching tools used in academic settings.

Rewards. Although there may be no direct monetary compensation received either from the academic programs or from the health care setting within which they work, CTs do feel that there are rewards for participating in clinical education programs. Primary rewards are those of personal satisfaction and professional development. One factor of personal satisfaction was expressed this way:

> It's a nice feeling to teach someone something; it's satisfying. Maybe that's ego building, but it is a nice feeling to pass on knowledge you have to someone else. (Field Note)

Sometimes the CT experiences satisfying professional growth:

> I am a beginning clinical teacher. I was told I was going to have this 'super' student. I was ill at ease, but I enjoyed her very much. I learned so much looking things up to have her do and finding answers together on questions she would ask. Students get you out of your rut. They sharpen your curiosity. (Field Note)

The student program can have more than just an influence on individual CTs. It can have an enriching effect on the total department. For example, the student evaluation process has been noted to have a positive effect on the staff in general:

> Doing evaluations on students are important for the staff and students. It's a good teaching tool for the staff. It reminds the staff of qualities and techniques we are looking for in the students and therefore reminds the staff of skills and characteristics they should possess. Student evaluations help in staff self evaluation. (Field Note)

In addition to personal satisfaction and professional growth of the staff, there is a very practical advantage explained as follows by a chief therapist:

> It's good to have a student program in our department. It brings exposure to our department. It allows our department to be known by the students. This, in turn, helps us with recruitment of staff. (Field Note)

Hardships. If students are to be guided to professional competence, they must have an opportunity to assume responsibility for the patients' treatments. This opportunity for students results in a severe hardship for physical therapists in the clinical teaching situation—a loss of patient contact.

> I like my patients and having students all the time. I turn their treatments over to them.... I get bored when students have the responsibilities for the patients' treatments. (Field Note)

Another hardship experienced by CTs, especially if a student is just beginning, is conflict in the use of time.

> Time is the greatest hardship I have in working with students. I have so many patients to treat and when I have a student, particularly a beginning student, to work with, it takes me twice as long. I need more

time because I have to stop and explain or demonstrate what I mean. It's even longer when the student has a lot of questions. (Field Note)

A third hardship expressed by CTs was loss of privacy.

When you have a student, there is just no time during the day to call your own. (Field Note)

This loss of privacy is particularly apparent to CTs in high-risk patient care areas, considered by either the student or the CT as situations filled with potential opportunities for something to go wrong.

It's like having a shadow; I can't even go to the bathroom and not be followed; this may be more true in my area (an acute surgical recovery area) than in other clinical teachers' areas. Being here, in a situation where anything could go wrong very quickly, where there is a lot of unfamiliar equipment and a lot of very sick patients, the students will not stay here alone. Even if I just go next door to get some supplies they trail after me. (Field Note)

Student Professional Maturity

Various degrees of student capabilities in knowledge and performance of skills are recognized, tolerated, and worked with by CTs. Optimism is expressed that deficiencies in performance competencies often can be overcome with increased time and experience in clinical education. However, variations in professional maturity are less tolerated, and pessimism is expressed as to whether the CT can do anything to develop a student's professional maturity. One CT expressed it this way:

'The student has it or he doesn't have it.' Another said, 'The student comes with it, even the beginning student.' (Field Note)

What are these characteristics that CTs consider indicative of professional maturity? The most critical characteristic appears to be the student's ability to work with people. As one academic clinical coordinator noted on a visit to the clinical setting,

The greatest reason for the student to fail in the clinical setting is his inability to work with people. (Field Note)

This characteristic of professional maturity appears to have one major criterion: the student's ability to gain the respect and cooperation of the patient. How this is done by the student, or the therapist for that matter, is not clearly understood. However, evidence of this ability is often measured by the CT by observing reciprocal behavior of the patient and the student. For example, one CT commented,

This is only the second time he has seen the patient and the first time he had the responsibility for her

treatment, but look at the way the patient responds to him. (Field Note)

Other characteristics that demonstrate professional maturity are a willingness to try, an eagerness to learn, and a quickness in learning. When students are judged not interested or slow in learning, the CTs are placed in a dilemma. Should they use precious time to work with the patients who need the treatment or with the student who requires a great deal of time to get the education needed to reach the goals of professional competency?

In addition to the above characteristics of professional maturity, a necessary complementary behavior is the student's ability to act as a good guest-in-the-house previously described under "House Rules."

RESULTS: TEACHING TOOLS USED BY CLINICAL TEACHERS

The process of pacing a student to professional competence—that is, guiding a student by way of individualized planning toward professional competence—begins with the student in the role of an observer and ends with the student in the role of a temporary staff member. Thus, the students' early clinical days are spent following CTs around, observing what they do, who they talk to, how they talk, how they conduct patient treatments, and how they evaluate patient care outcomes. In their final days of clinical internship, students are expected to assume a role of nearly full, but still sheltered, participation in patient care.

During this process, the CT uses a variety of tools to assess, guide, and promote the student. Because they must be used within the context of the environmental ground rules, the CT's belief in patient primacy, and the student's level of professional maturity, these teaching tools are extremely flexible and have only two consistent properties. First, they must yield student learning with minimal risk to the patient, the learner, the teacher, the institution, and the profession. Second, they must advance the student toward clinical competency. Thus, they are characteristically unlike most academic teaching tools. Even the CTs using the tools appear to be unaware of their unique and specific characteristics.

Diagnosis of Readiness

The first tool used by CTs as their student enters the teaching setting is diagnosis of readiness. Working with limited knowledge of the students' backgrounds, teachers seek information on which to build clinical programs and to have some control over risks involving patient primacy. All CTs, however, use some form of questioning and verbal exchange in their appraisal of students. Verbal exchanges were of particular importance and used frequently on acute patient care services. One CT on a postsurgical unit explained it this way:

> We have to judge the student's capabilities. We do this by watching for his responses when we are talking with him or asking him questions. If we get a lot of blank stares we know we have a lot of work to do. . . . We just can't let a student go out and suction a patient or use some of the respiratory equipment without knowing what he can do. (Field Note)

In addition to using verbal exchanges, CTs often use performance "tests." One CT on a rehabilitation unit explained her appraisal techniques as follows:

> I usually start a student off by having him do a patient evaluation, including range-of-motion and manual muscle tests. He does this with me. How he does it and how he handles himself with the patient usually tells me a *lot* about the student. If he should flub he will not hurt the patient. (Field Note)

Often CTs ask students to help in determining their performance readiness. This may be done informally by observing and questioning the student or in a more formal manner usually early in the clinical teaching program.

> On the first day in the clinic, at an orientation session the supervisor of the student program asked the new students to rank their performance skills. They did this by identifying those skills they thought they could perform independently, those they only needed to be checked out on and those in which they thought they needed considerable practice. (Field Note)

Diagnosis of readiness by CTs is usually individualized to each student. However, all physical therapy clinical units visited during this study had written objectives describing what all students should accomplish during their clinical education program in that unit. Thus, although CTs work with students with varying degrees of readiness, they must help all their students to accomplish the same minimal level of competency.

Selection of Clinical Problems

The selection of knowledge-oriented activities is not as difficult as the selection of patient treatment activities. Knowledge-oriented activities are often routinely scheduled in the hospital's clinical teaching program. They generally take the form of a lecture series, and in most cases, students are expected to attend all the lectures regardless of their readiness level. However, ensuring student success in patient treatment activities while adhering to patient primacy concerns requires a great deal of individualized pacing. Clinical teachers control student activities by the types and number of patients assigned. Assignments are increased as student competency increases.

Another consideration is the selection of "interesting patients." This can mean selecting "textbook patients" exhibiting classical symptoms the student has learned about in the academic setting, or a "variety of patients." Preventing boredom was the reason most often given for the selection of a variety of patients.

Just as in diagnosing readiness, students were often asked to participate in the selection of clinical problems. This opportunity was usually extended to all students in the selection of their topics for an in-service program. Student participation in the selection of patient problems, however, was often reserved for the "good" students; they were allowed to choose patients with whom they would like to work or were encouraged to take responsibility for an increased number of patients.

Supervision: Use of Time, Coaching, and Shifting Status

Supervision is the major clinical teaching tool used by CTs. Paraphrasing Margaret Wilson's definition,[9] supervision is a dynamic enabling process by which student physical therapists are helped by a CT to make the best use of their knowledge and skills and to improve their abilities so that the job is completed more effectively and with increasing satisfaction to themselves, their CTs, and their profession. Supervisory responsibilities of CTs are both supportive and instructive and shift rapidly as student knowledge and skills grow. Three interrelated aspects of supervision are used by CTs to pace students to competency: time, coaching, and the student's status.

Time is an important dimension of the clinical teaching situation. The timing of the students' arrival at the facility and the length of time they spent in the facility are ground rules over which the individual CTs have little control. Time for student education that is taken from time allocated for patient treatment or that is added to work hours is considered one of the hardships of being a CT. Teachers attempt to minimize this hardship by manipulating time in three ways: stretching it, saving it, and finding it.

Time is stretched by using time not ordinarily set aside for clinical teaching. For example, the CT suggested to a student who was having difficulty performing manual muscle tests,

> Don, why don't you stay after you are finished with your patient treatments today and you can practice your muscle testing on me. (Field Note)

Another way to stretch time is to ask the student to prepare for future activities.

> Tomorrow we will be treating a patient with a new hip replacement. There is a book in the library here that describes the surgery. Why don't you take a look at it before coming in tomorrow. (Field Note)

Time is saved by having students participate formally or informally in their own diagnosis of readiness. It can also be saved if ways can be found for the student to learn more quickly or by teaching students in groups, for example, orientation sessions and lecture series.

Time is found by using slower periods of the day or patient cancellations for instructional periods. Time is also found by shifting priorities and subsequently changing activities of the student and teacher. For example, the CT on a surgical floor wanted the student to have more time to prepare her in-service lecture and suggested, "If you want to have some time to work on your case study, I can do some of your patients for you."

Coaching, as a technique of supervision, varies with the rate of development of student competence and with immediate patient primacy concerns. Coaching may occur before, concurrent with, or after the student's performance. Coaching concurrent with performance, or coaching-on-the-spot, is usually employed at a beginning level of pacing. Thus, it is used with a new student or a student whose readiness is either unknown or unacceptable for the potential risks in the situation. Coaching-on-the-spot takes one of two forms. In the first form the CT performs while the student observes and responds to directions given by the teacher to "look" or "feel." The opportunity to "feel" differentiates this type of coaching from the academic laboratory demonstration, in the eyes of many CTs. Questions such as "Why do you think I am doing such and such?" are often asked of the student. These questions, delivered when the CT is performing and the student observing, are usually direct queries and made in front of patients. This form of coaching when not indicated by the student's readiness level or the risk of the situation may be viewed negatively by the student:

> This experience was a waste of time. I didn't get to do anything. The only way to learn skills is to practice them and all I did was watch. (Field Note)

The second form of coaching-on-the-spot occurs when the student is performing and the CT is close by. Patient primacy is again of major concern, this time both from the standpoint of patient risk and of establishing and maintaining the patient's confidence in the person (student) who is administering the treatment. For this reason, clues, questions, and directions to students are generally given with more indirectness than in the former coaching situation. A slight clearing of the throat by the CT, questioning looks, and instructions directed through the patient are commonly used techniques of indirect coaching. In addition, while coaching-on-the-spot in this way, CTs often position themselves in such a manner that they can be seen by the student but not by the patient.

In situations where student error is imminent and risk is high, indirectness is superseded by direct action of the CTs such as in the following incident:

> The student had completed the exercise program for a patient on the mat table and was transferring the patient to her wheelchair. The student had forgotten to raise the footpedals on the wheelchair before beginning the transfer. The clinical teacher seeing this immediate danger to the patient did not take the time to tell the student of his error but quickly raised the footpedals with much force as the patient was in the midst of her transfer. (Field Note)

Two other forms of coaching, coaching ahead of performance and coaching after performance, can be used to minimize the directness of the CT's coaching-on-the-spot or to replace this close form of coaching when the student is ready. Coaching-ahead assures the teacher of the student's readiness, and coaching-after provides a check. These coaching forms usually take place in hallways, in corners of treatment areas, or while waiting for elevators as student and teacher proceed from one patient to the next.

As students increase their competence to the point of being placed in the role of temporary staff, all forms of coaching are decreased. If during this time the CTs are not available or time is not set aside for discussion, questioning, and guidance, the charge may be leveled by the students that they were not given the opportunity for learning and they were only "being used as another pair of hands." To allow the students the opportunity to practice and also to receive the proper amount of supervision without coaching, CTs employ a technique of "being on call." The following incident illustrates how this is done:

> The clinical teacher had divided her patient load so the student now had some of the patients on a ward service to herself. The clinical teacher made a point to inform the student of the patients she would be treating and in what part of the hospital she would be during the morning, explaining to the student 'just in case you run into trouble.' (Field Note)

A third supervision tool is shifting the student's status from student to therapist. This shift may be difficult for clinicians to use in a systematic way and its use is often a source of confusion and frustration to students. The confusion students feel in the clinical setting is easy to understand in the context of the environmental ground rules and the role of patient primacy discussed earlier. The behavior of CTs in clinical teaching situations may shift instantaneously depending on their perceptions of the situation, their receptiveness to the student, and their assessment of the student's competency. The following illustration demonstrates the tightrope the student walks between learner and treater, student and therapist:

> The clinical teacher and student were discussing the total hip replacement procedure that was being done

on the service. She gave the student a handout and said, 'We will see two of these patients this afternoon. I probably will give you one to treat.' The student responded that she was anxious to get started.

After reviewing the x-rays of the two patients and the student having some difficulties with the questions the clinical teacher asked her about the x-rays, they went off to see the two patients. Upon arriving at the patients' room, the clinical teacher said, 'I think it would be best if you just help me and observe today.'

When I (the investigator) asked the clinical teacher why she had changed her plans about the student working with the second patient with the hip replacement, she answered, 'It was just the feeling I had about the situation once we were in it. After the discussion of the x-rays with the student, I felt I had made her uncomfortable by asking her some questions she had difficulty answering. Maybe I shook her confidence. Once we were in the patients' room, I realized I had been treating both patients before. What would it seem like to the second patient if she saw me treating the first patient and giving instructions to the student, then after this lesson having the student treat her. Wouldn't the second patient feel cheated? The situation just didn't feel right. I had to change my plans for the student.' (Field Note)

The actions of the CT determine the status of the student not only for patients but also for other professional and nonprofessional personnel within the clinical setting. How the student is introduced to others and the amount of decision making conferred on the student in front of others are actions that enhance or detract from the student's status.

The clinical teacher and the student were walking down the hall of an orthopedic service. They were stopped by a nurse on the service with the question, 'Do you think it would be all right for Mr. H to sit up in a chair today?' . . .The clinical teacher did not answer the question, but turned to the student and asked, 'What do you think, Pam?' (Field Note)

Evaluation

Evaluation as a teaching tool used throughout the pacing process is usually individualized to the student and to the situation and appears in two forms: private and public. Ongoing private evaluations are necessary to assess student readiness, to select clinical problems, and to indicate the type and amount of supervision. Private evaluations are characterized by two notions. First, errors in performance need to be pointed out to the student in such a manner as not to cause undue psychological stress. Clinical teachers may soften the blow of unsatisfactory student performance by assuming some of the fault themselves with such statements as, "Maybe I didn't ask the right question" or "Perhaps I didn't demonstrate that very clearly."

The second notion that characterizes private evaluations is that students are not expected to know everything. Certain mistakes are permissible. However, students must be aware of what they do not know and be honest in their self-appraisal so as not to cover up errors. To support and encourage this honesty, CTs practice being candid. Clinical teachers use candor to point out to students their own errors in patient treatment performance or in their knowledge.

After a clinical teacher had treated a patient with a student observing, she told the student, 'My sterile technique was not the greatest. I wasn't prepared. Today you saw what not to do, tomorrow I'll show you what to do. I will read up on it and practice tonight.' (Field Note)

When CTs were asked why they were candid with students in admitting their own shortcomings, many answers were given similar to the following:

It's a model for students to learn. They begin to think, 'See, they don't know everything either.' I think this is very good because students are under a great deal of pressure. They feel they need to know everything before they finish their affiliations and get their jobs. The therapist's candor helps them realize learning is an ongoing process. (Field Note)

Clinical teachers are expected to participate in public judgments. One of the ground rules emanating from academic programs is that a final written report be sent to the program at the close of the student's clinical education program. The evaluation requires CTs to recount and document their impression of the student's behavior and progress on selected variables. Clinical teachers express ambivalence about complying with this external organization ground rule because of the difficulties inherent in completing written evaluations. First of all, it is a time-consuming process that infringes on patient care responsibilities and often on personal time of CTs. When the preceptor has students from different academic programs, requiring the use of different evaluation forms, the process is even more time-consuming as different sets of instructions and form idiosyncrasies must be sorted out. Second, the form itself often presents a problem because it is standardized, and students' behaviors in vastly different clinical settings, such as a pediatric unit and a burn unit, must be translated to fit the generalized format. Third, if students have spent time in several units of a hospital, their specific behaviors, as appraised by several different CTs, must be synthesized into one form. The variable being evaluated may be seen very differently by different CTs in these different settings.

Despite these difficulties, clinical educators comply with the public evaluation ground rule. They are aware that the academic programs have a public institutional and professional responsibility to certify that students have successfully completed their program of study in physical therapy including the clinical education component. Clinical educators also feel the weight of this responsibility.

It's a professional responsibility. If the student is successful in graduating and in practice does not live up to professional standards, this question may be raised, 'How did he ever get through his clinical education experiences? I was responsible for this clinical education program here.' (Field Note)

DISCUSSION

The findings in this grounded theory exploration of the clinical education process from the vantage point of CTs allow for many areas of discussion. The authors will confine this discussion to the uniqueness of clinical teaching and how that should affect preparation of CTs.

Philip Jackson has suggested that unless we accept a very limited definition of teaching we must be willing to examine everything a teacher does.[10] When one observes CTs in the field, one is observing interactive teaching activities. The data in this study suggest the following characteristics of interactive teaching in clinical settings.

Clinical teaching is conducted by clinicians. Clinical teachers never lose sight of themselves as clinicians. Highest priority is given to the individual patient's welfare. This appropriate professional ethic may constrain activities that otherwise may be desirable from the standpoint of student education. The question, "Is clinical teaching centered around patient needs or student needs?" was answered by CTs who suggested that no conflict existed between their roles as physical therapy clinicians and CTs. Students' educational needs are met by CTs who pace them to professional competence by using teaching tools such as individual diagnosis of readiness, careful selection of patients, various forms of coaching, and ongoing performance evaluations. This guidance method simultaneously protects and serves the patient. This method also suggests that clinical teaching has a strong pragmatic orientation, and therefore only limited educational experimentation can be condoned, particularly if it means interrupting or modifying patient treatment and departmental and institutional procedures.

Clinical teaching takes place in a situation in which clinical teachers have little control. Health care organizations are designed for patient care activities. The structure and function of these patient care settings affect the availability, content, and delivery of clinical educational programs. Organizational factors essentially beyond the control of CTs include the treatment-teaching settings, patient care factors (such as diagnoses, length of stay, and fluctuation in patient load), institutional policies and procedures, and physical therapy department ground rules (such as rotation schedules). These factors make it difficult to make generalizations in planning clinical learning experiences. In academic teaching many of the factors that operate as variables in the learning experience can be planned for and controlled by the teacher. The rapidity, complexity, and uncertainty of events in interactive clinical teaching make decisions among alternative courses of action more spontaneous. Clinical teachers need to know their teaching environments and what effect it has on their behaviors to gain a greater understanding of their teaching strategies.

Clinical teaching is individualized and personal. Therapist-patient activities are highly individualized and are usually conducted in a private setting. The CT-student relationship is also highly individualized and relatively private. Although this mode of teaching may occur occasionally in the classroom setting, it is a way of life for CTs and their students. In private teaching, student and teacher behaviors are continually mutually responsive. For example, many teachers' behaviors are in response to students' "diagnosis of readiness" and their questions or lack of them. This immediate teacher behavior is very difficult to preplan. In private teaching, the CTs do not stand in front of a classroom in a face-to-face confrontation with students. They are more often at a student's side, and instead of confronting each other, they are confronting a common clinical problem.

Preparation of clinical teachers. In the authors' opinion, educational experiences designed to prepare CTs have overemphasized planning for teaching activities, many of which have limited applicability in the clinical teaching setting.[11] From the data presented here, interactive teaching activities that occur in clinical settings have unique characteristics that have not been fully defined. Defining the uniqueness of clinical teaching from both the students' and CTs' viewpoints should help in designing educational programs appropriate to preparing CTs.

The authors suggest that follow-up research in clinical education include validation of the described clinical teaching situation and clinical teaching tools in various clinical education settings. There should be further qualitative research studies to expand the model through grounded theory, field studies of students' and patients' perspectives on clinical education, and further explanation of how specific teaching tools are used so that programs to train physical therapy CTs are meaningful.

SUMMARY

The clinical teaching environment is perceived by CTs as a setting in which students are moved toward professional competence. The environment demands that professional competence be accomplished with the least risk to the patient, the learner, the institution, and the profession. The clinical teaching program and CTs' actions are constrained by ground rules emanating from academic programs, the health care institutions, and the physical therapy department within those institutions. Clinical teachers' belief in and adherence to the concept of patient primacy and the students' level of professional maturity are givens that influence the form and quality of education within clinical settings and result in the use of teaching tools that are vastly different from those used within academic settings. These clinical education teaching tools include diagnosis of readiness; selection of knowledge-oriented and patient treatment-oriented clinical problems; supervision through the use of techniques such as time manipulation, coaching, and shifting status; and ongoing private and public summary evaluations.

REFERENCES

1. Patton MQ: Qualitative Evaluation Methods. Beverly Hills, CA, Sage Publications Inc, 1980, pp 121–194
2. McCall GJ, Simmons JL: Issues in Participant Observation: A Text and Reader. Reading, PA, Addison-Wesley Publishing Co Inc, 1969, p 61
3. Glaser BG, Strauss AL: The Discovery of Grounded Theory. Chicago, IL, Aldine Publishing Co, 1967
4. Glaser BG: Theoretical Sensitivity: Advances in the Methodology of Grounded Theory. Mill Valley, CA, The Sociology Press, 1978
5. Glaser BG, Strauss AL: Awareness of Dying. Chicago, IL, Aldine Publishing Co, 1966
6. Glaser BG, Strauss AL: Time for Dying. Chicago, IL, Aldine Publishing Co, 1966
7. Stern PN: Grounded theory methodology: Its uses and processes. Image 12:20–23, 1980
8. Glass HP: Teaching Behavior in the Nursing Laboratory in Selected Baccalaureate Nursing Programs in Canada. EdD Dissertation. New York, NY, Teachers College, Columbia University, 1971, p 129
9. Wilson M: Supervision: New Patterns and Process. New York, NY, Associated Press, 1969, p 19
10. Jackson PW: The Way Teaching Is. In: Report of the Seminar on Teaching: The Way Teaching Is. Washington, DC, Association for Supervision and Curriculum Development and the Center for the Study of Instruction of the National Education Association, 1966, p 12
11. Shepard KF: Clinical and academic education: Two different phylums. Section for Education, American Physical Therapy Association, Washington, DC, Fall, 1979, pp 5–6

Clinical Teaching in Physical Therapy: Student and Teacher Perceptions

Many practicing physical therapists participate in the most crucial phase of a student's education by serving as Clinical Instructors. The purposes of this study were to identify the clinical teaching behaviors perceived as most effective and most hindering by students and CIs and to compare the response rates of students in bachelor's and master's degree programs. A published 58-item questionnaire was completed by 172 participants from eight physical therapy education programs. The results were analyzed by multivariate analysis of variance. The perceived most helpful teaching behaviors pertained to providing information through feedback. The perceived most hindering behaviors were intimidating questioning and correcting student errors in the presence of patients. The different student and CI ratings for the item "leaves student alone until asked to supervise" has important ethical and educational implications. Master's and bachelor's degree students' ratings differed significantly on four teaching behaviors. Different instructional methods might be necessary for educating these students. [Jarski RW, Kulig K, Olson RE: Clinical teaching in physical therapy: Student and teacher perceptions. Phys Ther 70:173–178, 1990]

Key Words: *Education: physical therapist, clinical education/teaching methods; Education, professional; Teaching.*

Robert W Jarski
Kornelia Kulig
Ronald E Olson

Clinical instruction constitutes a major portion of the physical therapy curriculum. Clinical teaching involves exposing a student to conditions, usually in an active patient setting, where the probability of learning clinical information is high. The process uniquely involves a student, a Clinical Instructor, and patients. The conditions include the physical environment as well as the behaviors and attitudes of all people in the clinic where the teaching takes place. The learning outcomes may be intentional or unintentional, positive or negative. Because students in clinical education programs learn behaviors that influence their lifetime professional performance, improvement of physical therapy professional services depends to a great degree on maintaining a high quality of clinical education.

Many practicing physical therapists in hospitals as well as outpatient settings are involved in the clinical phase of student education. Effective clinical instruction in these settings is believed to require a unique subset of teaching skills,[1-5] and specific teaching behaviors should be identified and evaluated[1,2] for at least three reasons.

The first reason is to promote and help ensure a positive and constructive learning experience[6,7] so that appropriate skills, behaviors, and attitudes for future professional practice are not only learned but also assimilated. The clinical phase is where the theoretical and practical educational components are integrated into real-life situations with actual patients

R Jarski, PhD, PA-C, is Associate Professor of Health Sciences, Oakland University and Meadow Brook Health Enhancement Institute, School of Health Sciences, Rochester, MI 48309-4401.

K Kulig, PhD, PT, is Assistant Professor of Physical Therapy, Oakland University, and Staff Physical Therapist, Oakland Physical Therapy and Rehabilitation, PC, Novi, MI 48050.

R Olson, PhD, is Dean and Professor, School of Health Sciences, Oakland University.

Address all correspondence to Dr Jarski at Program in Physical Therapy, Oakland University, Rochester, MI 48309-4401 (USA).

This project was funded in part by a grant from the Oakland University Educational Development Fund.

This article was submitted February 23, 1989, was with the authors for revision for 14 weeks; and was accepted November 8, 1989.

brought into the instructional process. Clinical Instructors serve as role models for students and should facilitate the integration of the educational components. Clinical Instructors, therefore, should exemplify the highest caliber of cognitive, interpersonal, and humanitarian qualities.

Second, physical therapy education is moving toward a master's degree-level curriculum for entry-level professional graduates.[8] It is not known, however, whether students entering bachelor's and master's degree programs actually differ in their instructional needs or whether specific teaching practices are required to meet these needs. This knowledge may be especially important in clinical instruction because of its preponderance of personal interactions. Different prerequisites are usually required for admission to graduate programs. Admissions committees, therefore, might select applicants differently, and applicants might also select programs differently.

Third, many CIs have not had formal preparation in education and have been selected, not because of their teaching abilities, but because of their professional skills.[9] Because the qualities that constitute effective clinical teaching in physical therapy education are not well publicized, CIs may lack information and direction in planning their professional development activities. Currently, it is often not possible to accurately assess clinical instruction.

The primary purpose of this study was to identify the teaching behaviors perceived to be the most effective and those perceived to be the most hindering by students in physical therapy clinical education programs and by CIs. The secondary purpose was to compare teaching behavior ratings of students in bachelor's and master's degree programs. Our null hypothesis was that there would be no difference between bachelor's and master's degree student ratings.

Method

A list of 58 teaching behaviors thought to be effective or ineffective have been identified by Gjerde and Coble[3] based primarily on the theoretical work of Stritter et al.[5] Gjerde and Coble developed a questionnaire for use in family medicine.[3] The questionnaire items address four areas important in clinical education: communication skills, professional skills, interpersonal skills, and andragogic (adult education) skills. With the authors' permission, we adapted the questionnaire for use in allied health education by changing some of the terminology. For example, we changed the word "resident" to "student." Two questions regarding student or CI status and professional degrees were added at the beginning of the instrument. To investigate the role of CIs in clinical practice, an additional item was added at the end of the instrument: "Is actively and regularly engaged in clinical practice."

The five-point (1–5) rating scale of the original instrument was expanded to a seven-point scale to increase the numerical choices for rating behaviors. The ratings were weighted as follows: 1 = very helpful, 2 = moderately helpful, 3 = slightly helpful, 4 = neither helpful nor hindering, 5 = slightly hindering, 6 = moderately hindering, and 7 = very hindering. Results were analyzed for 1) the entire group of respondents, 2) the differences between student and CI ratings, and 3) the differences between ratings by students in bachelor's and master's degree programs.

To help increase the accuracy and general applicability of the findings, two physical therapy programs were selected from different states in each of four different geographical regions of the United States: Northwest, Northeast, Southwest, and Southeast. By chance, four programs were bachelor's degree programs and four were entry-level master's degree programs. For the purposes of this study, this distribution of bachelor's and master's degree programs was retained in the sample.

Questionnaires with instructions and postage-paid return envelopes were mailed with an accompanying letter to the program directors. The program directors were asked to distribute a questionnaire to each CI who was actively involved in clinical teaching and to each student who had completed at least one clinical rotation. In the questionnaire, the CIs were asked to indicate the length of time they had been involved in clinical teaching and the students were asked to indicate the duration of their clinical learning experience in their present program. A cover letter attached to each questionnaire explained the general purpose of the study and that participation was voluntary. The project was approved by the Oakland University (Rochester, Mich) Institutional Review Board.

One hundred thirty-nine students and 33 CIs returned completed questionnaires. The characteristics of the subjects are shown in Table 1. The percentage of questionnaires returned by each program varied from approximately 14% to 100%. It was not possible to determine the exact percentage returned because questionnaires were distributed by the program directors.

The various return rates possibly could have affected the results of the study. In an unpublished 1988 study on physician assistant students using the same survey instrument and sampling method, we tested for possible rating differences among 10 physician assistant programs with high and low return rates. Instrument ratings from the programs having the two highest return rates (94% and 60%; n = 38) were compared with the responses from the five programs having the lowest return rates (28%–33%; n = 34). A comparison of mean ratings by t tests showed no significant difference for any of the 58 questionnaire items. We concluded that the different return rates did not significantly affect the results. We expected that the different response rates would not affect the results of the present study because 1) the allied health professions have many shared characteristics[8,10,11] and 2) the questionnaire items in both studies addressed educational issues generally applicable to all students in clinical education programs and were not emotional or personal items for which sampling biases would be highly probable.

The perceived most helpful and most hindering teaching behaviors were identified by ranking mean ratings. To test for behavior rating differences between CIs and students and between students in master's and bachelor's degree programs, the following procedures were used. Instrument ratings were analyzed by multivariate analysis of variance to detect overall item differences. Where a significant multivariate F statistic was found, a follow-up univariate F statistic was calculated to identify individual items that differed significantly. When testing for differences between students' and CIs' ratings, a conservative alpha level of .01 was used to decrease the probability of detecting chance differences. When testing for differences between bachelor's and master's degree students' ratings, the conventional .05 alpha level was used.

Results

The 20 behaviors perceived as most helpful by both students and CIs are rank-ordered and listed in Table 2. The mean ratings were between 1.20 ("takes time for discussion and questions") and 1.57 ("demonstrates sensitivity to student needs [eg, feelings of inadequacy, frustration]"). The most highly rated perceived helpful behaviors pertain to the teaching process, such as answering and discussing questions, providing constructive feedback, and facilitating practice and problem solving. Interpersonal behaviors such as "deals with students in a friendly, outgoing manner" were the next most highly rated category. The behavior "is actively and regularly engaged in clinical practice," which was added to the revised survey instrument, ranked 18th with a mean rating of 1.55. This behavior is one of only three professional skill behaviors included among the 20 teaching behaviors rated as most helpful.

The perceived most hindering behavior—"questions students in an intimidating manner"—had a mean rating of 5.88 based on the combined ratings of the students and the CIs. The other 9 behaviors perceived as most hindering were rated between 5.67 and 4.44 (Tab. 3). Like the behaviors rated as most helpful, the most hindering behaviors focused primarily on the teaching process. In addition to these behaviors, availability and negative interpersonal skill behaviors were perceived as hindering, especially those pertaining to behavior around patients.

Five behaviors were rated differently by students and CIs. The significantly different behaviors are shown in Table 4 along with their univariate F statistics and significance levels. The greatest difference was found in the mean ratings for the behavior "leaves student alone until asked to supervise." Students, with a mean rating of 3.36, considered this behavior helpful (ie, less than 4, the neutral rating on the seven-point scale); CIs, with a mean rating of 5.09, considered this behavior hindering.

Four behaviors were perceived differently by bachelor's and master's degree students. Table 5 lists the behaviors and their univariate F statistics and significance levels. These behaviors related to student supervision, behavior around patients, and basing judgments of students on indirect evidence. Interestingly, all of the behaviors were rated significantly higher (ie, more hindering or less helpful) by the master's degree students compared with their bachelor's degree counterparts.

Discussion

The primary purpose of this study was to identify the teaching behaviors perceived to be the most effective and those perceived to be the most hindering by students in physical therapy clinical education programs and by CIs.

Table 1. *Description of Subjects (N = 172)*

Variable	Total
Number of programs represented	8
Bachelor's degree	4
Master's degree	4
Number of states represented	8
Number of student respondents by program	139
Bachelor's degree	82
Master's degree	57
Number of student respondents by geographic region	139
Northwest	28
Northeast	58
Southwest	37
Southeast	16
Duration of clinical instruction (mo)	
$\bar{X}$	5.64
s	6.01
Mode (N = 30)	2
Number of Clinical Instructor respondents	33
Physical therapists	31
Other[a]	1
No response	1
Duration of clinical teaching (yr)	
$\bar{X}$	7.22
s	5.27
Bimodalities (N = 4,4)	1,8

[a]Respondent indicated only Bachelor of Science degree.

Most Helpful Behaviors

Gjerde and Coble identified 58 behaviors believed to be important in clinical instruction.[3] These behaviors were classified into four skill domains: communication skills, professional skills, interpersonal skills, and andragogic skills. The mean ratings in our study indicate that andragogic skills—behaviors pertaining to providing information through feedback or through discussion and answering questions—were perceived as most helpful. Seven (35%) of the 20 behaviors rated as most helpful pertained to providing information. There was also strong support for CIs to provide

Table 2. *Teaching Behaviors Identified as Most Helpful*

Rank	Rating[a] X	s	Behavior[b]
1	1.20	.50	Takes time for discussion and questions
2	1.26	.51	Answers questions clearly
3	1.26	.65	Provides constructive feedback
4	1.33	.55	Provides students with opportunities to practice both technical and problem-solving skills
5	1.37	.61	Is willingly accessible to students
6	1.37	.62	Discusses practical applications of knowledge and skills
7	1.38	.64	Shares his or her knowledge and experience
8	1.40	.66	Creates practice opportunities for students
9	1.41	.62	Asks questions that stimulate problem solving
10	1.47	.69	Deals with students in a friendly, outgoing manner
11	1.48	.71	Emphasizes problem-solving approaches rather than solutions per se
12	1.49	.74	Asks questions in a nonthreatening manner
13	1.50	.75	Demonstrates a genuine interest in the student
14	1.52	.69	Demonstrates enthusiasm for teaching
15	1.52	.72	Demonstrates sensitivity to patient needs
16	1.52	.69	Summarizes major points at the conclusion of the teaching session
17	1.52	.75	Demonstrates skills for students
18	1.55	.75	Is actively and regularly engaged in clinical practice
19	1.55	.69	Actively promotes discussion
20	1.57	.72	Demonstrates sensitivity to student needs (eg, feelings of inadequacy, frustration)

[a]Based on combined ratings of 58 teaching behaviors by 139 students and 33 Clinical Instructors. (1 = very helpful, 2 = moderately helpful, 3 = slightly helpful, 4 = neither helpful nor hindering, 5 = slightly hindering, 6 = moderately hindering, 7 = very hindering.)

[b]Adapted from Gjerde and Coble.[3]

practice opportunities with active participation in patient care.

Six (30%) of the 20 behaviors perceived as most helpful (30%) were interpersonal skill behaviors such as friendliness toward students, enthusiasm for teaching, and sensitivity to patient needs. Behaviors relating to providing information and discussing questions, however, were consistently rated as more helpful. Few professional skill behaviors were rated among the 20 behaviors perceived as most helpful. Even though certain affective behaviors were regarded as important, teaching skills were considered more important in facilitating learning.

Our results are generally consistent with the findings in the family medicine study by Gjerde and Coble.[3] A similar survey instrument was used, and the mean ratings of the 18 teaching behaviors identified as most helpful by family practice CIs and residents-in-training were reported. The results of our physical therapy study differed from those of Gjerde and Coble's[3] family medicine study on only two items ("willing to admit when he or she does not know" and "is well prepared for teaching sessions"). Apparently, physical therapy and family medicine respondents do not differ widely in their perceptions of effective clinical teaching. This finding would be expected because

both physical therapists and family physicians are health care professionals having intensive patient care responsibilities during the clinical education phase of their respective programs.

Our results are also consistent with those reported in the ethnographic study of physical therapy CIs by Scully and Shepard,[2] but different from the results reported by Moore and Perry[9] and by Emery,[1] who found that physical therapy students rated interpersonal relations as more important than teaching behaviors. This difference in results is not explained by our study, which found only five significant differences between student and CI ratings. One possible explanation is the overlap between the categories used in Emery's[1] investigation. For example, "communication" and "teaching behaviors" cannot always be clearly differentiated. Using exact definitions of the categories might have increased the precision in categorizing the behaviors in Emery's valuable study.

Most Hindering Behaviors

In our study as well as in the study by Gjerde and Coble,[3] the same two teaching behaviors were rated as most hindering (ie, "questions students in an intimidating manner" and "corrects students' errors in front of patients"). Students and CIs did not differ in their perceptions of intimidating behavior in our survey, which called upon subjects to imagine or recall clinical teaching behaviors. Their perceptions, however, might differ in actual practice. For example, a CI might think his or her feedback is helpful, whereas the student might think the CI's teaching behavior is intimidating. Future studies should test for differences between ratings for imagined versus observed teaching behaviors. Videotaped interactions might be instrumental, and rating assessments should consider the teacher, the learner, and the patient.

Table 3. *Teaching Behaviors Identified as Most Hindering*

| Rank | Rating[a] | | Behavior[b] |
	$\overline{X}$	s	
58	5.88	1.60	Questions students in an intimidating manner
57	5.67	1.50	Corrects students' errors in front of patients
56	5.37	1.54	Bases judgments of students on indirect evidence
55	5.05	1.36	Fails to adhere to teaching schedule
54	4.92	1.61	Fails to recognize extra effort
53	4.81	1.75	Discusses medical cases in front of patients
52	4.71	1.34	Is difficult to summon for consultation after hours
51	4.69	1.32	Appears to discourage student-faculty relationships outside of clinical areas
50	4.58	1.68	Gives general answers to specific questions
49	4.44	1.52	Fails to set time limits for teaching activities

[a]Based on combined ratings of 58 teaching behaviors by 139 students and 33 Clinical Instructors. (1 = very helpful, 2 = moderately helpful, 3 = slightly helpful, 4 = neither helpful nor hindering, 5 = slightly hindering, 6 = moderately hindering, 7 = very hindering.)

[b]Adapted from Gjerde and Coble.[5]

Different Ratings by Students and Clinical Instructors

Of the five behaviors rated differently by students and CIs, the greatest difference was for the item "leaves student alone until asked to supervise." Students consider this behavior helpful, whereas CIs considered it hindering. This finding poses interesting insights into the educational process; students may prefer to develop their own clinical skills without constant, direct supervision—the "discovery-learning" mode. This finding could also represent students' fear of teacher criticism. That CIs considered this a hindering behavior is possibly due to ethical as well as didactic concerns. Do students know when their learning might jeopardize the quality of health care or patient safety? Can students recognize when they really need supervision either for learning or for ensuring patient safety?

These judgments should be the prerogative of the experienced clinical professional who is also able to use educational strategies that help students learn. It must be recognized, however, that students and teachers have opposite perceptions of this potentially critical behavior. With this difference in mind, the CI should allow discovery learning only when it has been ascertained that the activity will be safely performed by the student.

Different Ratings by Bachelor's and Master's Degree Students

The secondary purpose of this study was to compare teaching behavior ratings of students in bachelor's and master's degree programs. Four behaviors were rated differently by these two student groups. Differences in mean ratings show that master's degree students considered as more hindering 1) discussing medical cases in the presence of patients, 2) having their errors corrected in the presence of patients, and 3) having judgments made about them based on indirect evidence. Interestingly, bachelor's degree students rated "leaves student alone until asked to supervise" more helpful than did master's degree students. One possible explanation for these results might be that master's degree students consider graduate-level education a more serious endeavor than undergraduate education. Further studies might help further explain these findings and add further credence to adopting the master's degree as the entry-level degree.

Table 4. *Behaviors Clinical Instructors and Students Rated Differently[a]*

| Behavior[b] | Rating | | F | p |
	CI ($\overline{X}$)	Student ($\overline{X}$)		
Leaves student alone until asked to supervise	5.09	3.36	39.44	.001
Fails to recognize extra effort	5.81	4.71	14.45	.001
Fails to set time limits for teaching activities	5.00	4.31	9.59	.002
Answers questions clearly	1.03	1.31	8.16	.005
Discusses medical cases in front of patients	5.48	4.66	7.28	.008

[a]$\alpha = .01$.

[b]Adapted from Gjerde and Coble.[5]

Conclusions and Recommendations

From these data, we conclude that clinical teaching behaviors rated as most helpful pertain to the instructional process. Facilitating a favorable learning environment depends on instructor availability and positive

Table 5. *Behavior Ratings that Differed Significantly[a] Between Students in Master's and Bachelor's Degree Programs*

	Rating			
Behavior[b]	Master's Degree Students ($\bar{X}$)	Bachelor's Degree Students ($\bar{X}$)	F	p
Leaves student alone until asked to supervise	3.91	2.88	11.24	.001
Discusses medical cases in front of patients	5.09	4.03	7.92	.006
Corrects students' errors in front of patients	6.11	5.33	6.08	.016
Bases judgments of students on indirect evidence	5.93	5.22	5.78	.019

[a] $\alpha = .05$.

[b] Adapted from Gjerde and Coble.[3]

interpersonal relationships with the student, patients, and other personnel. Professional skills appear to play a less important role in effective clinical teaching.

As physical therapy programs move toward the master's degree entry level, CIs might need to change some of their behaviors to meet the needs of their new students. The results of this study should help CIs to 1) assess their own clinical teaching behaviors and 2) identify and practice educational skills found to be most effective.

Many graduate physical therapists are called upon to be CIs sometime during their careers, and all physical therapy practitioners should participate in educating patients. Continuing education planners are encouraged to make education-related sessions available to graduate physical therapists, and practicing physical therapists are encouraged to select continuing education courses in related disciplines.

For students, mastering instructional skills should be an educational program objective. It may be achieved by learning essential instructional theory, and then practicing by making classroom presentations and assisting in laboratory sessions with proper faculty guidance and supervision. This level of education is consistent with the master's degree level of preparation. Using instructional methods known to be effective should enrich the clinical education of our students and help enhance future physical therapy services for patients.

References

1 Emery MJ: Effectiveness of the clinical instructor: Students' perspective. Phys Ther 64:1079–1083, 1984

2 Scully RM, Shepard KF: Clinical teaching in physical therapy education: An ethnographic study. Phys Ther 63:349–358, 1983

3 Gjerde CL, Coble RJ: Resident and faculty perceptions of effective clinical teaching in family practice. J Fam Pract 14:323–327, 1982

4 Irby DM: Clinical teacher effectiveness in medicine. J Med Educ 53:808–815, 1978

5 Stritter FT, Hain JD, Grimes DA: Clinical teaching reexamined. J Med Educ 50:876–882, 1975

6 DeCecco JP, Crawford WR: The Psychology of Learning and Instruction. Englewood Cliffs, NJ, Prentice-Hall Inc, 1974

7 Knowles MS: Andragogy in Action: Applying Modern Principles of Adult Learning. San Francisco, CA, Jossey-Bass Inc, Publishers, 1985

8 Tammivaara J, Yarbrough P, Shepard KF: Assessing the Quality of Physical Therapy Education Programs. Alexandria, VA, American Physical Therapy Association, 1986

9 Moore ML, Perry JF: Clinical Education in Physical Therapy: Present Status/Future Needs. Washington, DC, American Physical Therapy Association, 1976

10 Schafft GE, Cawley JF: The Physician Assistant in a Changing Health Care Environment. Rockville, MD, Aspen Publishers Inc, 1987

11 Hislop HJ: Tenth Mary McMillan Lecture: The not-so-impossible dream. Phys Ther 55:1069–1080, 1975

Perceived Importance and Frequency of Clinical Teaching Behaviors: Surveys of Students, Clinical Instructors and Center Coordinators of Clinical Education

MICHAEL EMERY   CATHERINE PERRY WILKINSON

INTRODUCTION

Preparing physical therapy clinicians to become clinical instructors is a concern of both the academic and clinical communities in physical therapy. A primary need in this preparation process is for a clear understanding of clinical instruction competencies. Several studies in physical therapy have been done to identify what clinical instruction characteristics are necessary for effective clinical education to occur.[1,2] Further work has been done in identifying which previously identified characteristics clinical instructors may already possess and which will be necessary to develop.[3]

We wanted to survey Clinical Instructors (CI) and Center Coordinators of Clinical Education (CCCE) to determine which clinical teaching behaviors were being used by CIs, and to determine which behaviors needed to be taught to CIs. We also wanted to compare our survey results with data from a previous study on students' perceptions about clinical teaching behaviors.

We believe the results from these two studies could be helpful in identifying appropriate clinical teaching behaviors for CIs and in identifying teaching behaviors needing improvement. Study results could also be helpful in developing appropriate clinical instruction training materials.

METHOD

A literature review was done to determine appropriate teaching behaviors for clinical instructor.[1,2,4-6] Descriptions of appropriate teaching behaviors were refined into statements of observable behavior. We organized these behaviors into four categories: communication, teaching, professional and interpersonal behaviors (Appendix). Communication behaviors were defined as those where direct verbal or non-verbal interaction occurred. We categorized teaching behaviors as those pertaining to the activities of supervision, instruction or evaluation. Professional behaviors we defined as including the cognitive, affective and psychomotor competencies of physical therapy practice. Interpersonal behaviors were those that focused on establishing a learning environment and developing a relationship between the clinical instructor and the student.

We developed a questionnaire and asked the respondents to rate each behavior twice; first for the "importance" of the behavior in facilitating effective clinical education and, secondly, for how "frequently" they believed the behavior occurred in the clinical education environment. Our rating scales for scoring "importance" and "frequency" were adopted from work by Frank Stritter in his assessment of the clinical education process of medical students.[7] On our scale for rating "importance", a rating of 1 represented "significant importance", a 2 meant "moderately important", a 3 meant "somewhat significant", and a 4 represented "not significant". For ranking "frequency", a ranking of 1 represented "frequent" (75 to 100% of the time), a 2 represented "more than not" (50 to 75%), a 3 meant "occasionally" (25 to 50%) and a 4 meant "seldom" (0 to 25%).

In a previous study by Emery, these questions on perceptions of "importance" and "frequency" of clinical teaching behaviors had been administered to 102 senior physical therapy students.[3] Subjects were from three undergraduate programs of physical therapy in the New England area. The questionnaire was given to students following their completion of all clinical education requirements. In this study, students rated communication behaviors as being most important for clinical instructors to have. Students thought interpersonal behaviors were the second most important behavior for clinical instructors, followed by teaching and professional behaviors. All clinical teaching behaviors were found to be reasonably frequent and evenly distributed across the four categories of behaviors. Sixteen teaching behaviors had near random correlations between "importance" and "frequency"; suggesting that these students believed these behaviors should be the focus of clinical instructor development.[3]

For this follow-up study, we asked the same questions (as in the Emery study) of a mixed group consisting of 67 CIs and CCCEs from various clinical education facilities in the New England area. These subjects represented many, but not all, of the clinical facilities in which the students

in the previous study received their clinical education. All subjects were attending a Clinical Faculty Institute meeting on clinical instructor development, sponsored by the University of Vermont. The questionnaire was administered in person. Subjects were questioned prior to any discussion regarding the findings of Emery's earlier study on student perceptions. All conference participants completed the questionnaire and all data were usable for analysis. A profile of the respondents is found in Table 1.

PROFILE OF CLINICAL INSTRUCTORS AND CENTER COORDINATORS FOR CLINICAL EDUCATION SURVEY RESPONDENTS

Present P.T. Position In Clinical Education:	N	%
CCCE	40	60.6
CI	14	21.2
Director	1	1.5
CCCE & Director	9	13.6
CI & Director	2	3.0
NR	1	0.1
Provide Clinical Education Program For:		
PT Students Only	32	47.8
PT and PTA Students	35	52.2
Years Working With PT Students:		
One or Less	6	9.0
Two-Three	12	17.9
Four-Five	20	29.9
Six-Ten	13	19.4
More than Ten	16	23.9
PT Employment Setting:		
General Hospital	33	49.3
Teaching Hospital/Medical Center	10	14.9
Rehabilitation Center	9	13.4
Out-Patient Clinic	1	1.5
Nursing Home/ECF	1	1.5
Home Health	4	6.0
Private Practice	1	1.5
Specialty Center	8	11.9

Table 1

Subjects in the mixed CI/CCCE group were asked to rate the clinical teaching behaviors from the perspective of "importance" and "frequency" within their own clinical settings. An optical scanner answer sheet was used to facilitate computer tabulation and statistical analysis. Frequency distribution and mean scores were tabulated for each behavior for both "importance" and "frequency". Clinical teaching behaviors, with the greatest discrepancy between "importance" and "frequency", were identified. Data from the mixed

29

CI/CCCE group were compared with previous data from students. The relationship between student and CI/CCCE data was also studied for both behavior "importance" and behavior "frequency".

Data from the student study and the CI/CCCE study were combined. When combined, data were organized to study the relationship between "importance" and "frequency" in the combined group. Statistical analysis was done using the Statistical Packages for the Social Sciences programs for Pearson Product Moment correlation studies and the Sign and Mann-Whitney tests for correlation data.

RESULTS

We identified thirteen behaviors that were rated by both the CI/CCCE and student groups as being very important but occurring less frequently in the between groups analysis. Of these thirteen high "importance"/low "frequency" behaviors, six were communication behaviors, five were teaching behaviors and two were interpersonal behaviors (Table 2).

**THIRTEEN HIGH IMPORTANCE/
LOW FREQUENCY BEHAVIORS**

Communication Behaviors:

— Is an active listener
— Makes himself/herself understood
— Provides timely feedback
— Provides useful feedback
— Communicates in a non-threatening manner
— Openly and honestly reveals perceptions that the clinical instructor has of student performance

Teaching Behaviors:

— Is available to the student
— Plans effective learning experiences
— Provides positive feedback on performance
— Makes the formal evaluation experience a constructive process
— Allows the student progressive, appropriate independence

Interpersonal Behaviors:

— Provides support for student's concerns, frustrations, and anxieties
— Establishes an environment in which the student feels comfortable

---

Table 2

From the CI/CCCE group data, four of the thirteen behaviors demonstrated weak positive correlations between "importance" and "frequency" (Table 3). The remaining nine behaviors were clearly in discrepancy as suggested by both groups. Although both groups stated all thirteen behaviors were highly "important" but less "frequent", a between groups correlation test

for "importance" of the behavior yielded only two weak correlations (Table 4).

**BEHAVIORS DEMONSTRATING POSITIVE
IMPORTANCE/FREQUENCY
CORRELATIONS: CI/CCCE GROUP**

Teaching Behaviors:	R
— Allows student progressive, appropriate independence	.22
— Makes the formal evaluation a constructive process	.24
Interpersonal Behaviors:	
— Provides appropriate support for the student's concerns, frustrations, and anxieties	.39
Communications Behaviors:	
— Provides positive feedback on performance	.32
P .05	

Table 3

A review of the data indicated that students had scored the behaviors consistently higher in "importance" than did the CI/CCCE group members. The correlations between student and CI/CCCE ratings of "frequency" were much higher.

**BEHAVIORS DEMONSTRATING
CORRELATION BETWEEN STUDENTS
AND CI/CCCEs FOR FREQUENCY**

Communication Behaviors:	Z
— Provides timely feedback	-2.13
Interpersonal Behaviors:	
— Establishes an environment in which the student feels comfortable	-2.85
P .05	

Table 4

This finding suggested that both groups agreed on the relatively low "frequency" with which these behaviors occurred in the clinical education setting (Table 5).

When we combined data from the student and CI/CCCE studies and analyzed the relationship between "importance" and "frequency", we found that all behaviors were scored as more "important" than "frequent" in the clinical education setting (Table 6).

DISCUSSION

This approach to analyzing data allowed us to select from the previously studied student rating of behaviors, those in which there appeared to be a discrepancy between "importance" and "frequency". As a result of our data analysis, we made several conclusions.

**BEHAVIORS DEMONSTRATING
CORRELATION BETWEEN STUDENTS AND
CI/CCCEs FOR FREQUENCY**

Communication Behaviors	Z
— Provides timely feedback	-2.31*
— Provides useful feedback	-3.13**
— Is an active listener	-4.19**
— Makes himself/herself understood	-5.75**
— Communicates in a non-threatening manner	-5.19**
— Provides positive feedback on performance	-5.24**
Teaching Behaviors	
— Plans effective learning experiences	-3.03**
— Is available to the student	-2.82**
— Makes the formal evaluation a constructive process	-3.89**
Interpersonal Behaviors	
— Establishes an environment in which the student feels comfortable	-4.65**
— Provides appropriate support for student's concerns, frustrations, and anxieties	-3.23**
*P .05	
**P .01	

Table 5

**BEHAVIORS DEMONSTRATING
SIGNIFICANT DIFFERENCE BETWEEN
IMPORTANCE AND FREQUENCY**

Communication Behaviors	Z
— Is an active listener	6.32
— Makes himself/herself understood	8.94
— Provides timely feedback	6.57
— Provides useful feedback	6.16
— Communicates in a non-threatening manner	6.99
— Openly and honestly reveals perceptions that the clinical instructor has of student performance	6.97
Teaching Behaviors	
— Is available to the student	4.00
— Plans effective learning experiences	7.17
— Provides positive feedback on performance	5.46
— Makes the formal evaluation experience a constructive process	4.31
— Allows the student progressive, appropriate independence	6.07
Interpersonal Skills Behaviors	
— Provides support for student's concerns, frustrations, and anxieties	6.00
— Establishes an environment in which the student feels comfortable	4.98
P .01	

Table 6

A general agreement exists between students and CI/CCCEs on the "importance" and "frequency" of the forty-three clinical instructor teaching behaviors examined. Of the thirteen high "importance"/low "frequency" behaviors identified, we found four relevant results: 1) students scored these behaviors higher in "importance" than did the CI/CCCE group; 2) the CI/CCCE group perceived greater consistency between "importance" and "frequency" of the thirteen behaviors than did the students; 3) both groups agreed on the relatively low "frequency" of the thirteen behaviors, and 4) both groups agreed there were differences between the perceived "importance" of the thirteen behaviors and the "frequency" with which they perceived these behaviors to occur in the clinical education setting.

We suggest that while both the student group and the CI/CCCE group perceived discrepancies in the performance of the clinical instructor relative to these behaviors, the CI/CCCE group members did not interpret the discrepancies to be as great as did the students. This may cause the student and the CI/CCCE to view problems in regard to these behaviors somewhat differently as they arise during the clinical education experience. Even when these differences are acknowledged, there remains significant agreement in the views of the students and the CI/CCCEs regarding these behaviors. These results offer credibility to our concern that these teaching behaviors may well be in need of further development for our clinical instructors.

CONCLUSIONS

This study has yielded additional information regarding the training needs of clinical instructors. By comparing the data of this study with a previous study from the students' perspective on clinical instructor behaviors, several clinical instructor behaviors have been identified which both groups agree are important but are not being consistently demonstrated in the clinic. We suggest that these clinical teaching behaviors are in need of further development by clinical education instructors. Further research is needed to consider other key perspectives on clinical instructor behaviors including those of the Academic Coordinators of Clinical Education. We recommend the use of these forty-three clinical instructor teaching behaviors, and that they be used to develop an individualized clinical instructor evaluation form. Also, we believe that formal programs for training clinical instructors must be developed and implemented.

Mr. Emery is an Assistant Professor and the Academic Coordinator of Clinical Education at the University of Vermont, Burlington, VT 05401. At the time of this study, he was a Clinical Assistant Professor at the university and an Advanced Clinician at the Medical Center Hospital of Vermont in Burlington.

Dr. Wilkinson is an independent consultant in physical therapy, White River Junction, VT 05001. At the time of this study, she was an Associate Professor and the Academic Coordinator of Clinical Education at the University of Vermont, Burlington, VT.

APPENDIX
Clinical Instructor Behaviors

Communication Behaviors

1. Makes himself/herself understood
2. Provides useful feedback
3. Is an active listener
4. Provides positive feedback on performance
5. Communicates in a non-threatening manner
6. Openly and honestly reveals perceptions that the clinical instructor has of the student
7. Provides timely feedback
8. Is open in discussing issues with the student
9. Teaches in an interactive way; encourages dialogue
10. Provides feedback in private

Interpersonal Relations Behaviors

11. Establishes an environment in which the student feels comfortable
12. Provides appropriate support for student concerns, frustrations, anxieties
13. Empathetic
14. Demonstrates a genuine concern for patients
15. Presents student as a professional to others
16. Demonstrates positive regard for student as a person

Professional Skills Behaviors

17. Employs PT practice with competence
18. Demonstrates professional behavior as a member of the health care team
19. Demonstrates systematic approach to problem-solving
20. Explains physiological basis of PT treatment
21. Explains psychological basis of PT evaluation
22. Demonstrates appropriate role of PT as part of total health care
23. Serves as an appropriate role model
24. Manages own time well
25. Demonstrates leadership among peers

Teaching Behaviors

26. Allows the student progressive, appropriate independence
27. Is available to the student
28. Makes the formal evaluation a constructive process
29. Makes effective learning experience out of situations as they arise
30. Plans effective learning experiences
31. Provides a variety of patients
32. Questions/coaches in way to facilitate student learning
33. Points out discrepancies in student's performance
34. Provides unique learning experiences
35. Makes relationships between academic knowledge and clinical practice
36. Is accurate in documenting student evaluation
37. Helps student define specific objectives for the clinical education experience
38. Observes performance in a discreet manner
39. Schedules regular meetings with the student
40. Plans learning experiences before the student arrives
41. Manages student's time well
42. Timely in documenting the student's evaluation
43. Is perceived as a consistent extension of the academic program

REFERENCES

1. Moore, Margaret: Clinical Education in Physical Therapy; Present Status/Future Needs. Section for Education, American Physical Therapy Association, 1976.

2. Scully, Rosemary; Clinical Teaching of Physical Therapy Students in Clinical Education. Unpublished Doctoral Dissertation, Columbia University, March 18, 1974.

3. Emery, Michael: Effectiveness of the Clinical Instructor; Students' Perspective. Phys·Ther 64:1079-1083, 1984.

4. Dickenson, Ruth, et al: Handbook for Physical Therapy Teachers. New York, NY, American Physical Therapy Association, 1967.

5. May, Bella J: Interactive Strategies in Supervision and Education. Center for Allied Health Instructional Personnel, College of Education, University of Florida, 1977.

6. Perry, Jan: Handbook for Clinical Faculty Development. Division of Physical Therapy, Department of Medical Allied Health Professions, University of North Carolina at Chapel Hill, 1977.

7. Stritter, Frank: Clinical Teaching Re-examined. J Med Educ 50:876-882, 1975.

Methods of Clinical Instruction in Physical Therapy

Beatrice Whitcomb, Capt., WMSC

INTRODUCTION

Clinical instruction in physical therapy education represents the laboratory portion of the student's training and may well be considered the heart of the curriculum. Considered in its entirety, the subject of clinical instruction is a broad one, worthy of detailed study of its many aspects. The present discussion will be limited to methods of instruction in the clinical practice phase of the undergraduate program, especially as they relate to the teaching supervisors. Staff qualifications, specific objectives, content, orientation to the facility, and student evaluation will not be included, although their great importance cannot be disregarded.

Clinical practice should be offered for the sole purpose of teaching the student and it must be organized and administered as is any other laboratory course. It should be under the direction of physical therapists who are well qualified both personally and professionally and who are also qualified for university appointment. These instructors should have sufficient freedom from routine duties to permit optimum time for preparation, instruction, and student supervision.

It is assumed that the student in the clinical practice phase of his education has a foundation in the basic sciences and the technics of physical therapy. It is the general function of the clinical practice supervisory staff to create, continually, learning situations which will supplement, integrate, and vitalize classroom instruction. In addition to helping the student make correct application of scientific principles, it is generally agreed that an equally important responsibility of the clinical practice staff is the continuous, persistent teaching of desirable personal and professional attitudes and conduct and emphasis upon their application.

Each school of physical therapy has in writing its own specific aims, policies, and procedures based on a careful analysis of the particular school and its student body. It is needless to say that teaching supervisors must be familiar with the

Medical Field Service School. Brooke Army Medical Center, Fort Sam Houston, Tex.

course outlines, understand and accept the objectives and policies for clinical practice which have been formulated by the school, and know the procedures by which the students are taught in the didactic phase of their instruction.

In any educational program the most important single factor for success is the instructor. The satisfaction and effectiveness of the students in their clinical practice experience, as well as many of their future attitudes toward their work, will depend almost entirely upon the quality of supervision. It is the function of the clinical practice instructor to assist, guide, and inspire the student toward self-development; his role is that of a senior student or a more experienced friend. In addition to a broad knowledge of the subject, and certain personal traits, it is essential that the teaching supervisor have a liking for and a degree of skill in teaching.

PRINCIPLES OF LEARNING

There is developing at this time a more comprehensive theory of instruction, each principle being based on psychological knowledge gained from the observation of overt behavior that accompanies learning. The teaching supervisor needs an understanding of these well-recognized principles of learning and teaching in order to avoid the common pitfalls which lead to error, waste, or heartbreak.

Learning must be purposeful, and goal centered, with experience growing out of a recognized need. We learn best those things which have meaning, and the learning process is stimulated when the how and why are known. It is the responsibility of the clinical instructor to guide students in selecting worthy objectives and to point out constantly the reasons which lie behind requests, methods, and activities.

Interest is an important factor in learning and new interests usually grow out of the old. Learning occurs largely in terms of past experience and through association, the knowledge of which fact brings out the value of helping the student create a rich background of experience. There should be constant utilization in learning situations of that background which already has been acquired. Frequent reference to related classroom experience will promote increased interest and learning.

Satisfaction and success must attend the act of learning because we learn most rapidly that which gives us satisfaction. It is important that the assignment of work be kept within the learner's training, experience, and maturity. The student needs guidance in maintaining a level of aspiration which is consistent with his power of attainment. The instructor should endeavor to make the learning process pleasant, and this can be done without lowering the standards.

Individuals vary in their interests, needs, and capacities. There is a difference in the ability to learn, the rate of learning, and the performance after learning. It is essential that the instructor know each student well and that he attempt to satisfy, in so far as possible, the variations in interests, needs, and capacities.

The whole individual, emotionally, physically, and intellectually engages in the learning process and he reacts in a unified way to whole situations or total patterns. With this principle in mind, the instructor will consider the student a feeling and doing, as well as thinking, person. He will also realize that items within any learning situation should be related to each other and that all should have some relation to a central core or purpose. He will summarize frequently the many facts and concepts, emphasize certain points, and tie them together in the proper order.

Learning is a process of experiencing, reacting, and doing. The learner is a behaving organism in whom activity is primary and continuous. One learns by such self-activities as listening, visualizing, recalling, memorizing, reasoning, judging, and thinking. The greater the active participation encouraged on the part of the learner, the more effective will be the learning.

We learn as we respond to stimuli. We remember the longest those things which are accompanied by the strongest stimuli or the things which stimulate the greatest number of our senses. It is said that the average person learns about 75 percent through sight, 13 percent by hearing, 6 percent by touch, and 3 percent each from taste and smell. The instructor should know the various teaching aids and use as many avenues to learning as possible.

Learning must be specific and to the point, and not general or haphazard, since a transfer of training in a knowledge or a skill does not occur in a general way. The instructor must teach a skill or fact specifically and should not rely on the student's success in one activity to carry over to a similar activity unless the elements are identical. Knowledge of the nature of transfer of training also reveals the fallacy that one must do unpleasant tasks or learn the hard way. It has been proved that forced learnings do not carry over into life and do not beget perseverance and discipline. Utilizing "student purpose" does not mean letting students do as they please nor avoiding the unpleasant, but it does stress the need for making acts sensible and meaningful for the learner.

The amount of learning and the level of skill usually can be increased by distributing the learning over a long period rather than concentrating it into a short period. It also has been found that shorter sessions of training with time allowed in between for other activities produce better results than do long sessions, in terms of the amount learned, the level of skill acquired, and the retention. This principle has practical significance for the supervisor in planning his teaching units in that he will provide shorter sessions of a given activity extended over a longer period of time as contrasted to the "shot in the arm" procedure.

There is value in over-learning. Studies show that skills and knowledge once learned are soon lost. For example, it has been found that the average college student forgets more than two thirds of what he has learned in a course within two years, and the typist who has attained a rate of sixty words a minute drops to forty words or less within a year without practice or retraining. The answer to the problem in physical therapy is either to retrain periodically or to train in clinical activities to such a high standard of proficiency that, when the usual loss has taken place, the physical therapist will have retained sufficient professional knowledge, habits, skills, and attitudes as are required for superior performance in her work.

People learn only as they are given adequate incentives. The best types of motivation are those which are intrinsic or inherent in the learning situation, the most desirable being those purposes growing out of the needs, interests, and activities accepted by the student. The student's increasing insight into the problem to be solved or the skill to be mastered has a favorable effect on learning. A very desirable intrinsic motive and an important factor in effective learning is the knowledge of one's own progress. Extrinsic incentives such as marks, rewards, and punishment not functionally related to the learning situation, as well as such motives as sarcasm, rivalry, and strong personal influence, may also beget learning, but learning of a kind soon lost or often accompanied by detrimental learning outcomes. Social motives of co-operation, deserved recognition by one's peers or supervisor, and participation in planning and deciding have beneficial effects on learning. It has been conclusively proved that praise and respect are more conducive to desirable learning than are criticism and fear. On the basis of this principle, the clinical instructor will let the student know periodically how he is getting along and he will give praise generously and with discrimination.

Studies have been made which show that learning is more rapid and effective where there is uniformity among instructors as to approach, content, and emphasis, especially during the early stages of learning. After a skill is mastered, variations may be introduced without confusion to the learner. This principle indicates that teaching supervisors should be familiar with the technics and procedures followed during the preclinical phase. As the student becomes more advanced he may be exposed to other methods and, before his graduation, must be made to realize that there is more than one adequate way of administering most physical treatments.

PRINCIPLES AND METHODS OF TEACHING

Teaching is a highly variable performance and there are wide limits within which the instructor may select his activities and still be reasonably successful. To suggest a single technic in teaching which will apply generally is impossible since, of necessity, it will vary with the situation, the purpose of the instruction, the personality and the ability of both the instructor and the student, the material available, and the policy of the particular school. The important point for the instructor to remember is that effective teaching is planned specifically and that it is based on well-established principles of learning and teaching. Because people learn in much the same manner, the usual procedure in teaching any skill or subject includes five steps—namely, get ready to instruct, prepare the student, present the information, encourage sufficient practice, and evaluate results. Each step will be considered in greater detail.

Step I. Get ready to instruct.

Have a time table so you know how much the student is to learn and by when. To clarify any task in your own mind, break it down into key points. Review any additional material necessary. Have everything in readiness, including equipment and material to be used, and make sure it is arranged exactly as you expect the student to keep it. The significance of this is seen clearly in the use of some of the more complicated electrical equipment. If desirable, make preliminary arrangement with patients to be involved.

Step II. Prepare the student.

Obtain the interest and attention of the learner. It is assumed that the physical therapy student will have interest in most cases, so it becomes a matter of showing him how much the acquisition of knowledge and skill enhances the value and benefit to be derived from his work. It has been shown that even the most routine jobs may be "psychologically enlarged" for the worker and interest sustained when attention is given to an explanation of the purpose and importance of the job and its relation to the whole. For this reason, among others, the student should be reminded frequently of the values obtainable from such treatments as whirlpool, infra-red, diathermy, and ultraviolet. As the student increases his knowledge of the various technics and of the equipment and can relate their use intelligently to patient care, interest will develop and be maintained.

Where possible, the student should be given an opportunity to read the patient's chart in advance of the treatment he is going to observe or with which he is to assist. The instructor must find out what the student already knows so he may integrate new information with the old. Needless to say, the student should be put at ease during this period.

Step III. Present the information.

The new information must be presented on the border of the learner's knowledge since learning is largely a matter of association. The material must be presented in a logical way. If, for example, patients were expected for treatment with such conditions as Marie-Strumpell arthritis, rheumatoid arthritis, fibrositis, and multiple sclerosis, a logical way would be to consider with the student the diagnosis, etiology, signs and symptoms, pathological changes, general disability caused, and the prognosis. Possible treatments could then be mentioned along with the prescribed treatment and its specific aims. Lastly, the technics of treatment would be reviewed including all the key points such as the proper steps in the operation of the equipment, physics involved in the procedure, and the details to be observed in carrying out the prescription. Explanations should be given clearly, completely, and patiently at the right rate for the learner, since too rapid a presentation leads to dissatisfaction and one which is too slow may lead to boredom.

Present the information through as many avenues of learning as possible. Tell the student and show him and use training aids freely, as for example, X rays, charts, pictures, films, diagrams, slides, models, etc. Repeat the demonstration and explanation as necessary, remembering that the average person can grasp only a few ideas at a time. Allowance should be made for the answering of questions.

Step IV. Encourage sufficient practice.

Encouragement should be given, regardless of how poor the initial performance, as this is the critical point in learning. Have the student tell you and show you. Mistakes should be corrected a few at a time since mentioning a few does not cause discouragement. All suggestions should be kept positive, and they should be given in a constructive and kindly, yet firm, manner. Have the student make suggestions for her own improvement where possible. Seek accuracy first and speed later. Continue the practice until you know your student knows. It should be emphasized that during the practice period the instructor's mental attitude will affect considerably the results of learning.

If a patient is to be included in the lesson, rapport must first be established by introductions and suitable explanations to the patient. Patients usually are very willing to participate when they understand they are helping the student to learn improved patient care. The center of teaching is always the patient, remembering that he is a feeling as well as thinking person. The teaching supervisor must be ever mindful of her two-fold responsibility in safeguarding the patient and in giving security to the student. If the student is to give the treatment, any anxiety which the patient may have can be allayed quickly by letting him know that the student has had the advantage of the most recent instruction and by the confidence the supervisor displays in the student.

The supervisor should draw the attention of the student to signs and symptoms which may be present. For example, the student observes the stiffness and deformity of the spine and the rigidity of the thoracic cage of the patient with Marie-Strumpell arthritis. He palpates the nodules and listens to any crepitus which the patient with fibrositis may have. Swelling and inflammation of an arthritic joint are noted and pain during movement or tenderness to pressure may be observed. The instructor indicates muscles which are weak and spastic in the patient with multiple sclerosis. With the help of the supervisor the student may elicit a reflex as the patient wills a movement in a weak muscle group. While exercises are given to decrease incoordinate movement and

tremor, the supervisor carefully explains the procedure and reasons. The student learns to observe and to question with tact and understanding.

Step V. Follow-up.

The last step in any teaching is follow-up and evaluation. The student is placed on her own. The supervisor must check frequently to avoid the formation of bad habits. Taper off extra coaching when the student can work under normal supervision. Designate to whom he is to go in case he needs help. Various methods of evaluation will not be discussed. However, suffice it to say that "If the student hasn't learned, the instructor hasn't taught."

Increasing emphasis in the student program is being placed on the subject of patient-teaching since this is recognized as an important responsibility of all physical therapists. During the clinical practice phase, provision should be made for the planning of method and content in selected teaching situations and for practice in teaching under supervision. There should be a critical evaluation of the procedure and outcome by the supervisor and the student. The following is one effective way by which a preoperative meniscectomy patient may be taught quadriceps setting:

I. The student prepares himself. The student studies the patient's chart. He has clearly in mind the objective of the lesson and the key points which he wishes to stress.

II. He obtains the interest of the patient. He introduces himself and calls the patient by his name. He explains the purpose of his visit to his ward. He points out why it is important that the patient know about his treatment in advance of his surgery.

III. He presents the information. The student finds out what the patient already knows about the structure and functioning of his knee and he proceeds accordingly to tie in new information with his previous knowledge. A picture of the knee joint may be shown as the explanation is given. The patient feels the muscles as the principles of muscle setting are described. The principles may be demonstrated with the brachioradialis or biceps muscle. The student is careful to proceed at the right rate for the patient and to use suitable terminology. He encourages the asking of questions.

IV. He provides sufficient practice. The patient sets his quadriceps, trying out the various ways suggested until he finds the way he can do it best. The student shows interest in the patient's results and gives him encouragement and recognition as he does well.

V. He checks the results. The patient is asked questions to make sure he understands the importance, purpose, and procedure. The patient demonstrates various technics giving an explanation as he does so. The student concludes his instruction in a friendly way, wishing the patient well in his surgery and allaying any fears he may have. The patient is left knowing that his physical therapist has confidence in his ability to carry out the exercises and realizing that it is up to him to do an important job well for the best results from his surgery.

METHODS FOR THE DEVELOPMENT OF DESIRABLE PERSONAL AND PROFESSIONAL ATTITUDES

It is generally agreed that attitudes may be developed through direct intellectual processes, through the emotional effects of particular experiences, and by the process of assimilation from the environment. While the entire learning situation should be conducive to the development of proper attitudes and their promotion should permeate all teaching, there are several ways in which the teaching supervisors can contribute immeasurably. Three methods will be considered briefly.

The Philosophy of the Supervisor

First, every member of the supervisory staff should have the "personnel point of view." The personnel point of view is identical with the guidance point of view and is an integral part of the modern educational philosophy.

The personnel point of view considers the student as a whole. The emphasis is upon understanding the student as a person, rather than upon his intellectual training and his professional skill alone. The supervisor with the personnel point of view accepts the principle of individual differences, believes in the importance of providing a means of participation for each according to his ability and seeks to develop each to his maximum potentialities. The supervisor recognizes the significance of human needs, interests, and inner motivations in determining behavior and knows that the ability to make satisfactory adjustment and to develop desirable attitudes is conditioned by the total personality development in a total environmental situation.

One with the personnel point of view regards education as a continuing process in which helping individuals to develop insight and to work out their own solutions to their problems is more effective than the exercise of strong personal power. He understands that the survival of democracy is dependent upon self-imposed discipline and the development within the individual of a sense of personal and social responsibility. He believes in the inherent soundness of cooperative endeavor and knows that the most desirable learning takes place when individuals share in the planning of their own activities and where they are encouraged to use their own judgment, ingenuity, and initiative.

The supervisor with the personnel point of view maintains a balanced perspective, keeping in mind the good of the individual as he looks at the school as a whole. He has the capacity for compromise, knowing that both the institution and the individual must make intelligent adaptations to a rapidly changing social order.

Finally, the supervisor recognizes that every individual has intrinsic worth and dignity as a person. Student personnel work is based on faith in the improvability of the human personality. This philosophy prevents labeling persons without seeking the natural causes which are behind all behavior and it also prevents the giving up of any student as hopeless.

The Supervisor as an Example

It is well known that students tend to reflect and perpetuate the beliefs and practices of their teachers and supervisors. Particularly with advanced students when supervision is less close, teaching becomes largely a matter of suggestion and example in many situations. The importance of attitude, kindly manner, tone, and bearing as among the most effective teaching tools is often overlooked.

By the supervisor's example the student learns his own relationship with patients. He observes the objective yet friendly and sympathetic manner of the supervisor. He notes the mutual respect, courtesy, and trust shown at all times and he soon comes to regard each patient as a person rather than a case.

From the supervisor the student learns a sense of responsibility. He observes how conscientiously all details of treatment are carried out, such as the careful following of the prescription and the continuous supervision of the patient during treatment. He copies other such habits of his supervisors as keeping the treatment room orderly, economic use of supplies, cleanliness of linen, and the prompt meeting of all appointments.

The student is quick to sense how his supervisor reacts to authority, his loyalty to the institution, and his cooperation with other members of the staff. The attitude of the supervisor becomes reflected in the behavior of the student and has considerable effect upon his sense of security in his work and upon his morale in general.

The Individual Conference

The individual conference between the supervisor and the student is a most effective tool in guiding student growth and there is no substitute for it. "The modern trend is to recognize that good personal adjustment is primarily the responsibility of the supervisor." (Gipe and Sellew, "Ward Administration and Clinical Teaching," Chapter 6) A conference does not necessarily presuppose that matters of unpleasantness or dissatisfaction are to be discussed. It becomes a way for the supervisor to know each individual better, a way for him to evaluate the student's experience and accomplishments, to spur him to achieve in accordance with his potentialities, and to bolster his weaknesses. It may be looked upon further as a means of keeping open the two-way channel of communication.

The supervisor should follow well-established interviewing technics in conducting the conference. Arrangements should be made to allow for privacy and freedom from interruption. The supervisor should cultivate an approachable and understanding attitude and should provide an atmosphere in which the student feels at ease and free to talk. The approach should be adapted to suit the nature of the situation and the individual. The supervisor listens attentively and tries to understand what the student says and what lies beyond that which he does not or cannot say. The supervisor does not argue, take sides, probe with questions, display anger, or censor. He does not jump at conclusions, but gathers all the facts, with possible causes, before arriving at a decision. If corrective advice is to be given, the attention is on the work rather than the person. Often, in matters involving dissatisfaction, "talking out" the problem by the student clarifies his own thinking. It should be remembered that a conference can be required but that counseling need not be accepted. The conference should end in a friendly fashion with the student feeling secure in his relationship with his supervisor, stronger in his understanding of himself, and more confident of his own ability to cope with future situations.

CONCLUSIONS

In a consideration of methods of clinical instruction, the following six points deserve emphasis:

(1) Where there is a student training program the teaching supervisors should be selected carefully on the basis of personal and professional qualities and should receive academic status in accordance with the faculty organization of the university of which the physical therapy school is a part.

(2) Clinical practice should be related in so far as possible to the didactic instruction which the student is receiving.

(3) An in-service training program should be provided for all instructors, wherever possible, in order to provide an opportunity to review occasionally the principles of learning and teaching, to discuss policies, methods, and problems, and to evaluate the results of teaching.

(4) Many problems of teaching will be avoided if the one instructing will remember that there is often more than one solution to a problem and that competence in teaching is possible only as there is an ardent desire to grow and improve both personally and professionally.

(5) It should be remembered that good personal and professional attitudes and conduct in students are of equal importance to the amount of knowledge and skill which they may possess.

(6) For the best results in teaching, every instructor should seek to develop the student personnel point of view, a philosophy which is in keeping with our democratic way of life.

BIBLIOGRAPHY

1. Bellows, Roger M., *Psychology of Personnel in Business and Industry.* Prentice-Hall, Inc., New York, 1949. Chapter 8.
2. Brown, Amy Frances, *Clinical Instruction.* W. B. Saunders Company, Philadelphia, 1949.
3. Burton, William H., *The Guidance of Learning Activities.* D. Appleton-Century Company, New York, 1944.
4. Gipe, Florence Meda and Sellew, Gladys, *Ward Administration and Clinical Teaching.* The C. V. Mosby Company, St. Louis, 1949.
5. Hellebrandt, F. A., Duvall, E. N., *Organizing for Clinical Practice in Physical Therapy.* Edwards Brothers, Inc., Ann Arbor, Michigan, 1948.
6. Medical Department, United States Army. *Clinical Practice for Physical Therapy Students.* 1949.
7. Nahm, Helen, *An Evaluation of Selected Schools of Nursing: With Respect to Certain Educational Objectives.* Stanford University Press, Stanford, California, 1948.
8. Triggs, Frances O., *Personnel Work in Schools of Nursing.* W. B. Saunders Company, Philadelphia, 1945.
9. Vitelles, M. S., "Psychological Methods for the Improvement of Training." Reprint, *American Psychological Association.* 1949.
10. Wagner, Margery L., "Patient Instruction," *The Physical Therapy Review.* February 1950.
11. Wolf, Lulu, "Clinical Teaching." *American Journal of Nursing.* 1949, page 494.

Clinical Environment and Resources

"As the end of the twentieth century draws near, it is clear to all, that the health care environment is changing. Along with impressive scientific and technological advances and changing practice patterns, we also are confronted with changing characteristics of the population, notably aging, and new diseases, notably AIDS. Above all, these forces have combined to fuel the acceleration of health care costs, and cost containment has been a driving force affecting us all—the payers, the providers, the professors, and the patients. Clinical education is under assault. Thus, we are gathered here to confront the challenge of how to pay for clinical education in an era of rising costs as the health care system undergoes substantial, possibly even startling change."

Joseph E. Johnson, III, M.D.
Dean
University of Michigan
Medical School

Trends in Compensation and Benefits Provided to Physical Therapy Students During Clinical Education

PAULETTE M. KONDELA, MS,
and RICHARD E. DARNELL, PhD

Many facilities offering physical therapy clinical education for full-time affiliation students also provide some sort of compensation or benefits to students. Fiscal policy trends within health care institutions have influenced the extent to which these benefits are provided. The purpose of this study was to examine trends in providing specific benefits, namely, stipend, housing, meals, and uniform laundry, to students in full-time clinical education at the University of Michigan from 1967 through 1977. Data from annual facility information forms showed that, in general, these benefits have decreased during the years examined.

Key Words: *Education; Students, health occupations.*

Physical therapy education consists of three major elements: 1) basic foundations in the social, psychological, physical, and biological sciences; 2) didactic components of physical therapy; and 3) clinical skills acquired through carefully planned and monitored clinical education experience. Of these, clinical education may be the element most sensitive to societal values and trends. Current emphasis upon the control of operating health care costs through cost effectiveness, accountability, and the separation of the costs of patient care from the costs of education has caused rapid change in support systems for clinical education.

In keeping with this rapid change, directors of physical therapy services that provide clinical education have become increasingly concerned with operating costs and have had to document costs in ways understandable to those responsible for allocating budget, space, and personnel. Among the more recent costs under consideration have been those associated with clinical education. These costs have been studied by many researchers and results of these studies are summarized by Moore and Perry.[1] The cost-benefit ratio of physical therapy clinical education has been studied by Porter and Kincaid.[2] More recently, Evans has predicted that the trend in physical therapy clinical education is for fiscal administrators and governmental agencies to take a closer look at health education costs in clinical centers and raise questions about them.[3]

The purpose of this study was to examine the financially identifiable benefits (stipend, housing, meals, and uniform laundry) provided by clinical centers affiliated with the Curriculum in Physical Therapy at the University of Michigan in Ann Arbor for the full-time clinical education experience (three six-week postgraduate experiences) from 1967–1977 in order to determine: 1) the overall trend in provision of benefits by clinical centers; 2) the trend in the provision of benefits by new clinical centers in the first year of affiliation; and 3) the overall trend of changes in provision of benefits over the entire 11-year period.

METHOD

Facility information forms completed by 40 clinical centers affiliated with the Curriculum in Physical Therapy at the University of Michigan were studied for each of the years 1967 to 1977; data for 1972 were not available. Ninety-seven percent of the 40 institutions were within a 350-mile radius of Ann Arbor; 3

Ms. Kondela is Instructor in Physical Therapy and Coordinator of Clinical Education, Curriculum in Physical Therapy, Department of Physical Medicine and Rehabilitation, University of Michigan, Ann Arbor, MI 48109.

Dr. Darnell is Associate Professor in Physical Therapy and Director, Curriculum in Physical Therapy, Department of Physical Medicine and Rehabilitation, University of Michigan, Ann Arbor, MI 48109.

This article was submitted June 8, 1978, and accepted November 16, 1979.

TABLE 1

Clinical Centers Providing Student Benefits

	1967, % (n = 8)	1968, % (n = 9)	1969, % (n = 14)	1970, % (n = 13)	1971, % (n = 18)	1972[a] %	1973, % (n = 20)	1974, % (n = 22)	1975, % (n = 26)	1976, % (n = 29)	1977, % (n = 34)
Stipend	50	67	50	38	39	44	45	45	38	28	18
Housing	50	44	43	54	50	48	45	32	38	38	35
Meals	63	44	50	62	55	48	40	45	42	41	35
Laundry	50	44	50	31	28	31	35	23	19	17	15

[a] Figures extrapolated arithmetically.

percent were 750 miles away. The majority (80%) of these facilities were continuously affiliated with the University throughout the 11-year period. Data on stipends, housing, meals, and laundry were tabulated for each year and the data for 1972 were extrapolated arithmetically. The number of clinical centers offering stipends, the amount offered to students for each clinical affiliation, and the number of centers providing housing or reimbursement to the students for full or partial cost of noncenter housing were recorded. The number of affiliating agencies providing one or more free meals was tabulated, but those clinical centers providing the regular employee discount were excluded from these figures. Lastly, the number of clinical centers providing the student with free uniform laundry for all uniforms or special uniforms (some indicated cotton only) was determined.

The percentage of clinical centers offering each benefit for each year was calculated. Also, the percentage of new clinical centers offering a benefit during the first year of affiliation was ascertained. Finally, the overall trend of changes during the 11-year period was determined by identifying the individual trend for each clinical center, calculating the percentage of centers sharing that trend for each benefit described, and then using these calculations to establish the trend throughout the years.

RESULTS

Throughout the 11-year period the percentage of clinical centers providing housing and meals was relatively higher than the percentage of those providing stipend and uniform laundry (Tab. 1). (The advent of modern wash-and-wear fabrics, which require special care in an institutional laundry, was thought to result in a decrease in the percentage of centers offering this benefit).

Between 1967–1973, there was some fluctuation among all of the benefits provided. Since 1974, however, stipend, meals, and laundry provisions decreased while the percentage of facilities offering housing increased initially and then decreased slightly (Tab. 1).

The percentages of new clinical centers offering stipends during the first year of affiliation for the last four years of the study were generally lower than for the previous years (Tab. 2). The percentage of new clinical centers offering the other benefits fluctuated.

For each benefit, most clinical centers maintained a steady trend in providing the benefit over the years; that is, once they established whether or not they would provide the benefit, they did so continuously throughout the 11-year period (Tab. 3). Of the centers demonstrating a steady trend, the majority never offered all types of benefits. Table 3 shows that when benefits provision fluctuated, more centers showed a negative trend for stipend, meals, and laundry benefits and slightly more centers showed a positive trend for housing. Table 3 also shows that the trend for stipends, meals, and laundry was moderately to strongly negative while the trend for housing was strongly negative for those facilities that never offered the benefit and moderately positive for those facilities

TABLE 2

New Clinical Centers Offering Benefits During First Year of Affiliation

	1967[a]	1968, % (n = 4)	1969, % (n = 5)	1970[b]	1971, % (n = 3)	1972[c]	1973, % (n = 5)	1974, % (n = 1)	1975, % (n = 5)	1976, % (n = 5)	1977, % (n = 4)
Stipend	...	75	60	...	33	...	80	0	20	20	0
Housing	...	25	20	...	66	...	40	0	20	40	0
Meals	...	25	40	...	66	...	0	0	60	40	25
Laundry	...	25	60	...	33	...	20	0	0	0	25

[a] Baseline year.
[b] No new clinical centers used that year.
[c] No data available for that year.

TABLE 3
Overall Trend of Changes in Benefits Provision During 11 Years (N = 40)

	Steady Trend			Fluctuating Trend		
	Steady (%)	Offering Benefit (%)	Not Offering Benefit (%)	Positive Trend (%)	Negative Trend (%)	Interpretation
Stipend	70	18	82	10	20	Steady, strongly negative trend Fluctuating, moderately negative trend
Housing	85	29	71	10	5	Steady, strongly negative trend Fluctuating, moderately positive trend
Meals	82.5	36	64	0	17.5	Steady, moderately negative trend Fluctuating, strongly negative trend
Laundry	72.5	10	90	5	22.5	Steady, strongly negative trend Fluctuating, strongly negative trend

that fluctuated over the years. In summary, the overall trend was negative.

DISCUSSION

The data from the facility information form must be considered in light of several factors operating within the clinical education program during 1967–1977. Among the most germane were the following:
1) Three different coordinators of clinical education were responsible for selecting and retaining clinical facilities. Each may have brought a different sense of importance to the value of student benefits.
2) The university had no policy statement on student benefits that could guide both those in the clinical facilities and those in the educational program. Benefits that had been negotiated as a condition of affiliation may not have been taken advantage of by the student. The university could have placed more or less emphasis on selecting affiliation sites that offer benefits, inasmuch as the provision of benefits often influences the student's request for placement.
3) During 1976–1977, the Curriculum in Physical Therapy was planned to increase the number of clinical facilities offering specialized clinical education experiences. Because of the scarcity of such affiliations, the school placed little emphasis on student benefits as a criterion for site selection.
4) During the period 1975–1976, Michigan, a highly industrialized state, was suffering from the worst economic condition since the Depression. The health care institutions of the state were seriously affected and this influence on health care may have contributed to the trend of decreased student benefits.

The results of this study have direct implications for clinical facilities as well as professional preparation programs in physical therapy. The immediate effect of reducing most benefits since 1974 has been to increase costs to students. This increase in costs is compounded by the higher rents charged for short-term leases (less than 12 months). Increased cost to students could reduce the attractiveness of the field to the economically disadvantaged or increase the debt load of many students. Some might find it necessary to continue employment in varying degrees while in professional programs. For a few students, this additional time commitment precludes full concentration on their studies and might influence them to elect a professional program on a part-time basis.

CONCLUSIONS AND IMPLICATIONS

In this study, the financially identifiable benefits provided to physical therapy students from the University of Michigan during clinical education were examined for the years 1967–1977. The results showed a general trend toward decrease in student benefits during these years.

In order to help provide student benefits most effectively, those in educational programs must offer in-service education programs to teach those in clinical programs how to determine cost effectiveness of clinical education. Institutionally defined cost-benefit ratios should become a major consideration in the increase, maintenance, or possible reduction of benefits when clinical contracts are negotiated between the sponsoring educational institution and the clinical facility. The personnel in professional preparation programs should explore methods by which additional benefits may accrue both to clinical facilities and to individual clinical educators in recognition of their contribution. The personnel in educational programs should vigorously undertake this task to offset a small but increasing tendency for clinical education facilities to require payment of a fee by the student or the sponsoring educational institution. The widespread adoption of this fee would have catastrophic effects on the costs of professional preparation in physical therapy. Although local conditions and practices vary from region to region, some process by which student benefits are ascertained is of vital significance to the future viability of the field of physical therapy.

REFERENCES

1. Moore ML, Perry JF: Clinical Education in Physical Therapy: Present Status/Future Needs. Section for Education, American Physical Therapy Association, Washington, DC, 1976, 3-34 to 3-39
2. Porter RE, Kincaid CB: Financial aspects of clinical education to facilities. Phys Ther 57:905-909, 1977
3. Evans P: Future trends in clinical education. Physical Therapy Education 19:1, 28, Winter, 1978

Financial Aspects of Clinical Education

Financial Model to Determine the Effect of Clinical Education Programs on Physical Therapy Departments

ROSALIE B. LOPOPOLO

The purpose of this study was to develop a financial model to help administrators determine the financial effect of physical therapy clinical education programs on facilities. I developed the model from an analysis of actual field data collected on the financial and time variables involved in the clinical education process. Therapists with and without students were matched in six (three large, three small) physical therapy departments. Each completed a modified time-motion study for a sample of typical days during 2 six-week student affiliation periods and for a one-week period without students. I identified and field tested five factors that can be integrated into a simple financial model. The field results also supported the concept that a clinical education program was profitable, producing an $89 per day per student net benefit, even though therapists working with students spent less time in income-generating activities.

Key Words: *Cost benefit analysis, Education, Hospital departments, Physical therapy.*

Education in the clinical setting is an essential part of the basic education of any health-care practitioner. In 1971, Mills identified the linkage between education and patient care when he said, "Education determines the quality of patient care and patient care determines the quality of education."[1]

Researchers have developed models over the years to determine the financial effect of clinical education programs on the health-care facilities that house them. The findings from published research on the cost of clinical education have differed widely. For example, a study of two British hospitals showed increases in weekly inpatient costs after these facilities became part of a teaching institution.[2] A study of Hartford, Connecticut hospitals, however, demonstrated that the costs of hospital services in facilities with hospital-wide educational programs were less than the costs in facilities that maintain the same level of services without these programs.[3]

Disparate findings also are apparent when the costs for specific health-care disciplines are analyzed. Porter and Kincaid determined that clinical education of full-time physical therapy students resulted in a financial gain for the facilities involved.[4] This finding was supported by Kushner's study[5] of nurse practitioners that showed an average benefit of $3,623 per student from having a clinical education program and by Pobojewski's study[6] of 10 radiological technology students over a 12-month period that indicated a net benefit of $46,186. On the other hand, Smith and Malcolm[7] demonstrated an average yearly cost of $5,100 for the clinical education of medical technology students. Pawlson et al[8] demonstrated a cost range from $5 to $112 per day per student for the clinical training of medical students in ambulatory-care settings, and Hammersberg[9] demonstrated an average daily cost of $14.55 for the clinical education of physical therapist assistant students.

Many researchers have proposed mathematical models to calculate the cost-benefit ratio of having students in a facility during the clinical training period.[8,10–12] Several factors, however, limit these models in general application. First a single standard used to compare patient-care productivity during periods with and without students presents problems because the standard itself may vary widely throughout the year as a result of changes in patient mix and work-load levels. Second, the numerous systems proposed to determine the income generated from patient-care activities are based on a variety of fee schedules: some on individual treatments performed, others on time, and still others on a combination of these two factors. Comparisons among facilities are almost impossible because of this variety. Third, no models have accounted for the usual ratio of time spent in income-generating, patient-care activities to nonincome-generating, patient-care activities in a facility when students are not present. Some authors, however, have postulated that a clinical education program reduced the income-generating, patient-care time and therefore reduced the income generated.[7,10] In one cost-analysis study, Ramsden and Fischer estimated that generally 40 percent of a therapist's time was spent in income-generating, patient care, and an additional 40 percent was spent in nonincome-generating, patient-care activities.[13] Fourth, no model has been proposed to determine if the work volume produced by students within a single facility is an addition to the work volume usually produced by the therapists or if it is a transference of the work volume from the therapists to the students.

In addition to these factors, researchers have raised a question in the literature relating to the relative accuracy of the use of "estimated figures" for determining time spent in clinical education.[4,8,12] Some researchers believe that the time spent in clinical training is underestimated by the clinical instructor; others believe that the time allocation between education and primary functions is extremely subjective.[8,12,14]

Ms. Lopopolo is Director, Department of Physical and Occupational Therapy, Stanford University Hospital, Stanford, CA 94305 (USA).

This study was supported by a grant from Lifemark, Inc. through the Foundation for Physical Therapy.

This article was submitted October 18, 1983; was with the author for revision four weeks; and was accepted April 16, 1984.

A cost analysis is not valid without accurate, factual data. The purpose of this descriptive study was to develop a simple model that departmental administrators can use to determine the financial effect of clinical education programs within any health-care facility. Furthermore, these results can serve as a basis for comparison among facilities.

METHOD

I chose physical therapy departments in six acute-care facilities in the San Francisco Bay Area for the study. Of these facilities, three were large (over 500 beds) and three were small (under 350 beds). All facilities had clinical education programs and students during the six-month study period.

Data Collection Schedule

The study period included 2 six-week affiliation periods during which physical therapy students were present and one week during which no physical therapy students were present in the facility. I designed the data collection schedule to sample progressive time periods during each affiliation period and to provide comparative data between the early and late affiliation period. Data were collected twice a week during the second, fourth, and fifth week of each six-week affiliation. I also collected data for two days during a period when no students were in the facility to represent the typical work volume and schedule. The days for actual data collection were randomly selected from typical work days, which meant that the department had a regular staff complement, a full caseload for that period of time, and a routine schedule of patient-care and nonpatient-care activities. I omitted days during the first and last weeks of the affiliation. These weeks were considered to be atypical student-activity periods because of new student orientation during the first week and phasing out of old students during the last week.

Matched Sample

I used a matched sample of physical therapists (one with a student—teaching therapist; one without a student—control therapist) within each facility for the study. The criteria used to match the therapists included 100 percent patient-care responsibility, similar clinical area or patient mix, a minimum of one year of clinical experience, previous supervision of at least one full-time student (for the therapist with a student), and the therapist scheduled to work the period used for data collection.

I oriented department directors, clinical education coordinators, and all therapists involved in the study to the study procedure and the use of the appropriate data collection forms. Therapists participating in the study were modestly reimbursed on a daily basis to maximize complete and accurate data collection.

Format

The therapists recorded the use of their time using a modified time and motion analysis format that I pilot tested before the study period (Fig. 1). The modifications of the time and motion analysis format included the following: five-minute increments to track the variety of brief duration activities during the day; seven specific categories to provide consistency in the listing of activities by the therapists; and a section to indicate the number of patients treated by the therapist alone, by the student alone, or jointly by the student and the therapist. I required the therapist to place the number of the appropriate category of activity adjacent to the time and to account for all of the time spent at work or on work beyond regular hours each day. Therapists without students used the same data collection form and merely omitted using categories 5, 6, and 7, which related to student education.

TIME	CATEGORY	TIME	CATEGORY
:00		:00	
05		05	
10		10	
15		15	
20		20	
25		25	
30		30	
35		35	
40		40	
45		45	
50		50	
55		55	
:00		:00	
05		05	
10		10	
15		15	
20		20	
25		25	
30		30	
35		35	
40		40	
45		45	
50		50	
55		55	
:00		:00	
05		05	
10		10	
15		15	
20		20	
25		25	
30		30	
35		35	
40		40	
45		45	
50		50	
55		55	

INSTRUCTIONS

Place the appropriate number of the category next to the time interval.

USE CATEGORIES 1-4 for time spent by you in performing the activity without a student present.

USE CATEGORY 5 for time spent by you with a student for education without a patient present.

USE CATEGORY 6 for time spent by you and a student jointly in direct patient care.

USE CATEGORY 7 for time spent by you observing or assisting a student in an indirect patient care activity.

CATEGORIES

1. DIRECT PATIENT CARE
   (Charged time)
2. INDIRECT PATIENT CARE ACTIVITY
   (Non-charged patient care time)
   Conferences/rounds/consults
   Chart review
   Documentation (include third party forms)
   Telephone calls
   Personnel teaching for specific patient
   Waiting for patient
   Travel to/from patient
3. ADMINISTRATIVE ACTIVITIES
   Self development
   Staff development/training
   Meetings/discussions
   Research
   Scheduling
   Completion of charge documents
4. PERSONAL TIME
5. STUDENT EDUCATION
   Preparation/orientation
   Teaching/coaching
   Evaluation/review
   Discussion
   Coordination
6. COMBINED STUDENT/THERAPIST DIRECT PATIENT CARE
7. COMBINED STUDENT/THERAPIST INDIRECT PATIENT CARE
   Conference/rounds/consults
   Personnel teaching for specific patient
   Telephone calls

NUMBER OF PATIENTS TREATED BY THERAPIST ALONE: ________

NUMBER OF PATIENTS TREATED BY STUDENT ALONE: ________

NUMBER OF PATIENTS TREATED JOINTLY BY THERAPIST AND STUDENT: ________

Fig. 1. Clinical education time analysis form.

I allocated the time reported by the therapist for each activity category (1 to 7) on the data collection form to one or more of the four time variables (income-generating patient care, nonincome-generating patient care, administrative and personal time, and student education), based on the category's contribution to that variable and whether the therapist had a student (Tab. 1). For a therapist without a student, the time recorded as direct patient care was allocated entirely to income-generating patient care. For a therapist with a student, the time recorded as combined student and therapist direct patient care was divided equally between income-generating patient care and student education. In this manner, I prorated the effect of having a student on a therapist's time between the two simultaneous activities—patient care and student education.

I obtained from the department director the financial costs, including direct clinical education costs, salary and benefits of the therapists and the clinical education coordinator, and financial benefits, including the number of patient visits and the income per visit. I used these to develop the financial variables for the data analysis. The Appendix identifies the formulas used to calculate these variables.

Data Analysis

I analyzed the data using the statistical Package for the Social Sciences on the IBM 3033. The statistical analysis included descriptive data, analysis of variance (ANOVA), and the multiple classification analysis (MCA). The MCA provides more specific information on the pattern of effect of the variables in a multiple factorial design such as the ANOVA. In other words, the MCA helps to identify the proportionate contribution each variable makes to the significance found with the ANOVA. The results produced formed the basis of the model presented.

RESULTS

Table 2 displays a comparison of the demographic data for the large and small facilities. The mean income per visit is almost identical for large ($35.58) and small ($35.51) facilities. The total visits per day are somewhat proportional to the mean staff size. The small facilities, however, generated an average of 1.9 more visits per therapist per day, which resulted in a greater income per therapist per day during nonstudent periods.

Financial

Figure 2 displays mean financial and time data for the study period and all facilities in histogram format. No significant difference existed in any variable between a teaching therapist during the nonstudent period and a control therapist. Differences were found, however, between the teaching therapists and the control therapists during the student period. Teaching therapists generated a $20 per day greater cost and a $109 per day greater benefit than control therapists. The net benefit was therefore $89 per day per student. The one-way ANOVA used to test the significance of having a student found the differences for the independent variable, student, to be highly significant ($p \leq .001$) for cost, benefit, and net benefit (Tab. 3).

When I compared facilities by size, the large facilities had a significantly higher cost per student than the small facilities ($p \leq .01$), but small facilities generated a significantly greater benefit ($p \leq .001$). A two-way ANOVA for the dependent variable of benefit demonstrated that the effect of having a student varied significantly between large and small facilities ($p \leq .01$). The pattern of effect, as determined by the MCA, demonstrated that the size factor (small) explained 23 percent of the variation, and the student factor (teaching) explained 15 percent of the variation. The net benefit also showed a similar significant two-way ANOVA ($p \leq .01$) and MCA with 25 percent of the variation explained by size and 9 percent by student.

Over the 12-week affiliation period, the differences in costs remained approximately the same when I analyzed the financial differences between teaching and control therapists. Benefits and net benefits appeared, however, to increase during each affiliation and from

TABLE 1
Allocation of Therapist's Time from Activity Categories to Time Variable Groups

Category	Allocation for Therapist Without a Student	Allocation for Therapist With a Student
1. Direct patient care	100% to income-generating patient care	100% to income-generating patient care
2. Indirect patient care	100% to nonincome-generating patient care	100% to nonincome-generating patient care
3. & 4. Administrative & personal	100% to administrative & personal	100% to administrative & personal
5. Student education	NA	100% to student education
6. Combined student/ therapist direct patient care	NA	50% to income-generating patient care 50% to student education
7. Combined student/ therapist indirect patient care	NA	50% to nonincome-generating patient care 50% to student education

TABLE 2
Comparison of Means and Standard Deviations for Demographic Data for Large and Small Facilities

Facility	Large X̄	Large s	Small X̄	Small s
Professional staff size	16.9	2.3	12.3	2.5
Visits per day per therapist	9.3	4	11.2	3.4
Total visits per day	112	49	86	14.4
Income per visit	$35.58	$3.60	$35.51	$2.13
Income per day per therapist	$330.89	. . .	$397.71	. . .
Number of students in facility	3	1.3	2.4	1.2

the early to the late affiliation period (Fig. 3).

Caseload

A significantly greater percent of the caseload was carried by the teaching therapist than the control therapist ($p \leq .01$). The two-way ANOVA demonstrated that the effect of having a student on percentage of caseload varied significantly between large and small facilities ($p \leq .05$) with facility size again accounting for a greater percentage of the variation (21%) than student (9%).

Time

The control therapist spent a significantly greater percentage of time overall in income-generating activities than the teaching therapist ($p \leq .001$). Therapists in small facilities spent a significantly greater percentage of time in these activities than therapists in large facilities ($p \leq .001$). A two-way ANOVA, however, identified no significant differences in the interrelationship between having a student, facility size, and the dependent variable of income-generating time.

The percentage of time spent in non-income-generating, patient-care activities was not significant between or among any of the independent variables. The percentage of time spent in administrative and personal activities was not significant for the independent variable, student, alone but was significant for both size (large) and time (late) ($p \leq .01$). A two-way ANOVA was significant for student and size combined ($p \leq .05$).

The magnitude of the difference between the control therapist's and the teaching therapist's use of time over the 12 weeks was not significant; however, it is interesting and is shown on Figure 4. The difference in the percentage of time spent in income-generating activities and student education progressively decreased. The difference in the percentage of time spent in administrative and personal activities progressively increased.

A final interesting, yet not significant, factor was the effect of the department-wide activity level (number of visits per month) on the percentage of the caseload carried by the control and teaching therapists. In facilities that were at or above the typical activity level during the data collection period compared

Mean Data for Financial, Caseload and Time Variables

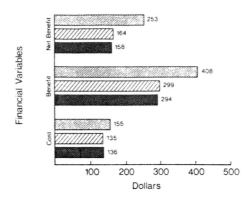

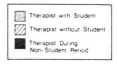

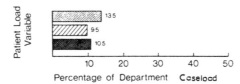

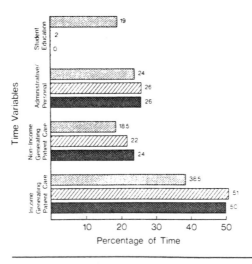

Fig. 2. Mean data for financial, caseload, and time variables.

with the previous 12-month period, the percentage of the caseload carried by all therapists remained fairly constant. The teaching therapist carried a slightly larger load than the control therapist and the control therapist carried a load nearly equal to the load of the therapist when students were not in the facility. In facilities where the activity level was below the previous 12-month average, however, the percentage of the caseload carried by the teaching therapist increased, and the percentage of the case-

load carried by the control therapist fell below the percentage of the caseload of the therapist when students were not in the facility.

DISCUSSION

Through the collection of actual field data using a matched sample of therapists, over the full-time affiliation period, study results support the concept that the net financial effect of having a clinical education program was profita-

TABLE 3
Summary of Analysis of Variance and Multiple Classification Analysis of the Significance of Independent Variables on the Financial, Caseload, and Time Dependent Variables

Dependent Variable	Independent Variable	ANOVA	MCA	
		p*	β^2	Direction
Financial				
Cost	student	.001	.42	teaching
	size	.005	.06	large
	time	NS		
Benefit	student	.001	.15	teaching
	size	.001	.23	small
	time	NS		
Net benefit	student	.001	.10	teaching
	size	.001	.25	small
	time	NS		
	student/size	.002		
Caseload				
Caseload	student	.003	.10	teaching
Percent	size	.001	.21	small
	time	NS		
	student/size	.024		
Time				
Income-	student	.001	.15	control
Generating	size	.001	.18	small
patient care	time	NS		
Nonincome-	student	NS		
Generating	size	NS		
patient care	time	NS		
		NS		
Administrative &	student	NS		
personal	size	.002	.10	large
	time	.008	.08	late
	student/size	.040		
Student	student	.001	.64	teaching
education	size	.056	.02	large
	time	NS		

* $p \le .01$ = highly significant; $p \le .05$ = significant.

ble.[4, 10] The study results also verify that in time, net benefit and percentage of time spent in income-generating activities by the teaching therapist progressively increase as the percentage of time spent in student education progressively decreases. The study results support the concept of longer affiliation periods to maximize the income-generating potential of the therapist-student unit and to minimize the effect of the teaching time on patient-care productivity.

The data also indicate that during the affiliation periods, therapists without students spend a progressively greater proportion of time in administrative and personal activities. This finding supports the concept that having students in a facility can actually free time for therapists to perform activities other than patient care.

The effect of size was significant in all financial and time factors with a positive inclination toward small facilities in all factors related to higher patient-care productivity (benefit, percentage of time in income-generating activities, percentage of caseload carried, and average patient visits per therapist per day). There also was a positive inclination toward large facilities on all factors related to lower patient-care productivity (cost, percentage of time in administrative and personal activities, and percentage of time in student education). Based on these findings, I might speculate that the potential variation in the cost of clinical education among facilities of different sizes found in the Porter and Kincaid study may have been more reflective of the effect of size rather than the effect of the clinical education program itself.[4]

Pobojewski[6] and Halonen et al[10] present a simple financial model (Direct Costs + Personnel Costs + Overhead-Benefits = Program Costs). Their model can be used effectively to determine costs and benefits to individual facilities and to compare these variables among

facilities if the following factors and findings from this study are integrated into the model:

1. The collection of actual sample time data during varying periods, as demonstrated in this study, can be a simple and inexpensive technique to determine how time is being used and what is the financial effect of the clinical education program. This methodology can help to eliminate the inaccuracy produced by estimates of time that have been previously reported.[4,12,13]

2. The formulas developed for this study to calculate costs, benefits, percentage of caseload, and allocation of time to income- and nonincome-generating variables can be used in any setting.

3. The cost per day per therapist with and without a student remained relatively constant; this figure needs to be determined only once a year for each facility.

4. The number of patient visits can be used within a facility and as a common factor among facilities to calculate the income generated regardless of the specific fee schedule because department directors commonly use income per patient visit in statistical reporting. From this, the financial benefit over an entire affiliation period can be calculated directly from the number of patient visits recorded by the therapist or therapist-student unit.

5. Using a matched sample of therapists and the reporting of work volume as a percentage of the department total can decrease the possibility of error when comparing productivity levels from different clinical areas or periods of time.[6,9,10]

Determining the effect of the total number of students present at one time within a facility was beyond the scope of this study. Because the greatest cost factor, however, is the clinical education coordinator's salary based on the percentage of time spent in clinical education activities, I would expect this percentage to increase with an increase in assigned students. Whether this change occurs in a linear or step-wise manner might be determined through the use of a time and motion study similar to the one presented here. In a practical sense, however, other variables, such as space and available staff, probably play a more significant role in determining the total

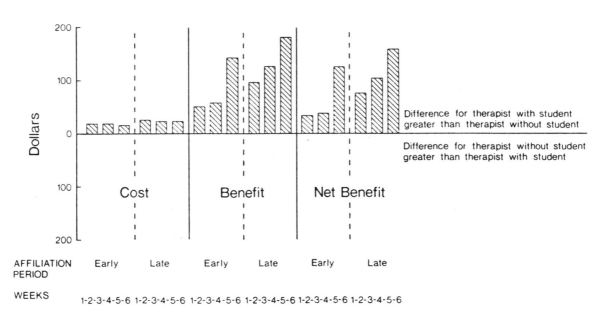

Fig. 3. Difference between therapists with students and therapists without students on financial variables.

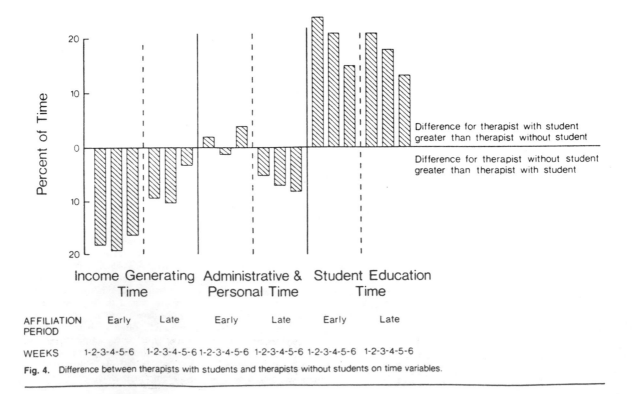

Fig. 4. Difference between therapists with students and therapists without students on time variables.

number of students that can be trained in a facility at one time.

The linear relationship between staff size and patient treatments postulated by Leiken also may not be valid for all facilities.[11] Data from this study, although not significant, pointed to the existence of a shift in caseload from therapists without students to therapists with students rather than increasing the total caseload as noted in facilities that were functioning below the typical departmental activity level. In clinical terms, this shift often is referred to as "keeping the students busy."

Finally, this study presents findings based on the actual collection of sample field data. Bias may exist relative to the area of the country, clinical education period studied, or the facilities selected. My intent, however, was to substantiate speculation from previous studies and, more importantly, present a simple model that all clinical administrators can use to determine the financial costs and benefits of a clinical education program.

CONCLUSIONS

In this study, clinical education was found to be a profitable program although factors such as facility size, level of experience of students, and the department activity level had an influence on the extent of the profitability. I identified five factors from this study that, when integrated into a simple financial formula, could be used by department directors to determine the financial effect of the clinical education program within the facility. This model can be used among facilities to compare data, improve profitability of programs, or justify the inclusion of a clinical education program in a new site.

Acknowledgments. I express my appreciation to Dr. Katherine F. Shepard

and Dr. Dianne Dutton for their consultation and assistance during the design and statistical analysis phases of this project.

APPENDIX
Formulas Used for Variable Calculation

Cost Formula
1. Clinical Education Coordinator (CEC)
   Hourly Salary + Benefits × Hours Worked × Percentage of Time for Clinical Education ÷ Number of Students per Day = Total CEC Cost/Day/Student   (1)
2. Therapist Salary
   Hourly Salary + Benefits × Hours Worked = Total Therapist Cost/Day   (2)
3. Direct Student Costs
   Cost Identified by the Clinical Education Coordinator ÷ 60 Days ÷ Total Number of Students = Direct Student Cost/Day   (3)

Cost Per Day
1. Therapist with a Student
   Use Formulas 1+2+3
2. Therapist without a Student
   Use Formula 2

Benefit
1. Income per Patient Visit
   Identified by the Department Director and Based on a 12-Month Period
2. Benefit (Income) per Day
   Number of Patient Visits × Income per Patient Visit

Caseload
1. Percentage of Caseload Treated by Therapist with a Student
   Number of Patients Treated by the Therapist + Number of Patients Treated by the Student + Number of Patients Treated Jointly by the Therapist and Student ÷ Total Number of Department Treatments
2. Percentage of Caseload Treated by Therapist Without a Student
   Number of Patients Treated by the Therapist ÷ Total Number of Department Treatments

REFERENCES

1. Mills JS: A Rational Public Policy for Medical Education and Its Financing. A Report to the Board of Directors. Cleveland, OH, National Fund for Medical Education, 1971
2. Editorial. Br Med J 2:1405–1406, 1966
3. Freymann JG, Springer JK: Cost of hospital based education. Hospitals 47:65–74, 1973
4. Porter RE, Kincaid CB: Financial aspects of clinical education to facilities. Phys Ther 57:905–909, 1977
5. Kushner J: A benefit-cost analysis of nurse practitioner training. Can J Public Health 67:405–409, 1976
6. Pobojewski TR: Case study: Cost benefit analysis of clinical education. J Allied Health 7:192–198, 1978
7. Smith JS, Malcolm GT: Education costs for medical technology programs in hospital laboratories. Am J Med Technol 40:273–276, 1975
8. Pawlson LG, Watkins R, Donaldson M: The cost of medical student instruction in the practice setting. J Fam Pract 10:847–852, 1980
9. Hammersberg SS: A cost/benefit study of clinical education in selected allied health programs. J Allied Health 11:35–41, 1982
10. Halonen RJ, Fitzgerald J, Simmon K: Measuring the costs of clinical education utilizing allied health professionals. J Allied Health 5(4):5–12, 1976
11. Leiken AM: Method to determine the effect of clinical education on production in a health care facility. Phys Ther 63:56–59, 1983
12. Stoddart GL: Effort-reporting and cost analysis of medical education. J Med Educ 48:814–823, 1973
13. Ramsden EL, Fischer WT: Cost allocation for physical therapy in a teaching hospital. Phys Ther 50:660–664, 1970
14. Thomas AL: Reporting of faculty time: An accounting perspective. Science 215:27–32, 1982

Method to Determine the Effect of Clinical Education on Production in a Health Care Facility

ALAN M. LEIKEN

Regression analysis was used to assess the effect of a clinical education program on production, that is, on provision of services, in a health care facility. This method enables one to determine the effect of students on the "quantity of patient care" provided by using data, which were readily available, on number of treatments. Application of this method to a physical therapy department in a 650-bed teaching hospital in suburban New York revealed that students contributed positively to the facility's capacity to provide patient care.

Key Words: *Education, clinical; Health facilities, productivity.*

There have been a number of studies undertaken to determine the effect of clinical education on the hospital or other health agency that provides a clinical education setting. Pressure to control health costs and the reluctance of third-party payers to reimburse institutions for clinical educational expenses have contributed to the urgent need to understand the effect of clinical education on health care costs. Most studies have focused on examining the costs and benefits of these programs.[1, 2] Costs that have been considered include 1) the use of equipment and supplies by students, 2) breakage caused by students, 3) the amount of staff time devoted to student education, and 4) stipends (if applicable). Benefits considered include 1) recruitment advantages, 2) the availability of students for part-time work during periods of heavy need, and 3) a stimulating environment that helps keep the permanent staff more alert.

Although these costs and benefits are important, the most important impact of clinical education is the net effect on the hospital's productivity (capacity to provide care). Carney and Keim attempted to evaluate the effect of students by interviewing students and clinical instructors.[3] The results indicated that both students and clinical instructors believe that students increase the productivity of the department. Pobojewski actually quantified the costs and benefits. He calculated the increased work time required by a staff person to perform one hour of departmental work when students are present.[4] This cost was calculated

and added to the additional costs of supplies purchased for students, providing a total cost figure. Students kept daily records of procedures observed, procedures performed alone, and procedures performed with staff assistance. Total benefit was calculated by multiplying a dollar figure per procedure by the number of procedures the student performed alone. A comparison of costs and benefits revealed a net benefit to the hospital.

Halonen and associates attempted to measure the effect that students have on productivity by examining the hospital department in months when students were not present.[5] They assigned relative value units to the procedures performed by the department. This value was used to measure, in dollars, the productivity of a clinical department. Productivity figures for the months when students were present were then compared with months when students were not present. A productivity increase was found during months when students were present. However, when the total expense of having students was added in, the hospital incurred a net cost of $208.25 per student.

These techniques have provided useful information regarding the effect of students on the hospital; however, applying them to a clinical setting requires interviewing, keeping student logs, or assigning relative values. The following technique offers an alternative to these approaches. All that is needed to determine the net effect of students on productivity is data that are readily available in most hospital departments and other health-related facilities.

THEORETICAL MODEL

Economic theory tells us that there is a relationship between a firm's number of units of input (employees) and the number of units of output. The theory further explains that for a given state of technology, the

Dr. Leiken is Assistant Professor of Health Sciences, Department of Allied Health Resources, School of Allied Health Professions, and Assistant Professor of Economics, Economics Department, State University of New York at Stony Brook, Long Island, NY 11794 (USA).

This article was submitted February 4, 1982, and accepted April 1, 1982.

addition of a variable factor of production, such as a new staff member, when other factors of production are fixed, will yield increasing marginal returns per unit of the variable factor added until a certain input point is reached; beyond this point, further additions of the variable factor will yield diminishing marginal returns per unit of the variable factor added.[6] We will assume (and the data confirm) that marginal returns are constant; that is, each additional staff member's contribution to output is the same.

When students are the variable factor, however, the yield of other "factors of production" (the staff) does not remain fixed. One effect of students is to lower the productivity of the staff because of the time staff members must spend on instruction rather than on patient care. Students, however, also perform services. If their direct contribution to output is greater than the corresponding reduction in staff productivity, a net increase in production is realized. If their direct contribution to output is less than the reduction in staff productivity, however, the result is a net decrease in production (Figure). Total production therefore depends on students, staff, and interaction effects.

The net effect of students on production can be obtained by constructing a regression line and estimating a linear regression equation. Regression analysis is a method of studying the effects and the magnitudes of the effects of one or more independent variables on one dependent variable.[7(p 603–605)] A simple linear regression will give us the relationship between output (patient treatments) and input (number of staff members):

Number of Patient Treatments

$$= a + b \cdot (\text{Number of Staff}), \quad (1)$$

where *a* is the intercept of the line (the point where the line crosses the axis of the dependent variable) and *b* is the regression coefficient, which tells us the change in the number of patient treatments in response to a unit change in the number of staff members. To compute this line, we need to collect data on a daily basis concerning the number of patient treatments and the number of staff. Using this data, we

TABLE 1
Contrived Patient Data Used for Regression Analysis

Day	No. of Staff (X)	No. of Patient Treatments (Y)	X²	XY
1	4	20	16	.80
2	5	24	25	120
3	6	27	36	162
4	4	19	16	76
5	3	18	9	54
Summation	22	108	102	492

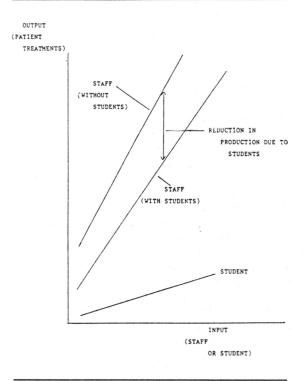

Figure. Production function with and without students.

can then compute the regression line. The formulas and examples are available in most introductory statistics books,[8] and most university computer centers have statistical packages, such as Statistical Package for the Social Sciences SPSS,[9] which can easily be used to obtain regression lines.

The contrived data listed in Table 1 will be used as an example, with X being the number of staff, and Y, the number of patient treatments. We use the following formula to compute *b*, the regression coefficient:

$$b = \Sigma xy / \Sigma x^2, \quad (2)$$

where $\Sigma xy = \Sigma XY - (\Sigma X)(\Sigma Y)/n$ and $\Sigma x^2 = \Sigma X^2 - (\Sigma X)^2/n$. From the summations in Table 1, $\Sigma xy = 492 - (22)(108)/5 = 16.8$, and $\Sigma x^2 = 102 - (22^2)/5 = 5.2$. Therefore, $b = 16.8/5.2 = 3.23$.

We compute the intercept, *a*, according to the following formula:

$$a = \bar{Y} - 3.23 \, \bar{X}, \quad (3)$$

where $\bar{Y} = \Sigma Y/N$ and $\bar{X} = \Sigma X/N$. Referring again to Table 1, $\bar{Y} = 108/5 = 21.6$, and $\bar{X} = 22/5 = 4.4$. Therefore, $a = 21.6 - 3.23 (4.4) = 7.38$.

The regression line is Treatments = 7.38 + 3.23 · (Number of Staff).

The *t* statistic in this case (7.51) indicates that an increase in the number of staff has a statistically significant positive effect on the number of treat-

TABLE 2
Contrived Data for Predicted and Observed Number of Treatments

Values of $\hat{Y}$ for each X[a]		Difference Between Predicted ($\hat{Y}$) and Observed (Y)	
Day	($\hat{Y}$)	(Y–$\hat{Y}$)	(Y–$\hat{Y}$)^2
1	20.30	−.30	.09
2	23.53	−.47	.22
3	26.76	−.24	.06
4	20.30	1.30	1.69
5	17.07	−.93	.86
Summation			2.92

[a] $\hat{Y} = 7.38 + 3.23\ X$.

ments. In this example, a t value greater than 3.74 means that the results are statistically significant ($p < .01$). The t statistic was computed as follows:

$$t = \frac{b}{\sqrt{\Sigma(Y - \hat{Y})^2/(n - 2)}/\sqrt{\Sigma x^2}}, \quad (4)$$

where (Y − $\hat{Y}$) was the difference between the predicted and the observed number of patient treatments. When computed from the data in Table 2, $t = 3.23/\sqrt{2.92/(5 - 2)}/\sqrt{5.2} = 7.51$. The coefficient 3.23 indicates that a unit change in the number of staff will result in an increase of 3.23 treatments provided per day.

This analysis can be expanded from determining the effect of staff to determining the effect of students on the number of patient treatments provided. We can accomplish this by estimating the following multiple linear regression:

Number of Patient Treatments = a + b · (Number of

Staff) + c · (Number of Students), (5)

where c tells us by what amount the number of patient treatments will change in response to a unit change in the number of students when the number of staff is maintained at a given level, that is, the net effect of

TABLE 3
Use of Students in the Physical Therapy Department

Students (no.)	Days in the Department (%)
Physical therapist	
0	36
1	42
2	9
3	9
4	4
Physical therapist assistant	
0	59
1	19
2	22

students on productivity. A positive c means that students increase productivity, and a negative c indicates a net reduction in productivity. The manual computations required to compute b and c[7 (p 611–616)] are more burdensome than when one only computes b. The task is simplified greatly, however, when one uses the computer to perform these calculations. Nonetheless, the method of computation is as follows, with X being the number of staff, Y being the number of patient treatments, and Z being the number of students.

$$b = [\Sigma(Y - \bar{Y})(X - \bar{X})][\Sigma(Z - \bar{Z})^2]$$
$$- [\Sigma(Y - \bar{Y})(Z - \bar{Z})] \quad (6)$$
$$[\Sigma(X - \bar{X})(Z - \bar{Z})]/$$
$$[\Sigma(X - \bar{X})^2][\Sigma(Z - \bar{Z})^2]$$
$$- [\Sigma(X - \bar{X})(Z - \bar{Z})]^2$$

$$c = [\Sigma(Y - \bar{Y})(Z - \bar{Z})][\Sigma(X - \bar{X})^2]$$
$$- [\Sigma(Y - \bar{Y})(X - \bar{X})] \quad (7)$$
$$[\Sigma(X - \bar{X})(Z - \bar{Z})]/$$
$$[\Sigma(X - \bar{X})^2][\Sigma(Z - \bar{Z})^2]$$
$$- [\Sigma(X - \bar{X})(Z - \bar{Z})]^2,$$

where $\bar{Y} = \Sigma Y/N$, $\bar{X} = \Sigma X/N$, and $\bar{Z} = \Sigma Z/N$, with N being the sample size.

APPLICATION TO A PHYSICAL THERAPY DEPARTMENT

A study was undertaken at a physical therapy department in a 650-bed teaching hospital in suburban New York. The department had an average of 11.5 staff members working each day. Table 3 provides information about the use of students in the physical therapy department. There were two types of students: those studying to become physical therapists (student PTs), who were in a four-year baccalaureate degree program, and those studying to become physical therapist assistants (student PTAs), who were in two-year associate degree programs.

Table 3 indicates that most of the time there was either no student PT present or just one present and that on most days included in the study (59%) there were no student PTAs present. This information is provided so that the reader can compare his department with the department used in this study. If the circumstances in the reader's department are different and the results not applicable, he can duplicate the study with the appropriate data by using the method described above.

The two student variables (PTs and PTAs) and the staff variable (Staff) will be used to explain variations in the number of treatments given each day. A treatment was defined as a half-hour of direct patient contact. If the patient was given an hour's worth of treatment, then it was recorded that two treatments were given. An average of 140 treatments were performed in this department each day. One reason we chose treatments as a measure of the output of the department was that these data were available. Other measures, such as the number of patients seen or the making of orthotic devices, could just as easily be used if the data are available.

Data were collected from the middle of September until the middle of May. December and the summer months were excluded because of the alteration of hospital operations during these months. A total of 124 days were used to estimate the regression model:

Treatments
$$= a + b \cdot Staff + c \cdot PTs + d \cdot PTAs \quad (8)$$

The results are Treatments = $83 + 4.06 \cdot$(Staff) + $1.57 \cdot$(PTs) + $1.2 \cdot$(PTAs), where t values for Staff (3.44) and PTAs (5.46) are significant ($p < .01$).

These results indicate that increases in the number of staff, student PTs, or student PTAs will result in an increase in the number of patient treatments. The t value corresponding to the coefficient for PTs is insignificant, however. The significant effect of student PTAs and the insignificant, although positive, effect of student PTs is due to the productivity measure (number of treatments) that has been used in this example. Besides providing direct patient care, student PTs give in-service lectures, make adaptive equipment, design home programs, do research, compile patient records, and make patient evaluations. Student PTAs are not permitted to make evaluations and are involved in these other activities to a lesser extent than are student PTs. Although the difficulties inherent in measuring these other productive activi-

ties preclude their inclusion in the analysis, they should be considered significant benefits that students provide in the clinical setting.

SUMMARY AND CONCLUSIONS

The effect of students on productivity has been a major issue whose quantification has in the past required burdensome data collection and arbitrary value judgments. We have presented a statistical method of assessing the effect of a clinical education program on production in a health care facility and applied this method to a physical therapy department in a teaching hospital in suburban New York. The available data enabled us to assess the impact of students on productivity by quantifying their effect on the number of patient treatments delivered by the physical therapy department.

The results indicated that students do contribute to the production of patient care in this particular setting. The other costs and benefits should also be taken into account, however. Costs might include the use of equipment and supplies by students, breakage caused by students, and stipends. Other benefits are that students might be future employees who can be observed now at no cost, they can be hired for part-time work during periods of heavy need, and they create a stimulating environment that helps keep the permanent staff more alert. Significant variations in costs and benefits across institutions require each institution to decide for themselves the relative importance they place on all the factors. By using regression analysis to determine the effect of students on productivity along with a discussion of the other factors, administrators will be better able to make decisions about the fate of clinical education programs at their institutions.

REFERENCES

1. Freyman JG, Springer JK: Education and the hospital-cost of hospital based education. Hospitals 47 (5):65, 1973
2. Wing P: Clinical costs of medical education. Inquiry 9 (4):36–44, 1972
3. Carney M, Keim S: Costs to the hospital of a clinical training program. J Allied Health 7:187–191, 1978
4. Pobojewski TR: Case study: Cost benefit analysis of clinical education. J Allied Health 7:192–198, 1978
5. Halonen RJ, Fitzgerald J, Simmon K: Measuring the costs of clinical education on departments utilizing allied health professionals. J Allied Health 5:5–12, 1976
6. Spencer MH: Contemporary Economics, ed 3. New York, NY, Worth Publishers, Inc, 1977, pp 394–395
7. Kerlinger FN: Foundations of Behavioral Research, ed 2. New York, NY, Holt, Rinehart & Winston, Inc, 1973
8. Duncan RC, Knapp RG, Miller CM: Introductory Biostatistics for the Health Sciences. New York, NY, John Wiley & Sons Inc, 1977, pp 99–109
9. Nie N, Hull H, Jenkins J, et al: Statistical Package for the Social Sciences, ed 2. New York, NY, McGraw-Hill Inc, 1975

Financial Aspects of Clinical Education to Facilities

REBECCA E. PORTER, MS,
and CYNTHIA B. KINCAID, MS

The financial aspects of clinical education for full-time junior and senior physical therapy students as related to facilities offering clinical affiliations were determined. A questionnaire concerning supervisory expenses, student support, direct and indirect costs returned by 35 facilities of all types provided the basic information. Comparisons of costs and revenues were made for junior and senior students separately and for facilities according to type, size, and personnel involved in student supervision.

An increasing concern of clinical educators in all allied health fields is the potential cost of providing clinical experience for student affiliates. With hospital expenses climbing at a rate of approximately 19 percent per annum, administrators are carefully analyzing departmental teaching commitments.[1]

In a recent article in the *Journal of Allied Health*, a mathematical model was presented for determining the costs of clinical education for allied health students. The model indicated that the cost or benefit of providing clinical education could be derived by comparing revenues (student paid tuition, room and meal charges, and patient revenues accountable to the student) with expenses (stipend to student, administrative costs, costs of providing room and board, and patient treatment costs). The calculation of patient revenue and patient treatment costs was based on a complex formula designed to derive relative value units based on comparison of the productivity during a month with students and a month without students. The article did not contain actual data but applied the mathematical model to a fictitious physical therapy department.[2]

A review of literature failed to reveal any direct analyses of data regarding the financial aspects of clinical education of physical therapy students. This study reports the comparative costs and revenues related to the clinical education of 273 full-time physical therapy students in 42 facilities offering affiliations with the Indiana University Physical Therapy Program during a one-year period. These institutions, located within approximately a 450-mile radius of the Indianapolis Medical Center Campus, include 29 general hospitals, 6 pediatric hospitals, 4 rehabilitation centers, and 3 skilled nursing centers.

The Physical Therapy Program at Indiana University consists of two years of preprofessional courses followed by two years of professional courses. At the completion of the first year of professional courses (the junior year of college), the students participate in one eight-week full-time clinical affiliation. The second semester of the senior year is devoted to three clinical affiliations, each consisting of a full-time six-week period. Facilities providing clinical education experiences receive no monetary compensation for tuition from either the students or the University, nor are the facilities which provide room and board compensated. Since the purpose of the study was to look at the total financial aspects of clinical education to the facility, data were gathered for all full-time students in the facility during the reporting period.

Mrs. Porter is Assistant Professor, Indiana University, Physical Therapy Program, Indianapolis, IN 46202.

Ms. Kincaid is Senior Staff Physical Therapist, Veterans Administration Hospital, Allen Park, MI 48101.

This study was conducted by the authors in partial fulfillment of requirements for the Master of Science Degree in Allied Health Education.

METHOD

A questionnaire was developed to elicit information related to the fiscal experience of each facility's clinical education program. To receive information from a broad sample of facilities, the questionnaire was directed to the supervisor of the physical therapy department rather than to the facility's financial officer or accountant. In order to develop a workable tool which could be answered by the supervisor, the questionnaire was limited to an examination of those costs which would be directly related to the budget of the physical therapy department. Hospital overhead costs were not included in this study.

The supervisor of the department was asked to provide the following information to determine the expenses involved in the program: percent of staff time involved in clinical education; salary of staff members involved in clinical education; amount of the stipend provided to the student; expense of providing housing or meals or both for the student; the cost of any fringe benefits provided to the student (laundering of uniforms, insurance, or health care); and any increase in the direct and indirect costs such as damaged equipment, increased use of linen, increased consumption of expendable supplies or increased use of secretarial time attributable to the student. The respondents were asked to provide estimates of information in categories where actual data were not available.

The expense of providing supervision for the clinical education of physical therapy students was determined for each person involved based on his salary multiplied by the percent of his time spent exclusively in the clinical education of physical therapy students. Clinical education was defined as time spent in clinical education meetings as well as student-related activities such as preparation, evaluation, orientation, reading of student notes, and the demonstration of techniques.

The total expenditure was balanced against the facility's estimation of the revenue generated by the student. The revenue was limited to the patient care services provided by the student. The determination of the revenue generated by the student was made by the facility based on the student's average patient load. Because treatment of patients by students frees the staff to provide supervision for the clinical education program (the expense of

which is accounted for by this study), provide direct patient treatment to other patients, or participate in other clinical or administrative functions, it is justifiable to attribute patient treatment revenue to the student.

The clarity of questionnaire items was tested in a pilot study of 36 facilities in March 1975. A revised questionnaire was then sent to 42 facilities which represented the total number of affiliating institutions for Indiana University full-time physical therapy students from July 1974 to January 1976. Because the questionnaire requested responses in terms of the most recent fiscal year, this time period was selected to encompass facilities working on a variety of types of fiscal years.

Based on the information obtained from each questionnaire, the financial expense/gain of clinical education for each facility was calculated for both junior and senior students. The calculations were based on the median affiliating period of eight weeks for junior students and six weeks for senior students to determine the expense/gain per student per affiliating period. To allow comparison between junior and senior students, the results for the senior students were projected for an eight-week period by breaking down the figure for the six-week period into a per diem figure and multiplying by 40. The financial expense/gain for all facilities was calculated as well as for various categories of facilities.

This study did not include consideration of the qualitative aspects of a clinical education program such as student contributions in terms of updating staff with new theories or techniques or staff contributions to the student in terms of practical experience. The influence of the number of students in a facility on the cost/gain ratio was not analyzed.

RESULTS

Of the 42 facilities surveyed, 35 returned completed questionnaires resulting in a response rate of 83 percent. Within the span of a fiscal year, 10 facilities were involved in the clinical education of juniors only, 10 with the education of seniors only, and 15 facilities dealt with both junior and senior students. Of the 273 students reported by the facilities, 59 were juniors and 214 were seniors.

The expense/gain of clinical education per junior student per eight-week affiliation spread from a loss of $3199 to a gain of $6001 per

TABLE 1

Financial Aspects of Physical Therapy Clinical Education to Facilities Affiliating with Indiana University

Analysis Categories	Mean Expenses/Gains per Student per Affiliation Period		
	Junior	Senior	
	(8 weeks)	(6 weeks)	(8 week equivalent)
I Supervisory Costs			
A. Clinical Education Coordinator salary costs	$ 341	$ 437	$ 583
B. Staff Physical Therapists salary costs	1290	794	1059
II Expenditures			
A. Student Support Costs (stipend, housing, etc.)	617	475	633
B. Indirect Costs (expendable supplies, equipment loss, etc.)	117	106	141
TOTAL EXPENSES	$2365	$1812	$2412
III. Reduction in expenses due to student productivity	3560	3335	4447
GAIN	$1195	$1523	$2031

student. Five facilities with junior students experienced losses. The mean figure for a junior was a gain of $1195 with the median falling at $2424. The spread of the results for a senior six-week affiliation ranged from a loss of $210 to a gain of $5840. Three facilities with senior students experienced losses. The mean was a gain of $1523 and the median was $1951.

Table 1 explains the details used in the determination of the mean expense/gain per junior and senior student per affiliation. The figures are reported for the eight-week junior affiliation, the six-week senior affiliation, and the calculated equivalency of an eight-week senior affiliation. The mean expense per student was determined by calculating the supervisory costs and the expenditures by the facility related to the student. Supervisory costs were examined in terms of the salary costs of the staff therapists involved in the clinical education process as well as the salary costs of the clinical education coordinator (if applicable). Other expenditures were divided into two cate-

gories: 1) student support costs (stipend, housing, meals, and fringe benefits) and 2) indirect costs (expendable supplies, equipment losses). Thus, the total mean expenditure for the clinical education of a junior was $2365 with a spread from $436 to $6925. The mean expenditure for a senior student was $2416 with the results ranging from $328 to $3852.

Student generated revenue was compared with the expenditures for clinical education to determine the net results. Based on equivalent eight-week periods, a mean revenue of $3560 was generated by a junior student (ranging from $240 to $6720); a senior produced an income of $4447 (ranging from $975 to $6000). When the total expenses were compared with student revenue, the figures for an eight-week period revealed a mean gain—$1195 for a junior student and $2031 for a senior student.

The gain per student per affiliation fluctuated depending on the type of facility (Tab. 2). A gain was noted with senior students in

TABLE 2

Mean Gain of Clinical Education in Different Types of Facilities

Type of Facility	No. of Facilities Responding		Mean Gain per Student per Affiliation		
	Junior	Senior	Junior	Senior	
			(8 weeks)	(6 weeks)	(8 week equivalent)
General Hospital	18	16	$1779	$2140	$2853
Pediatric Hospital	0	3	—	1810	2413
Rehabilitation Center	2	2	−478	2893	3857
Skilled Nursing Facility	3	0	4071	—	—

general hospitals, pediatric hospitals, and rehabilitation centers. The clinical education of junior students resulted in a gain in general hospitals and skilled nursing facilities; but their education resulted in a financial loss to rehabilitation centers. This finding was based on the report of two centers whose individual results spread from a gain of $2712 to a loss of $3190. The reason for the wide spread was not investigated. No data were available for junior students in pediatric settings or senior students in skilled nursing facilities due to lack of response to the questionnaire.

Another potential variant in the cost of clinical education is the size of the facility. The facilities were grouped into three categories based on bed capacity: small (0–300 beds), medium (301–600 beds), and large (over 600 beds). Junior affiliations resulted in a gain in all three categories—$2589 in small facilities, $1620 in medium facilities, and $1369 in large facilities. Senior affiliations also resulted in gains—$3611 in small facilities, $2469 in medium facilities, and $2587 in large facilities (all figures reported in terms of eight-week equivalent period). Affiliations in smaller facilities produced a greater gain than in the other two categories of facilities, but the difference was not statistically significant.

Fifteen of the facilities reporting had full or part-time clinical education coordinators, while twenty did not. The facilities with a clinical education coordinator experienced a mean gain of $2257 per junior student and $2188 per senior student. Facilities without a clinical education coordinator had a mean gain of $1714 per junior and $1624 per senior. By the median test (a test which uses the common median of the two groups to be compared to test for statistically significant difference), the difference between the median gain in facilities with and without a clinical education coordinator was not significant at the .05 level.

DISCUSSION

The results of this study revealed that the costs incurred by the affiliating clinical facilities were less than the revenue generated by the physical therapy students. The difference between junior and senior students' costs and revenues was predicted. Junior students spend more time (eight weeks) per affiliation than the senior students (six weeks), therefore, the expenditure would be greater. Based on the

eight-week equivalency for senior students as reported in Table 1, it is noted that the total expenditures vary by less than $50. The revenues attributed to junior students may be diminished by the student's lack of proficiency in technical skills and limited ability to provide patient care.

Comparison of the statistics for an eight-week junior affiliation with the projected figures for an eight-week senior affiliation should be done with a degree of caution. For example, many of the supervisory duties (orientation, midterm, and final evaluation) remain whether the student is present for a six- or eight-week period. Expanding the estimations for a six-week affiliation to an eight-week equivalency tends to distort these inherent costs. The limitation of the use of estimated figures should also be recognized.

The assumption that a clinical education coordinator may appear to be an additional expense to a facility did not prove to be valid. Apparently the cost in time to supervise a student remains equivalent regardless of the presence or absence of a clinical education coordinator in the clinical education supervisory structure.

The consistency of the findings of a mean gain, regardless of the variables of size or type of facility or type of supervisory personnel, supports the creditability of the study. Mean cost to rehabilitation centers which accept junior students requires further study since the figure was based on only two reporting facilities. Conjecture about the basis of this figure is not possible without a larger sample for this type of facility. Limitations to this study include the use of estimations in some data categories and the small number of responses from some types of facilities.

In order to further validate the data on the cost of clinical education, it is suggested that similar information be obtained from facilities other than those affiliating with Indiana University. It might be of interest to investigate the comparative costs of clinical education for different allied health disciplines in the same settings.

CONCLUSION

Assuming that the clinical education facilities affiliating with the Indiana University Physical Therapy Program are typical of facilities throughout the country, this study has indicated that the clinical education of full-time physical therapy students tends to be a financial asset to a facility rather than a liability. The type of facility and level of the student influence the financial aspect of clinical education and may be considerations when facilities accept students.

SUMMARY

The financial aspects of clinical education of full-time junior and senior physical therapy students were determined in 35 facilities affiliated with the Indiana University Physical Therapy Program. Consideration was given to supervisory, student supports, direct and indirect costs. Reduction in expenditures due to student productivity was calculated and subtracted from expenditures.

The results of this study revealed that the average outcome of the clinical education of full-time physical therapy students was not a deficit, but a financial gain regardless of the type, size, or clinical education supervisory structure of the facility. In this age of accountability, further research is needed to determine the financial aspects of clinical education in all allied health fields if student clinical education programs are to continue and expand.

REFERENCES

1. McFarland JB: Administrative profiles. Hospitals 49:38, July 1975
2. Halonen RJ, Fitzgerald J, Simmon K: Measuring the costs of clinical education in departments utilizing allied health professionals. J Allied Health 5:5-12, Fall 1976

Effects of Clinical Education on the Productivity of Private Practice Facilities

Elizabeth Coulson, MBA, PT
Dan Woeckel, PT
Rebekah Copenhaver, SPT
Tracey Gallatin, SPT
Jennifer Hawkins, SPT
Laurie Hixson, SPT
Carol Pruim, SPT

ABSTRACT: *The purpose of this study was to determine the effects of senior clinical affiliations on the productivity of private practice clinics. The monthly patient billing data of 18 students with their clinical instructors (CI) were collected and compared with similar data of the CI alone in a comparable month. Causal comparative and descriptive designs were used. While the students were present, an average daily increase of $216.77 was calculated, along with a daily increase of 3.25 patient visits. Both of these increases were found to be significant (p<.05). No significant difference existed in the average charge per patient. (p>.05). The results suggest that senior physical therapy students have positive effects on the productivity of private practice clinics while completing their senior clinical affiliations.*

INTRODUCTION

Clinical affiliations are an important part of a physical therapy student's (PTS's) education. Affiliations allow students to apply the knowledge they have gained in the academic setting to various types of patients. In addition to applying skills, students are also given the opportunity to establish working relationships with patients and various health professionals. A classroom setting can in no way provide the professional interactions afforded by clinical affiliations. Most importantly, the student is able to obtain these skills and interactions under the supervision

Ms Coulson is Assistant Chairman and Associate Professor, Department of Physical Therapy, University of Health Sciences/Chicago Medical School, 3333 Green Bay Rd, North Chicago, IL 60064. Mr Woeckel is a regional operations manager, Baxter Healthcare Corporation, Physical Therapy Division, 900 N State Pkwy, Ste 300, Schaumburg, IL 60173-5135. Ms Copenhaver, Ms Gallatin, Ms Hawkins, Ms Hixson, and Ms Pruim are senior physical therapy students, University of Health Sciences/Chicago Medical School.

of an experienced physical therapist. This allows for correction and guidance, enabling students to refine their skills.

Affiliations also provide students with the necessary exposure to identify their area of professional interest. It is important for students to be exposed to many different work settings so that, on graduation, they have a better idea of the type of setting in which they would like to practice. According to a 1987 American Physical Therapy Association active member survey, 24.2% of active physical therapists work in private practice settings. Physical therapy students, however, often graduate without the opportunity to experience a private practice clinical affiliation.

Until now, many private practice clinics have been unable or unwilling to provide clinical education programs. One of the concerns of private practitioners has been the possible decreased productivity that may result from time spent educating the student physical therapist.

Several studies have been conducted in hospital settings that have shown an increase in productivity of physical therapy departments while a PTS was present.[1,2] Likewise, studies done in acute care hospital, rehabilitation, and skilled nursing settings have shown financial gains.[3,4] No studies were found, however, concerning the effects of clinical education on the fiscal or patient volume aspects of private practice clinical instructors (CIs) or clinics.

To address this issue, one must first consider the concept of productivity. Economically, *productivity* is defined as the ratio of production to the resources required for the production. Labor is the most common factor used in measuring the required resources for productivity. From a health care point of view, the number of patient treatments per therapist and the amount of revenue generated are two of the most common measures of productivity.

Cebulski and Sojkowski measured productivity as the number of 15-minute units per day that were spent engaged in patient evaluation and treatment in a teaching hospital.[5] They noted an overall positive increase in productivity when combining that of the CI with that of the student for a one-month period.[5] Similarly, Leiken measured productivity as the number of patient treatments, and his study concluded that the net productivity of students combined with the productivity of the staff increased significantly.[2]

Using a mathematical model developed by Hanolen et al,[3] Porter and Kincaid compared costs and revenues associated with the clinical education of 273 full-time junior and senior PTSs in various rehabilitation, hospital, and skilled nursing centers.[1] This study found that regardless of the size or type of facility or the type of supervisory personnel, revenue generated by the students was greater than the costs incurred at the facility.[1] Lopopolo also considered the financial aspect of clinical affiliations by comparing two six-week periods with students to a one-week period with the therapist alone in an acute care facility.[4] The results indicated an $89-per-day net benefit of the clinical affiliation.[4] Clinical affiliations, therefore, seem to produce a net fiscal benefit rather than a cost to the affiliating acute care, rehabilitation hospital, and skilled nursing setting.

The purpose of our study was to discover the relationship between clinical affiliation programs and CI productivity in private practice outpatient clinics. Productivity was measured three ways: 1) as the average daily income, 2) as the average number of patient treatments per day, and 3) as the average charge per patient. It was hypothesized that a significant difference would be found in the average daily income and the number of patient treatments per day between the PTS and CI combined and the CI alone in a comparable month. It was also hypothesized that no significant difference would be found in the average charge per patient. We believed that in outpatient practice, having a senior PTS would increase the overall productivity in the private practice clinic.

METHOD

Subjects

Data were collected from 20 pairs of subjects consisting of one CI and one student each. Two of these pairs had incomplete data. A total of 18 pairs of subjects completed the study. One male and seventeen female senior PTSs participated. These students attended six different physical therapy schools. Each student's clinical affiliation lasted from four to eight weeks with a mean length of 5.39 weeks (s=1.33). The eighteen CIs (1 male and 17 female) who participated were from 14 private practice clinics owned by a single large parent corporation. This was a sample of convenience involving willing students and CIs who had affiliations between January and June of 1989. Verbal permission for participating in this study was given by the clinics, CIs, and students. All participants were informed that their daily logs and patient billings were being used for research; however, the exact purpose of the study was not revealed.

PROCEDURE

A formal meeting of CIs was held one month prior to the arrival of the students. During this meeting, the CIs were told how the daily logs should be filled out. The student log asked for a description of treatments completed by the student, the time spent on these treatments, and the time spent in other daily activities. The CI log requested information on the number of patients treated independently by the CI or PTS or jointly by the CI with the PTS and information on the time spent by the CI in supervision, discussion, or other activities with the student. The daily logs were used to verify computer billing and to identify other activities that the CI or PTS was involved in that may have affected their patient billings.

Also at this meeting, individual billing numbers were assigned to each student. The CIs were reminded that patient billing was to be computed in 15-minute intervals and that the student was required to perform at least two thirds of the treatment to bill for the patient. For this study, the students' patients were billed separately from those of the CI.

One day prior to the students' arrival, the CI was contacted to be reminded of the specific procedures.

The CIs and students were to fill out their logs and complete patient billing information on a daily basis. The daily logs, to be used to verify the computer information and in the descriptive portion of the research, were sent to the researchers on completion of the affiliation. Utilizing a comparative research design, monthly facility production reports were accessed from the facilities' computers after all affiliations were completed. The production reports were accessed for the months corresponding to the student affiliations and also for a comparable month of the CI alone within four months of the affiliations.

A comparable month was considered to be the month closest to the affiliation, excluding the months just before and just after the affiliations. These months were excluded because the researchers believed that productivity may have varied because of preparation for the student and readjustments in patient loads following the student's departure.

DATA ANALYSIS

The data were weighted to take into account the number of days the CI and PTS actually worked together. A paired data t test was used to determine whether any significant difference existed between the months when the CI worked independently and the months when the CI worked with the student. Three individual paired data t tests were performed to analyze average daily income, average daily patient visits, and average patient charges. An alpha level of 0.05 was chosen to minimize type II statistical errors.

RESULTS

Table 1 and Figure 1 summarize the data on a comparable month for the average income earned per day by the physical therapist with the student and the physical therapist alone. The paired data t test indicated that there was a significant increase in the average daily income when the PTS was in the facility (p<.05). Table 2 and Figure 2 summarize the data for the visits per day. This t test also showed a significant increase while the student was present (p<.05). Table 3 and Figure 3 summarize the data for the average charge per patient. The t test showed that there was no significant difference between the average charge per patient with the student present and that of the CI alone. (p > .05).

DISCUSSION

This study indicated that having a senior PTS in the clinic had a positive effect on the

Table 1

Average Number of Dollars Earned Per Day

Subject	X̄	SD	t	p
Clinical instructor and physical therapy student	1029.23	401.71	4.97	.000*
Clinical instructor	812.46	313.26		

*Significant (p<.05).

Figure 1

Comparison of subjects' average dollars earned per day.

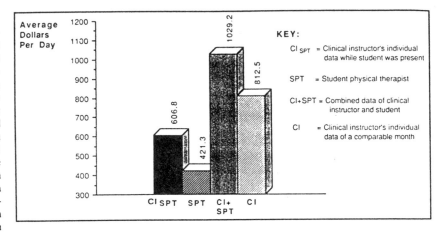

Table 2
Average Number of Patient Visits Per Day

Subject	$\bar{X}$	SD	t	p
Clinical instructor and physical therapy student	16.40	3.96	5.71	.000*
Clinical instructor	13.15	3.05		

*Significant (p<.05).

Figure 2
Comparison of subjects' average number of patient visits per day.

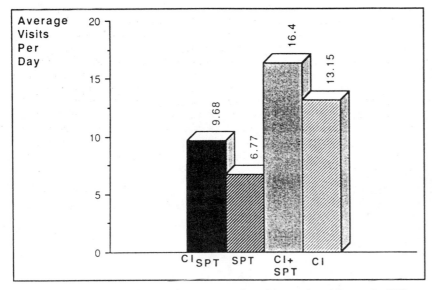

dents from the original sample of 20 was found to be inadequate. The first student's data were excluded because all of his quantitative data were unaccountably low. The corresponding CI was unable to determine whether this deviation was due to data entry errors or to problems with the student. The second student's data were excluded because the data from an entire month could not be located by the facility. These exclusions may introduce an element of experimenter bias; however, the researchers felt that they were justifiable alterations.

It should also be noted that the data of the CI practicing alone were taken from a different month. Therefore, the significant increase in productivity noted for the student and CI may have been influenced by extraneous factors such as monthly differences in productivity and patient load. This study attempted to control for these extraneous factors by using data for the CI alone from a comparable month.

The authors also found that in many cases there was a difference between the number of days worked by the CI and the number of days worked by the PTS. As a result, the monthly productivity averages for the CI were raised by the days he or she worked without the student, decreasing the accuracy of the comparisons. This necessitated the use of mathematical equations to properly weight the data to the number of days actually worked by the CI and student together.

Future studies concerning the effects of clinical affiliations on private practice clinics would be beneficial to the physical therapy profession. Quantitatively, improvements could be made by using larger and random samples from many different corporations. The student sample should consist of affiliations at all levels of physical therapy education. The control therapist may be a therapist with statistically comparable productivity to the CI, rather than the CI involved with the affiliation. This would allow the productivity of the control therapist to be compared with the productivity of the CI and student during the same time period, preventing extraneous variables of monthly fluctuation of productivity levels.

The data collected from the daily logs were reviewed for trends. One trend noted was that the number of patients treated jointly by the CI and PTS was greatest in the first two weeks of the affiliations for most of the subjects. Overall, the number of patients seen per week by the student alone appeared to increase from the first to the last week of affiliation. The inconsistent manner in which the daily logs were completed led to difficulty in interpreting some of the data. Future

average daily income as well as on the average number of patients that were seen per day. Thus the presence of a senior student results in an overall benefit to a facility's productivity. At the same time, there is no significant change in the average charge per patient, which shows that a facility generally does not alter patient treatment charges because a student is helping to perform the treatment.

No previous research has been conducted using exclusively private practice facilities; however, the authors' data corresponds to similar research that used acute care or rehabilitation facilities. Lopopolo[4] noted an $89 per day average increase in fiscal productivity in acute care facilities, which compares with the $216/day average increase in the private practice facilities. Therefore, private practice clinics may also have increased daily income resulting from the presence of a PTS.

The results of this study also correspond to those of a similar study performed by Leiken. His study found a net increase in the number of patient treatments performed by the physical therapy department while a student was present in a teaching hospital setting.[2] This is consistent with the average increase of 3.25

patient visits per day while a senior PTS was present in a private practice facility.

In the process of analyzing the quantitative data, several issues arose. Although a sample size of 18 pairs is adequate for causal comparative research, the authors believe that a larger sample would produce more valid generalizations about the total population of private practice clinics. In addition, the chosen sample may not be representative of all private practice clinics because it was not selected in a random fashion. Future studies could be conducted using larger as well as random samples. Also, all the clinics used were from one parent corporation. Therefore, any differences in productivity found in this research may have resulted from specific management policies of the corporation. All of these factors limit the authors' ability to generalize these findings to the entire population of private physical therapy clinics.

Furthermore, the sample of students consisted only of seniors. This limits the ability to generalize this study to all physical therapy clinical affiliations. The results can only be generalized to senior student affiliations. Finally, the quantitative data for two stu-

Table 3
Average Charge Per Patient

Subject	X̄	SD	t	p
Clinical instructor and physical therapy student	62.93	14.93	1.38	.186*
Clinical instructor	61.31	14.84		

*Not significant (*p*>.05).

Figure 3
Comparison of subjects' average charge per patient.

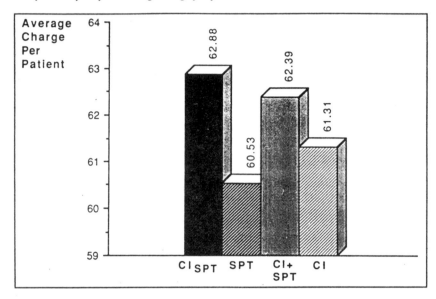

It is also our opinion that assessing the quality of patient care provided by the student would be of great value in evaluating the effects of students in a private practice facility.

A facility should also consider the positive effects that a student may have on the staff. A student comes to the clinic with current techniques and new ideas. With the help of the student, the staff can stay abreast of the latest developments and incorporate them into their treatment programs. In addition, instructing a student challenges the CI to keep his or her skills and knowledge current and refined. This helps to maintain a high level of competence in the CI and enhances the educational experience of the student.

CONCLUSION

This study addressed the effects of senior clinical affiliations on the productivity of private practice clinics. A significant increase in productivity was found. The findings of this study should provide incentive to the private practitioner to offer affiliations to PTSs. Future study of qualitative data is needed to gather information pertaining to the quality of care provided by the student.

researchers could remedy this problem by monitoring the completion of daily logs more closely throughout the affiliations. The major problem was the incompleteness of the data.

In addition, future studies could stress the assessment of qualitative data. Qualitative data should include demographic information such as age, grade point average, clinical experience, and nature of the affiliation. The influence of these extraneous variables on the student's effect on the CI's productivity could be determined. Future studies also could use semistructured questionnaires or checklists to decrease the inconsistency in the manner in which daily logs are filled out. This type of questionnaire would also be much easier to manipulate statistically and to apply to research.

REFERENCES

1. Porter RE, Kincaid CB: Financial aspects of clinical education to facilities. Phys Ther 57:905–909, 1977
2. Leiken AM: Method to determine the effect of clinical education on production in a health care facility. Phys Ther 63:56–59, 1983
3. Halonen RJ, Fitzgerald J, Simmon K: Measuring the costs of clinical education utilizing allied health professionals. J Allied Health 5(4):5–12, 1976
4. Lopopolo RB: Financial model to determine the effect of clinical education programs on physical therapy departments. Phys Ther 64:1396–1402, 1984
5. Cebulski P, Sojkowski M: Clinical education and staff productivity. Clinical Management 8(4):26–29, 1987

Cost of Clinical Instructors' Time in Clinical Education—Physical Therapy Students

GORDON G. PAGE
and JOYCE R. MacKINNON

The purpose of this study was to estimate the total clinical instructor time required to conduct the clinical education program of our physical therapy school. Clinical instructors in 12 of the 29 regional health care facilities providing clinical education programs described, through questionnaires and interviews, the instructional activities in their programs and the number of hours a week required for each activity. For each activity, the instructors indicated whether it served educational purposes only (a single purpose activity) or patient care and research purposes as well (a joint purpose activity), and they estimated the time that they spent with the student (direct contact time). The sample data were used to estimate the annual requirement for clinical instructor time for the physical therapy clinical program, totaling 10,264 hours. The methodology and the findings of this study can assist governmental agencies, educational institutions, and clinical facilities to define policy and funding agreements for clinical training purposes.

Key Words: *Data collection, Education, Physical therapy.*

As funding for health care agencies and health sciences schools becomes increasingly limited, the provision of clinical placements for students is becoming a serious problem. Both clinical facilities and schools now face the need to understand the costs (and benefits) of these placements to enable the preparation of statements of joint policy on the funding of clinical placements. In the 1982 to 1983 academic year, The University of British Columbia funded a study of clinical placements in its health sciences programs. The purpose of this study was to develop a database describing the time spent by health care facilities' staff members on activities related to teaching health sciences students. The data collected were to be used to develop a uniform university policy for the clinical placement of health sciences students. This article describes the methodology

of this study and estimates the annual clinical instructor time and costs to facilities providing clinical placement to physical therapy students at The University of British Columbia.

At the inception of this study, literature was reviewed relating to the costs and benefits of clinical placements. Many of the studies reviewed reported that health care facilities incurred financial loss and a decrease in productivity when students were present.[1-5] Friesen (V. Friesen, unpublished data, 1979–1981) and others[6-11] found that facilities gained financially and in productivity. The different methods used in these studies did not explain these apparently contradictory findings. The studies, however, did serve to highlight the diversity of clinical placement programs, the complexity of analyzing the costs and benefits of these placements, and the lack of adequate analytical methods. The analytical methods developed for this study were adapted from those developed by Gonyea.[12]

The purpose of this article is to describe the methodology and the results obtained in estimating the instructor time required to conduct a clinical education program for physical therapy students. The university study was undertaken to answer the following questions:

1. Of the total scheduled clinical time (for students), what percentage is given to single purpose activities as

compared with joint purpose activities? Scheduled clinical time is defined as the total number of hours that a student is assigned to a clinical facility. Single purpose activities are those whose sole purpose is to facilitate student learning (eg, instructor demonstrating, student reading). Joint purpose activities are activities that involve students for the purpose of learning but that also contribute to other purposes such as patient care and research (eg, case conferences, treatment of patients by students).

2. Of the total scheduled time, what percentage of this time is a clinician in direct contact with the physical therapy student? Direct contact time is the amount of time a practitioner is with a student to instruct or evaluate the performance of the student (eg, what percentage of the time is the instructor observing the student treat patients?).

3. Of the total scheduled clinical time that is direct contact, what percentage is given to single purpose activities as compared with joint purpose activities?

4. What additional time is spent by clinicians on behalf of the students?

5. How can the above information, drawn from a selected sample of facilities, be used to estimate the total clinical instructor costs to facilities providing placements for physical therapy students?

Dr. Page is Director and Associate Professor, Division of Educational Support and Development, Office of the Coordinator, Health Sciences, The University of British Columbia, Vancouver, British Columbia, Canada V6T 1W5.

Dr. MacKinnon is Associate Professor and Chairman, Department of Occupational Therapy, Faculty of Applied Health Sciences, The University of Western Ontario, London, Ontario, Canada N6A 5C1. She was Research Associate, Division of Educational Support and Development, The University of British Columbia, when this study was conducted.

Address all correspondence to Dr. MacKinnon.

This article was submitted September 3, 1985; was with the authors for revision 14 weeks; and was accepted April 25, 1986. Potential Conflict of Interest: 4.

METHOD

Procedure

Initially, basic descriptive information on the physical therapy program was collected through meetings with the director and clinical coordinators of the university's program. Information was obtained on the school's objectives for clinical placements. affiliation and financial agreements. numbers of students. length of clinical placements. and numbers and names of the facilities involved.

The next step was to meet with departmental directors and supervisors in the clinical training facilities to inform these individuals of the objectives of the study. to provide an instructional session on the completion of the form to be used to obtain. descriptive data on their program. to respond to anticipated problems with this form. and to elicit their views on clinical placement issues as these placements were organized currently in their facility. Forms were left with the clinical supervisor, and the expected date for their return to the investigator was established at the time of the meeting. Clinical supervisors were encouraged to collaborate closely with their clinical instructors in completing the form and to telephone the university if they encountered problems with it.

Letters of appreciation were sent to the clinical supervisors as the completed clinical placement forms were received. Incomplete or questionable forms were clarified by telephone contact.

Clinical Placement Form

Figure 1 displays the clinical placement form. In the fall of 1982. facilities completed a separate form for each placement of physical therapy students (eg. groups of second-, third-, or fourth-year students) in that facility between September 1. 1981. and August 31. 1982. All students of the same year were treated identically with no record kept of instructor or student absences or illnesses. Holidays were not included in the clinical hours.

As a basis for completing the form. facility personnel were asked to generate a list of 7 to 10 major activities that collectively encompassed all of the students' activities during their clinical placement. Typical activity categories recorded were orientation, evaluation. and instructor demonstration for single purpose activities and ward rounds, patient treatment, and in-service training

for joint purpose activities. Each of these activity categories then was to be classified as a single purpose activity or as a joint purpose activity based on the definitions provided and listed in Sections II (a) and (b) of the form. For each activity listed, data were elicited on the number of students grouped together during the activity, the number of scheduled hours each week (total. 35 hours) the students spent in each activity. and the percentage of time that a clinician was in direct contact with the student during the activity. Section III of the form elicited information on noninstructional activities and associated hours. Noninstructional activities included planning before the students' arrival and completing evaluation forms and letters after the students' departure.

September 1, 1981 - August 31, 1982

Hospital/Agency _____

Clinical Director _____

I Demographics of Students

Year of Student	Length of Placement	Number of Students
_____	_____	_____

II Instructional Activity

	Number of Students	Scheduled Hours/Student/Week	% Direct Contact
a) Single Purpose			
_____	_____	_____	_____
_____	_____	_____	_____
_____	_____	_____	_____
_____	_____	_____	_____
_____	_____	_____	_____
_____	_____	_____	_____
b) Joint Purpose			
_____	_____	_____	_____
_____	_____	_____	_____
_____	_____	_____	_____
_____	_____	_____	_____
_____	_____	_____	_____
_____	_____	35 hours	_____

III Non-instructional Activity (planning and preparing for students)

Activity	Time Spent/Student/Placement
_____	_____
_____	_____
_____	_____
_____	_____

Fig. 1. Clinical placement form.

Sample Size

Twenty-nine health care facilities provided clinical placement for physical therapy students between September 1, 1981, and August 31, 1982. Of these 29 facilities. 12 (41.4%) were included in the study sample. The criteria for selecting facilities were that they be within 50 miles of the university (for accessibility) and that they collectively provide placements to at least 50% of the students in our program. The study sample, therefore, did not include small rural facilities that provided placements for only a few students. Of the 12 facilities sampled. 9 provided placements for second-year students. 12 for third-year students, and 11 for fourth-year students. These facilities provided the placement required

TABLE 1
Percentage of the Distribution of Scheduled Time Between Single Purpose and Joint Purpose Activities Provided by Clinical Instructors

| Facility | Students | | | | | | | | | $\bar{X}$ | | |
| | Second-Year | | | Third-Year | | | Fourth-Year | | | | | |
	SP[a]	JP[b]	Total	SP	JP	Total	SP	JP	Total	SP	JP	Total
1	25.1	74.9	100	32.0	68.0	100				28.6	71.4	100
2				23.7	76.3	100	22.6	77.4	100	23.1	76.9	100
3	17.8	82.2	100	17.1	82.9	100	25.7	74.3	100	20.2	79.8	100
4	35.4	64.6	100	30.0	70.0	100	27.1	72.9	100	30.8	69.2	100
5				16.3	83.7	100	14.6	85.4	100	15.5	84.5	100
6	22.3	77.7	100	26.0	74.0	100	22.9	77.1	100	23.7	76.3	100
7	26.6	73.4	100	21.3	78.7	100	19.9	80.1	100	22.6	77.4	100
8				27.7	72.3	100	28.6	71.4	100	28.2	71.8	100
9	24.3	75.7	100	24.3	75.7	100	24.3	75.7	100	24.3	75.7	100
10	28.6	71.4	100	27.1	72.9	100	22.3	77.7	100	26.0	74.0	100
11	30.0	70.0	100	24.6	75.4	100	21.3	78.7	100	25.3	74.7	100
12	32.9	67.1	100	32.3	67.7	100	31.4	68.6	100	32.2	67.8	100
	n = 9			n = 12			n = 11			n = 12		
$\bar{X}$	27.0	73.0		25.2	74.8		23.7	76.3		25.0	75.0	
$\bar{X}$ (all years)	25.2	74.8										

[a] SP = single purpose activity.
[b] JP = joint purpose activity.

for 66.7% of the second-year students, 62.2% of the third-year students, and 68.6% of the fourth-year students. These 12 facilities also provided 65.1% of the clinical placement time for the entire population of students in the program, respectively providing 66.7%, 62.7%, and 67.3% of the clinical placement time for second-, third-, and fourth-year students. Although the study did not sample all facilities providing clinical placement for all students, therefore, it sampled the larger metropolitan facilities providing clinical placement to the majority of second-, third-, and fourth-year physical therapy students.

RESULTS

Scheduled Clinical Time

The total scheduled clinical time for students in the physical therapy program was calculated from the schedules provided by the clinical coordinator from the university's program.

Second-year students. In the 1981 to 1982 academic year, 39 second-year physical therapy students participated in a four-week placement at the end of the academic year. Each student spent a total of 140 hours (35 hr/wk × 4 weeks); the total scheduled clinical hours were 5,460 (39 students × 140 hr/student).

Third-year students. Each of the 37 third-year physical therapy students participated in a three-week and a six-week clinical placement. Each student spent a total of 315 hours (35 hr/wk × 9 weeks); the total scheduled clinical

hours for third-year students were 11,655 (37 students × 315 hr/student).

Fourth-year students. Each of the 35 fourth-year physical therapy students participated in a three-week and a four-week placement. Each student spent a total of 245 hours (35 hr/wk × 7 weeks); the total number of scheduled clinical hours for fourth-year students was 8,575 (35 students × 245 hr/student). The total scheduled clinical time for all students, therefore, was 25,690 hours.

Single Purpose and Joint Purpose Activities

For the facilities sampled, Table 1 describes the percentages of scheduled clinical time that were devoted to single purpose and joint purpose activities. The percentages were derived from the numbers of hours of such activities as reported on the clinical placement form completed by the agency personnel. Three significant observations can be drawn from these percentages:

1. Wide variations among agencies in the distribution of time between single purpose and joint purpose activities. At the extremes, Facility 4 reported a 35.4-64.6 division in the time between single purpose and joint purpose activities for second-year students, and Facility 3 reported a 17.8-82.2 division of this time.
2. The major proportion of scheduled clinical time was devoted to joint purpose activities. On the average, 75.0% of the scheduled clinical time was devoted to joint purpose activi-

ties, and 25.0% was devoted to single purpose activities.
3. The division of scheduled clinical time between single purpose and joint purpose activities essentially remained constant over the three years of the program.

Direct Contact Time

Table 2 describes the percentages of scheduled clinical time that was spent in direct contact hours. These percentages are reported for single purpose, joint purpose, and total direct contact time for second-, third-, and fourth-year physical therapy students. Three important observations can be drawn from these percentages:

1. Wide variations existed among facilities in the percentages of scheduled student clinical hours that were direct contact hours. The ranges of single purpose activities were from 44.1% to 100% for second-year students, 26.8% to 100% for third-year students, and 29.0% to 100% for fourth-year students. For the joint purpose activities, the ranges were not quite as large: from 45.6% to 86.9%, 27.0% to 83.7%, and 18.1% to 79.4% for second-, third-, and fourth-year students, respectively.
2. The average percentage of direct student contact time for single purpose activities was much greater than for joint purpose activities. These respective averages for all students were 70.8% and 48.8%.

TABLE 2
Percentage of Direct Contact Time Provided by Clinical Instructors

Facility	Second-Year			Third-Year			Fourth-Year			X̄		
	SP[a]	JP[b]	Total[c]	SP	JP	Total	SP	JP	Total	SP	JP	Total
1	87.5	73.3	76.8	87.5	65.5	72.6				87.5	69.4	74.7
2				66.3	59.2	60.9	64.6	50.9	54.0	65.5	55.0	57.5
3	100.0	86.9	89.2	100.0	83.7	86.1	76.0	79.4	78.5	92.0	83.3	84.6
4	72.6	45.6	54.4	81.9	44.1	55.4	82.7	42.4	53.8	79.0	44.0	54.5
5				80.7	46.8	52.3	74.5	31.1	37.4	77.6	40.0	44.9
6	75.6	45.6	52.3	74.7	30.9	42.3	77.5	21.5	34.3	75.9	32.7	43.0
7	57.0	66.1	63.7	53.7	52.3	52.6	50.6	22.4	27.9	53.8	46.9	48.0
8				26.8	41.9	37.7	29.0	31.2	30.6	27.9	36.6	34.2
9	44.1	68.7	62.7	44.1	48.4	47.3	44.1	48.3	47.3	44.1	55.1	52.4
10	90.6	64.8	72.2	89.5	45.5	57.4	87.2	25.7	39.4	89.1	45.3	56.3
11	52.2	49.8	50.5	55.6	41.9	45.5	64.4	38.9	44.3	57.4	43.5	46.8
12	100.0	54.5	69.4	100.0	27.0	50.6	100.0	18.1	37.7	100.0	33.2	52.6
	n = 9			n = 12			n = 11			n = 12		
X̄	75.5	61.7	65.7	71.7	48.9	55.1	68.2	37.3	44.1	70.8	48.8	54.1

[a] SP = single purpose activity.
[b] JP = joint purpose activity.
[c] Total = percentage of direct contact SP and JP hours from Table 1 (total assumed hours = 360).

TABLE 3
Percentage of the Distribution of Direct Contact Time Between Single Purpose and Joint Purpose Activities Provided by Clinical Instructors

Facility	Second-Year			Third-Year			Fourth-Year			X̄		
	SP[a]	JP[b]	Total	SP	JP	Total	SP	JP	Total	SP	JP	Total
1	20.7	54.9	75.6	28.0	44.6	72.6				24.3	49.8	74.1
2				15.7	45.1	60.8	14.6	39.4	54.0	15.1	42.3	57.4
3	17.8	71.4	89.2	14.7	71.4	86.1	19.9	58.7	78.6	17.5	67.2	84.7
4	25.7	29.4	55.1	24.5	30.9	55.4	23.4	30.4	53.8	24.5	30.2	54.7
5				13.1	39.1	52.2	10.8	26.6	37.4	11.9	32.9	44.8
6	16.9	35.4	52.3	19.4	22.9	42.3	17.7	16.6	34.3	18.0	25.0	43.0
7	15.1	48.6	63.7	11.4	41.1	52.5	9.9	18.0	27.9	12.1	35.9	48.0
8				7.4	30.3	37.7	8.3	22.3	30.6	7.9	26.3	34.2
9	10.7	52.0	62.7	10.7	36.6	47.3	10.7	36.6	47.3	10.7	41.7	52.4
10	25.9	46.3	72.2	24.3	33.1	57.4	19.4	20.0	39.4	23.2	33.1	56.3
11	15.6	34.8	50.4	15.5	33.2	48.7	14.7	32.8	47.5	15.3	33.6	48.9
12	32.9	36.6	69.5	32.3	18.3	50.6	23.1	12.0	35.1	29.4	22.3	51.7
	n = 9			n = 12			n = 11			n = 12		
X̄	20.1	45.5	65.6	18.1	37.2	55.3	15.7	28.5	44.2	17.5	36.7	54.2

[a] SP = single purpose activity.
[b] JP = joint purpose activity.

3. A consistent decrease was noted in the percentages of scheduled direct contact clinical time among the second-, third-, and fourth-year students. For single purpose activities, the mean respective percentages were 75.5%, 71.7%, and 68.2%; for joint purpose activities they were 61.7%, 48.9%, and 37.3%. Total direct contact time decreased from 65.7% to 55.1% to 44.1%.

Table 2 should not be interpreted to indicate that the majority of direct contact time provided by clinicians was given to single purpose activities. Al-though this table does report that a greater percentage of single purpose than joint purpose scheduled clinical time was direct contact time, Table 1 shows that the mean single purpose time represented a smaller percentage (25.0%) of the total scheduled clinical time. When these two factors were combined, the majority of direct contact hours were found to be associated with joint purpose activities. This relationship is clarified by Table 3, which reports the percentage distribution of total direct contact time over single purpose and joint purpose activities.

Direct Contact Time Compared with Single Purpose and Joint Purpose Activities

The data in Table 3 indicate the following:

1. Wide variations existed among facilities in the percentages of direct contact time for single purpose and joint purpose activities. For the single purpose activities for all students, the average direct contact time ranged from 7.9% to 29.4% for Facilities 8 and 12; for the joint purpose activities, from 22.3% to 67.2% for Facil-

ities 12 and 3; and for total time, from 34.2% to 84.7% for Facilities 8 and 3.

2. The average percentage of total scheduled time that was direct contact time was greater for joint purpose activities (36.7%) than for single purpose activities (17.5%).

3. A consistent decrease was noted in the percentages of direct contact time for both single purpose and joint purpose activities among the second-, third-, and fourth-year students. Mean single purpose direct contact time decreased from 20.1% to 18.1% to 15.7%, and mean joint purpose activities decreased more dramatically from 45.5% to 37.2% to 28.5%. The means for all students were 17.5% for single purpose time and 36.7% for joint purpose time for a total of 54.2% of the total time scheduled that was direct contact time.

Figure 2 depicts the division of the total scheduled clinical time into single purpose and joint purpose time and, within each, into direct contact time.

Related Activities

Table 4 summarizes the number of related activity hours clinicians estimated they spent with each student in planning for their arrival and reporting back to the university after their departure. On the average, 5.76 hours for each placement were devoted to each student, with a wide variation noted among agencies. Facility 7 reported 0.56 related activity hours, whereas Facility 6 indicated 13.64 related activity hours for each student.

Estimating Total Clinicians' Time

This section will provide an estimate of the total number of hours of facility staff time required to provide clinical teaching to the physical therapy students in the 1981 to 1982 academic year. The estimate incorporates data from the preceding sections describing scheduled clinical hours and direct contact hours, and it is based on two assumptions:

1. That the mean percentage distributions of single purpose, joint purpose, and direct contact time obtained from the facilities sampled in the study are representative of all facilities offering placements to physical therapy students.

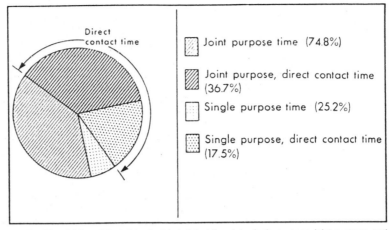

Fig. 2. The division of the total scheduled clinical time into single purpose, joint purpose, and direct purpose contact time.

Joint purpose time (74.8%)

Joint purpose, direct contact time (36.7%)

Single purpose time (25.2%)

Single purpose, direct contact time (17.5%)

2. That joint purpose activities address educational needs and clinical needs in equal proportions; hence, 50% of joint purpose hours represent educational time.

This second assumption addresses one of the most problematic issues in separating health care and education costs in a clinical setting. Neither the data collected in this study, nor the results of the studies cited earlier, provide an empirical basis for separating these costs. Furthermore, the division of these costs will be a function of several variables (eg, the level of training of the student, the type of joint purpose activity), which will vary greatly across different clinical teaching situations. Although other percentage figures could be used in this assumption, 50% was thought to be as representative as any.

Based on the second assumption, the total number of hours of agency staff time devoted to the teaching of students in the 1981 to 1982 academic year can be estimated by summing 1) the total scheduled clinical hours that were direct contact hours for single purpose activities, 2) 50% of the total scheduled clinical hours that were direct contact hours for joint purpose activities, and 3) the total related activities hours.

The total scheduled clinical hours for all students as reported previously was 25,690 hours. From the data in Table 3, 17.5% or 4,496 of these hours were single purpose direct contact hours, and 36.7% or 9,428 hours were direct contact joint purpose hours. Table 4 indicates that each agency provided an average of 5.76 hours of additional time for each student in each placement on

instructionally related activities, which, for a total of 183 placements, required 1,054 hours.

The number of hours of clinicians' time used for educational purposes by this program in the 1981 to 1982 academic year is estimated, therefore, to have been

$$4,496 + 0.5(9,428) + 1,054 = 10,264 \quad (1)$$

With a knowledge of the salary data of the facility staff members who teach the students, these hours can be converted into the dollar costs to agencies. The data reported in this study can be used by The University of British Columbia to estimate the annual facility staff costs of one student's clinical placements. For example, a third-year student has a three-week and a six-week rotation. During these nine weeks of 35 hours each week, the student will accu-

TABLE 4
Number of Related Activity Hours for Each Student Provided by Clinical Instructors

Facility	Hours Per Student
1	9.38
2	9.60
3	6.20
4	6.00
5	2.67
6	13.64
7	0.56
8	4.50
9	1.45
10	6.94
11	6.00
12	2.18
TOTAL	69.12
$\bar{X}$	5.76

mulate 315 scheduled clinical hours. Table 3 indicates that 17.5% of these hours (55.12 hours) are direct contact, single purpose hours, and 36.7% (115.60 hours) are direct contact, joint purpose hours. Recalling that clinicians spend an estimated additional 5.76 hours on instructionally related activities for each of the two placements, the number of clinician hours devoted totally to teaching this student is

$$55.12 + 0.5(115.60)$$
$$+ 2(5.76) = 124.44 \quad (2)$$

If a clinician's salary and benefits total $25,000 a year for a 200-working-day year, 7 hours a day, the clinician's hourly rate is $17.86 ($25,000/[200×7]). The cost to the agency for accepting one student for nine weeks, therefore, is $2,223 (124.44 hr × $17.86/hr). This amount represents an estimate of the most critical cost to a facility accepting a student for clinical placement.

DISCUSSION

The purpose of this study was to estimate the costs to facilities for clinical instructor time required to conduct a clinical education program for physical therapy students. The study did not address other costs associated with clinical education, that is, the use of equipment, supplies, and space, that were reported by Ramsden and Fischer[13] to be less critical. We also did not assess the short- and long-term benefits to the agency as a consequence of providing clinical placements or attempt to determine the amount of patient income generated by students. The study was conducted to assist The University of British Columbia to understand the instructional characteristics and the costs of clinical placement, as a basis for establishing joint policy and funding agreements with facilities.

The methodology for the study entailed conducting an in-depth analysis of the clinical placements in a sample of facilities, rather than generating a model of clinical placement[4,8,10] or conducting a comparative analysis of costs, productivity, and revenues of facilities with and without clinical placements.[11] The data provided from the facilities on single purpose, joint purpose, and direct contact time were obtained under conditions of careful direction and monitoring and, most often, after extensive consultations and collaboration with fa-

cility "teaching" staff members. The variation in these data from facility to facility was believed to reflect real differences in the instructional philosophy and activities of these facilities. This conclusion is supported by the descriptive information received during visits to and received in written form from the facilities, which explained many of the differences in the data. The accuracy of the data, however, was not assessed by formal reliability studies (ie. interrater reliability) of the data obtained on the clinical placement form.

The data describing the clinical placements have face validity. That is, the variation in single purpose, joint purpose, and direct contact times displays a pattern that would be expected on the basis of a general understanding of clinical placement programs. For example, about three quarters of the scheduled clinical time was reported to be devoted to joint purpose activities, which are the primary reason for sending students to clinical settings. In addition, the percentage of direct contact time, as we expected, is much higher for single purpose (learning) activities than for joint purpose (learning, patient care, research) activities. Also, a progressive and marked decline was seen in direct contact time for the more senior students, particularly in joint purpose activities in which the senior students require less clinical supervision.

This study is descriptive and, for the most part, it offers no basis for judging the quality of the students' clinical placement experience. Although the wide variations in the percentage of direct contact time for joint purpose activities (eg. clinical supervision) and in the number of hours of related activities (eg, planning activities) may suggest quality differences, such a conclusion would be premature. These findings, however, do provide an excellent base from which to approach issues of quality by collaborating with facilities in the analysis of their programs.

On a more far-reaching scale, the data from this study, in conjunction with the standards established by the American Physical Therapy Association, could be used to begin to build a model for clinical placement programs. For each level of students, the model could offer guidelines for 1) the percentage of the distribution of scheduled clinical time across specified single purpose and joint pur-

pose activities and 2) the percentage of direct contact (eg. supervision) activities required in each. Such guidelines would be welcomed by many physical therapy services.

CONCLUSIONS

The data collected in this study indicated that 10,264 hours of clinical facility staff time were devoted exclusively for the purpose of teaching The University of British Columbia's physical therapy students during the 1981 to 1982 academic year. This commitment by the facilities entails financial implications that are increasing greatly as government resources for both health care and education are being reduced. Through this study, the university and the facilities understand the scope of this commitment, and they can begin to establish policies for the organizational and fiscal management of the program. We recommend the methodology in this study to other educational institutions as a method of developing databases to be examined critically and cooperatively with health care agencies to develop guidelines for clinical placement.

REFERENCES

1. Garg ML, Elkhatib M, Kleinberg WM, et al: Reimbursing for residency training: How many times? Med Care 20:719–726, 1982
2. Light I, Frey DC: Dual responsibility for allied manpower training. Hospitals 47:85–90, 1973
3. Sheps GG, Clark DA, Gerdes JW, et al: Medical schools and hospitals: Interdependence for education and service. J Med Educ 40(Part II):1–169, 1965
4. Halonen RJ, Fitzgerald J, Simmon K: Measuring the costs of clinical education in departments utilizing allied health professionals. J Allied Health 5:5–12, 1976
5. Undergraduate medical education: Elements, objectives, costs. J Med Educ 49(Suppl):101–127, 1974
6. Chung YI, Spelbring LM, Boissoneau R: A cost-benefit analysis of fieldwork education in occupational therapy. Inquiry 17:216–229, 1980
7. Carney MK, Keim ST: Cost to the hospital of a clinical training program. J Allied Health 7:187–191, 1978
8. Leiken AM: Method to determine the effect of clinical education on production in a health care facility. Phys Ther 63:56–59, 1983
9. Moores B: The cost and effectiveness of nurse education. Nursing Times 75:65–72, 1979
10. Pobojewski TR: Case study: Cost-benefit analysis of clinical education. J Allied Health 7:192–198, 1978
11. Porter RE, Kincaid CB: Financial aspects of clinical education to facilities. Phys Ther 57:905–909, 1977
12. Gonyea MA: Analyzing and Constructing Cost. San Francisco, CA, Jossey-Bass Inc, Publishers, 1978
13. Ramsden EL, Fischer WT: Cost allocation for physical therapy in a teaching hospital. Phys Ther 50:660–664, 1970

Clinical Problem Solving in Clinical Education

Improving Physical Therapy Students' Clinical Problem-Solving Skills: An Analytical Questioning Model

The purpose of this study was to assess the effectiveness of a model for teaching problem-solving skills to first-year physical therapy students using the Watson-Glaser Critical Thinking Appraisal (CTA) and participant feedback. We used a pretest-posttest control group design. Subjects were 31 first-year physical therapy students divided into a Control Group (n = 15) and an Experimental Group (n = 16). Students in the Experimental Group used the problem-solving model during a four-week clerkship. No difference was found between the Experimental and Control Groups' performance on the CTA. Subjectively, students in the Experimental Group and their Clinical Instructors found the model to be an effective tool that aided students' understanding of patient assessment and treatment program planning. The need for an objective assessment tool of problem-solving models in physical therapy is discussed. [Slaughter DS, Brown DS, Gardner DL, et al: Improving physical therapy students' clinical problem-solving skills: An analytical questioning model. Phys Ther 69:441–447, 1989]

Diane S Slaughter
Debra S Brown
Davis L Gardner
Lea J Perritt

Key Words: *Clinical competence; Clinical protocols; Education: physical therapist, clinical education; Problem solving.*

A student's problem-solving ability is very often a concern among educators and clinicians.[1] With the current knowledge level required in physical therapy, giving students the didactic knowledge necessary to function as a physical therapist often precludes extensive teaching at the application level. The students' ability to shift the learning process from mere accumulation of facts to creative and critical analysis of those facts, however, is essential for adequate evaluation and treatment of our patients and for growth of our profession. Clinical Instructors of the University of Kentucky's physical therapy program expressed their concern regarding students' clinical problem-solving ability when assessing patient problems and designing treatment programs. In addition, Kentucky recently joined the growing number of states having direct access to patient care through Kentucky Law KRS327.010. These two factors prompted the design of a model to improve the problem-solving abilities of our students.

In reviewing the literature, we found many studies that addressed creative ways to teach problem-solving skills but none that were objectively evaluated. Because time is a premium in physical therapy education, we wanted not only to add a problem-solving model to the curriculum but also to measure any improvement in the problem-solving ability of our students resultant from our model. If improvement occurred, we would know we had developed an effective model. Conversely, if no improvement occurred, we would modify our model.

D Slaughter, MSEd, PT, is Director of Physical Therapy, University of Kentucky Sports Medicine Center, Medical Plaza, Rm D-103, Lexington, KY 40536 (USA). She was a student in the Curriculum and Instruction Clinical and College Teaching Program, University of Kentucky, when this study was completed in partial fulfillment of the requirements of her master's degree.

D Brown, MSEd, PT, is Assistant Professor and Academic Coordinator of Clinical Education, Physical Therapy Division, College of Allied Health Professions, University of Kentucky.

D Gardner, MEd, is Professor, Allied Health Education and Research Program, College of Allied Health Professions, University of Kentucky.

L Perritt, PhD, is a part-time assistant professor, Allied Health Education and Research Program, College of Allied Health Professions, University of Kentucky. Dr Perritt is also a licensed psychologist in private practice.

This article was submitted September 25, 1987; was with the authors for revision for 43 weeks; and was accepted February 10, 1989.

The purpose of the study was to evaluate our problem-solving model to determine whether it could assist first-year physical therapy students in developing more effective problem-solving skills. The model was evaluated by comparing the results of the pretest-posttest performance on the Watson-Glaser Critical Thinking Appraisal (CTA)[2] and posttest feedback gathered through a questionnaire. The null hypothesis was that no difference would exist between control and experimental groups' performance on the CTA.

Problem-solving Models in the Literature

Day states there is "an assumption that the ability to solve problems and to analyze new situations is paramount to good performance by a physical therapist."[3(p1555)] To this end, a collection of problem-solving strategies has been designed for use in physical therapy curricula and clinics.[1,4–8]

May and Newman describe problem solving as "an internal and sequential process that includes cognitive, affective, and psychomotor behaviors."[1(p1140)] They identify the following sequence of activities in their problem-solving model:

1. Problem recognition

2. Problem definition

3. Problem analysis

4. Data management

5. Solution development

6. Solution implementation

7. Outcome evaluation

Olsen[5] and Day[9] designed problem-solving models using a systems approach that requires each step to be analyzed in relation to other steps. Olsen states this approach "allows an instructor or clinical supervisor to monitor the student's problem-solving skills and facilitates feedback and

exchange of information" using a structured sequence of analytical assessments and decisions.[5(p526)] Other problem-solving models use case histories to simulate actual clinical experience.[7,8,10] Our model was developed using feedback from local CIs and information gained from the studies mentioned previously. In designing our model, *problem solving* was defined as the nine behaviors identified in the Blue MACS (Mastery and Assessment of Clinical Skill) skill #42.[11]

Assessment of Problem-solving Models

Problem-solving models generally are assessed by questionnaires and feedback from participants, a more subjective than objective assessment mode. Burnett et al developed a problem-solving model and concluded that

> although no statistical data were collected to demonstrate that the problem-solving skills of the students improved by using this educational model instead of a more traditional model of clinical experience, students and clinicians reported the experiences were worthwhile.[8(1–33)]

The authors of other problem-solving models stated similar conclusions. They found the models to be useful and effective[5,9] and cited positive feedback from students and clinical faculty.[5,7]

We hypothesized that the CTA would be an appropriate objective instrument to assess the effectiveness of our problem-solving model in this study. One use of the CTA postulated by its developers is "to measure gains in critical thinking abilities resulting from instructional programs in schools, colleges and business and industrial settings."[2] Studies have indicated that CTA reliability ranges from .85 to .87.[2] According to AJ Threlkeld (personal communication, November 1988), preliminary studies on validity at the University of Kentucky indicate a positive correlation between CTA scores of physical therapy students and grades students have earned in

required physical therapy clinical sciences courses. One of the CTA's primary uses, therefore, appeared to be compatible with our intent.

The University of Kentucky's Physical Therapy Division has used the CTA for eight years as one of several preadmission screening tools for applicants to the physical therapy program. The CTA was selected as an instrument to predict students' critical thinking and problem-solving abilities, and the CTA score currently represents 10% of the total criteria used to determine eligibility for admission.

All students accepted into the physical therapy program had CTA scores on file, and these scores were used as baseline data for the students in the study. We believed that the CTA data would provide objective, standardized assessment of a problem-solving model that other models in physical therapy have lacked.

Method

Subjects

This study was submitted to the University of Kentucky's Institutional Review Board and qualified for exempt status. Subjects were the 31 first-year physical therapy students enrolled in Clinical Clerkship I, a four-week clerkship beginning in the spring semester. The class consisted of 30 female students and 1 male student ranging in age from 20 to 36 years. Prior to Clinical Clerkship I, clinical experience for all subjects had been limited to preprofessional volunteer types of activities.

Procedure

In the University of Kentucky's physical therapy program, all first-year students are enrolled in Clinical Clerkship I. For this study, the class was divided into a Control Group (n = 15) and an Experimental Group (n = 16). The group assignments were based on a pre-existing random division of the class. Before attending the clinical clerkship, all students attended five lectures on various aspects of physical therapy. During the four-week clerkship period, all students attended one of seven general clinics for one-half day per week. In addition, students in the Control Group were required to observe 3 of 10 specialty clinics, and students in the Experimental Group were required to observe 2 of the 10 specialty clinics. Students in both groups were allowed to choose the specialty clinics.

Students in the Control Group generated an individual case study on a patient they had evaluated and treated according to an assigned format. These case studies were not discussed with the CIs, and no preclerkship or postclerkship meetings were scheduled.

Students in the Experimental Group met prior to the clerkship and were familiarized with the analytical questioning sequence that accompanied each of the five prepared case studies they would discuss with their CIs during the clerkship. They also generated an individual case study on a patient they had evaluated and treated. These additional case studies were discussed with the individual CIs and then with the other Experimental Group subjects during a postclerkship meeting. The total experiential span was six weeks.

The prepared case studies were designed for the Experimental Group and reflected typical patients seen in clinic. The case studies included 1) an inpatient with phlebitis, 2) a pediatric inpatient with a fractured fibula, 3) an outpatient with a sports-related knee injury, 4) an inpatient with a diabetic ulcer, and 5) a home care patient with a pinned fractured hip.

Each prepared case study was modeled after the physical assessment protocol students are instructed to use.[12] The evaluation consists of the following sections: 1) a patient history; 2) a subjective evaluation; and 3) objective findings consisting of inspection, function, palpation, neurologic, and special test sections. These prepared case studies were purposefully vague to

generate student questions about further information required.

At the conclusion of the clerkship, two assessment methods were used. The CTA again was administered to the students in both the Control and Experimental Groups. The preadmission CTA scores were compared with this second set of CTA scores to assess the effectiveness of the problem-solving model. Questionnaires were sent to the students in the Experimental Group and to their CIs, and the respondents' comments were reviewed.

The first questionnaire item rated the students' assessment of their own ability to use didactic information as the basis for clinical decisions. The remaining items were short-answer questions and focused on obtaining the respondents' perception of 1) the value of the questioning sequence and case studies, 2) the assessment of student-CI interaction resulting from case-study discussions, 3) the clinical applicability of the experiences, and 4) the ways in which problem-solving skills were affected. All respondents also were asked whether they recommended continued use of the model.

Implementation of the Model

Preclerkship. Using guidelines from existing problem-solving models,[1,4–9] we developed a questioning sequence to facilitate students progressing through any case study with the intent of developing uniform problem-solving thought patterns. Basic categories of the model included in the questioning sequence were 1) assessment, 2) problem identification, and 3) treatment planning. The questions were applied to each of the five prepared case studies developed for this study.

Answering questions about hypothetical patients in a step-by-step fashion would be useful, but not adequate, for developing effective problem-solving skills. To develop effective problem-solving skills in the clinic, the CIs' involvement was critical. This belief was based on May and New-

man's statement, "The role of the instructor is that of facilitator, rather than 'teller.' "[1(p1144)]

Before the clerkships began, we met for a two-hour session with the CIs to discuss the purpose of the study and the CIs' role. The CIs reviewed the five case studies and the questioning sequence design to be used with the Experimental Group. The final analytical questioning sequence shown in Table 1 incorporated their suggested revisions.

The CIs also generated a list of possible answers to each of the questions for each case study. A compilation of their responses was distributed to the CIs prior to the clerkships.

Strategies to facilitate student involvement through questioning were reviewed with the CIs.[13] These strategies were used during the weekly feedback sessions when the CIs and students discussed the case studies. The therapists were encouraged to use the same questioning strategies with the students to facilitate student involvement with other patients seen in the clinic.

Clerkship. During the orientation meeting, students in the Experimental Group reviewed Case Study 1 and completed the prescribed analytical questioning sequence. They then received Case Study 2, which they completed prior to beginning their clerkship. Students reviewed Case Study 2 with their CIs during the first week's feedback session. Students received Case Study 3 during the second week of the clerkship and again discussed it with their CIs. Students continued with Case Studies 4 and 5 during the third and fourth clerkship weeks, respectively.

During the third week of the clerkship, students wrote their individual case studies that were to be discussed with their CIs during the final week of the clerkship. Students also exchanged and discussed their case studies with another member of the Experimental Group group during the postclerkship meeting.

Table 1. *Analytical Questioning Sequence*

Category-Item Number	Question
Assessment	
1	What structure(s) may be involved?
2	Does the severity of the patient's condition limit your ability to perform a complete evaluation?
3	Is there any additional information you would need in making an assessment? If so, what?
4	Is there extraneous information? If so, what?
5	Are there any psychological or social factors that should be considered for this patient? If so, what are they?
Problem Identification	
6	Identify patient problems or complaints relevant to physical therapy.
7	What are the possible causes of these problems or complaints?
8	What do you perceive the primary problem to be? Why?
9	What data assist or support your analysis?
Treatment Planning	
10	What treatment(s) might you use to influence the problem(s) you identified in item 6?
11	How will the treatment(s) influence the problem(s)?
12	How will the treatment(s) influence the cause of the problems?
13	What do you think is the most appropriate way of delivering the treatment(s) you identified in item 10?
14	What modalities or equipment do you need to implement your solutions?
15	What is(are) your anticipated frequency(ies) and duration(s) of treatment?
16	What factors may change your frequency(ies) and duration(s)?
17	What is(are) your short-term goal(s)?
18	What is(are) your long-term goal(s)?
19	How can you assess the effectiveness of your treatment plan?
20	What might be an alternate plan?

Data Analysis

After completion of all Clinical Clerkship I requirements, all students took the posttest CTA. The scores from the posttest CTA were compared with the preadmission CTA scores and were analyzed using a two-way analysis of variance (ANOVA). One Control Group subject's posttest CTA score was not included in the data analysis because a pretest CTA score was not

available. Responses from the questionnaires also were reviewed.

Results

The three outlier CTA scores in the Experimental Group were considered in the data analysis. A Bartlett test for homogeneity of variance was performed to test the possibility that the three outlier scores on the posttest CTA in the Experimental Group skewed the results.[14] The range of

change in scores for the Control Group was from -6 to $+9$, whereas the range of change for the Experimental Group was from -17 to $+6$, with outlier changes of -17, -15, and -15. With the outlier scores included, the variances were heterogeneous ($\chi^2 = 8.73$, critical value = 5.02, $p < .05$). With the outlier scores removed, the range was from -12 to $+6$, and the Bartlett test showed the variances to be homogeneous ($\chi^2 = 1.34$, critical value = 5.02, $p < .05$). The three Experimental Group outlier scores, therefore, were omitted from the data analysis.

A two-way ANOVA was performed to determine whether there were differences in the overall performances of the two groups and whether there were changes in performance from pretest to posttest administration of the CTA.

There was no significant difference either between the two groups ($F[1,32] = 1.05$, $p > .05$) or in change in performance ($F[1,7] = 0.81$, $p > .05$). The interaction between the two groups and performance also was not significant ($F[1,43] = 4.92$, $p > .05$). The means and standard deviations for both groups on the pretest and posttest administration of the CTA appear in Table 2.

Participant feedback was gathered from the questionnaires returned by 7 Experimental Group subjects and by 7 of the 8 participating CIs. All respondents indicated they often or routinely used didactic information to make clinical decisions. The respondents commented that the questioning sequence was of value in several ways. Two sample comments were: "After I started answering the questions in sequence, solutions to the problems followed naturally" and "I feel I can better think things/ processes through in a more logical, orderly fashion."

Students' assessment of the feedback sessions with the CIs was very positive. Students stated: "I thought that this was a very valuable aspect of the

Table 2. *Watson-Glaser Critical Thinking Appraisal Pretest and Posttest Means and Standard Deviations for Control and Experimental Groups*

Group	Pretest		Posttest	
	$\overline{X}$	s	$\overline{X}$	s
Control (n = 14)	83.36	4.88	82.50	4.56
Experimental (n = 13)	82.69	4.25	80.08	3.85

course. The extra time spent on the discussion helped me get a perspective on how clinicians go about solving problems and served as examples that I will probably follow throughout my career" and "This was excellent. Not only did the case for the week get discussed, but other problems and possibilities were talked about. This made me feel more comfortable with the CI in other events."

Finally, students responded that the experience was clinically applicable. One respondent stated, "This experience will give me more confidence in deciding how a patient should be treated." The continued use of the model was recommended by the students in the Experimental Group.

Comments from the CIs' questionnaires indicated that they thought the case studies and questioning sequence were of value. For example, one CI stated the model "gave a focus to work with students on problem-solving, and gave students more insight on how they can be involved with patients in their first clinical exposure."

Clinical Instructors also responded that the experience was applicable clinically and had carry-over to other areas. One CI stated the model "helps students with what content should be in their note writing, (and) how to use objective measurements." Another CI commented, "Good system, (the) questioning sequence helped students design treatment programs with other patients they saw in the clinic." All CIs recommended that the model continue to be used with students in Clinical Clerkship I and further recommended the model to be used with second-year students.

Discussion

The CTA results did not allow for rejection of the null hypothesis. The problem-solving model, however, was found to be useful, effective, and generally worthwhile to both the students in the Experimental Group and to the participating CIs, as indicated by their questionnaire responses. Although the effectiveness of the model was not validated by the CTA, several explanations deserve discussion. As separate or combined factors, the study could have been affected by the assessment tool, student motivation, and the design and implementation of the problem-solving model.

The choice and administration of the assessment tool appear to have affected the results of the study. The baseline CTA scores had a mean of 83, which is relatively high. This mean corresponds to a percentile rank of 97% to 99%.[2] With initial scores this high, it is more difficult to show improvement, and there may be a tendency for regression toward the mean.

The application of skills tested by the CTA may not be as compatible with the specific problem-solving content that was intended in the model as it appeared to be. In the opinion of the Assistant Director of the University of Kentucky's Counseling and Testing Center, the CTA more appropriately tests the ability of students to work with abstractions in a reading situation (Peg Taylor, PhD; personal communication; July 1987). The questions for each case study required concrete reasoning, as opposed to the CTA's abstract reasoning mode. In addition, the CTA is intended to be an untimed test that usually takes at least an hour to complete. The preadmission CTA was untimed, but because of a class-schedule conflict, the postclerkship CTA was limited to 45 minutes.

Student motivation is an intangible, but influential, factor. The first time the CTA was administered to the students they were highly motivated to gain acceptance to the physical therapy program. That high level of motivation may not have been present during the postclerkship administration of the CTA. Additional required meeting times for the students in the Experimental Group also may have been a negative influence. The clerkship is a pass-fail course, and students knew that the outcome of the second CTA examination would not affect their clerkship grade.

Another uncontrolled factor was the CIs' participation. This was the first time the CIs had used the model; therefore, it is possible that their lack of experience with the model affected their ability to implement it. In several instances, because of work schedules and illness, the CI with whom the student met weekly changed. Some students in the Experimental Group, therefore, met with CIs who had not attended the two-hour preclerkship orientation session, had not been exposed to the purpose of the study, and had not been trained in the problem-solving analytical questioning sequence and student-involvement techniques. The study's design thus was disrupted, because the role of the CI was vital to the success of the model. In the implementation of the model, the variability of the CIs needed to be controlled to a greater degree than that of the students. The possibility also exists that our model was not effective.

At the time the junior physical therapy students began their clerkships, they had not been introduced to problem solving in the curriculum, and the four-week clerkship is the first time they are in the clinic. One-half day once a week is a relatively short time for students to adapt to the clinic and to acquire, assimilate, and use new information. Although the clerkship time is relatively limited, it is a very important part of their clinical education.

Attention to the development of problem-solving skills is essential early in students' clinical experience because initial thought patterns are established that become the foundation for entry-level practice. The quality of physical therapy services provided by the students during their clinical rotations can be affected positively if appropriate instructional methods are used that focus on problem-solving development.

Junior physical therapy students have no base of experience upon which to draw; they obviously lack professional experience and practice. Sanders and Ruvolo designed Mock Clinics primarily to develop students' awareness and insight into their own clinical knowledge, behaviors, and interactions with clients.[15] Although the Mock Clinics did not focus on developing problem-solving skills, the mock patient treatment sessions demonstrate one method to help students create a needed frame of reference for generating hypotheses and for enhancing the development of clinical problem-solving skills. The analytical questioning sequence applied to the six case studies with the Experimental Group represents our approach to simulating professional experience and practice.

Bruner states that effective instruction allows the learner to translate information into problem-solving efforts and that the goal of instruction should be to facilitate students to become self-propelled thinkers.[16] Elstein and associates studied how the translation of information occurred in medical practice and described the clinical reasoning process used by physicians

as cue acquisition, hypothesis generation, cue interpretation, and hypothesis evaluation.[17] Payton determined that experienced physical therapists used a clinical problem-solving sequence comparable to the physicians' sequence.[18] In both the Elstein et al[17] and Payton[18] studies, skilled practitioners began generating tentative hypotheses very early during patient contacts, hypotheses based on their experience prior to acquiring all the needed data from histories and physical examinations.

Elstein et al state that

> investigations of problem solving in chess, in logic, and in medicine are converging on the same conclusion. The differences between experts and weaker problem solvers are more to be found in the repertory of their experiences.[17(p276)]

An important component in the early clinical rotations is a structured problem-solving sequence of questions for data collection that initiates the creation of such a repertory. Successful instruction in problem-solving skills at the first-year level can provide a sound base for extended problem-solving development at the second-year level and at the professional entry level and can provide improved physical therapy services at all levels.

Positive participant feedback should not be discounted. The basis for evaluating other models to improve problem-solving skills have been participant feedback.[5,7] The feedback on our model was unanimously positive from those students who completed the questionnaire and those who did not.

Further research is needed in the area of problem-solving skill development in physical therapy students. The CTA and other standardized tools may be adjuncts to objectively validate many of the existing problem-solving models that have been assessed subjectively. In addition, studies of whether the CTA is a valid tool to assess changes in physical therapy students' critical thinking abilities are necessary.

Conclusions

Objective improvement in students' problem-solving skills as measured by the CTA was not apparent in this study. If the CTA is a valid instrument for measuring problem-solving skills, then the effectiveness of our model and its implementation may be questioned. Our participants strongly recommended that the model continue to be developed and used with our physical therapy students. In line with the recommendations, our model is being revised, but its degree of effectiveness will continue to be contingent on the CI's skill in its implementation.

If the CTA is not a valid instrument, other appropriate objective standardized assessment tools must be identified or developed to measure progress in physical therapy students' problem-solving abilities and skills as a result of clinical education. Valid assessment tools will ensure that we are providing our students with effective skills and future patients with effective evaluation and treatment.

Acknowledgment

We acknowledge the clinicians who gave of their time, experience, and expertise.

References

1 May BJ, Newman J: Developing competence in problem solving: A behavioral model. Phys Ther 60:1140–1145, 1980

2 Watson G, Glaser EM: Critical Thinking Appraisal Manual. Cleveland, OH, Psychological Corporation, 1980

3 Day JA: Graduate Record Examination analytical scores as predictors of academic success in four entry-level master's degree physical therapy programs. Phys Ther 66:1555–1562, 1986

4 Dunkle SE: Developing a Problem-Solving Approach to Teaching Physical Therapy Skills. Doctoral Dissertation. Nova University, Ft Lauderdale, FL, 1982

5 Olsen SL: Teaching treatment planning: A problem-solving model. Phys Ther 63:526–529, 1983

6 Barr J: A problem solving curriculum design in physical therapy. Phys Ther 57:262–270, 1977

7 van der Sijde PC, Sellink WJL, Wurms RJ: Developing audiovisuals for problem solving in physical therapy education. Phys Ther 67: 554–557, 1987

8 Burnett CN, Mahoney PJ, Chidley MJ, et al: Problem-solving approach to clinical education. Phys Ther 66:1730–1733, 1986

9 Day DJ: A systems diagram for teaching treatment planning. Am J Occup Ther 27:239–243, 1973

10 Henry JN: Identifying problems in clinical problem solving: Perceptions and interventions with nonproblem-solving clinical behaviors. Phys Ther 65:1071–1074, 1985

11 Mastery and Assessment of Clinical Skill. Developed by the Texas Consortium for Physical Therapy Clinical Education, Galveston, TX, 1980

12 Nitz AJ: Course Syllabus PT 807/846. Department of Physical Therapy, College of Allied Health Professions, University of Kentucky, Lexington, KY, 1987, p 6

13 Bowling B: Questioning: The Mechanics and Dynamics, TIPS (Teaching Improvement Project System). Department of Allied Health Education and Research, College of Allied Health Professions, University of Kentucky, Lexington, KY, 1978

14 Rosner B: Fundamentals of Biostatistics. Boston, MA, PWS-KENT Publishing Co, 1982, pp 435–438

15 Sanders BR, Ruvolo JF: Mock Clinic: An approach to clinical education. Phys Ther 61: 1163–1167, 1981

16 Bruner JS: Toward a Theory of Instruction. Cambridge, MA, Harvard University Press, 1966, p 53

17 Elstein AS, Shulman LS, Sprafka SA, et al: Medical Problem-Solving: An Analysis of Clinical Reasoning. Cambridge, MA, Harvard University Press, 1978, pp 273–302

18 Payton OD: Clinical reasoning process in physical therapy. Phys Ther 65:924–928, 1985

Problem-Solving Approach to Clinical Education

CAROLYN N. BURNETT,
PATRICK J. MAHONEY,
MARJORIE J. CHIDLEY,
and FRANK M. PIERSON

A problem-solving method to provide appropriate clinical learning experiences was developed for physical therapy students enrolled in their first year of professional course work. Clinicians from selected facilities were asked to participate in a clinical rotation over a two-quarter period. Using a problem-solving format, each clinician was responsible for a two-hour presentation relating to a disease or disability. Each rotation was repeated weekly for seven different groups of 10 students. During the rotation, the clinician presented a patient with a particular disability or disease and worked with the students to identify patient problems, establish treatment goals, and discuss methods used to achieve the goals. The difficulties encountered with the clinical experiences and the positive aspects of the experiences are discussed.

Key Words: Clinical competence, Physical therapy, Problem solving.

This article describes a series of structured clinical learning experiences that were developed for physical therapy students in their first year of professional course work at Ohio State University. A problem-solving format was used for the learning experiences. Before the development of these learning experiences, first-year students participated in clinical assignments that predominantly were assistive or observational. Clinicians in physical therapy practice settings served as preceptors.

Because of the large number of students and the limited number of clinical sites and preceptors, the academic faculty became interested in providing an experience that would serve as a common foundation for the treatment-oriented clinical affiliation during the second year. Faculty also were interested in improving the linkage and integration of classroom and clinical learning.

The problem-solving method was selected as the basis for the initial clinical experience because of its importance in the successful transfer of classroom information and skills to the clinical setting. Barr emphasized that transfer of information from one area to another is not automatic and complete unless teaching methods are used to facilitate it.[1] She also summarized, from several sources in the literature, that one of the benefits of the problem-solving method over more traditional methods of teaching appears to be a better application of knowledge to new situations. Barr defined problem solving as "a mental process whereby a person applies and/or transforms knowledge and understanding in order to arrive at a solution to a problem."[1]

Problem solving in physical therapy has been used as the basis for planning curricula or learning experiences in the classroom and clinical settings. May and Newman described a sequence of activities based on a behavioral model for improving problem-solving skills.[2] The sequence of activities (steps) used in the model was as follows: problem recognition, definition and analysis, data management, solution development and implementation, and outcome evaluation. In addition, the authors presented the problem-solver's cognitive, affective, and psychomotor behaviors for each step of the problem-solving process. A problem-solving model described by Olsen was used throughout an academic program as a teaching and evaluation tool.[3] Olsen's model was adapted from one described by Day to teach treatment program planning to occupational therapy students.[4] May described problem-solving clinical experiences in an integrated problem-solving curriculum that were initiated in the junior year and continued with increasing complexity throughout the curriculum.[5] That curriculum design seemed to enable students to understand interrelationships of content taught in different courses throughout the curriculum more effectively than in the traditional subject-oriented curriculum.

PLANNING

Clinicians from 12 clinical facilities were asked to participate in a series of patient-case presentations for the first-year students throughout the second and third quarters of their professional program. Each clinician was responsible for providing, through a problem-solving approach, a two-hour instructional presentation relating to a specific disease or disability. This presentation was to be repeated weekly for 7 different groups of 10 students so that each student attended 7 facilities each quarter. Clinicians from two of the facilities participated both quarters.

Academic faculty, in collaboration with the clinical faculty, determined which patient problems were to be studied during the clinical experience. Because the problem exercises the

Miss Burnett is Associate Professor, Division of Physical Therapy, School of Allied Medical Professions, Ohio State University, Columbus, OH 43210 (USA).

Mr. Mahoney is Instructor and Clinical Coordinator, Division of Physical Therapy, School of Allied Medical Professions, Ohio State University.

Mrs. Chidley is Staff Physical Therapist, Franklin County Board of Mental Retardation/Developmental Disabilities, Early Childhood Education Center, 2879 Johnstown Rd. Columbus, OH 43219. She was Program Specialist, Area Health Education Centers, Division of Physical Therapy, School of Allied Medical Professions, Ohio State University, at the time this approach was developed.

Mr. Pierson is Assistant Professor and Director, Division of Physical Therapy, School of Allied Medical Professions, Ohio State University.

This article was submitted May 28, 1985; was with the authors for revision 21 weeks; and was accepted March 5, 1986. Potential Conflict of Interest: 4.

clinicians developed included the process of problem solving and the content related to the problem, the clinicians were provided information about the course work the students had completed and were studying currently. Practical experience in solving real problems in the settings in which the problems occur is a learning activity that requires the use of all forms of content: specific facts and skills and basic ideas, concepts, and values.[1]

Related Course Work

During the first-quarter clinical experience, students had some knowledge of and skills in massage and techniques related to asepsis, basic transfer and assisted-ambulation activities, and active and passive exercise. Concurrent with their first problem-solving experience, they were developing knowledge of and skill in the use of therapeutic agents. During the second quarter of the problem-solving experience, they were gaining knowledge of and skill in the use of evaluation procedures that included muscle testing, goniometry, and screening for upper- and lower-extremity musculoskeletal conditions.

Objectives

The objectives of the clinical rotation for both quarters emphasized the problem-solving process. After successful completion of the clinical rotation sequence each quarter, the students would be able to
1. Describe the causes of the seven different disabilities and diseases selected for presentation.
2. List and describe the appropriate problems identified in the seven patients that would relate, directly or indirectly, to physical therapy intervention.
3. Discuss, in a group setting, the problems identified and establish realistic goals to solve or alleviate those problems.
4. Establish, with the assistance of the supervising clinician, an appropriate treatment program for the patients.
5. Discuss, in a group setting, factors other than direct patient treatment that would have an effect on the management of patients in that particular setting, such as health team interaction, physical setting, and facility philosophy.

Format

The problem-solving model developed for this clinical learning experience was a four-phase process:
A. Assess needs (determine the problem)
　1. Gather information
　2. Identify the problem areas
　3. Integrate the gathered information
B. Plan (design the solutions to the problems)
　1. Arrange the identified problems in the order of priority and list the potential solutions
　2. Determine the goals to resolve the identified problems
　3. Select alternative problem-solving strategies
　4. Determine action
　5. Select resources to implement the problems' solutions
　6. Determine how to observe and measure the effectiveness of the total plan
C. Implement (activate the plan)
　1. Apply or implement the plan using the selected solutions

D. Evaluate the plan (complete an outcome analysis of the implemented plan)
　1. Determine the effectiveness of the plan
　2. Determine the effectiveness of the problem-solving process

Guidelines

Guidelines for the two-hour session were established for the clinicians. The two-hour session was to be divided into different segments: 1) presentation of information that would enhance the students' understanding of the disability or disease of the patient being presented (overview), 2) demonstration of the patient's disability-disease characteristics and treatment program, and 3) problem solving by the students with the assistance of the clinical instructors. Any formal presentation of information was to be limited to 20 minutes and could be replaced by a less formal presentation of material throughout the patient demonstration and problem-solving periods. Each clinician was to determine the time required for the patient demonstration. Although a 30- to 45-minute demonstration was suggested, the clinicians were assured that even a 10-minute demonstration could be meaningful if problems that could be observed were emphasized. The clinicians were encouraged to allow communication between the patients and the students if it was appropriate for the specific patient and if the patient was willing.

The problem-solving component was considered to be the major purpose of the clinical experience, and the clinicians were requested to allow a minimum of 30 minutes for problem solving. Active participation by each student was to be emphasized.

IMPLEMENTATION

Facilities and Patient Conditions

The facilities used for the clinical rotations included general hospitals, a skilled nursing facility, a rehabilitation center, a children's hospital, a university-affiliated center, and a public school. Each setting and the patients' conditions are summarized in the Table.

TABLE
Patients Presented and the Facilities Used for the Problem-Solving Clinical Rotations

Setting	Patient Problem
General hospitals	low back pain
	periarthritis of shoulder
	knee problem
	total joint replacement
	myofascial pain syndrome
	sports injury
	myocardial infarct
Skilled nursing facility	hip fracture
Rehabilitation center	spinal cord injury
	cerebrovascular accident
	head trauma
Children's hospital	burn
	high-risk infant
University-affiliated center	Down syndrome
Public school	cerebral palsy

Role of the Academic Faculty Coordinator

The academic faculty coordinator of the clinical rotation experience provided preparatory information about the rotations to the students, assigned students to groups, arranged the rotation schedule, and assisted the participating clinicians to prepare for their presentations. The faculty coordinator accompanied a different student group each week to that group's clinical rotation site and returned to each site when a new clinician was the presenter. The faculty coordinator, in collaboration with the clinician, identified opportunities to improve the effectiveness of the experience.

Role of the Clinician

The clinician included in the two-hour clinical rotation a brief disability-disease overview and a summary of the patient's medical history. The patient was introduced to the students, who then had the opportunity to communicate with the patient and to observe the clinician identify signs and symptoms of the disease and demonstrate aspects of the physical therapy the patient was receiving. One clinical preceptor used a videotaped case study rather than an actual patient presentation. After the patient demonstration, each clinician was encouraged to assist the students in identifying problems of that patient, establishing goals, and discussing some of the therapeutic management techniques used to achieve the stated goals. The students were required to evaluate the experience at the end of the two-hour session by completing a prepared evaluation form. These forms were reviewed then by the faculty coordinator, and feedback was given to the clinician.

DISCUSSION

The clinical rotations provided consistency for the early clinical experiences for 70 first-year physical therapy students. Students had the opportunity to apply, in various clinical settings, a problem-solving process that focused on selected patient disabilities. Each student, throughout the two-quarter period, observed patients with similar disabilities. The clinical rotation also solved the problem of assigning a large number of students to a limited number of facilities and preceptors.

At the conclusion of each rotation, the students responded to three questions on a facility-appraisal form. Students were asked whether the clinical experience met the stated clinical objectives; whether the clinical rotation problem-solving format was followed; and whether the clinical supervisor encouraged group participation, with interaction between the students and the clinical supervisor to identify problems, goals, and programs. A majority (95%-99%) of the responses to the three questions indicated strong agreement or agreement with the statements. Clinicians also were positive in their assessment of the rotations as evidenced by their enthusiasm to participate in the experience.

Evaluation of the clinical learning experience to determine whether it optimized the application of classroom learning to the clinical setting and to patient care was not accomplished directly. The students, however, did have two opportunities to demonstrate their problem-solving abilities in writing. Each time, they were provided with a case history and were asked to use the problem-solving format to identify and arrange problems by priority, provide a rationale for the development

of goals, and indicate appropriate therapeutic intervention. Careful review and critique of the written exercises by the academic faculty coordinator provided feedback to the students about their abilities to use the problem-solving process in solving a simulated case study problem. The written exercises were designed primarily as learning experiences for the students, as opposed to an evaluation of their abilities for the designation of a grade. Some students demonstrated excellent critical thinking and application of the problem-solving process to simulated patient problems. Other students were not as accomplished in their problem-solving abilities, but they were able to demonstrate basic problem-solving skills.

Olsen's use of a problem-solving model throughout the curriculum emphasized the importance of students justifying or explaining their treatment decisions in writing or orally.[3] Our students, also, were asked to justify or explain their treatment decisions in their written exercises. Olsen, however, also used problem solving for evaluation, but this was not a major objective of our written exercise. May reported that therapists who supervised students from both the problem-oriented curriculum and the traditional subject-oriented programs indicated that students from the problem-oriented curriculum were less afraid to cope with new situations and were better able to identify and analyze complex problems. The same clinicians also stated that the problem-oriented curriculum enabled students to understand interrelationships of content taught in different courses in a more effective manner than the students in the more traditional subject-oriented curriculum.[5]

Because the faculty coordinator of the clinical rotation experience visited each facility and observed each presentation once during the quarter, she was able to identify and assess apparent benefits and problems of the experiences. These outcomes were discussed with each participating clinician. When the clinicians initially participated in the problem-solving experiences, they often were more content-oriented than process-oriented. This orientation was reflected by several events:

1. The clinician's comments about the specific characteristics of the disease sometimes were lengthy and presented formally in lecture format. Several clinicians thought that presenting all the necessary information in the two-hour session was difficult.
2. The clinicians did not encourage active participation by the students sufficiently.
3. The clinicians did not always allot an adequate amount of time for problem solving and frequently did not proceed past problem identification.

The clinicians, however, were receptive to suggestions by the faculty coordinator for improving the problem-solving sessions. With few exceptions, the clinicians who were content-oriented initially changed the experience in future sessions to allow for more student participation and more emphasis on problem solving.

Several positive aspects of the clinical rotation experience were noted by the faculty coordinator:

1. It provided a small group interactional experience for students who were part of a large physical therapy program.
2. It provided students an opportunity to practice a guided logical thought process that was designed to improve problem-solving skills.

3. It provided a foundation for treatment program planning and evaluation.
4. It provided an environment that allowed for immediate feedback to questions.
5. It provided the opportunity to observe the clinician's expertise. Most of the clinicians were outstanding when interacting with the patients. The clinicians served as excellent role models for the students.
6. The clinicians had the opportunity to develop instructional skills.
7. The students had an opportunity to communicate with the patients about aspects of their lives that did not relate directly to physical therapy but that were necessary to understand the patient's problems fully.
8. By exploring alternative forms of treatment, the students began to appreciate that there are few treatment absolutes and that several alternatives may exist for solving problems.

IMPLICATIONS

The need is growing to educate physical therapists to be problem solvers in diverse situations and environments. Although several educators have illustrated the use of problem solving in physical therapy curricula, the text *Clinical Decision Making in Physical Therapy* provides a clear mandate and guide for teaching the process of scientific inquiry through problem solving.[6] Hislop emphasized that developing educational experiences for clinical problem solving and clinical judgment is possible, so that scientific thinking will occur in the clinical setting.[7] She suggested that educators need to use more clinical role models from the practicing professional community to teach physical therapy students. Hislop views clinicians as tutorial directors of small groups of students in a patient care environment; as demonstrators in clinical skill laboratories on the campus; or as teachers of the process of patient evaluation, program planning, and treatment.[7] The clinicians responsible for the problem-solving rotations we discussed had an opportunity to participate as Hislop recommended.

CONCLUSION

Use of the problem-solving method to structure a clinical experience for first-year physical therapy students has been described. During the clinical problem-solving experience, a patient case study that related to a specific diagnosis was presented weekly to seven groups of 10 students. These students participated, with the help of a clinician, in identifying problems related to a specific patient, setting goals, and determining alternative treatment plans. Although no statistical data were collected to demonstrate that the problem-solving skills of the students improved by using this educational model instead of a more traditional model of clinical experience, students and clinicians reported the experiences were worthwhile.

Acknowledgment. We are grateful for the participation of the clinicians without whom these learning experiences could not have occurred.

REFERENCES

1. Barr JS: A Problem-Solving Curriculum Design in Physical Therapy. Doctoral Dissertation. Chapel Hill, NC, University of North Carolina, 1975, pp 27–48, 61–71, 86–91
2. May BJ, Newman J: Developing competence in problem solving: A behavioral model. Phys Ther 60:1140–1145, 1980
3. Olsen SL: Teaching treatment planning: A problem-solving model. Phys Ther 63:526–529, 1983
4. Day D: A systems diagram for teaching treatment planning. Am J Occup Ther 27:239–243, 1973
5. May BJ: An integrated problem-solving curriculum design for physical therapy education. Phys Ther 57:807–813, 1977
6. Wolf SL (ed): Clinical Decision Making in Physical Therapy. Philadelphia, PA, F A Davis, 1985
7. Hislop HJ: Clinical decision making: Educational, data, and risk factors. In Wolf SL (ed): Clinical Decision Making in Physical Therapy. Philadelphia, PA, FA Davis Co, 1985, pp 25–60

Identifying Problems in Clinical Problem Solving

Perceptions and Interventions with Nonproblem-Solving Clinical Behaviors

JILL NEWMAN HENRY

Students and practicing physical therapists are expected to be clinical problem solvers. The absence of clinical problem solving may result in decreased individuality of patient services. The purpose of this article is to assist clinical supervisors in identifying specific difficulties in clinical problem solving and to clarify confusions in the supervisor's perception of the problem-solving behaviors of students and therapists. I present a model by comparing the behaviors of the problem solver with the behaviors of the nonproblem solver at each step in the problem-solving process and then discuss sources of confusion in the perception of problem solving. I provide examples and suggest applications of the model for improving clinical problem-solving abilities.

Key Words: *Clinical competence, Education, Problem solving.*

The ability to problem solve has been described as an integral part of physical therapy practice.[1] Recent articles have detailed the steps and behaviors of clinical problem solving in physical therapy.[1,2] The behaviors of someone who is not problem solving or who is perceived not to be problem solving reflect the other side of the coin. I assume that all students and graduates of physical therapy programs are capable of problem solving. To survive from day to day in this complex world requires problem solving. What then limits use of problem-solving abilities in clinical settings? What are students and therapists doing when they are not problem solving? How is the individuality of patient-care services decreased when problem solving is limited or absent?

The purpose of this article is to answer these questions by closely examining the negative side of problem solving—its absence. Comparing clinical behaviors of the nonproblem solver with behaviors previously identified as problem solving will help specify the nature of the problem-solving difficulty.[1] Examining sources of confusion in the perception of problem solving will help the supervisor determine what type of problem exists. Further analysis of the absence of problem solving will assist the clinical supervisor in helping students or physi-

Ms. Henry is Assistant Professor and Academic Coordinator of Clinical Education. Department of Physical Therapy. Medical College of Georgia. Augusta, GA 30912 (USA).

This article was submitted February 21, 1984; was with the author for revision 15 weeks; and was accepted January 29, 1985.

cal therapists develop more consistent problem-solving skills.

BEHAVIORS OF THE NONPROBLEM SOLVER

The following is a fictitious case study of a student who is not using her clinical problem-solving abilities. Jane is a student who has successfully completed all her didactic course work and is on a clinical affiliation. Jane states that she does not like to treat a patient unless she has observed someone treating the same patient first. She often is unable to select appropriate evaluation procedures and prefers to evaluate patients when she can use one of the data-base protocols for evaluation developed by the department staff. Jane can plan general treatments for her patients but has few ideas of what to do if her patients are unable to participate in those treatments. Jane cares for patients very much and wants to be a good therapist to them. What are Jane's difficulties in problem solving? How can Jane's supervisor help Jane overcome her difficulties in problem solving?

BEHAVIORS OF THE NONPROBLEM-SOLVING STUDENT

The left-hand column in the Appendix summarizes the model of behaviors of the problem solver published by May and me.[1] The right-hand column identifies behaviors I have observed for students and therapists who are not problem solving. At each problem stage, the behaviors of the nonproblem solver will be discussed in relation to performance

in a clinical setting. Jane's case study will be used to illustrate a supervisor's application of the model.

Problem Presented

The nonproblem solver will not recognize a problem when it is presented. A person's ability to recognize problems depends on knowledge and experience background. A therapist who has not worked with children before may not initially recognize that parental overprotection may be a problem with a child who is relearning how to walk. By the time of graduation, students are expected to be able to recognize most patient problems. Initially in the course of student education, problem solving may not begin because the student was unable to recognize that a problem existed. Jane's inability to select appropriate evaluation procedures may be caused, in part, by a lack of experience or knowledge about certain types of patient dysfunctions. If Jane does not know that a patient who has chest congestion may have decreased ambulatory endurance because of a lack of oxygen exchange, she may not recognize chest congestion as a problem. Jane's supervisor may need to help Jane review her knowledge specific to cardiopulmonary dysfunction and its effects on endurance and ambulation.

Problem Defined

The nonproblem solver will have difficulty recognizing the scope of the problem. This difficulty is usually related to the student's or therapist's inability to view the patient as a whole entity composed of different systems. The student may tend to focus on only the physical aspects of the patient's problems and neglect the psychosocial and physiological problems resulting from physical disability. This lack of problem definition will influence later problem-solving processes.

In Jane's case, part of the ability to define a patient's problem requires reviewing all patient systems before deciding on evaluation techniques. Jane must recognize the effects of the pulmonary system on the musculoskeletal system. If Jane judges prematurely that her role as a physical therapist is to evaluate musculoskeletal function, not pulmonary function, Jane will be unable to recognize the scope of the problem. Jane's supervisor must discover, by questioning, whether Jane is viewing the patient as a whole entity or simply in terms of the musculoskeletal system.

Problem Analyzed

The nonproblem solver often skips this step entirely or judges the nature of the problem before collecting objective data. Instead of analyzing the components of the problem, the student or therapist jumps right into solution development. An example of this thought process is, "This patient has back pain. I read that heat was good for back pain. I'll give the patient a hot pack." The problem is solved before the therapist has discovered what the problem is. The solution is efficient, but not individualized to a patient's unique set of circumstances.

Jane's treatment plans, which are general instead of specific, may indicate her lack of problem analysis. If Jane determines that a patient has shoulder pain, she may decide that heat and exercise will help. If she had analyzed the problem of shoulder pain and selected appropriate evaluation techniques, she might have found that the pain was due to restriction of the inferior glenohumeral capsule and that ultrasound to that region followed by mobilization would be the most effective and individualized treatment. When Jane's supervisor realizes that Jane's treatment plans are usually general, the supervisor receives a clue that Jane may have an analysis problem. The supervisor must verify the existence of a problem in the analysis area by asking Jane to detail the components of the patient's problem and

explain the relationships that exist between the components. If Jane were analyzing the case by problem solving, the supervisor would expect Jane to say, "The patient's shoulder pain may be coming from several structures: the cervical spinal column, the muscles, the bursa, the capsule. In my evaluation, I need to check out all these areas before I can determine appropriate treatments."

Therapists tend to use their analytical abilities to a greater extent with patients who are unfamiliar to them or who display unusual signs and symptoms. The patient who presents a familiar picture often receives a routine treatment. Analysis takes time and the process may be eliminated in day-to-day routine patient care.

Data Collected

The major behavior of the nonproblem solver is to search for standardized evaluation protocols. Because the student or the therapist has not discovered in earlier steps what to look for, the student or therapist relies on a protocol to outline what to do. A nonproblem solver may be perceived as a great patient evaluator if told specifically enough what data to collect. One dilemma today in clinical education is how to provide the student with opportunities to select evaluation procedures and, yet, how to comply with the completion of standardized patient data base and evaluation forms. Completion of a form does not indicate either the presence or absence of problem solving. It simply indicates the student's ability to follow instructions. The problem solvers were the therapists who developed the original protocols. One department of physical therapy I know asks each student to develop his own evaluation protocol before he views those that exist in the department. In this way, the supervisor views the student's problem-solving abilities and the student receives feedback by comparing what he created with what the department uses. The data collection step is the first place the supervisor can observe the student's problem-solving abilities. The previous three steps are internal thought processes, and the supervisor can only discover through questioning what the student or therapist is thinking. Jane's preference for protocols may indicate difficulties in problem solving.

Solution Developed

The nonproblem solver cannot come up with unique and creative solutions. The student or therapist has not discovered what the problem is and so cannot identify a solution to resolve it. Even the person who has been problem solving may have difficulty in this situation. A tendency exists to separate evaluations from treatments. The nonproblem solver may think, "Whew, the evaluation is over; now what do I do for a patient with a fractured hip?" instead of thinking, "Mr. Jones has a fractured right hip, has pain on movement of his right leg, has an open wound at the surgical site, and lives on the third floor of a building with no elevator." The first thought is too general to develop anything but standardized treatments to resolve it. The second thought allows the student to think of possible treatments for each aspect of the problem. The student who generates general and nonspecific thoughts about goals and treatments either has not identified all the problems or has analyzed them but then disregarded the data. Jane's difficulty with problem analysis is reconfirmed here. Her treatments are general because she was unable to select her own appropriate evaluation techniques based on previous analysis of the problem. An additional clue to difficulty in this area is Jane's preference for treating patients only after she has observed someone else treating them first. If Jane has separated evaluations from treatments in her thinking, she must focus on how someone else would treat the patient to develop ideas of how she should treat the patient. The supervisor's major strategy to help Jane at this point is to refocus Jane's thinking on the evaluation data and away from how someone else would treat the patient.

Solution Implemented

The nonproblem solver may be able to implement a treatment correctly but probably will not be able to modify it. Modification requires an understanding of details and how one component of a problem influences another. The problem solver, however, has collected all the data necessary to individualize and modify treatments to a particular patient's unique combination of problems.

The solution implementation step is the second place the supervisor can observe the student's problem-solving abilities. Jane's lack of ideas of what to do when patients cannot participate in the treatment programs as planned reflects this inability to modify. A single goal can be achieved in many ways. If Jane's goal for the patient was to increase upper extremity strength in preparation for ambulation with assistive devices and her solution of treatment with weights did not work, she could substitute with other programs such as exercises with tubing, sitting push-ups, or manual resistive exercises. The supervisor's intervention can help Jane reanalyze the problem and specify clearly the goals and treatment options for each different patient.

Outcome Reevaluated

The nonproblem solver is unable to relate the actual outcome to the desired outcome because the student or therapist never had a clear idea of what was desired. If the original problem is never identified, the student or therapist must be told by someone else which aspects of the problem have been solved and which need further work. Because Jane has not completed the problem-solving steps, the supervisor expects Jane to have difficulty in this area. The supervisor can help Jane establish specific goals for the treatment based on thorough problem analysis and data collection. Once Jane clearly understands the nature of the patient's problem and the expected outcome of treatment, reevaluation becomes a matter of collecting data for comparison with the original patient evaluation.

In Jane's case study, Jane's supervisor has used the model in the Appendix to help Jane become aware of barriers that have blocked problem solving or the aspects of problem solving that have not been used. This awareness allows Jane to look at patient problems with a new understanding of self and responsibilities. Jane then can practice skill development in weak areas and gradually improve overall performance in the problem-solving process.

SOURCES OF CONFUSION IN THE PERCEPTION OF PROBLEM SOLVING

I have discussed problem solving with the assumption that the student or therapist is trying to problem solve but using inappropriate thought or action processes. At times, problem solving may

occur but not be perceived by the supervisor. At other times, the environment may prevent a student or therapist from initiating problem solving. Both situations may cause confusion for the supervisor in perceptions of problem solving. Bevis has reported four types of problems that elicit different responses in the problem solver.[3] Each type of problem will be discussed in relation to the problem solver's response and the supervisor's perceptions of that response.

Type One: Obscure Goal

In this first type of problem, the problem solver sets out to solve a problem without a clear goal in mind. The problem solver then generates multiple alternative solutions, but none seem consistent with each other. The supervisor may perceive that the therapist is "grasping at straws" and not able to problem solve. A stalemate will occur until both the therapist and the supervisor identify clearly the goal of the problem situation. The problem is not in the therapist's ability to solve problems but in the therapist's inability to identify the goal. Once the goal becomes clear, the problem solver will be able to demonstrate problem-solving abilities.

Type Two: Multiple Alternative Pathways to One Goal

One problem can be resolved many different ways. The supervisor naturally is pleased when the therapist chooses the alternative to solve the problem that the supervisor would have chosen. The supervisor may be more disconcerted if the therapist chooses an alternative that the supervisor had never considered or had used and discarded. New therapists may say that they could not do something their own way because the supervisor said, "But we don't do it that way here." A supervisor is not unreasonable in expecting a therapist to adhere to departmental standards. The difficulty comes if the supervisor perceives that the therapist is not problem solving because the therapist did not choose the same alternative as the supervisor.

Type Three: Barrier Between the Problem Solver and the Goal

Fear and anxiety are the greatest emotional barriers to problem solving. "What if I make a mistake?" and "What

if I do it wrong?" are thoughts every student has about a clinical affiliation. A clinical instructor may strengthen or weaken the anxiety barriers by the way that she interacts with the student. Rapid-fire questioning and putting students on the spot to "think on their feet" will decrease the students' ability to problem solve. Problem solving takes time and occurs most naturally in a punishment-free environment. If the assumption is that most students can problem solve, then the environment must be analyzed for barriers before the clinical instructor judges the student's problem-solving abilities.

In Jane's case, Jane cared very much about patients. An emotional barrier was created when Jane became afraid to do anything wrong, anything that might not let her be a good therapist. Jane felt she had to do what others did and would not trust her own problem-solving abilities to be a good therapist.

Type Four: Multiple Goals

The final type of problem is best explained by a story. Some years ago, a senior physical therapy student was on affiliation in a rehabilitation center. The student had assumed the clinical instructor's caseload. All the patients had been evaluated initially by the clinical instructor before the student arrived. The student's goal was to provide treatment consistent with what the clinical instructor had planned. The student was concerned about the effect on the patients of dramatically changing the treatments, but the clinical instructor's goal was for the student to show creativity and variety in treatments. The student worked hard on solving the problem of treating patients the way the instructor would have treated them. The instructor became frustrated at the perceived lack of problem-solving skills the student demonstrated. The instructor's initial conclusion was that the student was unable to problem solve. Once it was identified that the student was problem solving, but toward a different goal, the student's true problem-solving abilities were seen.

These examples illustrate that the student or therapist may be problem solving, but the supervisor may not perceive the approach as problem solving. A student or therapist may also be unable to use problem-solving abilities effectively in a clinical situation.

APPLICATIONS

The model in the Appendix was developed for and is being used in remediating the clinical performance problems of students. By the time students participate in full-time clinical affiliations, they have usually acquired the necessary knowledge and skills for physical therapy practice. Students have also developed problem-solving abilities to cope with everyday life situations. The students I work with in remediation have difficulty using problem-solving abilities in clinical settings. I use the model to increase student's self-awareness of what they do when they problem solve and what they may be doing in a clinical setting instead of problem solving. Students in clinical remediation in past years have gained insight into their problem-solving abilities and limitations by using this model. The students use the model in various ways. Some have written down their thoughts and developed elaborate diagrams of components of patient's problems and their relationships. The diagrams appear similar to computer-programmed simulations depicting "if . . . then" situations. "*If* a patient has pulmonary problems, *then* I will expect a decreased endurance and need to evaluate the patient for that." Some students are able theoretically to problem solve without difficulty, but they are reported by clinical supervisors to be nonproblem solvers. In these cases, the types of problems reported by Bevis[3] become a useful tool to determine why theoretical problem solving is not carried over into practice.

During the past several years, I have presented the model and ideas in this article to physical therapists in departmental in-services and clinical instructor workshops. I have received the following responses: "Yes, I see that in my students." "Oh, I see that in myself." "I'm going to use the model in my staff development program." A problem-solving physical therapist is expected to provide individualized patient care. Recognition of what we do when we are not problem solving permits further development of our problem-solving abilities. As a clinician, I find times when I do not problem solve. I believe that in providing the most individualized and effective care for the total patient, I am using problem-solving abilities to their fullest. The model and ideas presented in this article provide the structure necessary to facilitate the correction of deficits and the freedom to use problem-solving abilities in new ways.

SUMMARY

This article presented a model that compared the behaviors of the nonproblem solver with the behaviors of the problem solver.[1] I used a fictitious case study to apply the model to a clinical situation. I described student behaviors and supervisor interventions and discussed sources of confusion in the supervisor's perception of problem solving. The model and ideas presented are useful in developing student and therapist self-awareness to improve problem-solving skills and, therefore, increase the individuality of patient-care service.

REFERENCES

1. May BJ, Newman J: Developing competence in problem solving: A behavioral model. Phys Ther 60:1140–1145, 1980
2. Olsen SL: Teaching treatment planning: A problem-solving model. Phys Ther 63:526–529, 1983
3. Bevis EO: Curriculum Building in Nursing: A Process. St. Louis, MO, CV Mosby Co, 1978, pp 72–103

APPENDIX
Comparison between behaviors of problem solver and nonproblem solver at each stage of the problem-solving process.

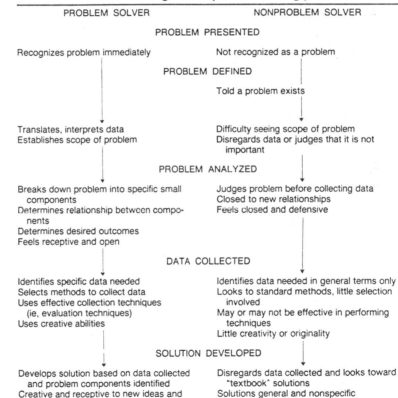

PROBLEM SOLVER	NONPROBLEM SOLVER
PROBLEM PRESENTED	
Recognizes problem immediately	Not recognized as a problem
PROBLEM DEFINED	
	Told a problem exists
Translates, interprets data	Difficulty seeing scope of problem
Establishes scope of problem	Disregards data or judges that it is not important
PROBLEM ANALYZED	
Breaks down problem into specific small components	Judges problem before collecting data
Determines relationship between components	Closed to new relationships
Determines desired outcomes	Feels closed and defensive
Feels receptive and open	
DATA COLLECTED	
Identifies specific data needed	Identifies data needed in general terms only
Selects methods to collect data	Looks to standard methods, little selection involved
Uses effective collection techniques (ie, evaluation techniques)	May or may not be effective in performing techniques
Uses creative abilities	Little creativity or originality
SOLUTION DEVELOPED	
Develops solution based on data collected and problem components identified	Disregards data collected and looks toward "textbook" solutions
Creative and receptive to new ideas and relationships	Solutions general and nonspecific
SOLUTION IMPLEMENTED	
Applies solution effectively	Solution implemented correctly, but little modification seen
Able to modify and adapt solutions to new data	Unable to make direct connection between solution and problem
OUTCOME REEVALUATED	
Relates actual outcome to desired outcome	Unable to relate actual outcome to desired outcome because never had a clear idea of what outcome was desired
Recognized components of original problem that have been solved and those that need further attention	Must be told what aspects have been solved and which need further work

Developing Competence in Problem Solving

A Behavioral Model

BELLA J. MAY, EdD,
and JILL NEWMAN, BS

Problem solving is an integral part of effective physical therapy practice. A model depicting the behaviors of the problem solver while solving problems is presented. The behaviors are related to each step in the problem-solving process and to cognitive, affective, and psychomotor functions of individuals. Guidelines for using the model in didactic and clinical activities are presented.

Key Words: *Cognition, Education, Thinking.*

Problem solving is an integral part of effective physical therapy practice as well as of everyday life. Even though people start solving problems almost from birth and continue throughout life, they rarely give the process thought. Individuals vary in their problem-solving styles: some are quite systematic, working through problems with step-by-step regularity; others appear to find solutions by intuition. Some individuals vary their approach with different types of problems, using a systematic approach for those problems requiring planning and organization, then using a trial-and-error approach for the more elusive problems.[1] Students enter physical therapy curricula with a developed approach to problem solving and unconsciously use that approach in solving problems related to physical therapy practice with varying degrees of success. If the student is able to solve the problems satisfactorily, little thought or consideration is given to the process. However, if the student encounters difficulty, the instructor is faced with the task of helping the student develop effective problem-solving skills to use in physical therapy practice. The purpose of this paper is to present a model for improving problem-solving skills in the classroom and the clinic.

Dr. May is Professor and Chairperson, Department of Physical Therapy, Medical College of Georgia, Augusta, GA 30912.

Ms. Newman is Academic Coordinator of Clinical Education and Instructor, Department of Physical Therapy, Medical College of Georgia.

This article was submitted August 13, 1979, and accepted December 31, 1979.

DEFINITIONS

The term *problem* is defined as "A stimulus situation for which an organism does not have a ready response."[2] What may be a problem for a young child may not be a problem for an adult. Determining the answer to "2 + 2" may be a problem the first time it is encountered, but it ceases to be a problem once the answer is learned. Discovering how to turn on a diathermy machine may be a problem the first time, but it does not remain a problem long, whereas determining the physical therapy needs of a patient with rheumatoid arthritis may be a problem with each new patient.

Problem solving can be defined as the process of finding a solution to the problem. Problem solving is primarily an internal and sequential process that includes cognitive, affective, and psychomotor behaviors.

Cognitive behaviors are intellectual activities, or thinking processes. These behaviors have been classified as thought processes, from simple to complex; they range from the ability to recall facts, through the ability to apply facts to new and different situations, to the most complex ability of making judgments and placing concepts in priority order[3] (Fig. 1).

Affective behaviors are emotional responses—attitudes and feelings. Affective behaviors range from the simple act of responding emotionally to a stimulus, through the more complex act of developing values, to the most complex act of categorizing one's value system[4] (Fig. 2).

Psychomotor behaviors are physical actions that range from the simple act of perceiving objects by touch or smell, through the more complex ability of performing habitual learned responses, to the most complex ability of creating new motor acts[5] (Fig. 3).

A *learning* experience is an activity or series of activities that lead to a change in behavior. A planned learning experience leads to a change of behavior in a predetermined desired direction. A learning experience is not usually limited to a single class, laboratory session, or clinical session but may include a series of such sessions. Throughout the paper, this entire definition of learning experience will be used.

THE PROBLEM-SOLVING MODEL

The problem-solving model in physical therapy is a tool to guide the individual in making, implementing, and evaluating decisions related to some aspect of physical therapy practice. As a tool, the process must be understandable and applicable to the prob-

---

1.0 KNOWLEDGE
Recall of specifics, universals, methods, patterns
2.0 COMPREHENSION
Lowest level of understanding
3.0 APPLICATION
Use of knowledge in a new situation
4.0 ANALYSIS
Breakdown of communication into constituent elements
5.0 SYNTHESIS
Putting together of elements to form a whole
6.0 EVALUATION
Making judgments on quantitative and qualitative bases

Fig. 1. *The Cognitive Domain, referring to intellectual abilities and skills.*

lems for which it is used. In developing the model described in this paper, the authors combined problem-solving and decision-making processes to delineate a sequence of activities that seems to encompass most situations in physical therapy. The sequence of activities used in the model is

1. Problem recognition
2. Problem definition
3. Problem analysis
4. Data management
5. Solution development
6. Solution implementation
7. Outcome evaluation

This sequence of activities was taught to students as a guide to help them improve their problem-solving skills. Some students were able to use the sequence to solve classroom and clinical problems with relative ease, whereas others encountered difficulty. The sequence was not detailed enough to help all students

---

1.0 RECEIVING
Awareness of the existence of emotional stimuli
2.0 RESPONDING
Willingness to pay attention and respond to emotional stimuli
3.0 VALUING
Consistent and stable responses to certain emotional stimuli
4.0 ORGANIZATION
Internalization and placing values in priority order
5.0 CHARACTERIZATION
Control of behavior by value system

Fig. 2. *The Affective Domain, referring to feelings, emotions, or degree of acceptance or rejection.*

develop effective problem-solving skills in physical therapy. To determine areas in which students encountered difficulty with the problem-solving sequence and to help students improve their problem-solving skills, the authors analyzed the problem-solving process to determine the cognitive, affective, and psychomotor behaviors in each step of the problem-solving sequence. A model was developed depicting the major behaviors expected of the individual as he goes through each step in the sequence of activities in the problem-solving process. The major thinking, feeling, and physical behaviors associated with each step in problem solving were outlined, and this delineation has been used to help students discover areas of difficulty. The model has also been used to plan and implement classroom and clinical learning experiences designed to help students improve their problem-solving skills.

The Table portrays the model and includes the major cognitive, affective, and psychomotor behaviors involved in each step of the sequence. The list of behaviors is not all-inclusive, nor do all people necessarily perform all behaviors to solve every problem encountered. Although the categories appear to be

---

1.0 PERCEPTION
Awareness of objects, qualities, or relations from sensory input
2.0 SET
Preparatory adjustment or readiness for action
3.0 GUIDED RESPONSE
Overt behavioral act following a model
4.0 MECHANISM
Learned response has become habitual
5.0 COMPLEX OVERT RESPONSE
Performance of complicated movement patterns
6.0 ADAPTATION
Alteration of motor activities to meet new situations
7.0 ORIGINATION
Creation of new motor acts

Fig. 3. *The Psychomotor Domain, referring to muscular or motor skills.*

TABLE

Behaviors of the Problem Solver in the Problem-Solving Process[a]

Process	Cognitive Domain	Affective Domain	Psychomotor Domain
Problem recognition	Realize that there is a problem	Be aware of own feelings of unease (constructive discontent)	Perceive sensory stimuli (auditory, visual, taste, tactile, smell, kinesthesia)
Problem definition	Translate and interpret all input received Establish problem boundary	Be aware of response sets Be willing to defer judgment	Perceive sensory stimuli and environmental input
Problem analysis	Break down the cognitive, affective, and psychomotor components of the problem Determine the relationships between elements Organize the principles involved Determine desired outcome	Be willing to defer judgment Be receptive to new relationships Be aware of own response sets Feel satisfaction	Perform habitual tasks related to thinking (write, pace, chew, read)
Data management Data-collection methods selection	Identify data needed Relate data to data-collection methods Select data-collection methods	Be receptive to new approaches Be aware of response sets Be willing to use creative abilities	Perform habitual tasks related to thinking (listen, read, write)
Data collection	Apply data-collection methods	Respond appropriately to internal and external cues Be aware of response sets	Perform appropriate complex overt responses
Solution development Data analysis	Organize data collected Classify data collected	Be aware of own response set Be willing to defer judgment	Perform habitual tasks related to thinking (read, pace, write)

discrete, in practice the behaviors from the cognitive, affective, and psychomotor areas influence each other both within each step and between steps. The words used to describe the specific cognitive, affective, and psychomotor behaviors for each step in the sequence of problem-solving activity were carefully selected to reflect the type of behavior related to the domain of function. A brief discussion will clarify the meaning of the words used and the relationships between domains.

Problem recognition is the first step in the problem-solving process. Before one can begin to solve a problem one must recognize that a problem actually exists. Recognizing that a problem exists usually requires that the individual respond to sensory perceptions and feelings of unease and translate these feelings into the cognitive recognition that there is a

problem. In situations in which the problem is given, this step is eliminated.

The second step, *problem definition*, requires that the person define the limit of the problem. The cognitive activity of translating and interpreting the stimuli coming in through all the senses from the environment is facilitated by the problem solver's attitude toward problem solving. An individual who has a positive attitude toward problem solving will usually be willing to defer judgment and work through the problem. Past experiences may influence a person's attitude toward problem solving and his willingness to defer judgment. Although making a quick decision and ending the problem-solving process at the beginning of the sequence may be a solution, it may lead to ineffective problem solving and an inappropriate solution. In this and the next several steps, the prob-

TABLE—*continued*

Process	Cognitive Domain	Affective Domain	Psychomotor Domain
	Relate data collected to problem components and desired outcome	Be willing to use creative abilities Be receptive to new relationships Feel satisfaction	
Alternative solution determination	Synthesize data into a series of alternatives related to the desired outcome	Seek out new ideas as beneficial to self Be willing to use creative abilities	Perform habitual tasks related to thinking (listen, pace, chew)
Solution selection	Evaluate all solutions and place in priority order Make judgment in terms of desired outcome	Be willing to make a decision Be aware of own ego Desire to be creative Feel satisfaction	Perform habitual tasks related to thinking (read, observe, pace)
Solution implementation	Apply solution to problem	Respond positively to risk taking Exhibit self-confidence Respond to internal and external cues Be willing to use creative abilities Feel satisfaction	Perform appropriate complex overt responses
Outcome evaluation	Relate actual outcomes to desired outcome	Be aware of own ego Be aware of own response set Be willing to respond objectively	Perform habitual tasks related to thinking (observe, listen, read)

[a] Copyright 1978, May and Newman.

lem-solving process can be aborted if the individual makes premature judgments.

The third step, *problem analysis*, is a very important part of effective problem solving. The analytical process is aided or hindered by the problem solver's emotional set, willingness to defer judgment, and willingness to discover new relationships between elements of a problem. The thinking behaviors include organizing all of the elements in the problem, determining relationships between elements, and beginning to outline desired outcomes. People generally perform physical actions while thinking. These physical activities may include doodling, pacing, drinking coffee, or writing notes. Although it may seem irrelevant to consider individuals' physical activities that may be related to thinking, many people have developed a strong association between habitual physical activities and intense thinking. The need to perform such physical activities may depend on the complexity of the problem and the degree to which solutions are or are not known. Recognition of the association between psychomotor and cognitive activities may help an individual become a more effective problem solver, partially through increased self-awareness.

Data management has been divided into two substeps, *data-collection methods selection* and *data collection*. Once the problem has been fully analyzed, the individual identifies the data needed to solve the problem, reviews the various methods of collecting data, relates the methods to the data needed, and selects the appropriate data-collection methods. The effectiveness of the cognitive processes involved in selecting appropriate data-collection methods is affected by the problem solver's willingness to find new approaches to data collection. The physical activities performed continue to be the individual's habitual tasks related to thinking.

Data collection includes remembering information previously obtained and gathering new data by reading, applying evaluative procedures, or talking with another individual. The psychomotor activities depend on the problem and the particular data-collection methods. The physical tasks may include manipulating tools, moving body parts, or pushing buttons on computers. Affectively, the person must respond to both internal and external cues. If the data collection involves interactions with another person, the individual's emotional response to that person may affect the accuracy of the data collected. Awareness of his own tendencies in responding to others and to different situations will help the problem solver be more accurate in data collection.

Solution development is divided into three substeps: *data analysis, alternative solution determination*, and *solution selection*. The process of data analysis is similar to problem analysis. Developing a list of alternative solutions and selecting the one solution that is most likely to succeed require complex cognitive functions as well as an affective willingness to be creative and to defer judgment. Physically, the person continues to perform those habitual tasks that enhance thinking. Developing alternative solutions requires that the individual take all the gathered data, organize them, and form them into a list of solutions. Intellectually, developing alternative solutions is the process of synthesis, the putting together of parts or elements to form a whole. Selecting the most appropriate solution requires the problem solver to evaluate each potential solution and make a judgment. The interrelationship between affective and cognitive function continues as the person's ability to develop and use high-level thinking skills is influenced by the degree of satisfaction he feels during the process. Previous positive experiences increase the likelihood that he will feel satisfaction and will desire to be creative in problem solving.

Solution implementation, like data collection, may require a variety of physical activities, depending on the problem and the solution. In physical therapy clinical practice, solution implementation will usually include the application of various treatment procedures that require complex overt psychomotor responses. Cognitively, the person is applying concepts to a situation. Affectively, his implementing a solution requires a willingness to take a chance. The degree of risk may be quite high in physical therapy if the solution involves making a decision that affects another human being. Emotionally, implementing the solution requires a degree of self-confidence, the awareness to respond to cues from oneself and the environment, and the ability to feel satisfaction in problem solving.

The final step, *outcome evaluation*, requires that the person relate the actual outcome to the desired outcome and determine the effectiveness of the problem-solving process. Affectively, evaluating the outcome of the problem-solving process requires that the individual have enough self-awareness and objectivity to determine the adequacy of the solution.

APPLYING THE MODEL

Instructors and students may apply the problem-solving model to all aspects of planning, implementing, and evaluating learning experiences in the classroom or clinic. The model may be a guide to both instructors and students for organizing, sequencing, and evaluating specific learning activities. This model may also be used to diagnose a student's difficulty with problem solving.

Learning experiences include the process the student goes through to achieve the desired outcomes and the content or subject matter concepts related to the problem situation. Problem-solving learning experiences include the process of problem solving and the content related to the problem. If a student is asked to determine the physical therapy needs of a patient with rheumatoid arthritis, the process of the experience will be the problem solving required to determine the needs of any patient, and the content will be the subject matter concepts related to rheumatoid arthritis and the evaluation procedures. In designing problem-solving learning experiences, the model can be used as a guide to the processes of the learning experience. The instructor selects and provides opportunities for the students to obtain the related subject matter concepts. In selecting content, instructors might differentiate between concepts necessary to solve the problem and concepts that are nice to know but not necessary. Students are frequently overwhelmed with an excess of facts and data that may be related to a particular situation but not necessarily helpful in solving the problem. Memory retention in such situations may be low, and students frequently spend more time memorizing facts than learning the process. Guiding students to select appropriate data from a variety of sources as well as to find necessary data should help students learn the process as well as aid them in remembering important facts.

Effective problem-solving skills are best learned in an environment in which the student is free to test thinking skills, explore alternatives, and discover solutions that may or may not match the instructor's solution. The role of the instructor is that of facilitator, rather than "teller." Not telling the student all the facts or exactly how to do something can be frustrating to both instructor and student; however, problem-solving skills are rarely developed by following step-by-step directions to a predetermined answer. Skill is required to evaluate a student's response, to recognize a student's frustration, and to respond to a student's needs in such a way as to strengthen his ability to think as well as his feelings of self-confidence in solving problems. The student's future attitude toward effective problem solving, his willingness to avoid making premature judgments, and his desire to seek creative solutions will depend to a great extent on the environment created during the learning experiences. The learning experience may be strengthened if the instructor and the student both recognize the student's entering level of problem-solving skills and attitudes. The model may be a useful tool in determining these skills and attitudes.

Developing a positive attitude toward problem solving in the relative security of the classroom is only the first step in the development of the student's effective ability to solve clinical problems. A student may feel very secure in solving patient problems in the classroom or laboratory setting, where the only penalty for failure may be a poor grade. The same student may have difficulty in solving patient-related problems when faced with a real patient. Testing problem-solving skills in the "real world" of the clinic is an important and necessary part of becoming an effective problem solver in physical therapy. This model can be used by the clinical instructor when developing problem-solving learning experiences that take the student through the critical steps of selecting a solution, implementing the solution, and evaluating the results.

Problems designed for physical therapy learning experiences may be simple or complex; the instructor determines the degree of complexity. A simple problem generally has few "unknowns" for the student to organize and classify and few alternative solutions. The greater the number of "unknowns" and the greater the number of alternatives, the more complex the problem. Instructors may simplify potentially complex situations to help students practice the problem-solving process. For example, determining the physical therapy needs of a patient can be structured as a simple or a complex problem by selecting a disability that involves only one area of dysfunction, such as a fractured tibia, or selecting one that involves many systems of the body, such as advanced peripheral vascular disease. The learning experience is simplified by providing a hypothetical patient situation in which there are only a few financial or emotional difficulties to deal with or made complex by selecting patients with a multitude of economic and emotional problems.

This model is a useful diagnostic tool for both instructor and student. A student having difficulty in problem solving may have omitted a step, may have made a premature judgment, may feel insecure, or may have difficulty performing necessary psychomo-

tor activities associated with a step. For example, a student who is unable to develop a complete list of goals for a patient, who does not seem to ask appropriate questions, or who is unable to recognize all the components of the problem may have omitted the step of *problem analysis*. By omitting problem analysis, the student may not have the appropriate base from which to select data-collection methods. In another example, a student who consistently uses the same approach to determine the physical therapy needs of patients with a wide variety of disabilities may be making premature judgments. Students who are insecure in their ability to solve problems may rely on standardized approaches to evaluation. If the student and the instructor can recognize areas of deficiency, then both can focus on remediating the specific weakness.

The model may be used as a guide to developing classroom and clinical evaluation instruments. Problem situations for practical examinations or paper-and-pencil tests can be developed to determine if students can solve problems. In evaluating a student's problem-solving ability, care must be taken to use tests that ensure the student focuses on the problem presented and does not guess the solution the instructor has in mind. Students need the freedom to create unique solutions, provided their solutions are logical and can achieve the desired goals. For the instructor, the key element is to develop problems that provide each student with the opportunity to use the model, rather than to recall predetermined steps and answers.

SUMMARY

This model depicts the cognitive, affective, and psychomotor behaviors of an individual going through the problem-solving sequence of activities. Identifying the intellectual, emotional, and physical activities of the individual in each step of the process provides a guide for students and teachers in helping students become effective at solving problems in physical therapy.

REFERENCES

1. Ewing DW: Discovering your problem-solving style. Psychology Today 69–73, Dec 1977
2. Davis GA: Psychology of Problem Solving: Theory and Practice. New York, Basic Books, Inc, Publishers, 1973, p 12
3. Bloom BS (ed): Taxonomy of Educational Objectives. Handbook I: Cognitive Domain. New York, David McKay Co, Inc, 1956
4. Krathwohl DR, Bloom BS, Masia BB: Taxonomy of Educational Objectives. The Classification of Educational Goals. Handbook II: Affective Domain. New York, David McKay Co, Inc, 1964
5. Simpson EJ: The Psychomotor Domain. Washington, DC, Gryphen House, 1972

Psychosocial Issues in Clinical Education

Counseling Function of Academic Coordinators of Clinical Education from Select Entry-Level Physical Therapy Educational Programs

PAULETTE M. KONDELA-CEBULSKI

This study describes the counseling function of academic coordinators of clinical education in the traditional physical therapy programs in the United States (N = 45) that grant a degree following satisfactory completion of 120 semester credit hours or an equivalent. An investigator-designed survey was administered to all of the available clinical coordinators (94%) from the type of program studied. Demographic data related to counseling functions are reported. Other results of specific research objectives showed most (97.9%) of the respondents indicated counseling is a part of their real and ideal roles and little more than half (53.2%) of these believed they were prepared for their counseling role. Real and ideal counseling functions of academic clinical coordinators are described. The means by which the counseling role of the respondents can be facilitated are also reported.

Key Words: Faculty counseling, Students, Physical therapy.

The Academic Coordinator of Clinical Education (ACCE) is the physical therapy faculty member who is primarily involved in coordinating clinical education of students with the entire educational program. As the professional intermediary between the academic and clinical faculties and as an advocate for the students, the ACCE works cooperatively with each of these groups.[1]

A review of the literature showed a few authors have commented on the role of the ACCE as counselor.[1-3] Two authors noted the counseling role of all physical therapy faculty.[4, 5] Worthingham reported in a national study that 76 percent of full-time academic physical therapy faculty (N = 255) had student counseling responsibilities. Most (93%) of the faculty members who had student counseling responsibilities indicated spending a range of from 1 to 10 hours a week counseling.[5]

Moore and Perry recommended that ACCEs have "advanced preparation in the areas of education, counseling, administration and interpersonal communication."[1] They also noted that counseling skills are beneficial in interaction with both students and clinical faculty. An extensive review of the literature showed, however, that little has been written about the counseling function of the ACCEs. Because only a few authors indicated ACCEs have important functions as counselors and inasmuch as no studies have been done describing this function, there was an apparent need to study this topic. I began by going directly to one group of ACCEs to ask them what they believed about this role. Several additional research questions were addressed. Did the ACCEs believe that counseling was part of their role? If so, for whom, on what occasion, and for what purposes was it a function of their role? Further, Did they believe they had been adequately prepared for this responsibility? If they did not think it was a part of their role, Why did they think this way? Finally, if one accepted the assumption that ACCEs should function as counselors, How could this role be facilitated?

The purpose of this study was to describe the counseling function of ACCEs from the largest homogeneous group of physical therapy educational programs in the United States. The research objectives were 1) to describe the respondents using demographic data related to counseling functions, 2) to describe the respondents' perceptions of their roles as counselors, 3) to compare the respondents' perceptions of their real and ideal counseling functions, and 4) to describe how the respondents believed the real role of counselor could be facilitated.

Dr. Kondela-Cebulski was Instructor and Academic Coordinator of Clinical Education, Department of Physical Medicine and Rehabilitation, Medical School, University of Michigan, at the time this study was done. She is currently Assistant Director and Center Coordinator of Clinical Education, Physical Therapy Division, University Hospital, Ann Arbor, MI 48109 (USA).

This article was submitted August 25, 1981, and accepted September 2, 1981.

METHOD

The population included all of the ACCEs from four-year baccalaureate programs in the United States that award the degree following satisfactory completion of 120 semester credit hours or their equivalent (N = 45). The ACCEs from other entry-level programs, that is, undergraduate programs that award a second undergraduate degree and entry-level master's degree programs were not included in this study. I assumed the counseling function of the ACCEs from these latter types of programs could be different than that for ACCEs from the traditional, first-degree awarding baccalaureate program. The programs represented in this study were identified from a list of universities published by the American Physical Therapy Association.[6]

I developed a 13-page questionnaire entitled *Counseling Function of Academic Coordinators of Clinical Education* to meet the objectives of the study. The questionnaire was made up primarily of closed-type, check-list questions and a few open-ended questions. It was organized into three major sections: 1) operational definitions (Fig. 1), 2) real and ideal counseling functions of the ACCEs, and 3) demographic data related to the counseling role. A pilot study was conducted during which four ACCEs from physical therapy educational programs other than the type studied were asked to complete the survey and offer recommendations for improvement.

After the questionnaire was developed, I called each of the physical therapy programs in the study. The names of primary or associate ACCEs (N = 50) were identified and I spoke with at least one of these individuals from each program to explain the nature of the study and to solicit his initial agreement to participate in it. Each ACCE was sent a questionnaire, a letter of transmittal, a stamped return envelope, and a postcard for the respondent's formal agreement or refusal to participate in the study. The questionnaire and postcard were coded for follow-up purposes and to assure confidentiality. About three weeks after the initial mailing, a reminder telephone call was made to nonrespondents. Two weeks after the final reminder telephone call was made, data analyses were begun. Descriptive statistics, including percentages, means, and standard deviations, were calculated to analyze the demographic data. Chi-square analysis was completed for the real and ideal counseling functions of ACCEs for each testable item on the survey.

RESULTS

Forty-seven (94%) of the total ACCEs in the United States (N = 50) were available to participate in the study and all of these ACCEs (100%) responded.

Counseling

Counseling is the relationship between two persons, in which the counselor attempts to assist the counselee in adjusting more effectively to himself and his environment. The goal of the counseling relationship is responsible and effective self-determination by the counselee.

Academic Coordinator of Clinical Education

The Academic Coordinator of Clinical Education is that academic faculty member who is responsible for relating the students' clinical education to the curriculum. This individual is responsible for planning and coordinating the students' entire clinical education experience, for scheduling students and clinical education sites, and for evaluating the student's progress.[1]

Clinical faculty

Clinical faculty include those physical therapists at the clinical education site who are involved in the provision of clinical education for students of a given school.

Academic Faculty

Academic faculty are those physical therapists at the academic institution who are primarily responsible for the didactic education of the physical therapy students.

"Should," or "should be functioning as a counselor," . . .

Phrases such as "should be functioning as a counselor" or "should provide counseling" and others using "should" mean that even though counseling services might be available to the students through some organized means on or off campus, you believe that you should still provide whatever services are being described as a part of your function as the coordinator of clinical education.

Fig. 1. Operational definitions included in questionnaire entitled "Counseling Function of Academic Coordinators of Clinical Education."

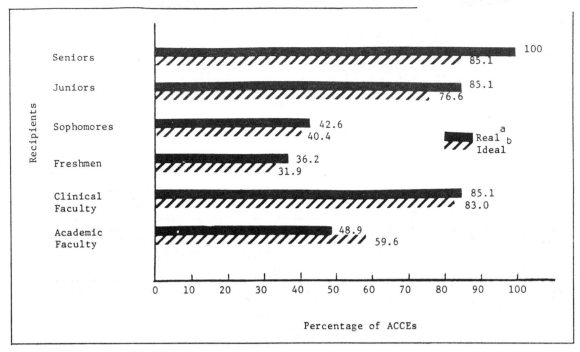

Fig. 2. Chi-square analysis of the real and ideal counseling for recipients of counseling. (Data on clinical faculty and academic faculty members is incidental to remaining study results.)
[a] "Real" counseling—counseling that had been provided by the ACCEs.
[b] "Ideal" counseling—counseling the ACCEs thought they should provide.

Demographic data. Thirty-six (76.6%) of the respondents held 12-month appointments; 7 (14.9%) held 9-month appointments; and 4 (8.5%) had other types of appointments. The greatest mean percentage of work time per year was spent on ACCE responsibilities ($\bar{X}$ = 44.7%, ± 22.4%), with teaching ($\bar{X}$ = 33.6%, ± 18.7%), and administrative duties ($\bar{X}$ = 10.5%, ± 12.3%) ranking second and third respectively. Other responsibilities including clinical practice ($\bar{X}$ = 6.0%, ± 7.9%) and general college or university responsibilities ($\bar{X}$ = 5.6%, ± 5.2%) were engaged in less frequently. Seven (14.9%) of the respondents worked 20 to 40 hours a week. Twenty-seven (57.4%) of the respondents worked 40 to 50 hours a week and 13 (27.7%) worked more than 50 hours a week. Twenty-three (48.9%) of the respondents indicated that they had received some assistance from other faculty members in the roles as ACCEs, but 17 (73.9%) of these respondents indicated that they had received assistance on an average of five hours or less a week each year. Analyses of descriptive characteristics of the group showed that 36 (76.6%) of the ACCEs had masters' degrees. The most frequently reported fields of graduate education were physical therapy education (14.9%) and allied health education and administration (12.8%). Sixteen (34.0%) of the respondents had taken formal graduate courses in counseling theory or technique. Thirty (63.8%) of the respondents

indicated they had attended short-term courses, workshops, or similar educational programs in which counseling theory or technique had been presented.

Role as counselor. All but one of the respondents (97.9%) reported they functioned as counselors in their roles as ACCEs. All but one of the respondents believed they should be functioning as a counselor in this role.

Function as counselor. Figures 2 to 4 show the results of the chi-square analyses of the real and ideal recipients of the ACCEs counseling functions, the locations of counseling, and when counseling had been or should be provided. Figure 2 shows that with each successive college year of the student, the counseling role of the ACCE increased. Figure 2 also shows no significant differences between the real and ideal counseling function of the ACCEs for the students.

Figure 3 shows that fewer ACCEs (χ^2 = 4.55, $p <$ .05) believed counseling should be provided in the classroom than those who had provided it there.

There were two differences between the real and ideal counseling functions when counseling was provided (Fig. 4). Fewer ACCEs (χ^2 = 3.92, $p <$ .05) thought counseling should be provided anytime they were available than those who had provided it then and fewer (χ^2 = 5.15, $p <$ .05) thought it should be provided anytime of the day or night than those who had provided it at those times. Figure 4 shows clearly

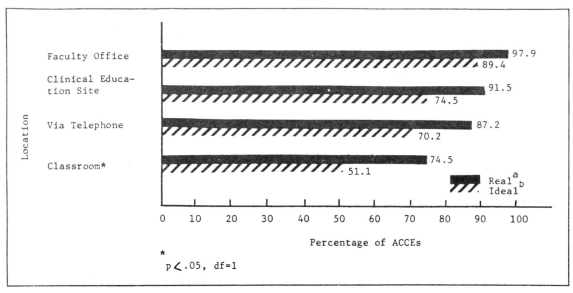

Fig. 3. *Chi-square analysis of the real and ideal counseling for the location of counseling students.*
[a] *"Real" counseling—counseling that had been provided by the ACCEs.*
[b] *"Ideal" counseling—counseling the ACCEs thought they should provide.*

a variety of times when counseling was provided by the ACCEs in this study.

Sixty-six physical therapy student needs or issues were identified by the ACCEs as being within their real and ideal counseling roles. Only those items that were most frequently reported or for which there was a significant difference between the real and ideal counseling roles are reported here. Provided are the chi-square analyses of the real and ideal counseling functions for the personal needs or issues (Tab. 1), for educational needs or issues (Tab. 2), and for professional needs or issues (Tab. 3).

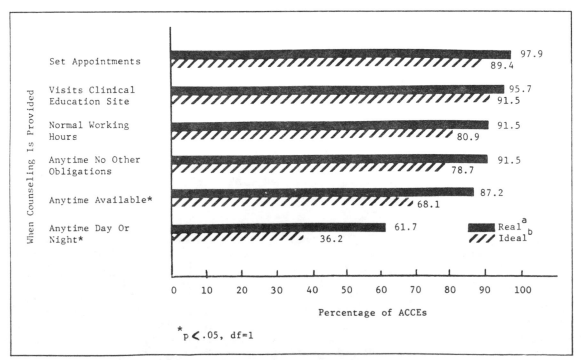

Fig. 4. *Chi-square analysis of real and ideal counseling when counseling is provided students.*
[a] *"Real" counseling—counseling that had been provided by the ACCEs.*
[b] *"Ideal" counseling—counseling the ACCEs thought they should provide.*

TABLE 1

Chi-Square Analysis of Real and Ideal Counseling for Personal Needs or Issues of Students

Need or Issue	Real[a]	Ideal[a]	p[b]
Emotional needs	96	70	NS
Become aware of an existing problem of which counselee is unaware	90	77	NS
Financial needs	85	64	.05
Psychosexual adjustment	15	30	.05
Acquisition of an ethical system	43	64	.05

[a] Percentage response.
[b] $df = 1$.

Three differences between real and ideal counseling functions of the ACCEs for personal needs or issues of the students were found (Tab. 1). Fewer ACCEs ($\chi^2 = 4.53$, $p < .05$) believed they should provide counseling for financial needs than those who had provided it for this counseling issue. More ACCEs believed they should provide counseling for psychosexual adjustment ($\chi^2 = 3.92$, $p < .05$) than those who had provided it for this counseling issue. Overall, relatively few ACCEs indicated that counseling for psychosexual issues was part of the real (14.9%) and ideal (29.8%) counseling role of the ACCE. More ACCEs ($\chi^2 = 5.17$, $p < .05$) believed they should provide counseling for a need to acquire an ethical system than those who had provided it for this counseling issue. It is unclear whether the ACCEs were referring to a personal or a professional ethical system, or both.

Table 2 shows that most of the educational needs or issues for which counseling had been provided by the ACCEs were directly related to clinical education. There were no significant differences between real and ideal counseling for educational needs or issues.

Table 3 shows that counseling intervention for professional needs or issues were reported by many ACCEs.

Preparation for counseling. Little more than half (53.2%) of the respondents indicated they believed they were adequately prepared for their counseling role. Each of these respondents commented that they believed they were adequately prepared as a result of personal experience and actual work in their role as ACCE.

Facilitation of counseling role. Eighteen ways in which the counseling role of the ACCEs could be facilitated were identified. The methods of facilitation most frequently identified by the ACCEs are reported in Table 4.

DISCUSSION

Response to this study was excellent. Of the three ACCEs who did not participate in the study, one had just resigned from the position and no replacement had been named, one ACCE had just gone on indefinite sick leave, and I was the third one so I excluded myself from participation in the study in an attempt to eliminate researcher bias.

Analyses of demographic data related to counseling function revealed no unexpected results. Because of the nature of ACCE responsibilities with regard to clinical education organization, planning, and implementation, it is not surprising that most of the ACCEs held 12-month appointments. It was also not surprising that a little more than 85 percent of the ACCEs worked more than 40 hours per week because many of the ACCE responsibilities require extra work time (eg, travel to or from clinic sites outside of regular work hours).

Only one ACCE responded negatively to the items asking whether the respondents believed they did and should function as counselors in the role of ACCE.

TABLE 2

Chi-Square Analysis of Real and Ideal Counseling for Educational Needs or Issues of Students

Need or Issue	Real[a]	Ideal[a]	p[b]
Adjustment to clinical setting	100	92	NS
Clinical competency issues	100	92	NS
Adjustment to clinical education as a means of learning skills	98	92	NS
Integration of knowledge and skill in clinical setting	98	89	NS
Appropriate professional behavior	94	89	NS
Grades	87	70	NS
Educational plans for future	87	77	NS

[a] Percentage response.
[b] $df = 1$.

TABLE 3

Chi-Square Analysis of Real and Ideal Counseling for Professional Needs or Issues of Students

Need or Issue	Real[a]	Ideal[a]	p[b]
Clinical performance	100	92	NS
Fear of clinical experiences	94	94	NS
Adjustment to different clinical education sites	94	92	NS
Overwhelming clinical responsibilities	94	92	NS
Adjustment to different supervisory styles	94	92	NS
Problems with interpersonal relationships in clinic	94	92	NS
Frustration from inability to help some patients	94	92	NS
Inability to recognize or understand personal problem in clinic	87	89	NS
Inordinate psychosexual attachment to patients	34	81	.001[c]
Transition from student to therapist role	51	85	.001[d]
Negative feelings about some patients	60	87	.01[e]
Acceptable goal and life purpose	49	72	.05[f]
Change of career goal	51	70	.05[g]

[a] Percentage response.   [c] $\chi^2 = 23.21$.   [f] $\chi^2 = 6.42$.
[b] $df = 1$.   [d] $\chi^2 = 14.15$.   [g] $\chi^2 = 4.46$.
[e] $\chi^2 = 10.68$.

Interestingly, this individual completed the remainder of the questionnaire and identified his real and ideal counseling functions.

Chi-square analyses of the real and ideal counseling function of the ACCEs for the types of students (Fig. 2), the location of counseling (Fig. 3), and the time of counseling provided (Fig. 4) revealed both expected and unexpected results. In Figure 2, it is unclear why not all of the ACCEs thought they should provide counseling to senior students when most seniors are involved in clinical education or help plan for it. This difference between real and ideal counseling functions may reflect, in part, that some of the associate ACCEs worked only with nonsenior students. In Figure 3, the difference between the real and ideal counseling in the classroom might reflect the fact that some ACCEs have used the classroom for group types of guidance and counseling activities in preparing students for clinical education and professional practice. Those ACCEs who believed counseling should not be provided in the classroom might have been reflecting a sound counseling process principle for one-to-one counseling, that is, that an

appropriate location to assure confidentiality and free, open discussion should be provided.[7]

Chi-square analyses of real and ideal counseling functions of the ACCEs for personal, professional, and educational needs or issues also revealed both expected and unexpected results. The difference between real and ideal counseling for financial needs of students (Tab. 1) could refer to the additional expenses related to clinical education. Student participation in clinical education results in additional expenditures beyond the usual college expenses for uniforms, housing, and transportation. Students often discuss these additional financial problems with the ACCE. In Table 1, the finding about the counseling by the ACCEs for psychosexual issues could reflect that only a few of the ACCEs found there were some students who were in need of assistance from the ACCE to help them through the normal psychosexual maturational stages at the college level.[8] It could also mean that only a few of the ACCEs felt comfortable dealing with this counseling issue with the students.

The implications from Table 2 are that as a group, the ACCEs believed the educational counseling they

TABLE 4

Respondents' Perceptions of Means by Which Counseling Role Could Be Facilitated

Means of Facilitation	Response	
	f	%
Qualified professionals should be available for referral	46	97.9
Atmosphere within physical therapy program should encourage student to seek appropriate counseling	46	97.9
ACCE and counselees should understand that confidentiality must exist unless permission is given to discuss issues	44	93.6
Financial resources should be available for ACCE's continuing education in counseling	43	91.5
Financial resources should be available to support ACCE's travel for purposes of counseling	42	89.4
Appropriate physical space should be available for counseling	42	89.4
Flexible time should be available to ACCE to travel outside regular work site for counseling purposes	41	87.2
Time should be available for ACCE to participate in continuing education in counseling	41	87.2

were providing was what they thought they should provide to the students. The reason for the differences between real and ideal counseling for the five issues at the bottom of Table 3 is unclear. Among many other possibilities, the appropriate opportunities for intervention may not have arisen. Or, the ACCEs may have been uncomfortable with the counseling focus or felt unprepared to deal with the issues in terms of counseling process and technique.

Inasmuch as only slightly more than half of the respondents reported feeling prepared for the counseling role, a need for participation in some other means of preparation for the counseling role seems to exist.

All of the most frequently reported means by which counseling could be facilitated (Tab. 4) are consistent with sound counseling principles.[9] Some of them show a definite need for support of the ACCE's continuing education in counseling and a need for appropriate resources for them to be effective counselors.

SUMMARY

The results of this study indicate that for the type of program studied, counseling is a function of the academic coordinator of clinical education. Demographic data related to counseling functions revealed no unexpected results. Some differences were found between real and ideal counseling functions for the location of counseling and for the time counseling was provided. Some differences were found between real and ideal counseling functions for personal and professional needs or issues of the student; no differences were found for educational needs or issues. About half (53.2%) of the respondents believed they were adequately prepared for the counseling role. Means by which the counseling role could be facilitated have been reported. All are consistent with sound counseling principles. All of these results are important to a broad population of individuals insofar as the ACCE's role is one of interaction with academic faculty, clinical faculty, and students among others.

Additional research needs to be conducted regarding the counseling function of ACCEs including: research describing the differences in the nature of the counseling functions of ACCEs from other types of physical therapy educational programs, research investigating the counselee's perceptions of the ACCE's role as a counselor, and research identifying the specific counseling needs of the counselee as perceived by the counselee. Further, research comparing the counseling function of ACCEs with other academic faculty members should be done. Related research should be conducted: 1) to identify who provides counseling to the students in the ACCEs' absence, 2) to describe the counseling function of center coordinators of clinical education and clinical instructors and their preparation for it, and 3) to describe what is needed to facilitate the counseling role of clinical faculty, if that role exists.

REFERENCES

1. Moore ML, Perry JF: Clinical Education in Physical Therapy: Present Status/Future Needs. Washington, DC, American Physical Therapy Association, 1976
2. Dickinson R, Dervitz HL, Meida HM: Handbook for Physical Therapy Teachers. New York, NY, American Physical Therapy Association, 1967, p 26
3. Ford CW (ed): Clinical Education for the Allied Health Professions. St. Louis, MO, The CV Mosby Co, 1978, p 117
4. Ramsden EL: Out-of-classroom responsibilities and the physical therapy educator. Phys Ther 50:513–516, 1970
5. Worthingham CA: The environment for basic physical therapy education: 1965–1966. Phys Ther 48:935–962, 1968
6. Careers in Physical Therapy. Washington, DC, American Physical Therapy Association, 1979
7. Benjamin A: The Helping interview. Boston, MA, Houghton Mifflin Co, 1981, pp 2–4
8. Hardee MD: Faculty Advising in Colleges and Universities. No. 9, Washington, DC, American College Personnel Association, 1970
9. Shertzer B, Stone SC: Fundamentals of Guidance. Boston, MA, Houghton Mifflin Co, 1981

Application of Client-Centered Counseling to Clinical Teaching*

W. Scott Gehman, Ph.D.

In the process of teaching individual adult students in the clinical situation, one question which faces the supervisor is, "How can we best help the individual develop his skills and technics to a near maximum degree?" One probable answer to this question lies in promoting the development of effective understanding of himself as a person, a student, and a clinician.

A. H. Maslow[1] has made much in his writings on motivation (the why of behavior) of the desirability of promoting the level of motivation referred to as that of *self-actualization*. It is assumed that if self-actualization is realized, the individual, in our case the student clinician, will benefit tremendously, as will the society of which he is a member. The self-actualized person, according to an interpretation from Maslow[2], is basically a satisfied person who is performing with the full use and exploitation of talents, capacities, and potentialities. He is fulfilling himself and is doing the best that he is capable of doing. In addition to this, he is also performing his tasks with serenity, peace of mind, and is creative. Maslow[3] says: "From the self-actualized person we may expect the fullest and healthiest kind of creativeness, or originality, or inventiveness . . . ."

Many of our students, particularly those in advanced training programs, have been thwarted in their satisfaction of self-realization and achievement needs because of our relatively stereotyped educational programs. One of the great rewards that can come to the supervisor is that of watching the student clinician improve in his application of old skills and seeing him develop new ones when he is free to *grow* in an atmosphere of security and emotional support.

In the individual teaching situation, first comes the experience of establishing a relationship, as in counseling and psychotherapy, between the student clinician and supervisor. How can the supervisor promote the development of a relationship that will lend itself toward self-actualization of the student clinician? To answer this question in general terms, it may be helpful to draw from the philosophical and theoretical formulations of such men as Rogers,[5,6] Snygg and Combs[8] and others who are described as phenomenologists or client-centered psychotherapists. The counterpart of the principles of psychotherapy from the client-centered frame of reference may be found in the teaching process and it is my purpose to stimulate your thinking to this end.

Rogers[5] describes two basic assumptions essential to the application of the client-centered method. In paraphrased form, these same assumptions apply to the supervisor who would adopt the client-centered frame of reference to the teaching of the individual student clinician. In paraphrased form as translated from counseling and psychotherapy to teaching these assumptions are:

(1) The supervisor or teacher must recognize the individuality of the student clinician, and within limits, recognize his need for freedom to make some of his own choices in treatment methods and technics. The clinician has had considerable basic training prior to the internship and is not a novice in the application of treatment methods. He is now ready for a limited "solo" flight when he arrives for internship training. As educators, we give a great deal of lip service to the principle of individual differences and most of us would swear on a "stack of holy bibles" that we fully believe that every person is different from every other one and yet behaviorally we set out to teach them in a manner that appears to be more of a recognition of similarities rather than that of individual differences. It would seem to me that with individual student clinicians to instruct, we have a "near" ideal situation in which to apply technics in keeping with the meaning of the concept of individual differences.

(2) A second basic assumption of client-centered counseling and psychotherapy which seems to have equal importance in its application

Associate Professor of Psychology in Education, Duke University, Durham, North Carolina; Fellow of American Psychological Association.

*Presented by W. Scott Gehman at Conference of Physical Therapy Supervisors held by Physical Therapy Department, Duke University Medical Center, November 24, 1958.

to the teaching of individual student clinicians is that the student has an enormous capacity for adaptation and growth. By this, is meant that the individual student clinician possesses within himself a motive or *need* (need for self-actualization) to arrive at a more satisfactory level of achievement in applying old skills and a further need to be creative in the development of new skills as well as to improve and sharpen old ones. These needs can be released in a situation in which he is relatively free of the usual educational impediments of being told "what to do, when to do it, and how to do it."

The character of client-centered psychotherapy has been described by Rogers [5,6] and Snyder [7] and one can translate the individual characteristics from the psychotherapeutic setting to the individual teaching situation.

Some characteristics of client-centered psychotherapy are:

(1) It aims directly toward the greater independence and integration of the person rather than hoping that such results will accrue if the counselor offers a solution to the problem. The focus is on the person and not the problem. The aim is not to solve one particular problem but to assist the person to *grow* so that he can cope with the present problem and with later problems in a more highly integrated fashion. If he can gain enough integration to handle one problem in more independent, more responsible, less confused, better organized ways, then it is hoped that he will handle new problems in that manner. It relies more heavily on the individual drive or need toward mental growth, and psychological adjustment in the social milieu. Therapy from this frame of reference is not a matter of doing something to the person or of inducing him to do something about himself. It is instead a matter of freeing him for *normal* growth and development, of removing obstacles so that he can again move forward.

When one takes these characteristics and translates them from the psychotherapeutic setting to the teaching situation, one can see how these same characteristics may promote the development of self-actualization. The supervisor's belief in the drive or motive for mental growth and psychological adjustment allows for the greater independence and integration of the individual student clinician. The clinician as a person and the patient as a person become the area of concentration and not the specific technics which are being taught to the clinician. The aim would not be to teach particular individual technics, since for the most part these have been taught

prior to the internship, but to assist the student clinician to grow psychologically so that he can further perfect his learning of the present technics and develop greater skills and technics in a better integrated fashion. If the student clinician can gain enough integration to master one or several technics in a more independent, more responsible, less confused, better organized way, then it is supposed that he will also handle the learning of new and more complex skills in a similar manner. As is true in therapy, teaching is not a matter of doing something to the student clinician or of inducing him to do something about himself. It is instead a matter of freeing him for *normal* educational growth and development by removing the "typical" education obstacles that were mentioned earlier so that he can continue to move forward toward a higher degree of self-actualization or self-fulfillment.

(2) Counseling from the client-centered frame of reference places greater stress upon the emotional or *feeling* aspects of the situation in addition to the emphasis upon the intellectual aspects.

In the educational process, this emphasis by the supervisor on accepting and reflecting the emotional needs of the student clinician should result in freeing the clinician for greater intellectual development. This is predicated on a well established principle that emotional disturbance can hinder learning. Thus, by meeting the emotional elements or feeling aspects of the learning situation, the student clinician's drive or need toward greater achievement is free to proceed toward greater mental growth and development.

(3) Client-centered counseling places greater stress upon the immediate situation than upon the person's past. In the individual teaching situation, the supervisor cannot rely heavily upon the student's past achievements but must consider the student clinician in the here and now, i.e., the present learning situation. This, in turn, will result in fewer negative attitudes toward the clinician in so far as what he or she should have known prior to entering the internship. If the supervisor proceeds with this point of view, the student clinician will feel less inadequate and again be free to proceed with the normal growth processes.

(4) Client-centered counseling lays stress upon the therapeutic relationship itself as a growth experience. In some other approaches, the person is expected to grow, change, or make better decisions after the psychotherapy session. From the client-centered frame of reference, the counseling session itself is considered to be a growth experience. Here the client learns to understand himself, to make significant independent choices, to

relate himself successfully to another person in a more adult fashion. Client-centered counseling is not preparation for change, it is thought to *be* change. The learning experiences of the student clinician can be interpreted in the same way, i.e., promoting change in behavior, and not merely preparation for change.

The client-centered psychotherapists hold that insight is the keystone of the process of therapy. Insight may be defined as the perception of new relationships to one's self and a fresh understanding of reality. Certainly educators give much emphasis to the need for the learner to experience insight if real learning is to take place.

How then, can the supervisor help the student clinician discover and use means of satisfying his need for self-enhancement and self-actualization? How can the supervisor help the student clinician develop to the full stature of which he is capable? As a supervisor and teacher, he can help the student clinician in the following ways:

(1) He can help provide the student clinician with the experiences and the physical resources which will make it possible for him to discover realistic and effective solutions to his personal and learning problems.

(2) He can help provide an atmosphere of acceptance in which the student clinician is free to explore his potential and to move toward a higher degree of self-actualization without fear of humiliation. In so doing, the supervisor should try to maintain an atmosphere in which the student clinician feels adequate and acceptable for the moment so that he can attend to the need for further and greater achievement. Even with failure, the student clinician needs to feel accepted in order to recognize the failure and deal with it so that he can move forward in the direction of further self-enhancement.

(3) The supervisor can act as a friendly representative of the professional society which the student clinician is expected to join in a responsible manner. As a representative of the profession, the supervisor can give the student clinician an opportunity to see himself realistically but acceptably for the time being so that further growth toward self-actualization is possible.

It has not been my purpose to suggest specific teaching technics. Certainly the technics are important but in the final analysis, the technics used by a supervisor will be determined by his self-concept, his concept of his supervisory duties, and his concept of the student clinicians.

It is my thesis that if we hope to allow for the development of more self-actualized clinicians we have much to learn from the principles of client-centered psychotherapy which can be applied to the teaching or educative process.

REFERENCES

1. Maslow, A. H.: A dynamic theory of human motivation, Psychol. Review 50: 370-396, 1943.
2. ————: Motivation and Personality, New York, Harper & Brothers, 1954.
3. ————: Self-Actualizing People: A Study of Psychological Health. Personality Symposium, No. 1. New York, Grune & Stratton, Inc., April 1950.
4. ————: Deficiency Motivation and Growth Motivation, in Nebraska Symposium on Motivation, Lincoln, U. of Nebraska Press, 1955.
5. Rogers, C. R.: Counseling and Psychotherapy, Boston, Houghton Mifflin, 1942.
6. ————: Client-Centered Therapy, Boston, Houghton Mifflin, 1951.
7. Snyder, W. U., et al.: Casebook of Non-Directive Therapy, Boston, Houghton Mifflin, 1947.
8 Snygg, Donald and Combs, A. W.: Individual Behavior, New York, Harper & Brothers, 1949.

How to Arrange to Borrow a Print of *The Return*

A complete listing of the film libraries where the Association's latest film is on deposit may be found on page 99ff. of the February, 1959, issue of the *Physical Therapy Review*. If the film library nearest you cannot supply you on the date you need *The Return*, look through the list to see if another library will service your state. National Office will send you a print if it is unavailable locally. In addition to the 38-minute version, there is a TV version running 28 minutes. There is also a 58-second TV spot with sound track, excerpted from *The Return*. Both of these are available for borrowing from the National Office. *The Return* was chosen by Howard Thompson of *The New York Times* as one of the 10 best nontheatrical films of 1958.

Comparison of Psychological Needs of Clinical Instructors and Physical Therapy Students: Implications for Communication While on Affiliation

Jeff Baker, PhD
Susan McPhail, MEd, PT
Janet Pfau, MS, PT

ABSTRACT: The purpose of this study was to assess the psychological needs of physical therapy students and clinical instructors and how these needs relate to the communication that occurs between the clinical instructor and physical therapy student. This study attempted to measure the differences between students' and clinical instructors' needs for inclusion, control, and affection using the Fundamental Interpersonal Orientation Relationship-Behavior assessment instrument. Six hypotheses were set forth to determine whether physical therapy students, when compared with clinical instructors, would have a higher need for inclusion, a higher need to be included, a lower need for control over others, a higher need for control from others, the same need to express affection, and the same need to receive affection. This study compares 73 clinical instructors' and 76 physical therapy students' differences in needs and discusses varying needs as a possible explanation of negative experiences on clinical affiliation. Differences in characteristics between the two groups were examined using a t test. Significant differences were observed between the groups for wanted inclusion, expressed control, wanted control, and expressed affection. The results suggest students and clinical instructors do have different needs. A discussion is included that addresses the degree of difference and how it could affect the students' experience on clinical affiliation.

During clinical affiliations, physical therapy students face a number of psychologi-

Dr Baker is Associate Professor and Director, Counseling & Student Services, School of Allied Health Sciences, The University of Texas Medical Branch at Galveston, Galveston, TX 77550. Ms McPhail is Assistant Professor and Academic Coordinator of Clinical Education, Department of Physical Therapy, School of Allied Health Sciences, The University of Texas Medical Branch at Galveston. Ms Pfau is Assistant Professor and Director, Physical Therapy Department, University of Texas Medical Branch Hospitals, Galveston, TX 77550.

cally challenging situations. Clinical instructors also are facing challenges while they attempt to provide stimulating learning experiences for students. Clinical affiliations call for using more than academic skills; students and clinicians must also rely on their interpersonal and communication skills to create a successful experience. Good communication skills usually involve the ability to listen and to be articulate, assertive, and enthusiastic.[1] Successful performance on clinical affiliation is often facilitated by a physical therapy student possessing these abilities and personality characteristics. There must also be an open channel through which communication may flow, and it is important that there be two-way communication. When the student has difficulty communicating with the clinical instructor, there is a strong possibility that there will be problems on the clinical affiliation. The clinical instructor may interpret the communication difficulty as a personal problem, a quirk, or an indication that a student is "not cut out to be a physical therapist." In addition, if the clinical instructor has a communication style that is different from that of the student, these issues may escalate or be even more complicated.

BACKGROUND

Determining when a communication problem exists is difficult for most clinical instructors. Not all clinical instructors are trained to be experts in the area of communication skills, nor are they trained to be supervisors and educators. Furthermore, not all clinical instructors become supervisors, because they are interested in teaching and assisting students to learn. In addition to the student having communication problems, these factors could also influence the affiliation experience. It may be difficult for clinical instructors to determine whether a student is experiencing a complex psychological problem or whether the difficulty stems from a

basic communication issue. It is important for the clinical instructor to keep in mind that psychological problems appear to be on the rise for the general population. They may also be interested to know that communication skills can be as much, or even more, of a problem on clinical affiliation as actual clinical skills knowledge.

The *Diagnostic and Statistical Manual of Mental Disorders* (3rd rev ed) (DSM-III-R)[2] provides specific information on the prevalence of psychiatric disorders.[2] The categories of disorders vary from rarities to "common occurrence" diagnoses. Some popular news programs estimate that 20% of the population will develop psychological disorders at some point in their lifetime. Because physical therapy students have to make many life adjustments in addition to those experienced by the general population, it is not surprising that these adjustments can frequently affect the experience of students on their affiliations. Some psychological difficulties can be related to specific problems that students are experiencing in their daily lives (eg, homesickness, marital problems, financial constraints). Problems may be manifested in a variety of ways and can range in severity from mild (eg, social anxiety, unassertiveness) to severe (eg, eating disorders, clinical depression). On clinical affiliation, these adjustments may show up as anxiety, nervousness, lateness, low motivation, anger, social withdrawal, or defensiveness. Any or all of these manifestations can lead to poor communication between the student and the clinical instructor, thereby jeopardizing the success of an affiliation.

Complicating the issue even further, students having trouble on an affiliation, specifically in areas other than knowledge and skill, may have a personality conflict with the clinical instructor. In an attempt to understand the problem, the instructor may then presume that the student was not adequately prepared in professionalism at the university or that the student's last affiliation had just passed them without regard to their interpersonal skills. Another possibility is that the student and instructor have different communication styles. There could exist a lack of clear understanding of the needs of the student or clinical instructor. The student has a need to learn and practice skills, whereas the instructor has a need to observe and provide a learning experience for the student. Additional needs that can affect communication include control, affection, and inclusion. When an individual's needs are not being met, he or she may choose to verbalize it or, more often, may choose to ignore it or may not even realize it. This situation can result in a deteriorating relationship between the instructor and the student. The student may respond with hurt feelings, stress, or withdrawal. The instructor may respond by assigning the student a failing grade on the affiliation or by feeling completely frustrated about the student's progress.

Student performance during an affiliation is tied to, and many times dependent on, communication. Thus, it is helpful for communication channels to be open and working. One method of achieving a better understanding of the communication style of both the clinical instructor and the physical therapy student is through a better understanding of their respective "wants and needs."

The clinical experience is a major part of the physical therapy student's education and will probably influence the kind of practice chosen for employment, the kind of facility at which employment is sought, and even the possible consideration of future employment at an affiliation site. A recent survey by Ciccone and Wolfner[3] revealed that 51% of their respondents actively sought employment at a previous clinical education site (CES) and that 29% were employed by a former CES.[3] Considering the current shortage of physical therapists and the fact that facilities are paying higher prices for recruitment, a better understanding of communication and how the student and clinical instructor interact is worth investigating. This article will investigate the differences in communication styles and suggest how these differences might affect communication styles and the relationship between a student and the clinical instructor.

FIRO-B

To obtain a better understanding of the wants and needs of students and clinical instructors, we used the Fundamental Interpersonal Orientation Relationship-Behavior (FIRO-B) assessment instrument in this study.[4,5] This inventory contains six basic

---

Table 1

Sample Items from the Fundamental Interpersonal Orientation Relationship-Behavior Questionnaire[a]

For each statement below, decide which of the following answers best applies to you. Place the number of the answer in the box at the left of the statement. Please be as honest as you can.

1. never   2. rarely   3. occasionally   4. sometimes   5. often   6. usually

_____ I try to be with people.
_____ I try to include other people in my plans.
_____ I try to be the dominant person when I am with people.
_____ I like people to include me in their activities.

For each of the next group of statements, choose one of the following answers:
1. nobody   2. one or two people   3. a few people   4. some people   5. many people   6. most people

_____ My personal relations with people are cool and distant.
_____ I let other people control my actions.
_____ I like other people to act close and personal with me.
_____ I try to have other people do things the way I want them done.

[a]Reproduced by permission from Consulting Psychologists Press Inc.

---

questions. Each question is repeated with a slight variation nine times, making a total of 54 items to be answered. The questionnaire is purported to measure three fundamental dimensions of interpersonal relationships.[6] Sample questions are presented in Table 1.

It is hypothesized that the FIRO-B, which measures both expressed and desired needs for interpersonal communication between individuals, can indicate when there are differences in communication styles. In the student/clinical instructor relationship, the FIRO-B could be used to identify communication differences that create friction between the student and the clinical instructor. Even though such differences were not the focus of this study, the instrument would help in facilitating a better understanding of the student's and the clinical instructor's needs if it indeed points out communication differences.

In the study of human interaction and communication, investigation of characteristic ways in which people respond to avoid anxiety or exposure has increasingly attracted attention.[7,8] Some theories of psychology assume that there are difficult and threatening aspects to everyone's personality, such as feelings of inferiority, inadequacy, or insignificance, hostile impulses, and strong lusts and desires. The FIRO-B provides an understanding of interpersonal orientation, which refers to a person's interpersonal frame of reference. A person who has a skewed interpersonal orientation may be said to be "out of community" in some sense. The individual's interpersonal life is impoverished, and he or she is withdrawn or cannot get along with family, friends, or co-workers. The interpersonal orientation is derived from an understanding of the individual's needs and wants.

The FIRO-B presents results based on three interpersonal needs and wants: inclusion, control, and affection. The inclusion dimension assesses the degree to which a person associates with others. The control dimension measures the extent to which a person assumes responsibility, makes decisions, or dominates people. The affection dimension score reflects the degree to which a person becomes emotionally involved with others.

The test assumes that these three areas are fundamental in understanding and predicting interpersonal behavior. The assumption includes the premise that communication styles and interpersonal behavior are measured in terms of how much people associate with others, the extent to which a person dominates others, and the degree of emotional involvement. The success of how well one communicates with another can be measured by these traits. Although many other factors will influence a person's actions, meaningful inferences can be made about an individual's behaviors if the person's stance regarding these three dimensions is known.

As a measure of interpersonal relationships, the FIRO-B's applications to human behavior are useful. The FIRO-B has been used in a number of situations for group and individual counseling,[6] a process that most often focuses on the individual's interpersonal skills. It has also been used with large groups of people for personnel selection or assignment, such as the selection of nuclear submarine crews, police officers, and firefighters and the assignment of teachers to "team-teaching" programs.[6] The FIRO-B was also used in living-group preferences[9] and family therapy.[10]

The FIRO-B has a number of advantages that made it appropriate for use in this research study. Unlike many other personality tests, for example, it obtains relevant

Table 2
Clinical Instructor Scores on the Fundamental Orientation Relationship-Behavior Questionnaire[a]
Survey (N=73)

| | Dimension | | | | | |
| | Inclusion | | Control | | Affection | |
Behavior	$\bar{X}$	SD	$\bar{X}$	SD	$\bar{X}$	SD
Expressed	4.7	1.9	3.4[b]	2.7	4.2[b]	2.3
Wanted	4.0[b]	3.4	3.4[b]	2.1	5.3	2.1

[a]Possible range=0–9; very high=8–9, high=6–7, moderate=4–5, low=2–3, very low=0–1.
[b] $P<.05$.

Table 3
Physical Therapy Student Scores on the Fundamental Interpersonal Orientation Relationship-Behavior
Questionnaire[a] Survey (N=76)

| | Dimension | | | | | |
| | Inclusion | | Control | | Affection | |
Behavior	$\bar{X}$	SD	$\bar{X}$	SD	$\bar{X}$	SD
Expressed	5.2	1.9	1.8[b]	1.7	4.5[b]	2.2
Wanted	5.4[b]	3.2	2.7[b]	1.8	5.5	2.5

[a]Possible range=0–9; very high=8–9, high=6–7, moderate=4–5, low=2–3, very low=0–1.
[b] $P<.05$.

information in a short period of time; an average of only 10 minutes is required to answer the 54 questions. The brevity of the test helps to avoid fatigue and the decrease in motivation that usually accompanies personality tests. The FIRO-B should not be regarded as the most statistically sound instrument according to Hurly[11] and Salminen.[12] In our experience, however, it can provide an excellent counseling tool when differences in communication exist.

Two scores are obtained for each of the three variables on the FIRO-B: (1) an "expressed-behavior" score and (2) a "wanted-behavior" score. The expressed-behavior score represents the person's manifest behavior: overt, observable behavior in the areas of inclusion, control, and affection. The wanted-behavior score refers to what the person wants from other people in the areas of inclusion, control, and affection. Wanted behavior is less directly observable than expressed behavior, and wanted-behavior scores thus provide valuable information for better understanding and predicting the person's behavior.

In order to illustrate the components and possible results of the FIRO-B, each variable will be briefly described and examples will be provided in the "Discussion" section to describe hypothetical problems physical therapy students and clinical instructors might have if they have vastly different needs and wants.

FIRO-B Inclusion Scores

Expressed inclusion can be defined as the psychological need to have other people around, to openly invite others to participate and to be a part of the group. *Wanted inclusion* is a psychological need to be included by others.

FIRO-B Control Scores

Expressed control can be defined as the psychological need to dominate a situation, to assume a decision-making role, or to be able to control the actions of others. *Wanted control* is a psychological need to let others dominate you, make decisions for you, or control your actions.

FIRO-B Affection Scores

Expressed affection can be defined as the psychological need to be close, personal, and warm with other people. *Wanted affection* is the psychological need to have others offer intimacy and provide close, personal, and warm feelings. People with high affection scores are seen as warm, friendly, and comforting. These characteristics are usually amenable to good patient relation skills and are commonly found among health care providers.[13]

In this article, the FIRO-B will be applied to the achievement of better understanding and improved communication between clinical instructors and physical therapy students.

The differences in the three traits measured by the FIRO-B is postulated to be a major determinant to the success of a student's clinical experience.

METHOD

The FIRO-B was administered to a group of clinical instructors attending a clinical instructor training workshop at Texas Woman's University in 1987 and to a second group attending the clinical training instructor workshop at The University of Texas Medical Branch at Galveston in 1988. A total of 73 physical therapists from these two groups, all employed in Texas, completed the FIRO-B. Their average length of professional employment was 4 years, and most were experienced clinical instructors. Seventy-six percent of the respondents were women.

The FIRO-B was also administered to two separate physical therapy classes of 40 students each from The University of Texas Medical Branch at Galveston. Both groups were enrolled as first-year professional school students and were tested within the 6-month period prior to their first full-time affiliation. A total of 76 students completed the FIRO-B questionnaire. The students' average age was 24 years, and 64% were women. The data were analyzed at the .05 probability level using t tests to determine whether a significant difference existed between the needs and wants of clinical instructors and those of students.

The scores on the FIRO-B range from 0 (very low) to 9 (very high). The closer the score is to the extremes of the range, the more applicable are the descriptions presented previously. An individual with very low scores (ie, 0–1) will exhibit compulsive behaviors. An individual with low scores (ie, 2–3) will exhibit behaviors that are noticeably characteristic of the person. Moderate scores (ie, 4–5) may indicate a tendency to demonstrate behaviors described for high or low scores. An individual with high scores (ie, 6–7) will exhibit behaviors that are noticeably characteristic of the person, and an individual with very high scores (ie, 8–9) will exhibit compulsive behaviors.[6] The six scores quantify the need to (1) express inclusion to others, (2) want inclusion from others, (3) express control to others, (4) want control from others, (5) express affection to others, and (6) want affection from others.

All participants responding to the questionnaire survey were volunteers. Each participant was presented with the same information regarding the use of the FIRO-B. Respondents were informed that results would be used only as group data. The hypotheses set forth were:

1. Students, when compared with clinical instructors, would have a higher need to express inclusion.
2. Students, when compared with clinical instructors, would have a higher need to receive (want) inclusion from others.
3. Students, when compared with clinical instructors, would have a lower need to express control.
4. Students, when compared with clinical instructors, would have a higher need to receive (want) control from others.
5. Students, when compared with clinical instructors, would have the same need to express affection.
6. Students, when compared with clinical instructors, would have the same need to receive affection.

RESULTS

The clinical instructors' and physical therapy students' mean scores (and standard deviations) are presented in Tables 2 and 3, respectively. There were no significant differences between male and female respondents for either group. The scores ranged from 0 to 9, with most scores moderate to low moderate (ie, 3–5). Significant differences were found between clinical instructors and physical therapy students for wanted inclusion, expressed control, wanted control, and expressed affection.

Analysis of the survey data resulted in the following:

1. The results indicated no significant differences between the students and the clinical instructors in the need to express inclusion, thus hypothesis 1 was rejected.
2. The scores indicated a significant difference between the students' need for inclusion and that of the clinical instructors. Students appeared to have a greater need for inclusion, thus hypothesis 2 was accepted.
3. The scores also indicated that the clinical instructors had a higher need for expressing control than the students, thus hypothesis 3 was accepted.
4. Clinical instructors exhibited a higher need for control compared with the students, thus hypothesis 4 was accepted.
5. Students were found to have a higher need than instructors to express affection to others, thus hypothesis 5 was rejected.
6. There were no significant differences between the students and the clinical instructors in the need to receive affection, thus hypothesis 6 was accepted.

DISCUSSION
FIRO-B Inclusion Scores

The finding that students have a higher need to receive inclusion compared with clinical instructors may indicate that students, who are at the threshold of becoming members of the physical therapy profession, are striving to meet the requirements for entry and thus may have a higher need to fit in. They may be striving to be accepted as members of their chosen profession. This finding may also be indicative of issues common to students, such as wanting to learn new information to be perceived as deserving of membership in this new group. When the student goes on an affiliation, the need to be included may even rise higher as they want to be accepted by the staff physical therapists who are in the role of providing clinical services.

A clinical instructor with a high need for inclusion and a physical therapy student with a high need for inclusion could manifest their needs in a close, professional relationship, which could be very positive. On the other hand, the clinical instructor with extremely high needs may give biased, uncritical feedback because of a reluctance to reject or feel rejected and risk losing inclusion by the student.

A clinical instructor with a low need for inclusion interacting with a physical therapy student with a high need for inclusion could result in the clinical instructor's perception of the physical therapy student as a very energetic, outgoing individual who wants to learn. Again, this perception could be positive. If the clinical instructor feels threatened by a physical therapy student with a high need to include others, however, the instructor may perceive the student as demanding, overconfident, or too personal. Conversely, a confrontation between a clinical instructor with a high need for inclusion and a physical therapy student with a low need for inclusion may result in the instructor's perception of the student as being disinterested in learning or interpersonally distant, because the student is demonstrating a need to move away from others.

Problems might also arise when a student's need for inclusion is considerably higher than that of the clinical instructor, as the clinical instructor might feel "crowded." The student's need may be so high that the clinical instructor's need for space may be challenged, especially if the clinical instructor has a very low need to express inclusion to others. A student's need may surface by wanting to spend every lunch hour with the clinical instructor. The clinical instructor might react by avoiding the student. This situation could lead to a significant conflict with miscommunication, possible hurt feelings or resentment, and an overall negative interaction with one another, all because the student and instructor did not understand one another's needs. This situation might be avoided if the clinical instructor and student had a clearer understanding of each other's needs, an objective that the FIRO-B is designed to accomplish.

FIRO-B Control Scores

The results also indicated that students have less need for expressing control than do clinical instructors. Students have less need for responsibility at this stage of their academic career, as they are possibly focused on being the learner. Clinical instructors, in their role, may feel a stronger responsibility for taking charge of the learning experience, protecting patients, abiding by policies and procedures of the facility, and so on.

A clinical instructor with a high need for control encountering a physical therapy student with a high need for control may result in conflict because of issues of dominance. A clinical instructor with a low need for control and a student with a low need for control might have less conflict, but learning may be inhibited without someone taking responsibility for direction. When a clinical instructor with a high need for control encounters a student with a low need for control, the result may be a dependent student who needs constant supervision. Such dependency may result in a student's inability to move on to the next affiliation or lack of success in a succeeding affiliation because of a small amount of independent experience. A student with high control scores and an instructor with low control scores may result in the student being too overwhelming or aggressive for the instructor to manage.

When the clinical instructor's control scores are higher than the students, a healthy atmosphere for an affiliation relationship may be created, as students are typically in the role of learning and clinical instructors are typically in the role of teaching. If the scores were reversed, however, there could be negative possibilities. The student would be uncomfortable being the one in control, and the instructor would not be in the role of providing adequate structure for the student's learning experience, especially a beginning experience.

If the needs of both the clinical instructor and the student are extremely high, a conflict over who is in control could be the result. When the conflict over control continues without resolution, the consequences can be very serious for some students. The instructor may build up resentment toward the student, which could lead to the student not successfully completing the affiliation.

FIRO-B Affection Scores

The Affection dimension scores in this study may indicate that students are still in the developmental stage of considering friendships, relationships, and lifelong partners. They may have a higher need, at this time, for exploration. The higher affection score may portray the student as friendly, sympathetic, warm, and caring. Students may also be experiencing a higher need for affection than instructors at this time in their lives. If the affection scores are extremely different, however, both the student and the clinical instructor may be uncomfortable during the affiliation experience because of unwanted or overly expressed affection. Jourard[5] points out that people who self-disclose too early will push people away from them for fear of too much intimacy too soon.

A clinical instructor with a high need for affection and a physical therapy student with a high need for affection may develop a close personal relationship. This scenario could provide an atmosphere that facilitates learning. This situation, however, could also create problems regarding the provision of objective critical feedback. A clinical instructor with a low need for affection and a physical therapy student with a low need for affection might experience problems in developing a relationship that is close enough to enable them to trust each other and to give objective critical feedback. When a clinical instructor with a high need for affection encounters a physical therapy student with a low need for affection, the clinical instructor may get the impression that the physical therapy student is cool, distant, unfriendly, or unhelpful. This situation, in turn, may push the clinical instructor away, leaving the student feeling unsupported. The last combination, that of the clinical instructor with a low need for affection and the physical therapy student with a high need for affection, could result in the student being perceived as too forward, pressing boundaries, and much too personal.

The highest mean score was obtained by physical therapy students on their want of affection. This need could be related to patient relationships and the willingness to involve oneself in another person's life. The lowest mean score was also obtained by physical therapy students for their need for expressed control. As stated earlier, the stu-

dents' need for control may be very low at this time, given their situation of being in the role of learner. Students who are eager to learn new ideas may have a tendency to give the dominant role to their teacher. The standard deviation scores were all ≤2.7 for both clinical instructors and physical therapy students, with the exception of the wanted inclusion standard deviation score (Tabs. 2, 3). This result may relate to the diversity of personalities among students and instructors, indicating that both groups contain individuals who may either feel very comfortable managing independently or have a need to be part of the treatment team.

CONCLUSIONS

The results of this study indicate that there are differences in the needs and wants of physical therapy students and clinical instructors in the areas of inclusion, control, and affection. Because some students eventually become clinical instructors, these identified differences may indicate that developmental stages exist as part of the professional identity process.

Communication styles are vital to understanding and learning in clinical education. When a communication problem arises on an affiliation, it may be prudent to evaluate communication styles with the FIRO-B or a similar assessment instrument. When the involved individuals' needs are understood, the result may be a better communication relationship.

In addition, it may be helpful to clarify individual needs in clinical education relationships before problems arise to prevent a breakdown in communication. Clinical instructors are usually not trained to be counselors; however, it is important for them to have a clear understanding of students' psychological needs and wants as well as their own. Incorporating the FIRO-B into clinical education may enable clinical instructors to more effectively clarify communication and psychological issues by developing a better understanding of expressed and wanted needs.

Testing all physical therapy students on affiliations or all clinical instructors employed at a site is not recommended solely for evaluation purposes. The FIRO-B, however, may be used as a helpful assessment tool for educational in-services or when communica-

tion problems or personality conflicts arise. The timely resolution of conflict through the use of this communication tool may assist in sparing clinical instructors and physical therapy students needless anxiety. Future studies may be useful to compare beginning students with new graduates or experienced professionals.

This study was limited because the studied population represented only one training program and two clinical education site workshops. A literature review of the reliability of the FIRO-B also indicated conflicting results, and caution should be taken not to apply this instrument as the only intervention in clarifying communication skills. Additional training would be required if the FIRO-B is an instrument to be applied to clarify an individual's wants and needs. Caution should also be applied when interpreting an individual's results. We would recommend a workshop or a consultant specifically trained and experienced in interpreting the FIRO-B.

REFERENCES

1. Jarski RW, Kulig K, Olson RE: Allied health perceptions of effective clinical instruction. J Allied Health 18(5):469–479, 1989
2. Diagnostic and Statistical Manual of Mental Disorders, 3rd rev ed. Washington, DC, American Psychiatric Association, 1987
3. Ciccone D, Wolfner ML: Clinical affiliations and postgraduate job selection: A survey. Clinical Management in Physical Therapy 8(3):16–19, 25, 1988
4. Schutz WC: FIRO-B. Palo Alto, CA, Consulting Psychologist Press Inc, 1957
5. Jourard: Self-Disclosure: An Experiential Analysis of the Transparent Self. New York, NY, John Wiley & Sons, 1971
6. Ryan L: Clinical Interpretation of the FIRO-B. Palo Alto, CA, Consulting Psychologists Press Inc, 1977
7. Maguire P: The case for improving communication skills . . . doctors, nurses, and other health professionals. Patient Counseling and Health Education 4(3):127–128, 1983
8. Raudsepp E: Seven ways to cure communication breakdowns. Journal of Nursing 20(4):132–142, 1990
9. Floyd NE: Interpersonal orientation and living group preferences: A validity check on the FIRO-B. Psychol Rep 62:923–929, 1989
10. Hafner R, Julian R, Ross M: The FIRO model of family therapy: Implications of factor analysis. J Clin Psychol 45:974–979, 1989
11. Hurly J: Dubious support for FIRO-B's validity. Psychol Rep 65:929–930, 1989
12. Salminen S: Two psychometric problems of the FIRO-B questionnaire. Psychol Rep 63:423–426, 1988
13. Egan G: The Skilled Helper. Monterey, CA, Brooks/Cole Publishing Co, 1975

education

Clinical Education: Interpersonal Foundations

ELSA L. RAMSDEN, Ed.D.
and HYMAN L. DERVITZ, M.A.

Clinical education has long been an integral aspect of physical therapy education though little attention has been given to the particular teaching-learning transactions involved. The clinical educator can better fulfill the important function of creating an environment conducive to learning by understanding the interpersonal bases of that transaction. In each clinical education setting the interpersonal relationship is negotiated by the clinical instructor and the student. The nature of this relationship is dependent upon the individualities of the student and the therapist as well as the characteristics of the clinical setting within which the learning takes place. Since the primary influence the clinical educator has on both other parties and on their relationship is his behavior, he should understand the effect of his behavior upon others. In this way, the needs of both the student and the clinic can best be served.

Clinical education has been an integral aspect of physical therapy preparation since the earliest days of the profession. Although the focal point has shifted from clinical centers to academic institutions, clinical experience is still heavily relied upon as a critical phase of physical therapy education. In recent years, attention has focused on the criteria for selecting clinical centers, on the establishment of goals,[1] and upon contract relationships between the academic institution and the clinical facility.[2] Little attention, however, has been devoted to the clinical educator and the

teaching-learning process within the clinical facility. In fact, that process is the key to effectiveness in clinical education and it is in the hands of every physical therapist who works with students.

The physical therapist may realize the importance of the clinical learning experience for the student who comes from the academic institution to the clinic in order to apply his knowledge.[3] That does not necessarily mean, however, that the physical therapist can assume the role and responsibilities of educator. Awareness of the importance of clinical experience is only the first step in developing an attitude toward the clinical education program that is facilitative for both teacher and learner. The profession's code of ethics suggests an educational function for its membership without specifically labeling it as such.[4] Academicians have a tendency to take advantage of the

Dr. Ramsden is Assistant Professor in the Department of Physical Therapy, School of Allied Medical Professions of the University of Pennsylvania, Philadelphia, Pennsylvania 19104.

Mr. Dervitz is Chairman and Professor, Department of Physical Therapy, College of Allied Health Professions of Temple University, Philadelphia, Pennsylvania 19140.

clinical institutions by assuming that they are willing to accept students in clinical education programs; however, even when willingness has been acknowledged, the academic institution also tends to take for granted the educational functions of the physical therapist in the clinical facilities.

What are the attributes of a good educator? Students and educators alike have been puzzling over that question for years. Educators have debated the issues in numerous publications. (For a summary of some of the major points, see Staats,[5] Highet,[6] Bruner,[7] Brown,[8] Klausmeier.[9]) In recent years, students have become active in the debate, evaluating teachers and courses and providing the information for incoming students. The National Students Association makes catalogs available from a variety of universities containing course evaluations and comments on instructor effectiveness. Students today are very concerned that their education be relevant and that their teachers provide a meaningful learning experience.

Perhaps one reason for so much discussion over the years is that the question as posed is really not answerable. Anyone who has known more than a few teachers knows that good teachers come with a wide variety of attributes. Recasting the question in terms of the transaction contract in the teaching-learning process is helpful. The basic components of this transaction are the teacher, the learner, and the setting (or environment) in which the learning takes place. Three questions can now be asked: 1) What does the students bring to the clinical experience? 2) What characteristics of the clinical setting are conducive to learning? 3) What behaviors of the supervising physical therapist facilitate learning?

WHAT DOES THE STUDENT BRING?

Everyone realizes that the physical therapy student comes to the clinical situation with a background of academic knowledge and some practice in clinical areas. The student very quickly makes assumptions about the potentials for his learning; these assumptions are based on his perception of the new learning situation, the teacher, and his past experiences. As a learner, he is concerned that the material for which he is to be responsible is not abstract and irrelevant. He is quite sensitive to the individual

called *teacher*, and he questions seriously the teacher's capability to understand and help him. His feelings of acceptance or rejection by the teacher are often critical to his ultimate sense of security. That sense of security is vital for effective learning in the clinical setting since, commonly, students entering it feel considerable anxiety.

As the student enters the clinical phase of his education, real causes exist for the apprehension which gives rise to his anxiety. He is unsure about his abilities with the patients. The actual physical and mechanical aspects of treatment are relatively new to him; the interpersonal relationship between patient and therapist is complex and often elusive. Further, the relationship between himself and the department staff is in the process of becoming defined, and he is aware that its character will greatly affect how much he enjoys the experience, as well as influence his learning experience—and grade. Anxiety may seriously hinder the student's ability to learn, as well as affect his ability to function in even routine activities.

For instance, in order to reduce his anxiety a student may be willing to settle for a passive role in learning. He is satisfied to sit and listen. The difference between this passive learning and active learning is similar to that between passive and active range-of-motion activities. The effect of a student's passivity is not only to reduce his learning, but also to encourage and perpetuate poor teaching. Alternatively, the student may defend himself from these anxieties by adopting a stance of, "You can't teach me; I already know."

Along with his anxieties, the student brings much to this new experience which is very positive in nature. He has the excitement of the explorer setting out on new terrain. The challenge this presents is stimulating and may be seen in the enthusiastic behavior that is so delightful to observe, and even envy. A strong desire to do well and to learn the prerequisites essential to attain the goal is typical. The quest for information and answers is strong and urgent in the attempt to fit the right treatment approach to the right patient problem in what seems to be a very complex puzzle.

Thus, motivations, perceptions, and attitudes have an important influence upon the student's approach and participation in the clinic. The student enters the learning transaction with his total personality, not merely with his intellect. If the education process is to succeed, therefore, it must involve him wholly, especially since the basic purpose of the clinical education program is to provide an opportunity for the student to develop skill in the application of knowledge to practical problems. The development of skill is a change in behavior.[10] Approaching a practical problem from new and different perspectives requires a change in behavior also. Suggesting appropriate changes is the point of the supervising therapist's comments. Many adults find it difficult or impossible to acknowledge deficiencies in their performance. Being placed in the position of having their deficiencies or inadequacies pointed out may be threatening or anxiety-provoking for physical therapy students, the majority of whom are emerging from the travails of adolescence to the responsibilities of adulthood.

Can the learning transaction be structured in such a way that the student may effectively use the resources without becoming defensive? Can the clinical educator help the student develop techniques of observation, experimentation, and creative therapeutic procedures? The answers to these questions can be "yes," but only when one recognizes that the most positive desires to learn may have an overlay of anxiety (the depth of the desire and the strength of anxiety-driven defensiveness will of course vary greatly among students).

WHAT CHARACTERISTICS IN THE CLINICAL SETTING ARE CONDUCIVE TO LEARNING?

The learning climate is dependent upon some factors not under the direct control of the individuals involved. They derive from the characteristics of the clinical setting itself. Although a facility may benefit by engaging in clinical education, this benefit clearly has its "costs." For this reason, time investment and cost are two critical issues that require attention, decision, and perhaps policy prior to any agreement to conduct an educational program.

The essential characteristic necessary for planning an effective clinical education program is the commitment of the department of physical therapy (and the institution or agency in which it is located) to the philosophy of clinical education and its importance for service and professional practice. Without this commitment, the clinical educator's task is compromised before he begins. The existence of a clinical education program within the department serves a dual purpose, with obvious benefits for the institution derived from each. One benefit is the service function provided by students in the direct provision of treatment to patients. This is an important benefit but must be viewed in the proper context. It should not be construed to mean a mechanism for obtaining cheap labor. Students in clinical education are learning by doing; however, an assembly-line process of administering treatment without supervision, feedback, and time for reflection is the antithesis of effective clinical education. The time factor that a clinical education program imposes on the department cannot be avoided.

The other benefit accrued from the presence of students in the clinical education program is the stimulus and impetus they provide the staff for maintaining and continually upgrading their own level of professional practice—in order to keep up with or ahead of the students. These bright young people come directly from an intensive academic program with a great deal of current information in their minds. They are looking for ways of applying this information. Many staff therapists find themselves learning from the students and are stimulated to pursue further this new knowledge. Even the staff therapist who tends to feel somewhat inadequate when presented with unfamiliar information and questions is often motivated toward self-improvement. In order to preserve his personal sense of competence and maintain the respect of the student, such a physical therapist often seeks to advance his professional education through self-study. This has the ultimate benefit of increased effectiveness in the provision of service to the patients—the primary concern of the institution.

The physical therapist in the health care facility may find a conflict between his responsibility to provide quality health care for his patients and, at the same time, meaningful learning experiences for the students. The demands upon his time and talent by the facility may be so heavy that educational functions necessarily receive scant attention. Should this person even attempt to maintain a clinical education program? The primary function of many service departments is patient care, and financial integrity is dependent upon effective and efficient use of personnel. The teaching function is usually a nonreimbursible expenditure of time for the physical therapist who must demonstrate fiscal responsiblity in allocation of time. In university-related facilities, on the other hand, often a three-fold focus exists of patient care, education, and research. An assumption of the past has been that at least a portion of the cost burden for research and education can be passed along to the patient in the per diem charge or in higher charges for specific services.[12] Currently, that particular practice is receiving careful scrutiny by insurance carriers, governmental agencies, and education institutions.

WHAT BEHAVIORS FACILITATE LEARNING IN THE CLINICAL PHYSICAL THERAPIST?

The clinical educator is an agent of change; that is, he helps students achieve changes in their behaviors.[13] He brings some degree of awareness of the interaction process between the teacher and learner. The process includes 1) diagnosing the change needs in the learner, 2) seeking and analyzing with the learner the information pertinent to the circumstances, 3) determining what new ways of thinking and acting the student might try, 4) applying those new behaviors independently, as appropriate, and 5) providing emotional support for the student to risk learning.

Diagnosing Change Needs

When the student enters the clinical education program of any given clinical setting, he should be asked to clarify his learning goals. What does he want to learn? By committing this to paper, the student and his supervisor can appraise them from the standpoint of the specific contributions and possibilities available in that particular clinical setting. They can then establish priorities. The next step is to determine the means by which the learning objectives are to be achieved.

Such a determination requires that the student first identify what he now knows, then specify what knowledge he needs to acquire in order to accomplish his learning objectives. At the same time, the student should designate the aspects of practice in which he feels some competence (what he can do), in order to determine those areas of practice in which he needs specialized attention. The individual skills that each student brings to the clinical situation should be identified so that they may be maximized and utilized most effectively. For example, a student may bring knowledge and experience in an unusual form of treatment not shared by the current staff. He should be encouraged to pursue this with appropriate patients. Furthermore, the student should be directed and assisted in presenting in-service education programs so that the staff may benefit from his particular assets. The student also should be able to designate those behaviors he would like to develop to the level of skilled performance. With this conscious process shared by the student and his supervisor, both individuals are more likely to work cooperatively toward the same goals for the learner. This is very similar to the treatment problem in which the physical therapist has one set of goals, but the patient has quite a different set. Utimately the treatment program is doomed to failure unless the discrepancy is clarified and resolved.

Analyzing Information

This process is basically similar in any particular treatment problem, although probably at less than a conscious awareness level for the experienced therapist. In the teaching-learning transaction, the supervisor needs to help the student learn the steps for solution of problems that are usually taken for granted. The first step is to look at the evidence in the form of clinical signs and symptoms. What does the student see when he observes? Specific focus of attention to this point will help the student develop his observational skills. The next step is to identify the information pertinent to the case. Some of this information will be available to the student in the form of knowledge he has already acquired; however, he may have to search for some information in various resources—the library, the chart, the supervisor, or a specialist.

Finally, with the several pieces of information assembled that might be pertinent to the particular clinical problem, that which is relevant to plan an adequate therapeutic program for the patient must be analyzed and sorted out. A look at the paraplegic patient with spasticity provides an example. What does the student see in the behavior of this patient? What of all that he sees is noteworthy? What raises questions? In the instance that reduction or management of spasticity becomes a priority in planning the treatment program for the patient, what is the pertinent information available on the topic?

Determining New Ways

If the example of the paraplegic patient is carried into this phase of the teaching-learning transaction one can perhaps understand what is meant by "determining what new ways of thinking and acting the student might try," referred to earlier. The data have been assembled; the supervisor and student can now apply the appropriate information to the problem at hand and establish a tentative treatment plan. The plan is tentative because it may need to be altered as new clinical evidence appears.

Several approaches are available in the management of spasticity in the paraplegic patient. After surveying the information and reviewing the available resources, the student may choose to apply an icing and brushing technique. The student is not knowledgeable in this particular treatment procedure but has listed it as one of his learning goals in the first phase of "diagnosing change needs." Part of the reason for that selection was that a therapist on the staff has proficiency in this procedure. The student has decided to acquire the necessary background information, coupling this with observations of the specific procedure performed by the staff therapist. The student is now ready to try it on his own, which leads to the next step.

Applying New Behaviors

The new treatment procedure is planned in detail, listing in advance the method, expected outcome, and possible difficulties that might be encountered by the student; this is reviewed with his mentor. The student probably will desire some supervision by the "expert" in his initial applications. As the student proceeds, the clinical educator should guide him to observe the behavior of the patient in order to determine the effects of the procedure. Over a period of time, such observations will form an important portion of the evaluation process. If, for example, the benefits are not of the magnitude hoped for, another procedure may be substituted or used in concert as deemed appropriate.

New behaviors are first tried with some hesitance and perhaps some expectation of failure. Success and the reward of achievement are the positive reinforcements that soon dispel those difficult feelings—and the new behavior is tried again. All of this is accompanied by the support and encouragement of the clinical educator who observes expectantly, assists only when necessary, and shares enthusiastically in the student's growth.

Providing Emotional Support

The entire teaching-learning transaction takes place in an emotional climate. If learning is to be facilitated this climate must be one of support and encouragement. Only in it can the student learn to identify his abilities and deficiencies. As the supervisor expects and encourages him to utilize his positive assets, the student is more able to confront his need to grow in the areas of deficiency identified in setting his learning goals. The crucial nature of such emotional support for learning must be understood, but equally important is the ability to recognize that it is provided by the climate of the relationship between clinical educator and student. The focus of that relationship must be the learning goals they have negotiated.

Thus, five phases are present in the interaction process in the work of the clinical educator with his student. If they are considered from the viewpoint of the interpersonal transaction between teacher and learner, it becomes clear that two fundamental features must be present for that transaction to be effective. One is the establishment and maintenance of relationships that result in reduction of defensive behavior and anxieties in the learner—thus facilitating the learning process. The second is the creation of the learning situation, with a resultant change in behavior. The learning environment is established by the physical therapy clinical educator, based largely upon the security base of that individual. The creation of a supportive climate within which learning can take place is necessary for the reduction of tension and anxiety in the learner.

In turn, these interpersonal developments depend greatly upon certain vital attitudes in the clinical educator. If the clinical educator is anxious about status or defensive because of imagined deficiency, the resultant tension will interfere with the creation of a supportive climate conducive to learning. The resultant behavior will intensify the student's feelings of insecurity and anxiety. An atmosphere or climate that is conducive to the learning process is one in which threat to the student's security is reduced; this should result in less defensive behavior.

The clinical educator must have the awareness of himself as the "expert" and awareness of the anxieties of the student as the "novice." The student's dependency upon the teacher conflicts with his growing desire to be independent. Changes may occur in the relationship as it develops which the supervisor needs to perceive in order to build and maintain rapport. The clinical educator may be viewed as a partner and co-worker in the transaction of learning; as such, he should be aware of his own needs and motivations as he engages in the teaching-learning process. For example, does he need to control people? Does he want people to be dependent upon him? Does he seek to give love and affection and derive satisfactions from this kind of interaction? Is he able to handle his authority effectively?[14] Does he fear his expression of hostility to the extent that it interferes with his function as a clinical educator? In this event, he will keep the learner at arm's length, thus reducing his effectiveness as a teacher. If the clinical educator understands his own motivations and the effect of his own personality upon others, he is better able to keep his behavior under conscious control and direction.

The educator should have the ability to accept the student as an individual, to respect and listen to him, separating the person from the possibly disliked aspects of his behavior. The therapist with a dislike for skin disease who also dislikes and rejects the patient who has the skin disease is not an effective therapist. Frequently, educators are unaware that they reject the learner because of his lack of knowledge or deficiency in abilities, or for lack of facility in relationship. The educator does not have to approve the current status and behavior of the learner in order to accept him as a person.

Building on these attitudes, the clinical educator will be able to use his own behavior to create the kind of learning situation in which the student will be able to manage his anxiety, set realistic learning goals, and utilize the clinic setting and the "teacher" to achieve them.

SUMMARY

As the student is involved in the difficult process of change in both thought and action, the learning climate should be one which provides emotional support as well as intellectual challenge. The clinical educator has the important function of creating a climate conducive to learning. In each clinical education setting, the interpersonal relationship is negotiated by the clinical instructor and the student, and is dependent upon the student, the instructor, and the clinic. The primary accountability of providing a good learning experience for the student belongs to the clinical instructor. He must, therefore, work to build a relationship with the student that will reduce initial anxiety and enable the development and achievement of appropriate learning goals.

REFERENCES

1. Committee on Basic Education: Education for physical therapy. Washington, American Physical Therapy Association, May 1968
2. Moore M: Institutional Agreements for Clinical Education in Physical Therapy. Paper presented at Fiftieth Annual Conference of the American Physical Therapy Association, Boston, Massachusetts, June 1971
3. Dickinson R, Dervitz HL, Meida HM: Handbook for Physical Therapy Teachers. Washington, American Physical Therapy Association, 1967
4. Standards for physical therapy services, adopted by the Board of Directors February 1971. Phys Ther 51:1315−1318, 1971
5. Staats AW, Staats CK: Complex Human Behavior. New York, Holt, Rinehart and Winston, Inc., 1964

6. Highet G: The Art of Teaching. New York, Vintage Books, 1959

7. Bruner JS: Toward a Theory of Instruction. Cambridge, Harvard University Press, 1967

8. Brown JW, Thornton JW: College Teaching: Perspectives and Guidelines. New York, McGraw-Hill Book Company, 1963

9. Klausmeier HJ, Ripple RE: Learning and Human Abilities. New York, Harper and Row, Publishers, 1971

10. Lippitt R, Watson J, Westley B: The Dynamics of Planned Change. New York, Harcourt Brace and Company, 1958

11. Dervitz HL: Advantages to a clinical facility in providing a program of clinical education. APTA-OVR Institute Papers, Washington, American Physical Therapy Association, April 1961, pp. 62–68

12. Ramsden E, Fisher W: Cost allocation for physical therapy in a teaching hospital. Phys Ther 50:660–664, 1970

13. Schutz W: Interpersonal Underworld. In The Planning of Change by Bennis W, Benne K, Chin R: New York, Holt, Rinehart and Winston, Inc., 1961

14. Ramsden E: Authority: professional responsibility. Phys Ther 51:418–421, 1971

Clinical Contracts:
A Method for Identifying and Resolving Student Clinical Performance Problems
JILL NEWMAN HENRY

INTRODUCTION

At one time or another students may encounter difficulties or problems in various aspects of clinical performance. One of the responsibilities of a clinical instructor is to assist students in resolving their performance problems. Proper resolution of student problems begins with problem recognition and definition[1] or determination and cause identification.[2] Recognition and definition is important because solutions developed without a clear understanding of the nature of the problem often fail to produce satisfactory results. Other authors have addressed problem identification[3] and use of learning contracts[4] in clinical settings. The purpose of this article is to present a systematic method that can be used by clinical instructors to identify and resolve student clinical performance problems. Detailed problem identification combined with the use of a student/instructor clinical contract may effectively resolve the majority of student clinical performance problems.

IDENTIFYING STUDENT PERFORMANCE PROBLEMS

Step I: Recognize the student's clinical performance behaviors and describe them using specific and objective terminology. The first step in identifying student performance problems is to describe the facts in the situation (intellectual response) and separate the facts from feelings about the facts (emotional response). Facts are objectively verifiable aspects of experience...information or data having no particular emotional connotation.[5] Feelings are emotional responses to experience; they are here and now reactions.[5] Attempting to respond at the same time on both a fact and feeling level may interfere with problem identification. Recording facts, not feelings, in a log or clinical diary can provide objective data to assist in making opinions and decisions (Table 1).

Step II: Develop a list of opinions or assumptions about the possible causes of a student's behavior. Opinions are beliefs or judgments that fall short of certainty and are oriented to the immediate situation; short-range ideas about what is happening, how others are behaving, what is being

said or proposed.[5] Two clinical instructors and the student may have three different sets of opinions about the possible causes of a performance problem.

STEPS IN IDENTIFYING STUDENT PERFORMANCE PROBLEMS

I. Describe the student's clinical performance.
II. Develop a list of opinions about causes of performance.
III. Analyze each opinion.
IV. Develop a problem list.

Table 1

For example, when a student fails to perform a thorough patient evaluation, one clinical instructor may believe the failure is due to the student's lack of preparation or knowledge. However, the second clinical instructor may believe that the student's attitude was a factor in the poor performance. For example, the student could have resented being assigned to that particular patient and therefore was not thorough. Finally, the student may believe that if she had been allowed more time, the performance could have been completed successfully. All three opinions are real, and include each individual's unique interpretation of facts and feelings, often based on different past experiences. In most cases, clear identification of facts (in Step I) will result in similar but not identical lists of opinions about the causes (in Step II).

In this step separate opinion lists are developed by the clinical instructor and the student. Then all lists are combined into one master list. At this phase of the process, everyone's opinions about the causes of the problem are viewed as being potentially true.

Step III: Analyze each opinion to verify or deny its truth. The purpose of this activity is to categorize each opinion as being either a fact or a fabrication.

For ease of analysis, opinions may be divided into three separate educational domains; 1) psychomotor, 2) cognitive, and 3) affective. For example, opinions about how the student uses her hands or body to perform a treatment would be classified as psychomotor.[6] Opinions about

what the student knows or how she thinks would be classified as cognitive.[6] Opinions about what the student believes or values would be assigned to the affective category.[5] After categorizing each opinion, the clinical instructor and student work together to examine and validate each opinion listed.

Psychomotor problems are often the easiest to analyze and resolve. If there is concern about a student's ability to do manual muscle testing correctly, the student needs only to demonstrate muscle testing on the clinical instructor. If performed correctly, and if manual muscle testing was identified initially as a possible reason for lack of thoroughness in patient evaluation, then the clinical performance problem may be resolved. If the student is unable to perform the muscle test, then muscle testing is noted as one aspect of the student's overall problem.

Problems pertaining to cognitive deficiencies are difficult to validate. Usual evaluation methods include asking the student questions about her knowledge or understanding of patient care. However, a difference exists between asking a student to describe the components of an evaluation process while a patient is waiting for treatment in the next room, and meeting with the student at the end of the day to discuss the evaluation process. The former situation demonstrates the student's ability to think on-the-spot, the later situation uncovers knowledge accessible to the student when time pressures are removed. Additionally, the clinical instructor should investigate the student's ability to make decisions and develop solutions for patient problems. Common methods for identifying cognitive domain problems are, use of paper and pencil tests, and the use of simulated or real patient situations. References are available describing how cognitive processes can be evaluated.[1,7-9]

Opinions about the motives underlying the student's clinical performance behavior are validated by exploring the student's values. According to Boshear and Albrecht, values are ideals; behavioral standards based on one's sense of propriety; they are relatively permanent ideas about what should be.[5] Students bring their own attitudes to the clinic but are also influ-

13

enced by role models they see around them. Value exploration must be done in an atmosphere of trust. Confidence and caring must exist between the student and clinical instructor. Often a student's clinical performance problems are the result of fears or beliefs. Detailed analysis of affective behavior should produce the final data necessary to identify all components of the student's performance deficit.

Step IV: Develop a problem list accepted as "true for now" by both the clinical instructor and the student. This final step in problem identification is the development of a problem list. Each problem should be stated broadly enough to allow flexibility in planning learning experiences and specifically enough to identify cognitive, affective, and psychomotor components expected in the student's performance. The problem list must be a product of the combined efforts of both the student and instructor. Because the list has been developed by both, it will be valued and used by both as the basis for developing a clinical contract to resolve the problem.

THE CLINICAL CONTRACT

Figure 1 illustrates the relationship between problem identification and the development of a clinical contract for problem resolution. A clinical contract is a written agreement between a student and clinical instructor outlining specific activities each will do to resolve a problem or reach a goal. The clinical contract presented is a modification of the work done by

Knowles[10,11] in the development of an adult self-directed learning contract. The purpose of a clinical contract is to clarify communication and identify the responsibilities of the student and clinical instructor during student problem resolution. The clinical contract should be developed by both the student and the clinical instructor, agreed upon by both, and the outcome evaluated by both. A third person may be useful in the development and evaluation phases to serve as a negotiator or to have an unbiased viewpoint on the terms of the contract.

COMPONENTS OF A CLINICAL CONTRACT

Goals. Goals are re-statements of the identified problems in a positive way. Problem statements are oriented to the past; "The student was unable to perform..." and therefore, have a negative connotation. Goal statements are oriented to the future; "The student will be able to perform..." and give a sense of hope and purpose in the problem resolution stage (Table 2).

COMPONENTS OF A
CLINICAL CONTRACT

1. Goals
2. Specific Objectives
3. Activities of the Student
4. Activities of the Clinical Instructor
5. Evaluation
6. Signatures

Table 2

Specific Objectives. In a thorough process of a problem identification, many smaller issues contributing to the overall student's problem may be identified. These smaller problems are again re-stated, in positive behavioral terms, as specific objectives to be accomplished by the student.

Activities of the Student. Participants outline the specific activities the student will do to meet the stated goals and objectives. Responsibilities and obligations of the student toward resolving her own problems are described in the clinical contract.

Activities of the Clinical Instructor. This section of the contract includes specifications on how the clinical instructor will help the student meet the affiliation goals. For example, if one student activity was that the student would: "Write the components of an evaluation plan for review by the instructor." The instructor's responsibility would then be to: "Provide references and feedback to the student on her evaluation plan."

Evaluation. The clinical instructor and student specify when and how the student will be evaluated. The student may be given practice time to improve performance, followed by the formal evaluation.

Signatures. The student and instructor should sign the clinical contract. Their signatures represent an agreement and commitment to fulfilling the terms of the contract and resolving the student's problems.

EXPERIENCE WITH THE PROCESS

This process has been used by me for the past five years. It has also been used by our clinical instructors. The format of the clinical contract has been adopted by the Department of Physical Therapy, Medical College of Georgia as a remedial plan for any student who fails either a didactic course or a clinical affiliation.

BENEFITS OF THE PROCESS

The problem identification phase has provided students with opportunities to express their own opinions about problem causes. Students who understand and accept their problems through the problem identification process appear more motivated to take responsibility to resolve problems than students who are told they have problems and are told what to do to resolve them. This process allowed students to take control of their own learning while still receiving instructor support dur-

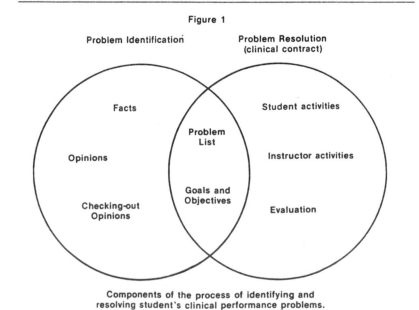

Figure 1

Problem Identification — Problem Resolution (clinical contract)

Components of the process of identifying and resolving student's clinical performance problems.

ing the process. Clinical instructors have reported positive results when using this clinical contract process. Students who have successfully completed the contract process have successfully completed later clinical affiliations in our program. Students who have been unsuccessful in completing their contracts have been encouraged to explore alternatives, such as taking time-off from the program for outside work, returning to repeat selected aspects of the program, or reconsidering their career goals.

LIMITATIONS OF THE PROCESS

Problem identification has been a time consuming process; requiring time for data collection, evaluation, and discussions between the student and the instructor. Contract negotiations require that an atmosphere of trust and mutual cooperation exist between the instructor and the student. Instructors must relinquish the role of "telling" the student what to do or "fixing" the problem for the student. The student must initiate action instead of waiting to be told. The student and the instructor must find enough common ground to become equal partners in the process.

The ultimate value of the process of problem identification and clinical contracting is in its identification and treatment of the problems affecting student performance. When the student and instructor have discovered the real problems, they experience a sense of relief, because then the student has a clear direction on how to facilitate change and growth.

Ms. Henry is an Associate Professor and the Academic Coordinator of Clinical Education in the Department of Physical Therapy at the Medical College of Georgia, Augusta, GA 30912-3100.

REFERENCES

1. May BJ, Newman J: Developing competence in problem solving, a behavioral model. Phys Ther 60(9):1140-1145, 1980.
2. Olsen SL: Teaching treatment planning, a problem solving model. Phys Ther 63(4):526-529, 1983.
3. Scully RM, Shepard KF: Clinical teaching in physical therapy education, and ethnographic study. Phys Ther 63(3):349-358, 1983.
4. Windom PA: Developing a Clinical Education program from the clinician's perspective. Phys Ther 62(11):1604-1609, 1982.
5. Boshear WC, Albrecht KG: Understanding People, Models and Concepts. San Diego, University Associates, Inc. pp 63-67, 1977.
6. Gronlund NE: Measurement and Evaluation in Teachingl. ed.3, New York, MacMillian, pp 28-33, 1976.
7. Shanahan PM: Methodology for Teaching Theory. JOTA 30(4):217-224, 1976.
8. Hoban JD: Simulation: A technique for instruction and evaluation. In Ford CW: Clinical Education for the Allied Health Professions. St. Louis, The CV Mosby Co., pp 145-157, 1978.
9. Henry JN: Identifying problems in clinical problem solving: perceptions and interventions with nonproblem-solving clinical behaviors. Phys Ther 65(7):1071-1074, 1985.
10. Knowles: Self-Directed Learning. Chicago, Follett Publishing Co., 1975.
11. Knowles MS: Some guidelines for using learning contracts. Presented at faculty workshop, Department of Physical Therapy, Medical College of Georgia, Augusta, GA, 1983.

special article

Clinical Education

Awareness of Our "Not-OK" Behavior

CAROL M. DAVIS, M.S.,
and ANN E. McKAIN, Ed.D.

The education of students in physical therapy is a complex process involving cognitive, affective, and psychomotor learning. One of the most perplexing challenges for clinical and didactic faculty is that of developing appropriate attitudes in students. We can look at the development of appropriate attitudes in several ways. First, Mager has stated that teachers must accept the responsibility of striving to ensure that their students leave their influence with as favorable an attitude toward the subject as possible. When this attitude is developed, teachers "maximize the possibility that [students] will *remember* what they have been taught, and will willingly learn more about what they have been taught."[1] We want our students to have a favorable attitude about our profession, to feel good about being a part of physical therapy.

Equally as important, however, is the realization that physical therapy educators must assume responsibility for students' learning how to "act" in the clinical setting. Part of the affective, or attitude, learning can take place with a cognitive approach in the classroom.

Lectures or seminars on the Code of Ethics or on defining quality of care in physical therapy help to accomplish this objective. The major extent of students' learning how to act as physical therapists, however, seems to take place in the form of modeling, acting like someone they admire.

Moon and Render have pointed out the importance of student-teacher interaction as a basis for the formation of student attitudes. The actual interaction between teacher and student, the personality characteristics of the teacher, the exchange of knowledge, and the feelings and behavior which reveal our value system all have a profound effect on the student's self-concept, values, and attitudes, especially as they relate to their professional goals.[2] Daily interaction with our students does more to develop their appropriate attitudes than any other form of teaching. In addition, the more prestige the teacher has in the eyes of the student, the more the student will tend to learn by imitation.[1]

The importance of learning "how to do" by watching others has long been recognized as a powerful teaching tool by clinical instructors in physical therapy. Jacobson revealed that new graduates of physical therapy curricula more significantly tended to model their behavior after one of their clinical instructors than after a classroom instructor or another staff therapist.[3] Physical therapy students in the clinic

Miss Davis is Assistant Professor and Coordinator of Clinical Education, Department of Physical Therapy, University of Alabama in Birmingham, Birmingham, AL 35294.

Dr. McKain is Assistant Professor of Educational Foundations, Georgia State University, Atlanta, GA 30303, and a licensed clinical psychologist in Atlanta.

watch what their clinical instructor does, and they tend to identify that behavior as being the right way or the best way to act as they imitate it. The clinical instructor is placed in a powerful position by the student. Ramsden and Dervitz pointed out that a clinical instructor must be aware that the student sees the instructor as the expert and himself as a novice.[4] With that power come some rather obvious responsibilities. In addition to the awareness of being the expert in the students' eyes, the clinical instructor must assume awareness and responsibility of his own needs and motivations as a teacher of young professionals. The better able a clinical instructor is to understand his own strengths and weaknesses as a teacher, the better able he is to understand and use his own power and the better able he is to respond appropriately to students.[4] Clinical instructors would do well to be aware of any need to control people or to have others be dependent on them. They should be able to handle the authority placed on them as teachers and to be aware of strengths or weaknesses in interacting with people.[5]

In other words, not only must we "behave the way we want our students to behave,"[1] we must be aware of our behavior and consciously choose to avoid acting in ways that we do not want our students to act. What can we, as clinical instructors, do to become more aware of all of our behavior?

Students will see us as total persons; we cannot avoid revealing "not OK" behavior, but we must work to ensure that students will be more apt to model our "OK" behavior.

"Not OK" behavior is often revealed when we become frightened and give up our power, when we become confused and feel powerless, or when we become angry and say and do things which we regret later.

To better understand our own behavior as teachers or developers of behavior, we should try to analyze these thoughts on paper:

I am "OK" (feel good about myself and what I do) when:

I am "not OK" (act in ways we do not want students to act) when:

Once the events and circumstances that result in "not OK" behavior are identified, listing what we do in each instance when we

feel "not OK" may be helpful. Patient care responsibilities keep us so busy that often we are unaware of the behavior we exhibit which we do not want students to model. Our goal should be to identify those behaviors. If a red flag goes up, we need to stop and consider what is happening. Are you aware of an increase in the speed or volume of your voice? Did you dismiss your patient or student with a short remark? Are you aware of sarcasm or defensiveness in your reply? Are you feeling guilty for not spending enough time with your patient who is terminally ill, or who has a bad odor, or whose mother irritates you? Are you leaving the clinical setting before the accepted time or before your work is completed for the day? Do you avoid talking to certain colleagues? Do you make too many demands on staff, patients, and students which you cannot really justify? Has physical therapy practice become an eight-hour drudgery for you? Are you consistently late for work, for rounds, or for staffing?

Once we are aware of incidences of "not OK" behavior, the next step is to identify the feelings that prompted our behavior. Then we must decide what to do about those feelings and decide what behavior we would rather demonstrate as a result of our feelings. The behavior we choose to exhibit should be behavior appropriate for our students to model.

It is OK to feel "not OK"! It is not OK to not be aware of it, to not be aware that students are going to model after us, to not be aware that we do exhibit behavior that we might not want students to exhibit. Setting aside the time to be aware of all of our behavior and to make choices about our behavior results in a good feeling about ourselves as teachers—as developers of behavior.

REFERENCES

1. Mager R: Developing Attitude Toward Learning. Palo Alto, Fearon Publishers, 1968
2. Moon C, Render G: Affective Concerns for Education in the Health Professions. Paper presented at the Annual Meeting of the American Educational Research Association, New Orleans, Louisiana, February 1973
3. Jacobson B: Role modeling in physical therapy. Phys Ther 54:244-250, 1974
4. Ramsden E, Dervitz H: Clinical education: Interpersonal foundations. Phys Ther 52:1060-1066, 1972
5. Ramsden E: Authority: Professional responsibility. Phys Ther 51:418-421, 1971

Using Feedback and Evaluation Effectively in Clinical Supervision

Model for Interaction Characteristics and Strategies

JILL NEWMAN HENRY

Feedback and evaluation are both integral parts of daily communications that supervisors and instructors use to help employees and students learn and grow. The purpose of this article is to provide guidelines for the effective use of feedback and evaluation in the supervision and performance assessment of students and staff therapists and assistants. I define feedback and evaluation and give examples of their uses. Reactions of students and staff to feedback and evaluation are identified. Carkhuff's phases of helping are described and integrated in a model with interaction characteristics and strategies that supervisors and instructors use when giving feedback and evaluation. I describe and suggest applications of the model for using feedback and evaluation to facilitate the development of independent and competent physical therapists and assistants.

Key Words: Education, Interpersonal relations, Physical therapy, Professional competence.

Feedback and evaluation are terms often confused in supervision and education. These terms appear to mean the same thing; however, their effects on the recipient are different. Feedback and evaluation are both integral parts of daily communication that instructors and supervisors use to help students and employees learn and grow. One process of helping another individual learn and grow has been described by Carkhuff[1] and interpreted by Gazda et al[2(pp9-21)] in a model for helping relationships. The purpose of this paper is to define feedback and evaluation in clinical supervision and to describe the use of feedback and evaluation in a model for helping relationships. The integration of feedback and evaluation in a helping relationship model will provide the supervisor or clinical instructor with guidelines for a systematic use of these communication techniques.

DEFINITIONS

Feedback

Feedback is operationally described in this model as a nonjudgmental communication to another individual for the purpose of facilitating self-aware-

Ms. Henry is Assistant Professor and Academic Coordinator of Clinical Education. Department of Physical Therapy. Medical College of Georgia. Augusta. GA 30912 (USA).

This article was submitted February 21, 1984; was with the author for revision 21 weeks; and was accepted September 25, 1984.

ness. Developing self-awareness is an essential component of functioning as an effective physical therapist or assistant. Carkhuff states that understanding of self helps an individual to act differently from the way he acted before, or in other words, to learn.[3] Self-awareness enables an individual to recognize the consequences of his actions. The individual may then choose to repeat his actions if the consequences are favorable or to modify his actions to produce more desirable results. The self-aware physical therapist or assistant can independently change, learn, and grow to provide more effective and efficient patient care.

Hanson describes the characteristics of feedback as being "direct, descriptive, accepting, respecting an individual's freedom, immediate, and focused."[4] True feedback is difficult to give because it is often confused with judgments made during evaluation. Feedback permits the recipient to act on his own because he chooses to, not because someone else judged that he should.

Evaluation

Evaluation is operationally described in this model as the judgment of an individual's behavior based on specified or unspecified criteria for performance. Evaluation of student performance occurs when the student's behavior is compared with a performance standard. Specified performance standards are written in the objectives of the affiliation and policies of the department. Unspec-

ified performance standards are held in the minds of clinical supervisors or instructors as expectations of what a student or employee should or should not do. A specified performance standard may be "The staff therapist or assistant should demonstrate interest in and commitment to quality patient care." An unspecified standard that is assumed and evaluated is "The staff therapist or assistant should be sensitive, flexible, enthusiastic, and respectful toward his patients and supervisors." Both standards are closely related to value systems against which the student and employee are judged.

Informal and Formal Feedback and Evaluation

Feedback and evaluation are further categorized as informal and formal in this model. Informal refers to communication given through words, tone of voice, body language, and other forms of nonverbal behaviors. Formal refers to communication documented in writing.

Informal feedback. Informal feedback is given through nonjudgmental oral communication. It consists of stating observations of behavior without inferring positive or negative attributes to the behavior. When giving informal feedback, a person assumes the role of a videocamera—recording and replaying observations. Statements of fact, such as, "When you came into the room, you hesitated for a minute," or "Do you realize that you have been working on that patient discharge summary for an hour?" constitute informal feedback.

Informal evaluation. Informal evaluation is given through judgmental oral communication and body language. Praise and blame are part of informal evaluation. Statements such as "Good work" or shifts in voice tone while stating, "Why did you do it *that* way?" imply comparison with a standard. Looks of disapproval given across a crowded gym from supervisor to student are part of informal evaluation.

Formal feedback. Any feedback given in writing is considered formal. The use of the critical incident technique of collecting and organizing direct observations of significant acts of student or staff performance is considered formal feedback.[5] The critical incident technique results in the recording of a "group of critical behaviors relatively free from bias."[5] A supervisor or instructor may further categorize these incidents as positive or negative and use them as a part of the formal evaluation process. In formal feedback, these incidents are used without value judgments to document observable events. An example of a critical incident used for formal feedback is as follows. While the student was helping Mrs. Jones exercise her leg, Mrs. Jones began to cry. The student stopped the treatment and talked with Mrs. Jones. The student resumed treatment after Mrs. Jones was no longer crying. The incident itself is a recording of the facts, an action, and its apparent results. An element of judgment is involved in deciding which behaviors to document as critical incidents. The judgment is toward a set of behaviors and their consequences and not what the student or staff member should or should not do. Whether the action and its results were "right" is an evaluation based on feedback given through the incidents themselves. Other examples of formal feedback include the following: nonjudgmental logs and diaries, listings of patients' problems, student or staff treatments, and descriptions of the effects of the treatments on problems. Formal feedback may be equated to the objective portion of a S.O.A.P. note. It is a recording of the facts of a given situation.

Formal evaluation. Written performance evaluations are the most comon form of formal evaluation. Check lists, student evaluation instruments, and any documentation that requires judgments between pass or fail or correct or incorrect are all part of formal evaluation. The assessment portion of the S.O.A.P. note corresponds to formal evaluation. The supervisor or clinical instructor states in writing that, in his opinion, based on observed facts and department standards or goals, the employee or student has strengths and weaknesses in certain areas. In addition, the supervisor or clinical instructor may make recommendations for future activities. Formal evaluations are an integral part of both preparation for and practice as physical therapists and assistants.

REACTIONS TO EVALUATION AND FEEDBACK

The recipient of the communication reacts differently to feedback than he does to evaluation. Evaluation implies a "should" and the power of the evaluator. Regardless of what the student or employee believes is appropriate, he must conform in some degree to the opinions of the evaluator. Nonconformance may result in failure of an affiliation or loss of a raise or even a job. Evaluation often creates feelings of anxiety, defensiveness, and helplessness. The person being evaluated has given another person permission and power (willingly or not) to judge his performance and sometimes his very being. The use of self-evaluation helps to diffuse the emotional reactions to evaluation. It equalizes the relationship between the people involved. Self-evaluation requires self-awareness and self-awareness is developed through feedback.

Feedback permits a choice on the part of the recipient. Because feedback is nonjudgmental, both people are on an equal basis in the communication. Casual feedback comes as easily as saying, "Did you know that whenever you work with a patient on the new exercise machine, you look worried and seem to get tense? It seems like your patients become worried with you." After receiving that communication, the recipient can say, "No, I didn't realize it. Thanks for telling me." The recipient can then reflect on the feedback and decide whether to modify his behavior. He is not obligated to change his behavior in the same way he would if evaluated. He is in control of his own response. A supervisor using evaluation in the above example would say, "Stop making your patients worried when you use the new exercise machine with them." Feedback usually contains more specificity than evaluation because it is a reporting of facts. Evaluation also uses facts as a basis for opinions, but often the facts are not directly expressed.

Recipients often confuse evaluation with feedback when the communication is factual, but the tone of voice is judgmental. Using the same example as before, a supervisor may say, "*Did you know that your patients look worried?*" implying that they shouldn't be and you better do something about it. Whether a communication is evaluative or offered as feedback depends on the purpose and intent of the communicator. The following model for a helping relationship can assist supervisors and instructors to clarify the intent of communication they use. The assumption made by including the helping model is that supervisors and clinical instructors wish to assume the role of an ally to their staff and students and not an adversary.

MODEL FOR A HELPING RELATIONSHIP

Carkhuff's model for helping relationships as interpreted by Gazda et al[2(pp9-21)] contains three distinct phases of helping. Each phase requires certain actions on the part of the helper (supervisor or instructor) to facilitate the helpee (staff member or student) in solving his own problems.

Facilitation Phase

The goal of this phase is helpee self-exploration. The helper uses empathy, respect, and warmth toward the helpee. To communicate empathy, the helper must listen to what the helpee is saying, think of words that represent the helpee's feelings and situation, and use those words to convey a level of awareness and understanding.[2(pp246-254)] The following is an example of an empathic response. Staff member to supervisor: "I know I have to go treat Mr. Jones, but it's late and I don't think I can do anything for him because he always refuses treatment anyway." Supervisor's empathic response: "You *feel* frustrated because Mr. Jones continues to refuse your treatments." A response that conveys empathy identifies a perceived feeling and places the feeling in relation to a particular situation, "You feel ... because ...."[2(pp9-21)] The helpee on hearing the response can validate his feelings by saying, "Yes, that's how I feel," or "No, I feel ...." The responses have

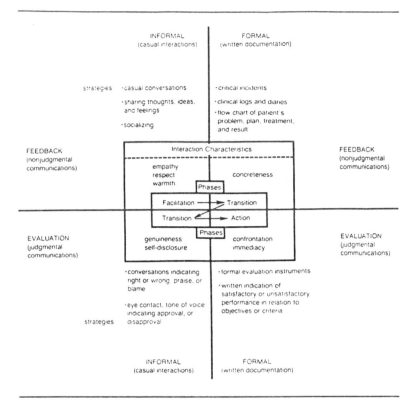

Figure. Integration of Carkhuff's phases of helping with interaction characteristics and strategies used by supervisors during informal and formal feedback and evaluation.

assisted the helpee to clarify his feelings and engage in self-exploration.

Respect means the belief in the value and potential of a person.[2(pp 9-21)] To communicate respect, the helper must have confidence in the helpee's ability to help himself. Respect is not "advice-giving": it is giving permission for the helpee to feel free to solve his own problems with support and confidence. Warmth is the degree to which the helper communicates his caring about the helpee.[2(pp 9-21)] Both warmth and respect are communicated through empathic responses and nonverbal communications such as gestures and voice tones.

Transition Phase

The helper begins to become gently evaluative in helping the helpee achieve a goal of better self-understanding. The helper uses concreteness, genuineness, and self-disclosure in his communications with the helpee to facilitate this phase.[2(pp 9-21)]

The helper uses concreteness to help the helpee focus on specific details of the problem to gain a better perspective of the problem situation.[2(pp 9-21)] The following is an example of concreteness and empathy combined in a single response. Student to clinical supervisor: "I wish that all my clinical instructors could agree on the way to write a S.O.A.P. note. One tells me that my note is OK, and the next one tells me it's wrong and I should redo it. I give up!" Clinical supervisor's response: "You sound confused and frustrated over the inconsistent evaluations by your clinical instructors. If they can't agree on what goes in a S.O.A.P. note, how can you tell when your note is satisfactory?"

Genuineness refers to the ability of the helper to communicate verbal and nonverbal messages that are congruent with how he feels.[2(pp 246-254)] Most people have had the experience of approaching someone who looks upset, asking if he feels all right, and receiving a sharp reply of, "Yes! I'm fine!" At times, the clinical

supervisor must be able to admit to the staff member that, yes, he is frustrated or disappointed or that something is bothering him. The ability to share the reason for a discrepancy between words and emotions is a part of self-disclosure.

Action Phase

In this phase, the helper uses confrontation and immediacy to judge the helpee and communicate his judgments. The goal of this phase is for the helpee to take appropriate action to solve his own problems.[2(pp 9-21)]

Confrontation is the ability of the helper to point out clearly discrepancies between actual performance and desired performance that the helper has observed.[2(pp 246-254)] Confrontation is the communication supervisors most often use during formal evaluations. An example of a confrontational communication is, "You are expected to be able to finish all your patient progress notes and enter them in the medical record by 5 PM. For the past two weeks, you have been here writing them until 7 PM. That is not appropriate. We will have to do something to help you solve this problem." Immediacy is the ability of the helper and helpee to discuss their interpersonal relationship as it exists at that moment.[2(pp 246-254)] A supervisor might say, "I know you're frustrated right now. So am I. We have to work through whatever anger we feel toward each other before we can help you improve your performance."

INTEGRATION OF THE PHASES OF HELPING WITH THE USE OF FEEDBACK AND EVALUATION

The model in the Figure illustrates the relationship between the uses of formal and informal feedback and evaluation and Carkhuff's phases of helping in a helping relationship. In the facilitation phase of helping, informal feedback is used to ask and answer questions, to communicate empathy, and to develop feelings of warmth and respect between the instructor or supervisor and student or staff member. Nonjudgmental, casual communication enables the supervisor to earn the role of helper and the student or staff member to accept the role of helpee. This role clarification is essential to prevent later misunderstandings. Premature use of evaluation creates one of two scenarios. If the student has ac-

356

cepted the clinical instructor as an authority figure already, then the student will spend his initial energy on figuring out what the clinical instructor thinks is "right." The student becomes focused on pleasing the authority figure, and his own original or creative ideas have less value and, therefore, less use. If, on the other hand, the staff member has not had the opportunity to get to know and respect the supervisor, and the supervisor becomes evaluative, then the staff member may refuse to take the evaluations seriously. The staff member thinks to himself, "He has no right to tell me what to do. I'll listen to him but I won't change. After all, it's his opinion against mine." Both responses described above prevent meaningful evaluations that facilitate growth.

The transition phase of helping includes formal feedback and informal evaluation. Formal feedback helps supply the data on which informal evaluations are based. The student or staff member learns that his performance was good because when he was treating Mrs. Smith, he did certain things, and those actions had certain good effects. The student or staff member begins to realize the effects of his own actions and to increase his own self-awareness. Self-awareness leads to better decision making, change, and growth. The quality of the performance in patient care, education, administration, and all areas increases.

In a helping relationship, the action phase occurs after facilitation and transition dimensions have been established. In this phase, written evaluations are used as the focus for confrontation. The evaluations are presented in here and now terms: "You may have been different last year, you may be different tomorrow, but as of right now, this is how you stand in relation to the expected performance." In clinical education, the action phase occurs primarily at student performance midterm evaluation and final evaluation sessions. In other patient care settings, the action phase comes at annual performance evaluation.

APPLICATIONS OF THE MODEL

The helping relationship model may be used as a self-evaluation tool for clinical instructors. Effective use of feedback and evaluation in clinical supervision requires attention to both variety and timing. Some clinical instructors may find themselves functioning predominantly in the informal evaluation mode—always praising or criticizing the student. Without a balance of feedback to help the student understand the source of the evaluation, interpersonal relations become difficult. If the initial facilitation phase is passed over because the instructor has no time for informal feedback, then the student may respond negatively to further attempts on the part of the instructor to help him learn. The use of formal feedback in the form of logs and clinical diaries helps the student anticipate the ratings on the formal evaluation instruments.

Use of this model requires self-awareness on the part of the supervisor. That is perhaps its greatest advantage and disadvantage. The development of self-awareness takes time and effort. When I began using the model, I found that my primary mode of communication was informal evaluation. The use of praise words like "nice work" and "good job" without specific feedback left my students wondering what they had done right and how they could do it again. In addition, certain aspects of formal evaluation came as a surprise to the students. Without feedback, they did not understand the basis for the opinions expressed in the evaluation. The monitoring of self and the use of interaction characteristics and strategies for the supervisor described in this model requires time. The priorities of each new day prevent all of us from following the model all of the time.

A balanced mixture of the techniques used in the helping sequence will often produce a student or staff member who is ready and able to take action on his own to resolve identified problems. The ultimate goal of the helping relationship and of clinical supervision is to facilitate the development of independent or self-dependent individuals capable of recognizing and resolving their own problems. The time spent in initial supervision will be regained in the efficiency and effectiveness of a self-dependent student, therapist, or assistant.

SUMMARY

This article has presented the integration of feedback and evaluation techniques with Carkhuff's phases of helping. The model provides guidelines for the clinical supervisor's effective use of both feedback and evaluation during clinical supervision of students and employees.

REFERENCES

1. Carkhuff RR: A human technology for group helping process. Educational Technology XIII:31–38, 1973
2. Gazda GM, Walters RP, Childers WC: Human Relations Development: A Manual for Health Sciences. Newton, MA, Allyn & Bacon Inc, 1975, pp 246–254
3. Carkhuff RR: Helping and human relations: A brief guide for training lay helpers. Journal of Research and Development in Education 4(2):17–27, 1971
4. Hanson, quoted in Boshear WC, Albrecht KG: Understanding People: Models and Concepts. San Diego, CA, University Associates Inc, 1977, p 237
5. McDaniel LV: The critical incident method in evaluation. Phys Ther 44:235–242, 1964

Design of Clinical Education

"It's the tunnel visions that keep us from looking at all the possibilities and options of a situation or opportunity that confronts us."

Laurence Smith
Vice President for University
Marketing and Student Affairs
Eastern Michigan University

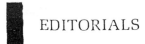 EDITORIALS

POST-GRADUATE EDUCATION:
The Internship

INCREASING CONCERN IS being expressed about the availability of physical therapy services—particularly as the backlog of patients with chronic disease grows and as commitments to acute care are broadened. At the same time there is a ground swell of concern about the quality of services being offered.

I doubt if the manpower gap will ever be closed, or high quality demands met if we continue to cherish our present-day notions of education and practice. Physical therapy must adapt to modern demands and this will require a revolution of attitudes as well as methods. It will require the development of persons whose approach to their professional service is that of a person who thinks and reasons . . . persons who will sift through the myriad of clinical problems with the approach of the scientist tempered with the finesse of the artist.

One of the first steps needed in the revitalization of physical therapy is the initiation of means of training a superior practitioner. To effect this in the most efficient manner and at the earliest time, revisions of current modes of clinical education should be explored.

Clinical affiliation, where the student spends a few weeks at each of several institutions, are inadequate to train in either scope or depth, the kind of physical therapist now in demand: a person who knows how to evaluate patients adequately, is decisive about treatment planning, who has a capacity for intense observation and who sees what he looks *at* as well as what he looks *for*. Present systems do not provide practitioners with a grasp of the rudiments of supervision or an insight into administrative problems.

The establishment of a unified, coordinated internship at the end of the academic program seems to be indicated. Inclusion of clerkship programs as an integral part of the academic program would supply the early desirable patient-contact. The internship should provide experience primarily in patient care, but could also offer exposures in supervision, administration and research as preferred by the student.

They should be 9 months to one year in duration and be stipend-supported.

Though this need is expressed at a time when medicine is considering the abolition of its traditional internship, the idea should not be cast aside because the education of physician and physical therapist is in no way comparable.

Development of clinical centers that can provide an internship of quality, establishment of standards, and accreditation procedures would all need to be part of the initial blueprint. The time to start imaginative planning is now.

The impetus and method of producing a physical therapist capable of satisfying the complex demands of modern patient care must come from within the profession. The internship would be a step in the right direction.

HELEN J. HISLOP, PH.D.
Editor

Receptivity to Full-Time Early Clinical Education Experience

PAULETTE M. KONDELA, PhD,
and RICHARD E. DARNELL, PhD

This report describes feedback from clinical instructors, academic faculty members, and students following a part-time to full-time change in the scheduling of early clinical education in the Curriculum in Physical Therapy at the University of Michigan. A questionnaire was distributed to all academic faculty members and students of the physical therapy program and to all center coordinators of clinical education and primary clinical instructors who worked with students during the trial year. Results of the study indicated strong support for the full-time schedule.

Key Words: *Clinical competence, Education, Physical therapy.*

A major challenge currently facing the profession is alteration of its educational practices to meet the needs of the future within the constraints of available resources. One of the foundations of the professional preparation of physical therapists is the collaborative relationship supporting clinical education. The purpose of this article is to describe outcomes related to the trial alteration of early clinical experience from a part-time to a full-time basis as reported by clinical instructors, academic faculty members, and students. Moore and Perry described this design as one of four possible clinical education scheduling patterns.[1]

NEED FOR CHANGE OF SCHEDULE

The Curriculum in Physical Therapy at the University of Michigan is an undergraduate professional preparation program in which all but one of the professional courses are currently taught in the senior year. Clinical education consists of three components: Clinic Observation, Clinical Education I, and Clinical Education II. Clinic observation is scheduled for about five sessions of two and one-half hours during the fall term of senior year. Clinical Education I is the early clinical experience of about 160 hours distributed into four 1-week periods scheduled in the winter term. Clinical Education II is the postgraduation experience of 18 weeks of full-time clinical ex-

perience, the satisfactory completion of which leads to the awarding of the Certificate in Physical Therapy from the Medical School.

Prior to 1979, the Clinical Education I experience had been scheduled as a part-time experience, that is, for two or three half-days a week throughout the entire winter term. Each student had four different rotations, each about two to three weeks in length. When the students were not in the clinic, they were in classes in which the content was organized in modules and units both within and across courses. Between 1973 and 1979, many problems related to the scheduling of this experience became apparent to academic and clinical faculty members as well as to students. Among these problems were

1) Limited number of clinical education sites available within a 30- to 40-minute drive from Ann Arbor. Placements could not be scheduled at a greater distance from the university because students were in class for the other half-days and time had to be allotted for inclement weather.

2) Local clinical facilities were used maximally. Clinical instructor fatigue as a result of almost continuous interaction with students was becoming evident. Having students affiliate with these facilities for the entire winter term allowed little or no break for clinical instructors during this period.

3) Student fatigue was evident, particularly at the end of the term. Rushing from clinic to class or vice versa often left the student physically exhausted.

4) Some students experienced difficulty in adjusting from class to clinic. The students' interest in didactic homework often took second place to or was substituted totally by their exploration of material related to the clinical experiences.

In 1978, acquiring the needed clinical placements in the immediate Ann Arbor area was difficult. In

Dr. Kondela was an Instructor and Academic Coordinator of Clinical Education, Curriculum in Physical Therapy, Department of Physical Medicine and Rehabilitation, the University of Michigan, Ann Arbor, MI, when this paper was written. She is now Assistant Director and Center Coordinator of Clinical Education, Physical Therapy Division, University Hospital, Ann Arbor, MI 48109 (USA).

Dr. Darnell is Associate Professor in Physical Therapy and Director, Curriculum in Physical Therapy, Department of Physical Medicine and Rehabilitation, University of Michigan, Ann Arbor, MI.

This article was submitted July 31, 1980, and accepted December 10, 1980.

TABLE 1
Years of Experience of Clinical and Academic Faculty Members

	Range	X̄	s
Clinical faculty member (n = 79)			
as physical therapist	0.5–36	7.4	6.8
as clinical instructor	0.5–25	3.9	4.1
Academic faculty member (n = 7)			
as physical therapist	6.0–23	12.9	6.5
as academic instructor	0.5–14	3.9	4.3
as clinical instructor	0–12	3.0	3.9

planning for the 1979 clinical education year, the faculty of the physical therapy program approved the trial of a new Clinical Education I schedule to alleviate some of the problems of the old schedule.

PLAN TO SOLVE PROBLEM

The schedule for the trial year consisted of four 1-week rotations, during which the students were to be in clinic full-time for the regular hours of service of that facility or agency. During the other weeks of the term, the students were in class full-time. As discussed in the report by Moore and Perry, the scheduling and the frequency of the assignments were influenced by the constraints associated with the academic phase of the program.[1]

EVALUATION OF PLAN

A questionnaire was designed to gather feedback from clinical instructors, academic faculty members, and students about the new schedule. Questions to obtain demographic information about each of the groups were included. The body of the questionnaire was the same for each of the groups: 1) a forced-response rating of effects of the new schedule as an advantage, a disadvantage, or neither, 2) rank ordering of listed possible advantages, 3) rank ordering of listed possible disadvantages, and 4) additional questions concerning the trial schedule and future planning.

Questionnaires were distributed to each of the groups following the completion of Clinical Education I, but before the students and clinical instructors became involved in Clinical Education II. Participants were asked not to discuss the contents of the survey or their responses until all respondents had had the opportunity to complete the survey. Surveys along with letters of transmittal were mailed to clinical instructors. Both center coordinators of clinical education and primary clinical instructors were asked to complete the questionnaire. Academic faculty members received their questionnaires at a regularly scheduled faculty meeting. Student copies were distributed at the end of a class session when there was sufficient free time for them to complete the instruments before leaving the classroom.

FINDINGS

Completed surveys were received from 79 clinical instructors, 7 (100%) academic faculty members, and 35 (97%) students. The total possible number of center coordinators of clinical education and primary clinical instructors was unknown; therefore, the percentage of returned surveys from this group could not be calculated. However, surveys were returned from representatives from 32 (96.9%) of the affiliating institutions.

Demographic Data

The number of years of experience of both the clinical and academic faculty members working as physical therapist, clinical instructor, and academic teacher are reported in Table 1. Forty-seven (59.5%) of the respondents from the clinical facilities had been a primary clinical instructor (PCI), 6 (7.6%) had been a center coordinator of clinical education (CCCE), and 25 (31.6%) had been both. One individual did not respond to this question. Thirty-eight (48.1%) of the clinical faculty members were from general, acute care hospitals, 17 (21.5%) were from rehabilitation facilities, 5 (6.3%) were from pediatric, acute care settings, 17 (21.5%) were from the Michigan educational system (public school districts), and 2 (2.5%) represented special types of experiences, namely sports medicine and the county health department. Seventeen (53%) of the institutions had been involved with Clinical Education I before 1979.

Seventy-three clinical instructors (92%) responded to the item that asked how many rotations the clinical instructor (CI) had supervised during the term. Thirty-four (46.6%) of the CIs had supervised for one rotation, 20 (27.4%) had supervised for two rotations, 10 (13.7%) had supervised for three rotations, and 9 (12.3%) had supervised for all four rotations. Twenty-four (30%) of the CIs had supervised University of Michigan students for Clinical Education II at some prior time. Thirty-nine (43%) of the CIs were graduates of the physical therapy program at the University of Michigan. A further analysis of groups of respondents from the clinical faculty showed that a total of 24 (30%) of the CIs had had some direct experience with the prior Clinical Education I schedule.

TABLE 2
Percentage of Participants Perceiving Trial Schedule Effects as Advantageous

Advantage	Clinical Instructor (n = 79) %	Academic Faculty Member (n = 7) %	Student (n = 35) %	Composite (N = 121) %
More typical workday experience	97	100	97	98
Block-type full-time scheduling as opposed to part-time scheduling	89	100	97	92
Increase in the number of clinical education sites	91	100	89	91
Increase in the number of specialized experiences	89	86	97	91
Fewer students at clinical education site at one time because more sites are available	78	100	60	74
Expansion of clinical education sites to larger geographic area	68	86	80	73
Full-time clinical experience interspersed with full-time didactic work	67	100	80	73
Increase in number of general acute-care experiences	80	86	51	72
Student can secure housing with family and friends	55	71	66	59
Student treated as Clinical Education II affiliate	29	14	63	38

During the trial year, two (28%) of the academic faculty members functioned as CCCEs, and one of these individuals was also a PCI for students. The PCI supervised two students for one rotation. Four (57%) of the academic faculty members had supervised University of Michigan students for Clinical Education I in the past, two (28%) had supervised the students for Clinical Education II, and one (14%) was a graduate of the physical therapy program.

Prior to their clinical education experience, only two (5%) students had ever worked in a physical therapy department when students from the University of Michigan were there on placement for Clinical Education I. Rating their knowledge of the advantages and disadvantages of the old Clinical Education I schedule of three half-days a week, 3 (9%) students indicated excellent knowledge, 27 (77%) indicated average knowledge, 4 (11%) indicated poor knowledge, and 1 (3%) indicated no knowledge of the scheduling of that experience.

Advantages and Disadvantages

Analysis of the forced-response rating about the effects of the new schedule as an advantage, a disadvantage, or neither showed that the effects listed were

TABLE 3
Rank[a] of Possible Advantages of Block-Type Preclinical Experience by Groups

	Clinical Instructor (n = 79)	Academic Faculty Member (n = 7)	Student (n = 35)	Composite (N = 121)
Continuity of patient care	1	5	1	1
Greater variety of experiences	2	1	2	2
More realistic picture of workweek	3	3	6	3
Students more confident	4	4	3	4
Minimizes students' "shifting gears"	6	6	4	5
Less stress on students	7	2	5	6
More realistic picture of Clinical Education II	5	8	7	7
Facilitates transition to modularized curriculum	8	10	8	8
Greater break for clinical instructors	9	7	9	9
More blocks of administrative time for academic faculty	10	9	10	10

[a] 1 is highest, 10 lowest.

considered to be advantages. The response rate of the perceived advantages by group and composite response are reported in Table 2.

The overall ranking of listed possible advantages of the new schedule was determined for each group and the composite group (Tab. 3). Additional comments from participants about advantages of the block-type early clinical experience indicated that several (9%) of the CIs believed the trial schedule made it easier for students to follow through with patient treatment and thereby gain more self-confidence in their abilities. Five percent of the CIs commented that evaluation of the student was facilitated by the trial schedule. Nine percent of the students stated that learning was facilitated by this schedule, inasmuch as there was better continuity of patient contact with a full-time experience.

Table 4 shows the overall rank of possible disadvantages of the block-type early clinical schedule by group and overall composite response. All academic faculty members and students responded to this section as instructed. Twenty (25%) of the CIs did not complete this section. Each of these CIs indicated that they disagreed with the premise that there were "possible disadvantages." They noted in the comment section that there are no disadvantages but only advantages to the one-week clinical schedule. Two (6%) of the students commented that an additional disadvantage not listed is that if the student is ill during a block scheduled experience, he might miss a great deal and sometimes all of a given experience. Two (6%) of the students also believed that the CIs had higher expectations of their performance than they should.

Additional Responses Related to Schedule Change

Eighty-two percent of all of the respondents indicated that they thought the Clinical Education I objectives could be achieved during the one-week block-type clinical experience. Eighteen percent responded negatively to this question and three percent failed to respond to the item. Ninety-four percent of all of the respondents concluded that the new clinical education schedule of one full week in the clinic at a time was a better way to schedule the early clinical education experience than the former schedule of three half-days a week.

DISCUSSION

The response rate for each of the groups was excellent, even though participation was optional. This willingness to provide feedback may have been influenced by the respondents' time investment and interest in the quality of this particular experience. Although on other occasions representatives from each of the participating groups had expressed a desire for earlier student clinical education, the former schedule made earlier clinical experience impossible. This fact seemed to intensify interest in the Clinical Education I experience and its maintenance as a high-quality experience.

Clinical Education Sites

Demographic data showed that only a little more than half (53%) of the clinical education sites had had

TABLE 4

Rank[a] of Possible Disadvantages of Block-Type Preclinical Experience by Groups

	Clinical Instructor (n = 59)	Academic Faculty (n = 7)	Student (n = 35)	Composite (N = 101)
Students more stressed during class time	1	4	1	1
Scheduling of classes in compact units is difficult	2	1	2	2
Difficult for student to "gear up" for classes	3	3	3	3
Academic faculty more intensely involved in teaching during nonclinic time	4	2	4	4
Clinical instructors "blitzed" by students for one full week	5	5	6	5
Lack of carry-through	6	6.5	5	6
Too short to give realistic picture of Clinical Education II	7	9.5	7	7
Too many specialized types of experiences	8	8	10	8
Students less confident	9	9.5	9	9
One week too short to give realistic picture of work at facility	10	6.5	8	10

[a] 1 is highest, 10 lowest.

students for Clinical Education I before 1979. The experimental schedule allowed the academic coordinator of clinical education to expand the number of Clinical Education I facilities by 47 percent, inasmuch as all of the facilities that had affiliated with us in 1978 also affiliated with us for Clinical Education I in 1979. The expansion permitted a greater variety of types of experience, opening up new types of exposure that had not been available before because of the limited travel time available to students on the half-day schedule and the limited numbers of facilities available in the immediate Ann Arbor area.

Clinical Faculty

The majority (91.9%) of the clinical faculty members had had direct experience supervising students during Clinical Education I in 1979, whereas 7.6 percent had had some experience with this trial schedule in their role as CCCE. Only 30 percent of the CIs had supervised University of Michigan students for Clinical Education I in the past. This latter group seems to be the group most qualified to make a judgment comparing the old and new schedule from the perspective of the CI. However, 54 percent of the CIs had supervised Michigan students for Clinical Education II. These individuals may have been fairly knowledgeable about the prior Clinical Education I schedule and the advantages and disadvantages from working directly with students. A little more than two-fifths (43%) of the CIs were graduates of the University of Michigan. These individuals had first-hand knowledge of the previous schedule and of its assets and deficits. Empirical study of demographic data reported on the questionnaire showed that the majority of CIs have some sound basis upon which to make a comparative judgment.

Academic Faculty

Data analyses from the academic faculty responses are based on results from a much smaller group (n = 7) than either of the other two groups. These results are significant, however, inasmuch as they represent 100 percent of this group. Two of the academic faculty members had also had direct clinical faculty responsibilities: both of them functioned as CCCEs and one of them functioned as a CI for Clinical Education I in 1979. Four of the academic faculty members had had direct experience in supervising students for Clinical Education I in the past. All but one faculty member had been on the faculty under both the old and new clinical schedule. The individual who had not been on the academic faculty had been a CCCE and a CI prior to the 1979 experimental year. Each faculty member had first-hand knowledge of the old early clinical education schedule.

Students

Very few students (5%) had first-hand knowledge of the former Clinical Education I schedule by working in a physical therapy department when students from the University of Michigan were on affiliation for this segment of their training. Knowledge of the old schedule was probably based on the students' interaction with upperclassmen in addition to the exchange of information among classes at both formal and informal events of the program. The information the students may have acquired about the former clinical education schedule might have been biased.

Overall Effects of Schedule Change

The change in the beginning clinical experience from part-time to a full-time, block type of experience interspersed with full-time academic classes was received favorably by academic and clinical faculty members as well as by students. This did not surprise us because the alteration of schedule appeared to address and subsequently alleviate the four major problems outlined earlier in this report. Among the advantages noted by those who provided feedback were 1) greater student exposure to the typical work day and week, 2) an increase in the number of clinical education sites available for student experiences, 3) an increase in the number of available specialized learning experiences, and 4) better continuity of patient care by the student. Although no formal follow-up measures of participants' satisfaction with the block schedule has been done, the authors have observed ongoing satisfaction with the block scheduling of the early clinical experience.

IMPLICATIONS FOR FURTHER STUDY

The results of this report indicate a definite need for further comparative investigations of the problem. The study should be replicated in other educational programs located in different geographical locations and using different curricular designs. If possible, such investigations should include a longitudinal component, allowing comparisons prior to, during, and after alterations in scheduling. Considering current trends in the field, another major focus for future investigation lies in the area of comparisons between professional preparation programs leading to undergraduate and graduate degrees. Finally, some further analyses of associated costs to both educational and clinical facilities appear appropriate, as well as comparative objective measures of influence on patient care.

REFERENCE

1. Moore ML, Perry JF: Clinical Education in Physical Therapy: Present Status/Future Needs. Washington, DC, American Physical Therapy Association, 1976

Comparison of 1-Day-Per-Week, 1-Week, and 5-Week Clinical Education Experiences

Cecilia L Graham, MMSc, PT
Pamela A Catlin, EdD, PT
Johnnie Morgan, MEd, PT
Elizabeth Martin, PT

ABSTRACT: *This retrospective study was conducted to compare efficiency and effectiveness of 1-day-per-week, 1-week, and 5-week clinical education experiences. Efficiency of experiences was measured by cost-effectiveness and productivity variables. Effectiveness of experiences was measured by student-performance and perception data. All data were measured through review of existing records. Subjects were 33 entry-level, Master of Physical Therapy Degree students. Student performance and student-perception data (N=33) and cost-effectiveness and productivity data (n=8) were collected. Cost-effectiveness and productivity were highest in 5-week experiences and lowest in 1-day-per-week experiences for the combined student-clinical instructor team. Clinical instructor productivity was significantly higher without students, versus with students, in comparative 1-day and 1-week periods. However, productivity of the combined student-clinical instructor team was significantly higher than that of the clinical instructor alone in comparative 5-week periods. Departmental productivity was not significantly different with students, versus without students, in comparative 1-day and 1-week periods, but was significantly higher without students in comparative 5-week periods. Study of larger samples of students and clinical facilities is indicated.*

Educational and financial issues regarding the clinical education component of physical therapy preparation have become a major focus of the profession of physical therapy in recent years.[1] The advent of the postbaccalaureate entry level and the increasing reality of direct patient access have sparked discussion of lengthening the entire clinical education process to allow adequate preparation for changing responsibilities in health care.[2] At the same time, as clinical facilities are subject to increased financial constraints, the type and length of clinical education experiences have become significant factors in the cost-effectiveness of clinical education.[1] The combination of educational and financial issues has created a need for research directed toward analyzing the effectiveness and efficiency of the current clinical education process. This study focused on the following question: As students progress through the curriculum, do efficiency and effectiveness of learning experiences differ between 1-day-per-week, 1-week, and 5-week clinical education experiences?

Current patterns of clinical education may be either concurrent or nonconcurrent.[3] Clinical education experiences within these patterns may be part-time or full-time. In part-time experiences, a portion of each day or week is devoted to didactic instruction, and the remainder is spent in clinical education.[3] In full-time experiences, the entire time period is spent in clinical education. Concurrent patterns always include part-time experiences and full-time experiences may be included in the middle or end of the curriculum or interspersed throughout the curriculum.[3] In nonconcurrent patterns, all clinical education experiences are full-time assignments.[3]

A concurrent pattern with final full-time experiences was the most frequently used pattern in physical therapy curricula in the 1970s.[3] However, a trend toward inclusion of multiple full-time experiences throughout the curriculum and expansion of the length of individual clinical rotations was noted in a 1985 study.[4] The clinical education experiences in the present study followed the concurrent pattern of 1-day-per-week experiences with several 1-week experiences interspersed throughout the curriculum and with three, 5-week experiences scheduled at the end of the basic preparation component of the curriculum.

Efficiency of clinical education experiences in the medical professions has been examined through cost-benefit analysis and cost-effectiveness studies.[5,6] *Cost-benefit analysis* may be defined as "an estimation and evaluation of net benefits associated with alternatives for achieving defined public goals."[7] Various methods have been used by health care professionals to conduct cost-benefit studies. One example is a retrospective approach, in which respondents estimated percentage of time spent in patient care, education, and research to determine costs in a multidisciplinary family-practice teaching unit.[5]

Financial and time variables were used by Lopopolo[8] to determine financial effects of clinical education in a matched sample of physical therapists with and without students. Time spent in various activities, including teaching and patient care, was recorded by the therapists. Therapists with students were found to generate a $20-per-day greater cost and a $109-per-day greater benefit than therapists without students, or a net benefit of $89 per day. In another study,[9] comparative costs and revenues of junior and senior physical therapy students were assessed through questionnaires regarding supervisory expenses, student support benefits, and direct and indirect costs to the clinical facility. Mean expense-gain figures

Ms Graham is Assistant Professor and Academic Coordinator of Clinical Education, Physical Therapy Program, The University of Texas Health Science Center at San Antonio, 7703 Floyd Curl Dr, San Antonio, TX 78284-7781. She was a student in the Master of Medical Science Degree Program, Division of Physical Therapy, Department of Rehabilitation Medicine, Emory University School of Medicine, Atlanta, GA, when this study was conducted. Dr Catlin is Associate Professor and Director, Division of Physical Therapy, Department of Rehabilitation Medicine, Emory University School of Medicine. Ms Morgan is Assistant Professor and Academic Coordinator of Clinical Education, Division of Physical Therapy, Department of Rehabilitation Medicine, Emory University School of Medicine. Ms Martin is Clinical Instructor, Division of Physical Therapy, Department of Rehabilitation Medicine, Emory University School of Medicine. She was Director, Physical Therapy Department, Georgia Baptist Medical Center, Atlanta, GA, when this study was conducted. This study was completed in partial fulfillment of the requirements for Ms Graham's Master of Medical Science Degree, Emory University.

were computed, revealing that costs incurred by the clinical facilities were generally less than the revenue generated by both junior and senior physical therapy students. To date, the relative efficiency of part-time and full-time experiences, incorporated across the curriculum, has not been reported in the literature.

Effectiveness of clinical education experiences has been studied by assessment of feedback from physical therapy students, clinical instructors, and academic faculty after a change from part-time to full-time early clinical education experiences.[10] Results indicated that the effects of the early full-time experience were considered advantageous by all groups. An increase in some student concerns following a nearly concurrent clinical education assignment has also been cited.[11] The concerns expressed most often regarded interpersonal interactions, the students' knowledge, and treatment procedures.[11] In the present study, both student perceptions and student performance in various types of clinical education experiences were studied to gain a wider perspective of effectiveness of the experiences.

The following null hypothesis was tested: There will be no statistically significant difference in 1) the productivity of the combined student-clinical instructor team and the physical therapy department, 2) cost-benefit ratios, 3) student perceptions of the clinical experience, and 4) student performance among 1-day-per-week, 1-week, and 5-week clinical education experiences.

METHOD
Subjects

The study utilized a retrospective research design. Sampling was nonrandom and exhaustive of all students who enrolled in and completed the entry-level, Master of Physical Therapy Degree curriculum at Emory University during a 2-year period. Sample size for the student perception and student performance variables was 33 subjects. A subsample of 8 students, who completed clinical education experiences at a 523-bed acute care hospital, was used for study of productivity and cost-benefit variables.

Measurements

The entry-level curriculum sampled in the study was composed of three, sequential symptom complexes. The first of the three symptom complexes was the Nutrition complex, which centered around medical and physical therapy management of problems of basic life systems (eg, pulmonary and cardiac systems). The Nutrition complex was followed by the Mobility complex, which emphasized management of problems of the musculoskeletal system. The final symptom complex was the Excitability complex, which focused on problems of the central nervous system.

Clinical education experiences included in the study consisted of 1-day-per-week experiences throughout each of the three symptom complexes, a full-time 1-week experience at the end of each complex, and three full-time 5-week experiences at the completion of the basic preparation component of the curriculum (ie, after the final symptom complex).

Methods for measuring productivity and cost-benefit variables were adapted from methods previously described by Lopopolo[8] and Porter and Kincaid.[9] *Productivity* was defined as the mean number of patients treated per day, mean number of treatment units provided per day, and mean revenue generated per day by the combined student-clinical instructor team and by the physical therapy department as a whole. One treatment unit was defined as 15 minutes of evaluation or treatment. Revenue generated per day was calculated by multiplying the dollar amount charged for each treatment unit by the number of treatment units provided.

Costs were determined by multiplying the hourly salary of the clinical instructor by (1) the total time the student or the clinical instructor were in the clinic per day and (2) the time spent by the student or clinical instructor in direct patient care per day. Total time spent in the clinic per day was considered to be 7½ hours, based on a 8½-hour workday with a 1-hour lunch break. Time spent by the student or the clinical instructor in direct patient care was determined in hours and minutes by multiplying the number of treatment units provided by 15 minutes for each unit. Two cost-benefit ratios were then calculated: 1) costs (total time)/revenue generated (CBTT) and 2) costs (time in direct patient care)/revenue generated (CBPC). Costs were determined for the combined student-clinical instructor team and for the clinical instructor alone in comparative time periods when no students were present in the clinic.

Student perceptions of the clinical experience were defined as student responses on a form entitled "Student Evaluation of the Clinical Experience," which had been completed by all 33 subjects for each clinical education experience throughout the curriculum. Although the validity of the items on this instrument has not been established, the items are derived directly from established elements of the teaching-learning process.[12] The form consisted of 15 statements for the 1-day-per-week and 1-week experiences and 19 statements for the 5-week experiences (Figure). The statements were directed toward the student's perceptions of the experience in terms of time allotted to accomplish objectives, responsiveness and accessibility of the clinical instructor, amount of supervision, and general conditions of the learning experience. Students responded to the questions by marking YES, NO, or NA (not applicable). The percentage of positive (YES) responses was calculated for each clinical experience.

Student performance was defined as student scores (in percentages) in each evaluated clinical education experience throughout the curriculum. Validation of the behaviors on the clinical evaluation instrument used in the study was reported in 1987.[13] Students received scores in four categories: patient care skills, interpersonal skills, teaching-learning skills, and administrative skills. Each section of the evaluation form contained behaviors that were evaluated by the clinical instructors as YES, NO, LO (lack of observation), or DA (does not apply). YES responses were given if the student met the criteria for the behavior at least 80% of the time during the clinical experience.

A numerical score was derived for each performance category (patient care, interpersonal skills, teaching-learning skills, and administrative skills) by dividing the number of behaviors marked YES by the total number of evaluated behaviors in each category. A total score was also derived by averaging the scores across categories. Formal evaluations were conducted daily during the 1-day-per-week experiences, once during the 1-week experiences, and once during the 5-week experiences. Scores from informal evaluation sessions, including midterm evaluations, were not used in the study. Administrative skills were evaluated only during the Excitability complex and during the three 5-week experiences.

Procedure

As the study was retrospective in nature, all data were measured through review of existing records. Written permission was obtained from the clinical facility for review of physical therapy department records. Anonymity of the students and clinical instructors was maintained by assignment of numbers to subjects. Intrarater and interrater reliability of measured variables, calculated as percentages of agreement, was established prior to data collection and maintained throughout the study (agreement=100%).

Productivity and cost-benefit ratio data were collected through review of daily departmental ledgers during the time periods the subsample of eight subjects were in the clinical facility. Of the eight subjects, one subject completed 1-day-per-week and 1-week experiences in the Nutrition complex. Two subjects completed 1-day-per-week and 1-week experiences in the Mobility complex. Three subjects completed 1-day-per-week and 1-week experiences in the Excitability complex. Two subjects completed 5-week experiences. The total number of 1-day-per-week experiences was 29 (number of students × number of days). The total number of 1-week experiences was 6 (number of students × number of 1-week periods). The total number of 5-week experiences was 2 (number of students × number of 5-week periods).

Departmental productivity and productivity of the clinical instructor alone were also calculated from daily departmental ledgers during comparative time periods when no students were present in the clinic. Days for data collection were randomly sampled from comparative time periods. For the 1-day-per-week experiences, comparative days (n=29) were selected from the period spanning 24 days before and after the student was present in the clinic. For the 1-week experiences, comparative 1-week periods (n=6) were selected from the period spanning 6 weeks before and after the student was present in the clinic. For the 5-week experiences, comparative 5-week periods (n=2) were selected from the period spanning 15 weeks before and after the student was present in the clinic. The average number of full-time–equivalent physical therapists employed by the physical therapy department during all data-collection periods was also recorded.

Student perception data were collected through review of "Student Evaluation of the Clinical Experience" forms completed by all subjects for each clinical experience. Student performance data were collected through review of "Evaluation of Student Performance" forms completed by the clinical instructors for all subjects in each evaluated clinical experience.

Data Analysis

Descriptive statistics (mean and standard deviation) were calculated for all measured variables. Data were considered collectively to compare all 1-day-per-week experiences, all 1-week experiences, and all 5-week experiences.

Table 1

Analysis-of-Variance Summary for Patient Visits, Treatment Units, Revenue, and Cost-Benefit Ratios for the Student-Clinical Instructor Team (1-Day-Per-Week Versus 1-Week Versus 5-Week Experiences)

Variable	df	F	P
Patient visits	2	19.47	.0001
Treatment units	2	27.44	.0001
Revenue	2	27.48	.0001
Cost-benefit ratio: CBTT[a]	2	16.18	.0001
Cost-benefit ratio: CBPC[b]	2	7.26	.0011

[a]Cost of total time in clinic/revenue.
[b]Cost of time in patient care/revenue.

Table 2

Means, Standard Deviations, and Paired t-Test Results for Comparisons of Productivity of Student-Clinical Instructor Team (SCIT) and Clinical Instructor Alone (CI) (1-Day-Per-Week Versus 1-Week Versus 5-Week Experiences)

Variable	SCIT		CI		Mean Difference	t	P
	$\bar{X}$	SD	$\bar{X}$	SD			
1 Day							
Patient visits	5.0	2.4	9.1	3.2	4.1	5.9	.0001
Treatment units	7.9	4.1	14.7	5.3	6.8	5.6	.0001
Revenue	$168.2	$ 94.9	$327.0	$131.40	$ 158.8	6.0	.0001
CBTT[a]	0.76	0.62	0.31	0.14	−0.45	−4.14	.0003
CBPC[b]	0.14	0.04	0.13	0.03	−0.01	−1.04	.3061
1 Week							
Patient visits	6.5	2.7	9.0	3.8	2.5	3.31	.0031
Treatment units	10.6	4.4	14.8	6.8	4.2	2.75	.0114
Revenue	$243.7	$108.1	$328.9	$143.7	$ 85.2	2.62	.0154
CBTT	0.41	0.22	0.39	0.53	−0.02	−0.15	.8837
CBPC	0.13	0.03	0.12	0.02	−0.01	−1.12	.2764
5 Weeks							
Patient visits	10.1	4.5	5.3	2.1	−4.8	−6.0	.0001
Treatment units	18.9	8.8	8.0	3.8	−10.9	−7.3	.0001
Revenue	$406.4	$177.6	$173.7	$ 76.2	$−232.7	−7.9	.0001
CBTT	0.29	0.12	0.66	0.3	0.37	0.05	.0001
CBPC	0.15	0.03	0.145	0.02	−0.005	−1.13	.2644

[a]Cost of total time in clinic/revenue.
[b]Cost of time in patient care/revenue.

Comparisons between types of clinical education experiences were tested by a one-way, repeated-measures analysis of variance (ANOVA). Although the number of subjects was small for some comparisons, the assumptions for the one-way ANOVA were met.[14] *Post hoc* analysis, using Tukey's test, was performed when applicable.[14] Paired *t* tests were used for comparisons of clinical instructor and departmental productivity with students, versus without students. An alpha level of .05 was the criterion for all statistical tests.

RESULTS
Productivity and Cost-Benefit Variables

The composite 1-day-per-week, 1-week, and 5-week experiences were significantly different from each other in terms of all productivity variables for the student-clinical instructor team (Tab. 1). Highest values for patient visits (10.1), treatment units (18.9), and revenue ($406.4) were found in the 5-week experiences. Lowest values for patient visits (5.0), treatment units (7.9), and revenue ($168.2) were found in the 1-day-per-week experiences (Tab. 2).

The cost-benefit ratio comparing cost of total time in the clinic with revenue generated (CBTT) was lowest for the 5-week experiences (0.29), indicating the most cost-effective situation. The CBTT ratio was highest for the 1-day-per-week experiences (0.76). The cost-benefit ratio comparing cost of time spent in patient care with revenue produced (CBPC) was lowest in the 1-week experiences (0.13) and highest in the 5-week experiences (0.15) and 1-day-per-week experiences (.14) (Tab. 2).

Clinical Instructor Productivity

Results of comparisons of clinical instructor productivity with students, versus without students, are presented in Table 2. The clinical instructor generated significantly higher patient visits, treatment units, and revenue without the student in the clinic than were generated by the combined student-clinical instructor team during comparative 1-day-per-week and 1-week periods. Mean difference for patient visits was 4.1 for comparative 1-day-per week periods and 2.5 for comparative 1-week periods. Mean difference for treatment units was 6.8 for 1-day-per-week periods and 4.2 for 1-week periods. Mean difference for revenue was $158.8 for comparative 1-day-per-week periods and $85.2 for comparative 1-week periods. The CBTT ratio (cost-benefit: total time in clinic) was significantly lower for the clinical instructor alone in the 1-day-per-week periods (mean difference, −0.45), but was not significantly different from the combined student-clinical instructor team in the 1-week periods.

In comparative 5-week periods, patient visits, treatment units, and revenue generated by the combined student-clinical instructor team were significantly higher than those generated by the clinical instructor alone. Mean difference was −4.8 for patient visits, −10.9 for treatment units, and $−232.7 for revenue. The CBTT ratio produced by the student-clinical instructor team was significantly lower than the CBTT ratio produced by the clinical instructor alone in the comparative 5-week periods (mean difference, 0.37). No significant differences were found in the CBPC ratios between the clinical instructor alone and the combined student-clinical instructor team in the 1-day-per-week, 1-week, and 5-week periods.

Departmental Productivity

Results of comparisons of productivity of the physical therapy department without students, versus with students, are presented in Table 3. Patient visits, treatment units, and revenue produced by the entire physical therapy department were not significantly different during 1-day-per-week and 1-week periods when students were present in the clinic than in comparative periods when no students were present in the clinic. During comparative 5-week periods, patient visits, treatment units, and revenue produced by the physical therapy department were significantly higher when no students were present. Mean difference was 5.3 for patient visits, 9.3 for treatment units, and $235.5 for revenue.

Student Perceptions

Results of statistical analysis of the student perception data are presented in Table 4. No significant differences were found in student perceptions of the clinical experiences between composite 1-day-per-week, 1-week, and 5-week experiences.

Student Performance

Results of statistical analysis of the student performance data are presented in Table 4. Total scores, patient care scores, and teaching-learning scores were each significantly different between composite 1-day-per-week, 1-week, and 5-week experiences. For all scores, highest scores were found in the 5-week experiences, whereas lowest scores were found in the 1-day-per-week experiences. Mean values for total scores were 98.9 in the 5-week experiences, 95.5 in the 1-week experiences, and 92.1 in the 1-day-per-week experiences. Mean values for patient care scores were 98.9 in the 5-week experiences, 95.5 in the 1-week experiences, and 92.1 in the 1-day-per-week experiences. Mean values for teaching-learning scores were 98.1 in the 5-week experiences, 93.4 in the 1-week experiences, and 87.6 in the 1-day-per-week experiences. Interpersonal and administrative mean scores were significantly higher in the 5-week experiences than in the 1-day-per-week experiences. Mean values for interpersonal scores were 99.0 in the 5-week experiences and 96.5 in the 1-day-per-week experiences. Mean values for administrative scores were 99.4 in the 5-week experiences and 94.6 in the Excitability-complex 1-day-per-week experiences.

DISCUSSION

Because of the descriptive nature of this study and the small sample size, cause-and-effect relationships cannot be established between the length of the clinical experiences and the cost-effectiveness, productivity, student perception, and student performance variables. The intent of this study was to describe these variables during each type of experience across the curriculum for the sample studied. The discussion will focus on possible factors that could have contributed to the results and on implications for future studies.

Productivity and Cost-Benefit Variables

The issue of cost of clinical education in the medical professions has reached a critical point.[5,6] Although many researchers have studied the issue of cost-effectiveness of clinical education, no studies have specifically focused on the length of the clinical education experience as a significant cost factor.

Table 3

Means, Standard Deviations, and Paired t-Test Results for Comparisons of Productivity of Therapy Department Without Students Versus with Students (1-Day-Per-Week Versus 1-Week Versus 5-Week Experiences)

Variable	Without Students		With Students		Mean Difference	t	P
	$\bar{X}$	SD	$\bar{X}$	SD			
1 Day							
Patient visits	54.93	10.0	57.0	10.5	−2.07	−0.92	.3653
Treatment units	109.0	22.1	113.79	25.7	−4.79	−0.89	.3812
Revenue	$2,283.1	$351.0	$2,367.8	$425.6	$−84.7	−0.82	.4204
1 Week							
Patient visits	57.6	11.0	57.28	11.4	0.32	0.10	.9175
Treatment units	122.3	28.1	120.58	31.9	1.72	0.22	.8305
Revenue	$2,416.6	$472.0	$2,465.1	$568.0	$−48.5	−0.37	.7142
5 Weeks							
Patient visits	61.9	10.6	56.6	7.6	5.3	3.13	.0030
Treatment units	131.0	20.2	121.7	19.8	9.3	2.38	.0213
Revenue	$2,681.9	$412.4	$2,446.4	$328.6	$ 235.5	3.28	.0020

Table 4

Analysis-of-Variance Summary for Student Perceptions and Student Performance Scores (1-Day-Per-Week Versus 1-Week Versus 5-Week Experiences)

Variance	df	F	P
Student perceptions	2	0.46	.6359
Total performance scores	2	56.5	.0001
Patient care scores	2	56.49	.0001
Interpersonal scores	2	5.79	.0049
Teaching-learning scores	2	55.8	.0011
Administrative scores	2	4.72	.0127

Analysis of the cost-benefit and productivity data in this study generally indicated that cost-effectiveness of the clinical experiences was highest in the 5-week experiences and lowest in the 1-day-per-week experiences. One factor that may have contributed to the decreased cost-effectiveness of the 1-day-per-week experience is the introduction of new skills and concepts in each symptom complex. As the subject matter was new to the student, increased time may have been spent in non–patient care activities, including chart reviews, discussions, observation, and practice. Additionally, time was required for formal evaluation of the student at the end of each 1-day-per-week experience. The skill level of the student and the teaching-learning styles of both the student and the clinical instructor may also play a role in the cost-effectiveness of any clinical experience.

The finding of greatest cost-effectiveness in the 5-week experiences may be related to the student's ability to assume increased responsibility in managing a patient load and administrative tasks. In addition, the student's level of academic preparation was highest during the 5-week experiences. These factors may have enabled the combined student-clinical instructor team to carry a greater patient load in the 5-week experiences than in the 1-day-per-week and 1-week experiences. Additionally, in the 5-week experiences, the student was allowed increased time to accommodate to the daily routines of the clinical facility. Experimental studies, comparing students at the same academic level but with varying lengths of clinical experiences, are needed to verify this cost-effectiveness pattern.

The CBTT ratio (cost-benefit: total time in clinic) followed the pattern of greatest cost-effectiveness in the 5-week experiences and least cost-effectiveness in the 1-day-per-week experiences. The CBTT ratios, however, were generally favorable during all types and lengths of clinical education experiences. With the exception of the 1-day-per-week experiences in the Nutrition complex, all CBTT ratios were less than 1.0. This finding indicates that, except during early clinical experiences, the revenue generated by students outweighed costs to the clinical facility. Although the CBPC ratios (cost-benefit: time spent in patient care) were statistically different between the composite 1-day-per-week, 1-week, and 5-week experiences, the numerical variation was minimal (range=.02). The consistency of the CBPC ratios throughout the clinical experiences indicates that that cost of the time in patient care as compared with revenue generated varied minimally, regardless of the length of the clinical experience or phase of the curriculum. This finding is important in that it addresses concerns that patients may be overcharged when treated by students, particularly during early clinical education experiences.

The finding of greater productivity of the clinical instructor alone in 1-day-per-week and 1-week periods, as compared with the combined student-clinical instructor teams in comparative periods, may be based on a greater amount of time spent in non–patient care activities when the student is present. The finding of greater productivity of the combined student-clinical instructor team than of the clinical instructor alone in comparative 5-week periods may again reflect the ability of the student to handle a greater patient load in the 5-week experiences. This finding is consistent with Lopopolo's[8] finding of greater costs and benefits generated by therapists with students, as opposed to therapists without students, in 6-week affiliation periods.

No differences were found in departmental productivity with students, versus without students, in the 1-day-per-week and 1-week periods. This finding indicates that the department was able to accommodate students during these time periods without a significant effect on departmental productivity. The importance of this finding is that departmental productivity was not adversely affected by the presence of students, even during the least cost-effective (ie, 1-day-per-week) experiences. The finding of significantly lower departmental productivity with students, versus without students, in the 5-week periods is not consistent with other cost-effectiveness findings for the 5-week periods. This finding may reflect a seasonal decrease in patient load or greater use of vacation time by the departmental therapists, as the 5-week affiliation periods were scheduled during the summer months. Sampling of several comparative time periods may be needed in future studies. The CBTT and CBPC ratios were not calculated for the physical therapy department with students, versus without students, in this study. Calculation of the cost-benefit ratios for the physical therapy department is indicated in future studies to provide comprehensive data concerning the effect of student performance and perceptions on departmental productivity.

For all cost-benefit and productivity variables, study of larger samples of students and clinical facilities is indicated. The generalizability of the results of this study are limited by the small sample size.

Student Perception Variables

The general findings of positive student perceptions of all clinical experiences may

---

Figure
Items from "Student Evaluation of the Clinical Experience."

You understood what was expected of you from the objectives for the experience[a]
You were able to negotiate the objectives of the affiliation with the clinical supervisor[b]
Your preparation was consistent with the objectives for the experience[a]
Previous classroom and clinical experiences prepared you for the affiliation[b]
The objectives of the experience were met
The learning experiences were well-planned
The time available for this experience was sufficient for meeting the objectives[a]
The general conditions of the experience were conducive to your learning
The amount of supervision you received was sufficient
Explanations and demonstrations were adequate for your needs
The clinical instructor was accessible and responsive to your needs
The clinical instructor was an effective teacher[b]
You received sufficient feedback on your performance
You were encouraged to develop your own thoughts and ideas
You were encouraged to integrate information[a]
You were allowed to implement your ideas for treatment programs, when appropriate[b]
Adequate time was allowed at the end of the experience for evaluation[a]
The midterm evaluation helped you to improve your performance[b]
The evaluation at the end of the experience was helpful[a]
The evaluation conferences were comfortable and worthwhile[b]
The evaluation helped you identify your strengths and weaknesses[b]
You felt the evaluations were fair[b]
The clinical instructor was receptive to your evaluative comments and suggestions[b]
You were given an appropriate amount of responsibility[b]
An effort was made to provide the learning experiences you specifically requested[b]
Generally speaking, your time was spent in a good learning experience[a]

[a]5-week experiences only.
[b]1-day-per-week and 1-week experiences only.

---

indicate that the needs of the students were met by the clinical instructor and facility, regardless of the length of the clinical experience or the point at which the experience occurs in the curriculum. As the facility evaluation form is reviewed by the clinical instructor, however, the student may have a tendency to give all favorable responses. Another limitation may relate to the lack of established content validity of the items on the instrument. Further research may be needed using validated items and a process in which the student's evaluation is not reviewed by the clinical instructor. In that way, true student perceptions of the various types of clinical experiences may be measured.

Student Performance Variables

Student performance scores were generally found to increase as the length of the clinical experiences increased and as the student progressed through the curriculum. This finding is consistent with an expected gradual development of skill and competence throughout the entry-level physical therapy curriculum.

The range of student performance scores throughout the curriculum was relatively small. Mean scores ranged from 82.9 to 99.4. This finding is consistent with the design and passing criteria of the curriculum sampled in this study. Although new concepts, pathophysiology, and patient care skills are introduced throughout the curriculum, emphasis is consistently placed on process skills implicit in the provision of care, teaching-learning, and interpersonal skills. Also, a minimum score of 80% is required for success in each phase of the curriculum. Further research is needed to determine factors that affect student performance in the clinical

setting, the relationship of academic to clinical performance, and the effect of concurrent versus nonconcurrent experiences on the quality of learning.

CONCLUSION

Cost-effectiveness of clinical education experiences was found to be highest in 5-week experiences and lowest in 1-day-per-week experiences in this study. Productivity of the physical therapy department did not appear to be adversely affected by the presence of students during 1-day-per-week and 1-week periods.

Student perceptions of the clinical experience did not differ significantly in various types and lengths of clinical experiences. As might be expected with increasing knowledge and skill, student performance scores generally improved as the length of the clinical experiences increased and as the student progressed through the curriculum.

This study provided a comprehensive view of efficiency and effectiveness of clinical experiences in a limited sample. Further research, incorporating data from multiple clinical facilities, is needed to verify the cost-effectiveness patterns suggested by the results of this study. On completion of expanded research in this area, potential changes in the current patterns of clinical education in physical therapy may be suggested. The methods of this study may serve as a model to be used by academic and clinical educators for determination of efficiency and effectiveness of clinical education experiences.

ACKNOWLEDGMENTS

Appreciation is expressed to George Cotsonis, Department of Biometry, Emory University, for expertise and assistance in statistical analysis. Special thanks are extended to the administration and staff of the Department of Physical Therapy, Georgia Baptist Medical Center.

REFERENCES

1. Clinical Education in Physical Therapy: Considerations for Alternative Models. Alexandria, VA, American Physical Therapy Association, 1985
2. Physical Therapy Education and Societal Needs: Guidelines for Physical Therapy Education. Alexandria, VA, American Physical Therapy Association, 1984
3. Moore ML, Perry JF: Clinical Education in Physical Therapy: Present Status/Future Needs. Washington, DC, Section for Education, American Physical Therapy Association, 1976
4. Current Patterns for Providing Clinical Education in Physical Therapy Education. Alexandria, VA, American Physical Therapy Association, 1985
5. Stoddart GL: Effort-reporting and cost-analysis of medical education. J Med Educ 48:814–823, 1973
6. Freymann JG, Springer JK: Cost of hospital-based education. Hospitals 47:65–74, 1973
7. Sassone PG, Schaffer WA: Cost-Benefit Analysis: A Handbook. New York, NY, Academic Press Inc, 1978
8. Lopopolo RB: Financial model to determine the effect of clinical education on production in a health care facility. Phys Ther 64:1396–1402, 1984
9. Porter RE, Kincaid CB: Financial aspects of clinical education to facilities. Phys Ther 57:905–909, 1977
10. Kondela PM, Darnell RE: Receptivity to full-time early clinical education experiences. Phys Ther 61:1168–1172, 1981
11. Walish JF, Olson RE, Schuit D: Effects of a concurrent clinical education assignment on student concerns. Phys Ther 66:233–236, 1986
12. Gagne RM: The Conditions of Learning and Theory of Instruction, ed 4. New York, NY, Holt, Rinehart and Winston Inc, 1985
13. Catlin PA, Morgan J: Clinical problem-solving for the entry-level physical therapist. In: Proceedings of the Tenth International Congress of the World Confederation of Physical Therapy, Sydney, Australia, May 17–22, 1987
14. Neter J, Wasserman W, Kutner MH: Applied Linear Statistical Models: Regression, Analysis of Variance, and Experimental Design, ed 2. Homewood, IL, Richard D Irwin Inc, 1985

Effects of a Concurrent Clinical Education Assignment on Student Concerns

JANE F. WALISH,
RONALD E. OLSON,
and DALE SCHUIT

Students participating in a concurrent pattern of clinical education spend part of the day or week in didactic instruction and the remaining portion in clinical education. The purpose of this descriptive study was to identify concerns expressed by students before and after an early concurrent assignment and before a nonconcurrent assignment. Twenty junior level baccalaureate degree students participated in open-ended taped interviews before and after a concurrent assignment that occurred during the first six months of their professional program. The most frequently expressed concerns were about interpersonal interactions, the students' knowledge, and treatment procedures. The students expressed more concerns before the concurrent assignment than after the concurrent assignment and before a nonconcurrent assignment. We conclude that the concurrent assignment builds students' confidence in their affective and psychomotor skills.

Key Words: *Clinical competence, Education, Students.*

Moore and Perry defined two clinical education patterns within the total physical therapy education program.[1] In the concurrent pattern, students spend part of each day or week in didactic instruction and the rest receiving instruction in a clinical setting.[1] In the nonconcurrent pattern, students participate full time in clinical education.[1] An education program may intersperse concurrent and nonconcurrent patterns throughout the curriculum.[1]

The concurrent pattern of organization facilitates the transfer of learning between curriculum components, provides reinforcement for skill development, and promotes student interest in learning.[2] Problems, however, are encountered in the integration of the concurrent pattern into a clinical facility's education program.[1,2] Moore and Perry reported that clinical centers had difficulty managing overlapping schedules for full-time and part-time students.[1] Directors of the clinical centers were found to be more willing to accept full-time senior level students than they were part-time senior or part-time junior level students.[1] The selection of clinical centers and the availability of capable, interested clinical instructors were identified as additional factors that determined the success or failure of a concurrent pattern.[2]

Investigation into the problems encountered by students participating in the concurrent pattern of clinical education is needed. The purpose of this descriptive study was to identify and compare concerns expressed by junior level physical therapy students at a midwestern university before and after a concurrent assignment and before a nonconcurrent assignment.

METHOD

The design of clinical education in the baccalaureate physical therapy curriculum at our university consists of a concurrent assignment during the winter quarter of the junior year and multiple nonconcurrent assignments that begin during the summer quarter of the junior year and continue throughout the senior year. During the concurrent assignment, the students participate in clinical education experiences one half-day each week for five weeks. This assignment is designed to expose the student to patient and professional interactions and to provide integration and practice of didactic learning. The acute care hospital setting is the optimal clinical site choice, but placement of students depends on clinical center availability.

Subjects

We interviewed 20 junior level students of the class of 1984 before and after their concurrent assignments. We selected the students from a physical therapy class of 42 students by using a table of random numbers. All of the participants were women, ranging in age from 19 to 32 years ($\overline{X} = 23.8 \pm 3.29$). Twelve different clinical facilities were used as clinical education sites by the 20 students participating in this study. Sixteen students were affiliated with 11 acute care hospital settings, 3 with 1 rehabilitation hospital setting, and 1 with a private practice setting. All of the clinical education centers were located in the city and suburbs of Chicago, Ill. We obtained prior consent from each student to tape-record each interview. The students were identified by a numerical code to ensure confidentiality. Treatment of the participants in the study was approved by the Institutional Review Board of the university.

Ms. Walish is Teaching Associate, Department of Physical Therapy, The University of Illinois at Chicago. Chicago, IL 60612 (USA).

Dr. Olson is Professor of Psychology, Department of Occupational Therapy, The University of Illinois at Chicago.

Mr. Schuit is Teaching Associate, Department of Physical Therapy, The University of Illinois at Chicago.

This study was supported through a grant from the College of Associated Health Professions, The University of Illinois at Chicago.

This article was submitted September 14, 1984; was with the authors for revision 31 weeks, and was accepted August 21, 1985.

Procedure

Each student participated in two one-hour interviews. We conducted the first interview two weeks before the concurrent assignment. This interview followed an orientation lecture on various aspects of clinical education given by the Academic Coordinator of Clinical Education of the program. The students expressed preconcurrent assignment concerns during the first interview. The second interview took place one to two weeks after the concurrent assignment. During the second interview, the students expressed postconcurrent assignment concerns and concerns about their first upcoming nonconcurrent assignment. In the interviews, the students were asked to respond to a series of open-ended questions (Appendix) that had been developed to reflect the areas of student concern described in the literature.[1,3-5] A pilot study using the open-ended questions had been conducted during which the two investigators who were to conduct the interviews (J.F.W. or D.S.) each interviewed three subjects. These interviews were observed by the other investigator (R.E.O.). The two interviewers used feedback from this investigator and the individuals participating in the pilot study to standardize the interview technique. In this study, the order of the interview questions was randomized for both the first and second interview.

We reviewed each tape after the completion of the interviews and recorded preconcurrent, postconcurrent, and prenonconcurrent concerns for each student on an individual data sheet. Coding categories for the concerns had been established from the pilot study by the three investigators. Because two of us (J.F.W. and D.S.) participated in the data recording, the percentage of agreement between us in data recording was determined on a sample of 20 interviews. Each interviewer reviewed 10 interviews conducted by the other interviewer and recorded the students' concerns on a data sheet. We then compared the concerns recorded by the interviewers and found that agreement was 98%.

Data Analysis

We analyzed the data using frequency distributions.[6] The concerns were analyzed to determine if the same students expressed the same concerns before and after the concurrent assignment and before the nonconcurrent assignment, before and after the concurrent assignment, before the concurrent and the nonconcurrent assignments, and after the concurrent assignment and before the nonconcurrent assignment. Data were analyzed further to determine the preconcurrent, postconcurrent, and prenonconcurrent assignment concerns of students who participated in a concurrent assignment in rehabilitation and private practice settings.

RESULTS

Table 1 shows the distribution of concerns expressed by the students. Postconcurrent assignment concerns were problems that the students perceived had occurred during their concurrent assignment. The most frequently expressed preconcurrent assignment concerns were also the most frequently expressed postconcurrent assignment concerns. The concerns "clinical performance expectations of Clinical Instructor" and "transition from student to therapist" showed the greatest decrease in frequency of expression of all the concerns after the concurrent assignment as compared with before the concurrent assignment. The concerns "being unable to help a patient," "interacting with other students in clinical setting," and "transportation to clinical facility" increased in frequency of expression after the concurrent assignment as compared with before the concurrent assignment. The concerns "transition from student to therapist" and "adjusting to a clinical education pro-

TABLE 1
Preconcurrent and Postconcurrent Assignment Clinical Education Concerns of Physical Therapy Students

Concerns	Students Expressing Concerns (n)			
	Preconcurrent Assignment	Postconcurrent Assignment	Prenoncurrent Assignment	TOTAL
Transition from student to therapist	13	6	8	27
Interacting with patients	15	10	1	26
Administering exercise treatments	13	10	2	25
Interacting with physical therapy staff	11	8	1	20
Clinical performance expectations of CI	14	4	2	20
A particular diagnosis	9	4	0	13
Adjusting to a clinical education program	3	2	5	10
Being accepted as a person and colleague by physical therapy staff	7	2	1	10
Receiving verbal feedback about performance	8	2	0	10
Adapting to new location	4	4	1	9
Being supervised	6	3	0	9
Interacting with other health professionals	6	2	0	8
Interacting with other students in clinical setting	2	4	0	6
Transportation to clinical facility	2	3	1	6
Clinical responsibilities other than patient care	4	1	1	6
Using equipment	3	1	1	5
Being unable to help a patient	0	5	0	5
Treating the severely disabled patient	4	0	0	4
Overidentifying with patients	1	1	0	2
Grade received for clinical course	1	0	0	1

gram" were expressed more frequently as prenonconcurrent assignment concerns as compared with their frequency of expression as postconcurrent assignment concerns. For several coding categories, specific areas of concern were expressed by the students. Before the concurrent assignment, under the coding category "interacting with physical therapy staff," students expressed concern 11 times about interacting with licensed physical therapists. After the concurrent assignment, students expressed concern 5 times about interacting with licensed physical therapists, 2 times with physical therapist assistants, and 1 time with physical therapy aides. Before the concurrent assignment, under the coding category "interacting with other health professionals," the students expressed concerns 5 times about interacting with physicians and 1 time about interacting with registered nurses. After the concurrent assignment, students expressed concern 2 times about interacting with physicians. Before the concurrent assignment, seven students expressed concern under the coding category "being accepted as a person and colleague by physical therapy staff." Under the coding categories "interacting with patients," "administering exercise treatments," and "a particular diagnosis," the students expressed many concerns but we found no specific pattern of concerns between students.

Three concerns were expressed by the same students before the concurrent assignment, after the concurrent assignment, and before the nonconcurrent assignment. Two students were concerned about "administering exercise treatments," one student about "interacting with patients," and one student about "transition from student to therapist."

The concerns that were expressed by the same students before and after the concurrent assignment are shown in Table 2. Four concerns were expressed by the same students before the concurrent assignment and before the nonconcurrent assignment. The concern "transition from student to therapist" was expressed by four students; the concern "clinical performance expectations of CI," by one student; the concern "using equipment," by one student; and the concern "adjusting to a clinical education program," by one student.

Three concerns were expressed by the same students after the concurrent assignment and before the nonconcurrent

TABLE 2
Preconcurrent and Postconcurrent Assignment Concerns Expressed by the Same Students

Concerns	Students Expressing Concerns (n)
Interacting with patients	7
Administering exercise treatments	7
Interacting with physical therapy staff	4
A particular diagnosis	3
Transition from student to therapist	3
Clinical performance expectations of CI	2
Adapting to new location	1
Receiving verbal feedback about performance	1

assignment. The concern "adjusting to a clinical education program" was expressed by one student; the concern "being accepted as a person and colleague by physical therapy staff," by one student; and the concern "transition from student to therapist," by one student.

We studied the distribution of concerns expressed by the four students who participated in clinical education at the rehabilitation and private practice settings. Only one concern, "administering exercise treatments," was expressed by all four students both before and after the concurrent assignment. No further analysis was performed on this data because the sample size was small.

DISCUSSION

The high frequency of expressions of preconcurrent assignment concerns suggests the students lack confidence in their affective, cognitive, and psychomotor abilities and supports the opinion that the learning laboratory should not be a substitute for clinical experience.[2] The laboratory should serve instead as a bridge between didactic learning and clinical application. The fact that the five most frequently expressed preconcurrent assignment concerns were "transition from student to therapist," "interacting with patients," "administering exercise treatments," "interacting with physical therapy staff," and "clinical performance expectations of CI" supports the hypothesis that, before a clinical assignment, students are concerned most about interactions with CIs and patients and are insecure about their knowledge and about treatment procedures.[4] The finding that four of these five most frequently expressed preconcurrent assignment concerns were expressed by only 5% to 10% of the

students before the nonconcurrent assignment suggests that the concurrent assignment may build students' confidence in their affective and psychomotor abilities.

McCulloch and Thompson have suggested that a clinical assignment early in students' professional education resolves the students' personal concerns while developing more professional concerns. The concurrent assignment in our study was during the first six months of the students' professional program. The finding of a decrease in the frequency of expression of the prenonconcurrent assignment concern "being accepted as a person and colleague" and the increase in the frequency of expression of the prenonconcurrent assignment concern "transition from student to therapist" supports their hypothesis.

The finding of an increased expression of the postconcurrent assignment concern "being unable to help a patient" suggests that students may begin to experience frustrations in the practice of physical therapy during an early, concurrent clinical assignment. Clinical Instructors and ACCEs must be aware of this and be prepared to resolve this potential problem.

Approximately 50% of the students who expressed the preconcurrent assignment concerns "interacting with patients" and "administering exercise treatments" also expressed these same concerns after the concurrent assignment. Several factors may have contributed to this finding. One, because students spent only one half-day each week in the clinical facility, an establishment of an "open" relationship between CIs and students may have been prevented. An open relationship may be necessary for students to feel comfortable discussing their concerns at this phase of their professional preparation. Two, the students in an early phase of clinical education may be more passive than in later phases and, therefore, not make their concerns known to CIs. Three, the extent to which a student's personality may have contributed to this finding is unknown. Further investigation of these concerns is needed.

Clinical assignments can be simple observations or participations in the activities of the department and can involve simple tasks or problem-solving tasks.[1] The increase in the frequency of expressions of the concerns "transition from student to therapist" and "adjusting to a clinical education program" before the nonconcurrent assignment as compared with after the concurrent assignment may be a result of the students' perceptions that they might participate in more activities of the department and perform more problem-solving tasks during their upcoming nonconcurrent assignment. Additional investigation should determine the activities and tasks performed by the students during a concurrent versus a nonconcurrent assignment.

The expressions of the concern "administering exercise treatments" before and after the concurrent assignment by the students who participated in clinical education in rehabilitation and private practice settings support the hypothesis that a difficult factor of concurrent program planning is appropriate clinical site selection.[2] The practice in rehabilitation and private practice settings may have demanded more skill than the students possessed at that point in their professional education. Additional investigation should be done in this area.

Identification of student-expressed preconcurrent and postconcurrent assignment concerns is a necessary component in the evaluation of the concurrent model of clinical education. The concurrent assignment can be implemented better if student concerns and professional concerns are considered.

Related research could investigate the differences, if any, in prenonconcurrent assignment concerns between students who participate in concurrent assignments before a nonconcurrent assignment and those who do not participate in concurrent assignments before a nonconcurrent assignment. Additional research also could investigate the differences, if any, in concerns of students participating in a concurrent assignment early in the curriculum as compared with students participating in a concurrent assignment in the middle of or late in the curriculum.

CONCLUSIONS

Our findings suggest that an early concurrent clinical assignment builds students' confidence in their affective and psychomotor skills and develops more professional concerns among them. Those students participating in an early concurrent assignment, however, also begin to experience the frustration of being unable to help certain patients.

REFERENCES

1. Moore ML, Perry JF: Clinical Education in Physical Therapy: Present Status/Future Needs. Washington, DC, Section for Education, American Physical Therapy Association, 1976
2. Scanlan CL: Integrating didactic and clinical education: High patient contact. In Ford CW (ed): Clinical Education for the Allied Health Professions. St. Louis, MO, C V Mosby Co, 1978, pp 113–129
3. McCulloch J, Thompson B: Evaluation of student concerns. Abstract. Phys Ther 64:727, 1984
4. Ramsden EL, Dervitz HL: Clinical education: Interpersonal foundations. Phys Ther 52:1060–1066, 1972
5. Kondela-Cebulski PM: Counseling function of academic coordinators of clinical education from select entry-level physical therapy educational programs. Phys Ther 62:470–476, 1982
6. Mattson DE: Statistics: Difficult Concepts, Understandable Explanations. St. Louis, MO, C V Mosby Co, 1981

Utilization of Rotatory Clinical Faculty Members in Physical Therapy Education

MADELINE L. VERSTEEG   JOHN W. STREIN   DALE H. FITCH   RICHARD E. DARNELL

Members of our profession are committed to providing physical therapy education. Faculty shortages in physical therapy education programs across the nation[1,2] threaten the continued attainment of quality education. New, creative models are needed to meet the demand for qualified faculty in the physical therapy education programs. In 1986, in response to the need for more physical therapy faculty members, the American Physical Therapy Association's Board of Directors established the specific objective: "To increase the number of expert clinicians who hold faculty appointments."[3]

As faculty members in the Physical Therapy Program at the University of Michigan-Flint, we developed a model to address our faculty shortage problem. Rather than attempting to recruit new faculty from other physical therapy programs, we explored options for involving local clinicians as faculty members in our program. We believed that by including clinicians from the community as faculty members in our program there would be benefits to our program and to the community. By having clinicians as faculty members, we ensured the availability of clinical expertise at a time of great changes in the scope of physical therapy practice. This process would assist our physical therapy program to develop long-term relationships within the community. The process should provide community facilities with an additional incentive to use in recruiting, developing and retaining staff physical therapists. This exchange should result in a sharing of governance in the education of students between the clinicians and the program, thereby enabling the physical therapy program and the community to maintain a focus on the profession, rather than on the university. Joint governance by a physical therapy program and clinicians should serve to strengthen the concept of ownership of the program by members of the profession, rather than ownership of the program by the institution in which the program is housed.

We developed a faculty model we called the Rotatory Clinical Faculty Model (RCF). Our model was based on the assumption that therapists may be interested in assuming half-time faculty positions thereby allowing them to remain practicing half-time as clinicians. The purposes of this article are to describe the Rotatory Clinical Faculty Model, and to present the results of the evaluation of this model after its first year of operation.

THE ROTATORY CLINICAL FACULTY MODEL

In the RCF model, two physical therapists currently employed in two of the nine member institutions of the Greater Flint Area Hospital Assembly (GFAHA), were employed for a two-year half-time contractual basis as adjunct instructors in our physical therapy program. Half-time employment was defined as an average of twenty hours per week for eleven months (960 hours) for each year of the contract. During that two-year contract period, the RCF therapists also maintained half-time positions at their cooperating hospitals. Our university reimbursed each hospital a fee to cover salaries and benefits of their participating therapists. This payment probably did not cover the entire cost to the hospitals for the half-time positions. We required each RCF member to be an active participant in our governance proceedings. We agreed the RCF members would lose their governance privileges within the physical therapy program, the school and the university, if the hospitals would not release each therapist to work twenty hours per week in our program.

The RCF members were appointed as Adjunct Instructors. Possible duties and responsibilities included: classroom teaching, clinical education, student counseling, consultation, clinical practice, provision of continuing education courses, research and publication, professional activities, professional development (continuing education and in-service training) and faculty and program governance (including attendance at all faculty meetings and other designated meetings). The actual duties and responsibilities of the RCF member were determined by current program needs and the interests of the individual. The therapist's capabilities and experience were also factors in determining specific duties of the RCF member. Each RCF member assumed clinical duties and responsibilities as determined by the Director of their clinical facility.

Employing clinicians as part-time faculty members is a widespread practice,[4] however, the Rotatory Clinical Faculty Model represented a unique approach for addressing faculty needs in a physical therapy education program. The contractual basis of the RCF model provided a clinician the opportunity to assume a half-time faculty position while maintaining a half-time clinical position, and guaranteed the clinician could return to a full-time hospital position at the end of the contract period. Although the RCF members were not considered employees of the University, they were afforded all appropriate rights and privileges associated with being a faculty member at our institution.

QUALIFICATIONS OF THE RCF MEMBER

To be qualified for a RCF position, a therapist must be an employee of an institution in the GFAHA: be a graduate of an approved school of physical therapy, be licensed to practice in Michigan, possess expertise in a definitive area of clinical practice, demonstrate an interest in the RCF position, exhibit willingness to commit to a two-year period and demonstrate the ability to make academic contributions that strengthen and enhance our physical therapy program.

SELECTION OF RCF MEMBERS

The Chairperson of our physical therapy program notified all GFAHA hospitals of the availability of the RCF positions. Interested therapists made a formal application to a Selection Committee. This committee was composed of the Chairperson of our physical therapy program, a physical therapy faculty member, and a faculty member from our School of Health Sciences. Selection Committee members interviewed and ranked all qualified applicants, presenting the names of the two highest ranked applicants to the physical therapy faculty. The physical therapy faculty members endorsed the candidates. The Chairperson of our program forwarded the candidates' names to the Provost, who instructed the University's business office to negotiate a "Letter of Understanding" with the institutions regarding exchange of funds. After negotiations were finalized, the Chairperson informed the two RCF candidates of their selection.

21

The timelines for the completion of this selection process were established to provide sufficient time for the RCF members to prepare for fall classes.

In the absence of qualified candidates, the Chairperson may use the one full-time equivalent position (assigned for the RCF members) to employ a temporary full-time faculty member from other community resources, for up to a period of two years. Termination of a RCF member prior to the end of their contract period may be initiated by the RCF member, the hospital, or the physical therapy program, with a required three months notice.

LIMITATION ON SELECTION OF RCF MEMBERS

To ensure fair representation of all member hospitals, the University will not select both RCF members from the same hospital, unless only one hospital has qualified candidates available and offers to participate in the program. The University will not contract with the same hospital in successive contract periods, except when other qualified personnel are not available. Successive contracts are limited to one year on a renewable basis.

EVALUATION OF THE PROCESS

For the initial contract with our education program, both RCF positions were filled by two physical therapists from two hospitals in the area. At the end of the first year of the contract, an evaluation of the RCF program was conducted. A questionnaire was developed to identify: incentives to become involved with the RCF program, perceived advantages and disadvantages of the RCF program, impact of the program on all associated individuals and groups, extent to which the quality of education and patient care were perceived to be affected by the employment of RCF members, recommendations for continuance or discontinuance of the RCF program at the completion of the initial contract period, and applicability of the RCF program for other physical therapy education programs in the country.

The questionnaire was approved by the Human Subjects Review Committee at the University of Michigan-Flint. Questionnaires were mailed to numerous persons having interests in this process; senior physical therapy students, completing their full-time clinical education internships; physical therapy faculty members; hospital administrators, who supervise the physical therapy departments at the two participating hospitals; all physical therapists and physical therapists assistants from the two participating hospitals; and members of our Physical Therapy Program Community Advisory Committee (comprised of area physical therapists, physicians, and hospital administrators).

The questionnaire consisted of: checklist items to identify advantages and disadvantages, rating scales requiring judgments along ordered dimensions, and open ended questions to solicit additional comments and recommendations. The main text of the questionnaire was similar for all groups; however, several items were not applicable to all groups. The biases for the construction of the questionnaire were to obtain comparative data across groups where possible, and gather data from individual groups when such comparisons were not appropriate.

RESULTS

Data were tabulated and analyzed for: frequency (percent) for the checklist items; average (mean ± standard deviation) for the graphic rating scales; and listing of all comments and recommendations. Confidentiality was maintained throughout the study. Through meetings and written communication, separate evaluation information about the RCF program was received from the supervisors of the RCF members and from each RCF member.

Table 1. Percent of Respondents Perceiving RCF Program Effects as Advantages.

Advantages	Students (n = 32)	Faculty (n = 6)	Advisory Committee (n = 8)	Hospital Adm. (n = 2)	PT Dept. "A" (n = 12)	PT Dept. "B" (n = 4)	Composite (n = 64)
Access to university resources	NAa	NA	50	50	75	50	62b
Improves the quality of services	NA	67	38	0	25	50	38c
Strengthens PT Program faculty	91	83	100	NA	100	50	90d
Growth and development of RCF member	97	100	100	0	92	0	88
Educational program improved and strengthened	94	67	75	NA	83	75	85
Increases clinician's understanding of role in PT education	72	67	65	50	58	50	66
Strengthens relationship between PT clinicians and PT faculty	88	83	75	50	66	25	77
Clinician can assume faculty position and maintain clinical position	88	100	88	100	83	50	86
Clinician can enter and evaluate academic setting	97	83	100	100	100	50	94
Recruitment of physical therapists for hospital	31	50	25	100	42	75	39
Growth and development of PT profession	84	100	100	0	92	50	78
Financial incentive for hospital	NA	0	25	100	17	50	28c

a NA = item was not presented to respondent / b n = 26 / c n = 32 / d n = 62

Table 2. Percent of Respondents Perceiving RCF Program Effects as Disadvantages.

Disadvantages	Students (n = 32)	Faculty (n = 6)	Advisory Committee (n = 8)	Hospital Adm. (n = 2)	PT Dept. "A" (n = 12)	PT Dept. "B" (n = 4)	Composite (n = 64)
Only two half-time positions are available for RCF position	0	0	13	0	17	25	6
RCF members lack academic expertise to teach in PT Program	9	0	25	0	17	25	13
Time constraints impaired RCF member's ability to attend to all job responsibilities	50	50	88	50	83	75	63
Having a RCF member in PT department impaired ability to provide quality services	NAa	NA	25	50	42	0	31b
Availability and presence in hospital were based on PT Program schedule, not hospital schedule	NA	33	63	50	58	25	50c
Compensation from university for RCF member does not cover actual costs assumed by hospital	NA	50	50	50	0	25	28c

a NA = item was not presented to respondent / b n = 26 / c n = 32

Completed questionnaires were received from 32 (89%) senior physical therapy students, 6 (100%) faculty members, 9 (90%) community advisory committee members (one was not usable), 2 (100%) hospital administrators, 12 (80%) physical therapists and physical therapist assistants from Physical Therapy Department 'A' and 4 (80%) physical therapist and physical therapists assistants from Physical Therapy Department 'B'. This study yielded a composite response rate of 86 percent.

The response rates of the perceived advantages of the RCF program, by group and composite response, are reported in Table 1. Two strong advantages noted by all groups were the opportunity provided to clinicians to assume a faculty position while maintaining a clinical position and, the opportunity to experience working in an academic setting thereby assisting in planning personal career goals. Growth and development of the RCF member and the physical therapy profession were two strong advantages cited by all groups, except by the hospital administrators. Only the hospital administrators cited the financial incentive and the recruitment potential as strong advantages of the program.

The perceived disadvantages of the program are reported in Table 2. All groups identified time constraints imposed by the program on the RCF member as the most frequent disadvantage. Similarly, the second most frequently reported disadvantage was that the availability and presence of the clinician in the hospital were based on the physical therapy program schedule, and not the hospitals' schedule.

Hospital administrators in the participating hospitals, and members of the community advisory committee, who represented most of the remaining facilities that could potentially participate in this program in the future, identified factors for evaluating the feasibility of implementing the RCF program in a facility (Table 3). Both groups showed meaningful differences in the degree to which certain factors were or would be considered. The financial incentive was the strongest factor for hospital administrators because the RCF program provided money to cover salary and benefit costs of an employee. The second strongest incentives factor was the possibility of enhancing recruitment of new physical therapy graduates.

The community Advisory Committee stated a strong incentive was the opportunity to establish a definitive relationship between the community and our physical therapy program. Advisory Committee members also believed that the possibility of strengthening the community health care system and the physical therapy departments was another incentive for using this model.

Both students and academic faculty members responded that the RCF program had a positive impact on the education program (Table 4). Both groups agreed strongly that the quality of physical therapy education had been enhanced by the use of this model.

Table 3. Incentives for Participation in the Rotatory Clinical Faculty Program[a]

Incentives	Community Advisory Committee (n = 8)	Hospital Administration (n = 2)
Foster development of one PT staff member by providing this faculty position	2.5 ± 0.5[b]	2.5 ± 0.7
Utilize the financial incentive to cover salary and benefit costs of employee	2.9 ± 1.6	1.5 ± 0.7
Strengthen PT department by utilizing university resources	2.1 ± 0.8	2.5 ± 0.7
Enhance recruitment of new graduates for PT department	3.0 ± 1.7	2.0 ± 0.0
Establish definitive relationship with PT Program	1.6 ± 0.7	3.0 ± 2.8
Contribute to the growth and development of PT profession	2.5 ± 1.2	3.5 ± 2.1
Strengthen the Flint Community Health Care System by fostering a stronger relationship between PT clinicians and PT educators	2.0 ± 0.9	4.0 ± 2.8

a scale used: 1 = strongly considered
              6 = not considered at all
b mean ± standard deviation

Table 4. Impact of the Rotatory Clinical Faculty Program on the Educational Program

Educational Component	Students (n = 32)	Faculty (n = 6)
The RCF members have been reasonably accessible outside of regularly scheduled classroom time.[a]	2.4 ± 0.9[b]	1.4 ± 0.5
The RCF members were familiar with and appropriately worked within the collegial model.	1.6 ± 0.6	1.5 ± 0.5
Because of the presence and participation of the RCF members, the quality of education received by the students was enhanced.	1.6 ± 0.6	2.3 ± 1.0

a scale used: 1 = strongly considered
              6 = not considered at all
b mean ± standard deviation

Assumptions we made when developing the conceptual foundations of the RCF model were also evaluated (Table 5). All groups indicated the use of two half-time RCF members rather than one full-time faculty member strengthened the faculty. The groups did not believe that the academic expertise required to teach was sacrificed by employing clinicians. Academic preparation and terminal degrees held by the RCF participants did not appear to be criteria for selection that would be considered more important than clinical competency and ability to contribute to the education program.

All respondents were requested to give their opinions about the future of our RCF program (Table 6). Strong support was given for continuation of the RCF program. Respondents stated their facilities would consider participating in the program in the future. Respondents agreed that this program could be used by other physical therapy education programs in the country.

DISCUSSION

Faculty members and students indicated the program had a positive impact on our education program. Use of two RCF members, rather than one full-time faculty member, appeared to strengthen the faculty in terms of critical mass and with respect to gaining perspectives on various educational issues discussed by the faculty. Several students stated the use of RCF members helped them as they made the transition from the classroom to the clinic. This RCF program helped to address our problem of faculty shortages and appeared to maintain and enhance the quality of our education process.

The RCF program has begun to achieve our goal of developing a linkage between didactic education and clinical practice. In the future, this program may play an even greater role in bridging didactic work with clinical application as we explore and develop new clinical education models.

Key community individuals indicated strong support for the RCF program. Because the community is the arena from which our program intends to select future RCF members, we considered this support essential for the continuation of our program. In addition to strengthening our education program, the RCF program also addressed some community needs, such as: enhancing recruitment of physical therapists, contributing to the growth and devel-

Table 5. Evaluation of the Conceptual Foundations of the Rotatory Clinical Faculty Program.[a]

Concepts	Students (n = 32)	Faculty (n = 6)	Advisory Committee (n = 8)	PT Departments (n = 16)
The RCF Program provides for the utilization of clinicians with "clinical expertise" in the PT Program. In doing so, I feel the "academic expertise" required to educate was therefore sacrificed.	5.0 ± 0.9[b]	5.2 ± 1.2	4.8 ± 1.4	4.5 ± 1.2[c]
When selecting faculty members for a PT program, it should be considered that the individual's clinical competency and capacity to contribute is more important than the individual's academic preparation and degree level.	2.2 ± 1.1	3.3 ± 1.4	2.8 ± 1.2	2.6 ± 1.0
Employment of two RCF members helped to strengthen the faculty.	1.6 ± 0.6	1.5 ± 0.8	1.9 ± 0.6	2.3 ± 1.3[c]
One full-time faculty member, rather than two RCF members, could have better served the PT Program.	4.7 ± 0.9	5.2 ± 0.8	3.5 ± 1.6	NA[d]

a scale used: 1 = completely agree
6 = completely disagree

b mean ± standard deviation   /   c n = 15   /   d NA = item was not presented to respondent

Table 6. Evaluation of the Future of the Rotatory Clinical Faculty Program.[a]

Evaluation Items	Students (n = 32)	Faculty (n = 6)	Advisory Committee (n = 8)	Hospital Admin. (n = 2)	PT Dept. "A" (n = 12)	PT Dept. "B" (n = 4)
Based on my knowledge of and/or experience with the RCF Program, I believe this program:						
should continue to be offered by the UM-F PT Program	1.2 ± 0.4[b]	1.2 ± 0.4	1.6 ± 1.1	2.0 ± 1.4	1.8 ± 0.9	1.8 ± 0.5
could be incorporated within and utilized by other PT educational programs in the nation	1.3 ± 0.5	1.7 ± 0.8	1.9 ± 0.6	2.0 ± 1.4	1.7 ± 0.8[c]	1.8 ± 0.5
In the future, if feasible, the hospital/PT Department would consider participating in the RCF Program.	NA[d]	NA	1.9 ± 1.0	2.0 ± 1.4	2.1 ± 0.9[c]	2.8 ± 0.5

a scale used: 1 = completely agree
6 = completely disagree

b mean ± standard deviation   /   c n = 10   /   d NA = item was not presented to respondent

opment of the RCF members and the profession and, strengthening the health care system by fostering a positive relationship between physical therapist clinicians and physical therapy academic faculty.

Hospital administrators involved in making the decision to participate in the RCF program also responded favorably to the program. Each administrator had unique reactions. For example, the administrator in hospital 'B' indicated a less than favorable impact on the hospital by implement-

ing the program. One potential explanation of this response is that the RCF member from hospital 'B' was also the hospital's Director of Physical Therapy Services. For hospital 'B' administrators, an incentive for involvement with our RCF program was the fact that this hospital was experiencing excess man-hours in relation to its patient volume. Hospital 'B' administrators did not believe the compensation from the University covered the actual costs of the participating physical therapist.

Hospital 'A' administrators stated that the RCF program had a favorable impact, but also stated that their ability to provide physical therapy service was impaired. This perception of impaired service may have been related to the hospital having a shortage of physical therapy staff during the contract period. The hospital administrator from hospital 'A' stated participation in this program was a positive experience and indicated strong support for participating in the RCF program in the future.

Staff members in the physical therapy departments, where the RCF members worked, also had favorable evaluations of the program. The staff in physical therapy department 'B' stated an additional advantage of the RCF program was the enhanced potential for recruiting staff. Because this department is located in a rural community, it has less visibility among potential recruits than a large urban hospital. Staff at both departments identified the strongest disadvantage of the program as the constraints on participant's time which interfered with the RCF member's ability to attend to all job responsibilities, and thereby affected department functions. Again, the staff shortage at hospital 'A' and the administrative position held by the RCF member at hospital 'B' appeared to heighten this perception of time contraints as being a disadvantage.

On completion of the first year of this program, the academic and clinical supervisors of the RCF members provided evaluation information. A clinical supervisor provided information for the RCF member at hospital 'A' and the hospital administrator provided information for the RCF member at hospital 'B.' The clinical supervisor for RCF member at facility 'A' (who also served as the Director of Physical Therapy Services), stated the program provided an ideal opportunity for clinicians to enter and evaluate the academic setting without substantial risk to their employment and with no risk for a reduction of their current salary. We believe the RCF program should strengthen the hospital staff through the addition of high skilled, professional physical therapists. Although the Director stated the program contributed to the growth and development of the physical therapy profession, the Director indicated this factor was not considered a major incentive to hospital administrators who were more concerned with the fiscal viability of the hospital. The

Director believed the quality of services provided by the department in facility 'A' was not impaired but lower productivity was noted due to the variable workload duties of the RCF member. In general, the supervisor in facility 'A' concluded that the RCF program was excellent and provided a worthy professional experience for all parties involved.

The academic supervisor of the two RCF members is the Chairperson of our physical therapy program. In evaluating this program, the Chairperson believed there were many benefits for those who participated, such as: improving the quality of services provided to the students, and strengthening the relationship between the University and the community by reducing dissonance between clinical and academic aspects of the profession. The RCF program also provided for two additional faculty members to take part in governance of our physical therapy program. The Chairperson stated these members helped to assure that the academic faculty considered the clinical implications of any decisions made on education.

The two RCF members evaluated their experiences with this program as very positive. They believed their presence in both the clinical and academic settings positively influenced their functions in each setting. They calimed they gained better understandings of the coordinated functions of the University and the clinics with respect to physical therapy education. They believed there were other benefits such as: being exposed to academia; understanding the mechanism used by the faculty to deal with specific educational (professional) and general university (political) issues; strengthening interpersonal and management skills by participating in faculty governance and working in the collegial model; and, personal and professional growth enhancement by identification with faculty role models.

The first year required considerable adjustments so the RCF members could meet their academic and clinical responsibilities. For example, our class schedule prevented RCF members from practicing in the clinic daily. The irregular time schedule made it difficult for the RCF member to carry a regular patient load. In addition, because of the demands from the clinics and the University, the RCF members often felt as though they were maintaining two full-time jobs rather than two half-time jobs. We found that if not care-

fully monitored, the RCF members could be subjected to excessive work stress. We suggest holding frequent meetings between the clinical and academic supervisors and the RCF members. These meetings would maintain a clear line of communication that would serve to avoid potential problems, such as: misunderstanding about expectations, duties and responsibilities of all persons involved, scheduling conflicts which might be anticipated due to a heavy workload, or personal over commitment. In addition, these meetings would provide all participants with on-going evaluations of their performances in the program, as well as an evaluation of the RCF program in general. Modifications in job duties or performance expectations could be implemented immediately to assure the viability of participants and the RCF program.

IMPLICATIONS FOR THE USE OF THE RCF MODEL FOR THE PROFESSION

The benefits of this model to the profession are numerous. The model forces the physical therapy faculty to look at current practice patterns and incorporate these patterns into the education program. The model also has the potential for promoting and strengthening clinical research. Ideally, an RCF member brings clinical research ideas to the program to be pursued in collaboration with academic faculty members. This joint venture between RCF members and academic faculty members could further strengthen the tie between the university and the community, and ultimately benefit the profession. The employment of RCF members helps to release academic faculty members from excessive teaching loads so they can engage in other scholarly activities.

This model provides a mechanism to train and develop faculty members. Although each RCF member returns to the clinic on a full-time basis after the two year period, the hospital, the community, the education program and the profession are all strengthened by this individual's experience in the RCF program. With continued implementation of the RCF program, the community can acquire a large pool of trained and experienced RCF members who can further enhance the professional development of other therapists in the community, and promote the community as a center of excellence for the practice of physical therapy.

The RCF model demonstrates to the university the unique nature of a professional preparation program. The clinical foundations of the profession are the guidelines by which the physical therapy education programs are developed and maintained. This model reinforces the philosophy of "ownership" of the program in areas of mutual interest and concern.

This education model could be used by other physical therapy education programs in the country. Modifications can be made to accommodate the needs of a particular education program and community. The basic concepts on which this model was developed appear to be consistent with the educational philosophy of a professional preparation program, and appropriately address the concerns of the profession to meet the demands for faculty members to educate its future members.[5]

The potential for creative modification of the RCF model presents exciting possibilities. Two questions currently not addressed are: Should criteria for the clinical facilities which participate in the RCF program be developed? and; Should some form of reciprocation occur, so that regular full-time faculty members could assume a half-time position in the clinic? The use of the RCF model must be continually evaluated to ensure that the model is consistent with current and future trends in the profession. For example, the RCF model will need to be evaluated and perhaps modified as the profession continues to move toward post-baccalaureate entry-level, direct access and clinical specialization. This model could be a mechanism by which the profession can evaluate the criteria for faculty composition today, and in the future.[6,7] The fundamental question being addressed by the profession today is: Should the faculty of a physical therapy education program be composed of all doctoraly trained personnel, or master clinicians, or a mixture of both in some proportion?

The future success of the RCF model will depend upon the trust and flexibility between universities and clinical facilities, the satisfaction of the physical therapists involved in providing the RCF services and the degree to which the needs of the profession are met.

Acknowledgments. We wish to express our appreciation to Dr. Paulette K. Cebluski, PT, and Dr. Beverly Schmoll, PT, for their advice and assistance on this manuscript.

Ms. Versteeg is a physical therapist at the Providence Hospital, Cincinnati, OH. At the time of this study, she was an Adjunct Instructor in the Physical Therapy Program at the University of Michigan-Flint, and Clinical Research Coordinator for the Physical Therapy Services, McLaren General Hospital, Inc., Flint, MI.

Mr. Strein is an Instructor in the Physical Therapy Program at the University of Michigan-Flint, and is in private practice. At the time of this study, he was an Adjunct Instructor in the Physical Therapy Program and Director of Rehabilitative Services at Memorial Hospital, Owosso, MI.

Mr. Fitch is the Director of Physical Therapy Services at McLaren General Hospital, Inc., Flint, MI.

Dr. Darnell is a Professor and the Director of the Physical Therapy Program, School of Health Sciences, University of Michigan-Flint, Flint, MI.

REFERENCES

1. Physical Therapy Faculty Survey. American Physical Therapy Association, Department of Education, Fall, 1983.
2. The Plan to Address the Faculty Shortage in Physical Therapy Education: Final Report of the Task Force on Faculty Shortage in Physical Therapy Education; American Physical Therapy Association, September, 1985.
3. American Physical Therapy Association Board of Directors, Program 60, March, 1986.
4. Sherwin LN, Salzio K: The teacher/practitioner shared appointment: Making it work. Nurse Educator 8(2):30-33, 1983.
5. Accreditation Handbook: American Physical Therapy Association Commission on Accreditation in Education, 1985.
6. Developing the Physical Therapy Post-Baccalaureate Entry Level Degree Program: American Physical Therapy Association, 1985.
7. Yarbrough P: Questions and answers: Why raise entry level? American Physical Therapy Association Progress Report, April, 1983.

Development of Clinical Education Sites in an Area Health Education System

SHERRY L. CLARK, MS,
and STAN SCHLACHTER, BS

In 1974 the University of Kentucky was faced with two problems: 1) overburdening of local clinical facilities by students and 2) a large exodus of graduates from the state. The advent of the Area Health Education System offered the opportunity for the clinical education program to develop nontraditional clinical sites across the state. The development and use of these nontraditional sites in predominantly rural areas has become an integral part of the clinical education program. Local facilities are no longer inundated with students. The retention rate of graduates has improved in the seven years of the program from 36 percent in 1972 to 81 percent in 1979.

Key Words: *Clinical education, Physical therapy.*

In 1974, the Department of Physical Therapy at the University of Kentucky, which had 22 students in both the junior and senior classes, had two problems. One problem was that, because the clinical education experiences during the year were restricted to Lexington and a 30-mile radius, the number of clinical sites available was limited. As a result, the clinical sites in the area were overburdened with students.

The other problem at the time was the retention of graduates. The University of Kentucky was the only institution in the state educating physical therapists. In 1974, the retention rate of graduates was 36 percent. With the advent of the Area Health Education System (AHES) in the Commonwealth of Kentucky, the physical therapy program faculty members recognized the opportunity to expand the clinical education program as well as to reduce the exodus of graduates from the state. The purpose of this paper is to describe this component of the clinical education program.

AREA HEALTH EDUCATION SYSTEM

The AHES was developed and funded by the state legislature in 1974. It was a consortium of academic institutions and health care providers in a designated rural geographical area. There were seven geographical regions in Kentucky and they excluded the counties contiguous to the metropolitan areas of Louisville, Lexington, and Northern Kentucky (Cincinnati). The AHES provided a network of different health care facilities and providers in a region available for clinical sites of health care students. The resulting interaction between those in academic programs and providers of health care could contribute to a) more effective academic programs and better preparation of students, b) improvements in the distribution and effectiveness of health manpower, and c) improvements in the health care provision system. The goals of the new AHES appeared to relate to the problems of the physical therapy clinical education program.

As a result, a project for Physical Therapy Clinical Education was submitted to the state and funded for the 1974–1975 fiscal year. The goals of the project were 1) to place senior physical therapy students in health care settings in the AHES regions, 2) to improve the students' patient care skills through supervised patient treatment, 3) to provide an experience that would favorably influence a student's selection of employment within the Commonwealth, 4) to provide exposure of the student to the community and region through which they rotate, and 5) to enhance the patient treatment skills and teaching skills of clinical educators.

The funding of a project by the state provided monies to support the students off campus. Students placed in an AHES region were provided housing, an allotment for meals, and transportation expenses to the site. Alleviation of the financial burden to students encouraged participation of all students in the program.

Ms. Clark is Clinical Education Coordinator, Department of Physical Therapy, College of Allied Health, University of Kentucky, Lexington, KY 40536 (USA).

Mr. Schlachter was Clinical Education Coordinator, Department of Physical Therapy, College of Allied Health, University of Kentucky, when the AHES project was initiated. He is currently self-employed and can be reached at 938 University Ave, Sacramento, CA 95825.

This article was submitted December 27, 1979, and accepted September 15, 1980.

INCORPORATION OF AHES ROTATIONS INTO THE CLINICAL EDUCATION PROGRAM

The bulk of clinical education courses at the University of Kentucky curriculum occurred in the senior year. These clinical education experiences were referred to as "clerkships." Clerkships were 2- and 3-week blocks of time for clinical experience, interspersed with didactic material. There were two 2-week experiences and one 3-week experience, for a total of 7 weeks. The clinical blocks of time in weeks allowed students to go off campus for clinical education experiences. "Internships" were 4- to 6-week blocks of time following all didactic instruction and occurred following the senior year. The students chose three internship rotations, for a total of 14 to 18 weeks.

The types of clinical education experiences available in the AHES regions were varied. There were general hospitals and community hospitals ranging in size from 40 to 400 beds. In addition, there were home health agencies serving the rural areas, nursing homes, outpatient pediatric facilities, school systems, a rehabilitation center, and private practice. A student assigned to an AHES rotation could have worked in a community hospital and a nursing home and made home health visits. He could have observed and participated in many roles that a physical therapist can play in a community.

The initial project placed 15 students in four facilities located in AHES regions, for 23 student-weeks of activity. (Student-weeks = number of students times the number of weeks constituting a rotation.) The project slated for 1978–1979 (and still in effect today) placed all 32 students on AHES rotations for 243 student-weeks of activity. There are currently 23 sites available for physical therapy clinical education in seven regions. Students are placed in various facilities for two weeks, three weeks, and four to six weeks. Not all sites are used for the longer rotations.

While on rotation, the students were given four hours a week to become familiar with the region where they worked. The regional coordinator monitored the activities of all health students in the region and actively recruited students to become employed in the region. The off-campus rotation provided students with some time in an area in which they might settle as well as offered the region an opportunity to recruit prospective graduates.

Each facility was visited at least yearly by the Academic Coordinator of Clinical Education while the students were on rotation. Because of the distance and shorter rotations, students were not visited each rotation. If a facility was not visited, communication during the rotation was by telephone.

In order to facilitate the exchange of ideas and information, clinical educators from AHES regions came to Lexington for courses on improving patient treatment skills or teaching skills. Every two years a Clinical Educators' Symposium was held for all clinical educators in the physical therapy program. This program generally dealt with clinical teaching skills. In alternate years, the AHES clinical educators were sponsored at some continuing education courses in the state. These courses have generally dealt with some patient treatment skill. Academic faculty members were also available for consultation services with clinicians in AHES areas. For example, monthly visits were made by a faculty member to sites developing a pediatric program. This sharing of knowledge between University faculty members and clinicians enhanced the provision of health care to the children in the area and provided a new pediatric clinical site. Support for academic and clinical faculty members in these activities was funded by AHES monies. The AHES project exists today in the same form.

PROGRAM EVALUATION

The program was evaluated by students, clinical educators, University faculty members, and regional coordinators. The students completed forms on their learning experiences just as they did on all rotations. Questions regarding patient load (amount and variety), supervision, communication, professional growth, and good and bad experiences were shared between student, clinical educator, and the Academic

TABLE
Comparison of Placement of Physical Therapy Graduates

Location	Pre-AHES (%) 1967–1974	Post-AHES (%)					
		1975	1976	1977	1978	1979	Average
State							
Kentucky	36	75	68	58	60	81	68
Out-of-State	64	25	32	42	40	19	32
Setting							
Urban[a]	...	45	45	67	67	55	56
Rural[a]	...	55	55	33	33	45	44

[a]Figures include both in-state and out-of-state.

Coordinator of Clinical Education. Students rated their experiences in AHES facilities as high as they did rotations in larger centers. Also, when they entered the physical therapy program data had been collected from students on anticipated work preference and location. This information was compared to job acceptance after graduation. Students also reported on housing, reimbursement for meals, activities in the region, awareness of health care provision, and contact with other health students.

Clinical educators provided frequent feedback to the University on many issues. Changes were made in the length and spacing of clerkship rotations based on comments of both clinical educators and students. The academic faculty has made changes in the curriculum in order to accommodate the blocks of time needed for off-campus clinical education.

Because of the additional clinical education sites made available by AHES, the student enrollment has increased from 22 to 32 students in each class. Facilities in the Lexington area accommodate students as needed but are not constantly inundated with students throughout the year. The retention rate of graduates in the state has steadily increased. The retention rate for 1978–1979 was 81 percent—a definite improvement in the 36 percent retention rate from 1967–1974. Although some students continue to leave the state, many of them have chosen to practice in rural sites in other states (Table).

SUMMARY

The University of Kentucky Physical Therapy program has completed its seventh year of participation in the AHES. This program has afforded the physical therapy student the opportunity to gain clinical experience away from the Health Science Center during the last year of academic preparation. Clinical experience in AHES regions has enabled the student to see and practice physical therapy in predominantly rural, underserved health manpower areas. This experience has also demonstrated to the student the varied role that physical therapists and other health professionals must assume in a small community in contrast to their role in larger metropolitan or health science center areas. The quality of the experience in these regions was equal and complementary to the experience in metropolitan areas.

By arranging student clinical education experiences across the state, the burden of student overload in local facilities has been relieved. Exposure of students to rural practice has improved recruitment to underserved areas and decreased the exodus of graduates from the state. By our providing clinical experiences for students, communities and therapists across the state now have a direct link to the University.

Australian and American Clinical Education In Physiotherapy

The student-centred approach is designed to enhance student learning and prepare the student for clinical practice. It is the author's opinion that the clinical education in Australia adequately prepares physiotherapy students for clinical practice in Australia.

The clinical educator in Australia functions as a 'trailblazer'. A trailblazer is one who knows the territory and is able to blaze or lead the way for others to follow. Firstly, the skills needed to follow a trail are taught to students; these are the clinical skills. Secondly, the clinical educator selects the trail by carefully selecting patients for the student so that learning is facilitated; and thirdly, the clinical educator gives the student time to follow the trail and only functions to identify landmarks along the way. This pro-

duces a competent practitioner with good clinical skills in evaluation and treatment. The clinical educator lets the student discover the patient as new territory would be discovered. The culminating exam challenges all of the student's abilities in problem-solving.

This trailblazer model can be contrasted with the more traditional mentor model used in the U.S.A. In this model the student is often initially encouraged to follow the behaviour of the clinical educator. Since time is short it is often easier for the student to copy the behaviour of the clinical educator rather than use his own ideas. Students may be able to progress but only as the time and patient will permit. The clinical educator who is a mentor is often a clinician who does not understand how a student may learn most

efficiently. Some clinical educators inspire students to demonstrate initiative. It is the author's opinion that the mentor patient-centred model is appropriate to health care policies in the U.S.A. However, as an educator she prefers the student-centred, trailblazer approach which is so successful in Australia.

References

Matthews J (1988), Progress Report of the American Physical Therapy Association, September 1988.

Scully R and Shephard KF (1983), Clinical teaching in physical therapy education: an ethnographic study, *Physical Therapy*, 63: (3), 349-358.

Professor Nancy T. Farina
Program Director,
Department of Physical Therapy,
Russell Sage College,
Troy, New York, 12180.

Australian and American Clinical Education in Physiotherapy: A Comparison of Two Different Models†

The purpose of this paper is to compare the clinical education programmes in Australia as part of the physiotherapy education with programmes in the United States. As of May 1988 there were 121 Entry-Level programmes in physical therapy in the United States (Matthews 1988), while there are five in Australia. This difference in numbers is attributable to the difference in population size between the two countries. However, other differences exist which are attributable to differences in cultural views on health care and education. In Australia direct access physical therapy or, as the Australians say, 'first contact' physical therapy is practised throughout the country; it is the norm. However, in the U.S.A. this is not the norm, with less than 20 of the 50 States having direct access.

The academic education for the physiotherapist in Australia is approximately three and one-half years, with an average of 1000 hours of clinical education. In America all Bachelor of Science programmes are at least four years in length, with an average of 750 hours of clinical education. The academic programme in Australia consists of supporting sciences to the professional programme. In America, there is a liberal arts base of one and a half to two years which includes humanities as well as sciences. In spite of these differences the professional courses are quite similar. While the academic portion of the programme is similar in curricula in both countries, each country has distinct models of clinical education.

Scully (1983) has described the clinical education of physical therapists in the U.S.A. to be patient-centred. It is patient-centred because of the health care system as well as the reimbursement system for health care services. More recently the issue of professional malpractice and emphasis on patient's rights has pushed the clinical education even further in this direction. Additionally, physical therapy education in

the U.S.A. is modelled after medical education in which a separate faculty teaches academic courses as distinct from those faculties involved with clinical teaching. Recent literature published by the American Physical Therapy Association (APTA) indicates that students role-model after the clinical faculty and not after the academic faculty. The clinical educator in the U.S.A. works in a variety of health care settings such as: acute care hospitals, private practice settings, home care and rehabilitation centres. Patients all carry health insurance or if they are medically indigent they have federal insurance. In any case, fiscal resource constraints characterize health care in the U.S.A. today. The prospective health care reimbursement policies have reduced hospital stays for most of the diagnostic categories. Often, the time that the therapist can spend with the patient is determined by the patient's ability to pay for treatment. Time for patient treatment as well as time for student learning has become constrained. The clinical educator works as a mentor to one or two students at a time. She guides the student to cover her caseload, initially giving the student a reduced caseload and progressing to an increased level of responsibility. The clinical education experience may be a brief one to two days, two weeks or six weeks in duration. Longer clinical experiences are reserved for clinical affiliations after the student has completed the majority of professional courses. Students are evaluated against forms created by Schools or States or Regions. In New York State all the schools, and there are twelve, use the same form. Many parts of the United States use the Blue MACS evaluation form. The clinical education of the student is frequently evaluated separately from the academic education. Students failing clinical education experiences are expected to make them up with satisfactory and successful clinical experiences. Academic faculty are required by Accreditation Standards of the APTA to identify levels of clinical competency of students prior to the students' clinical experience.

On the other hand, a different model of clinical education is evident in most of Australia. This model is distinctly student-centred, not patient-centred. The clinical educator is also an academic 'tutor' who is employed by the physiotherapy programme. The tutor teaches in the academic portion of the curriculum teaching clinical skills. After the tutor teaches the skills she takes a group of four to five students into the clinic with her. In this student-centred model the tutor will select from all the patients at a facility some which will best meet student needs. If the rotation is in Orthopedics then a variety of orthopedic cases are selected so that students can see a variety of problems. Students are given ample time for evaluation, up to 90 minutes. Patients are tools to help students learn problem solving and master their clinical skills. As in the patient-centred approach, the student will take on a heavier patient load as time progresses through the clinical rotation. The student is evaluated by the tutor but has a final evaluation which involves patient assessment and treatment on a real patient. This 'viva' is evaluated by a tutor who comes from another facility and does not work directly with the student being tested. The student's grade on this examination is added to the other examinations that the student takes at the end of term. The combination of both will determine if the student passes the unit and thus the course or not. If there is no pass the student must repeat the clinical course again.

This seems possible because Australia has a Labor government in power which states that free education and health care are rights of its citizens. The health care system costs the patient little to be seen in a public hospital. Physiotherapy students, as other university students, pay a modest fee of approximately $263.00 per year, but tuition is free.* The average American student pays 9000.00 dollars per year in tuition. Since time is not a factor, students are given adequate opportunity to practice patient evaluation skills.

† Paper presented at the First World Congress on Allied Health sponsored by the American Society of Allied Health Professions at Elsinor, Denmark, June 1988.

* This will change in 1989 with the introduction of the Higher Education Contribution Scheme.

Journal of Advanced Nursing, 1991, 16, 101–107

A collaborative model for the clinical education of baccalaureate nursing students

H. Kirkpatrick RN MScN
Clinical Nurse Specialist, Hamilton Psychiatric Hospital and Assistant Clinical Professor,
School of Nursing, McMaster University

C. Byrne RN MHSc
Associate Professor, School of Nursing, McMaster University and Courtesy Appointment,
Hamilton Psychiatric Hospital

M.-L. Martin RN MScN
Clinical Nurse Specialist, Hamilton Psychiatric Hospital and Assistant Clinical Professor,
School of Nursing, McMaster University

and M.L. Roth RN MEd
Hospital Educator, Hamilton Psychiatric Hospital, and Assistant Clinical Professor,
Department of Psychiatry, McMaster University, Hamilton, Canada

Accepted for publication 22 May 1990

KIRKPATRICK H., BYRNE C., MARTIN M.-L. & ROTH M.L. (1991) *Journal of Advanced Nursing* **16**, 101–107
A collaborative model for the clinical education of baccalaureate nursing students
Quality clinical supervision is fundamental for the consolidation of knowledge and the development of a professional identity for baccalaureate nursing students. Problems in providing high-quality clinical supervision range from a lack of practitioner role models to inadequate or unsupportive learning environments. Collaboration between the education and service sectors allows for the development of enriched clinical learning experiences for students. This paper describes an innovative collaborative educational process developed by McMaster University School of Nursing and the Nursing and Education Departments at Hamilton Psychiatric Hospital, Hamilton, Ontario, Canada. Front-line nursing staff are the clinical supervisors, with support from clinical nurse specialists, the hospital educator and the university faculty member. When compared to more traditional approaches, this model ensures that the students receive more variety in placements and access to expert human resources.

INTRODUCTION

Quality clinical supervision to baccalaureate nursing students is fundamental for consolidating knowledge and developing a professional identity (Ford 1980, McPhail 1975). Problems in providing high quality supervision

Correspondence: Helen Kirkpatrick, Clinical Nurse Specialist, Hamilton Psychiatric Hospital, PO Box 585, Hamilton, Ontario L8N 3K7, Canada.

have been identified within the university (Wong & Wong 1987) and service sectors (Johnson 1980). These problems relate to difficulties in developing an appropriate learning environment and in establishing collaboration between the university and the service sector (McPhail 1988, Christy 1980).

An awareness of the difficulties in providing a positive clinical learning environment led the School of Nursing at

McMaster University and the Educational and Nursing departments at Hamilton Psychiatric Hospital to develop a collaborative approach for the clinical supervision of undergraduate students. McMaster University, Hamilton, Ontario was the first Canadian university to base its organization on a collaborative model (MacPhail 1988).

University's perspective

The major role functions of university faculty are to educate students and contribute to the discovery of knowledge. University schools of nursing face increasing pressure to provide both additional educational programmes and to simultaneously engage in scholarly activities. These demands on faculty are often in conflict. For example, high teacher–student ratios are essential to provide quality clinical supervision but drain faculty resources from the time needed to design and implement research.

The BScN programme at McMaster University is known for small group, problem-based and self-directed learning (Byrne *et al.* 1989). This focus provides a rich learning experience for the students but is labour-intensive for the faculty.

Hospital's perspective

Hamilton Psychiatric Hospital (HPH), one of 10 provincial hospitals in Ontario, is a tertiary-care facility with a three-fold mandate: service, research, education. HPH has been involved in educating nursing students for almost 80 years but has recruited few nursing staff prepared at the baccalaureate level. Clinical placements of baccalaureate nursing students provide an opportunity to attract potential staff members, but such placements in the past had resulted in few applications for employment. An enriched clinical placement was seen as a potential opportunity for recruiting baccalaureate-prepared nurses.

Arnswald (1987) questioned whether psychiatric mental health nursing is an endangered speciality, given that the proportion of nurses entering this field has been growing smaller compared to other areas of nursing over the past few years. Martin (1985) reported on an American national nursing survey which included non-psychiatric hospital-employed BScNs. A negative undergraduate practice experience was cited by over 50% of these nurses as the reason for not choosing to work in a psychiatric setting.

THE COLLABORATIVE PROCESS

Basic to a practice/education collaborative model is the recognition that practice and education are both essential and equal contributors to nursing. Collaboration implies that the contributions of both parties are separate but equal (Blazeck *et al.* 1982). Good communication, rapport, mutual trust and respect are cornerstones of effective collaboration. To develop these essential components, there must be a commitment to common goals. Participants must have opportunities for interaction and reap some benefits. Development of this collaborative model reflects the integration of several ingredients: elements which enhance clinical learning; knowledge about collaboration; appointments between the university and service setting; and the use of preceptorships.

The use of university/service setting appointments assists in bringing together the university and hospital systems. There are three types of university/service setting appointments: joint, clinical and courtesy. Nurses with joint appointments are employed by both the university and service setting. A less well-documented strategy is the use of clinical appointments, in which nurses are employed by one agency, but provide input to another non-paying agency. To obtain a clinical appointment, an individual must meet criteria set by the non-employing agency, and have the support of the employing agency. For the individual with a clinical appointment, this arrangement provides expanded opportunities to participate in clinical, research or teaching activities and to extend their network of colleagues with similar interests outside of the employing agency. The respective agencies benefit by having increased participation, cross fertilization of ideas and additional involvement in activities within the agency. Courtesy appointments permit individuals to utilize the human, audio-visual or library resources of a non-employing agency as an adjunct to their clinical practice, teaching or research.

Preceptorships

A strategy which enhances clinical learning is the use of preceptorships, whereby students work and learn with practising staff nurses in clinical settings (Davis & Barham 1989). These experiences usually occur on a one-to-one basis with the staff nurse functioning as a role model for a senior student (Clark 1981, Fuenson & Conhan 1980). Benefits to students, staff nurses and participating agencies include the professional socialization of students, personal growth, professional role enhancement for the staff nurses and increased recognition and sharing of resources for the agencies (Davis & Barham 1989).

In this collaborative model, the clinical nurse specialists at HPH have clinical appointments with the School of Nursing at McMaster University and the hospital educator has a

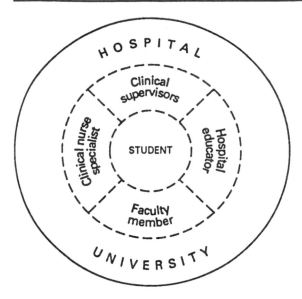

Figure 1 Student's learning environment.

clinical appointment with the Department of Psychiatry at the university. The faculty member from the School of Nursing has a courtesy appointment at HPH. The staff nurses function as preceptors in the role labelled clinical supervisor. The blending of the academic, nursing and educational services gives the students an appreciation for the unique roles played in this collaborative process.

Nursing student's learning in the clinical experience is strengthened through: assistance in identifying personal values; learning how to collaborate and solve problems; and encountering a positive attitude toward the faculty and students (Noonan 1979). Learning is enhanced when the teaching–learning methods are grounded in an understanding of the approaches used in the nursing programme and knowledge regarding issues specifically related to psychiatric–mental health nursing.

The process described in this paper addresses the above factors by providing students with direct clinical supervision from unit-based supervisors or staff nurses and input from clinical nurse specialists and the faculty member (see Figure 1). The hospital participants are committed to the teaching–learning process; they possess knowledge of the university programme and have participated in a workshop which the university provides for clinicians working with students. With the multifaceted assistance available, students learn to explore and clarify personal values in relation to psychiatric–mental health nursing. Participation in this collaborative process is new for the students and illustrates firsthand how to collaborate and solve problems. Students meet together weekly to discuss issues pertinent to

their clinical experience, such as: transference and counter-transference; therapeutic relationships; termination; and working in multidisciplinary teams.

In traditional clinical placements, students are assigned with one faculty member to a specific unit. However, in this collaborative model students are placed individually or in pairs on programmes where they are linked with a nurse who has knowledge and experience regarding the patients and the unit's functioning. The hospital educator, clinical nurse specialists and faculty member are resources who augment student learning. Details of the role played by each of the participants in this experience are described.

Hospital educator

The Educational Services Department co-ordinates student placements for all disciplines from bona fide educational institutions in the Hamilton region of Canada. The hospital educator assists and maintains an e. ational focus and climate without undertaking direct responsibility for education.

Educational Services and the Department of Nursing review requests for placements at the hospital. Considerations which affect placements include: major changes in the clinical programmes; the number of students the clinical teams can accommodate; learning experiences available; and the variety of roles nursing staff assume. When these negotiations are completed, clinical placement requests are forwarded to the programmes and the university. A contract is initiated by Educational Services to ensure that those involved in the clinical programmes are informed about their commitment to the School of Nursing. This strategy reinforces the commitment by the Department of Nursing and the clinical programmes to the education of future nurses.

In addition to orchestrating placements between the School of Nursing, HPH Educational Services, the Department of Nursing, and the clinical programmes, the hospital educator ensures ongoing communication and co-ordination by negotiating, monitoring and evaluating the overall clinical experience. The Educational Services Department also operates as a third party in interagency/student conflicts. This is rarely necessary due to the working relationship of key personnel in the hospital facility and faculty members at the university.

The students

Each term (13 weeks), approximately six third-year BScN students are placed at HPH for their first psychiatric nursing experience. Placements may include: admission units, long-term care units, an assessment team, and out-patient and community programmes. For 12 hours per week, students participate as members of the multidisciplinary team. Consistent with the self-directed learning approach, the students identify their individual learning needs and develop a learning plan. The learning plan, which reflects the student's learning needs and the course objectives, includes: (a) learning needs for the clinical placement; (b) methods to address these needs; and (c) evaluation criteria. Students also keep a journal in which they document the most important event which occurred each clinical day, their thoughts and feelings surrounding the event and consequent learning issues. This journal is shared with the faculty member.

Clinical supervisor

Individual clinical supervision is undertaken by a unit supervisor or staff nurse who has demonstrated: expertise in a specialized area of psychiatric–mental health nursing; in-depth knowledge of both the programme and patients; and an interest in teaching. The clinical supervisor has on-going responsibility for patient care and provides the day-to-day supervision of the student. The role of the supervisor is critical to the student's learning experience, assisting the student to acquire new knowledge and skills by functioning as a role model and supervising the student's clinical practice. Clinical supervision may include: observing student–patient interactions, reviewing process recordings, guiding the development of nursing formulations, and reviewing documentation such as nursing notes and care plans. The clinical supervisor and the faculty member are jointly responsible with the student for facilitating and evaluating the student's learning.

Faculty member

The faculty member has a background in psychiatric–mental health nursing as well as in-depth knowledge of the course goals and objectives, and the academic and clinical standards expected of students at this level. This knowledge is shared with both the clinical supervisor and clinical nurse specialists.

The students meet individually with the faculty member at regular intervals throughout the term. Initially, the faculty member facilitates development of the learning plan. Later, supervision focuses on the integration of theoretical knowledge and practice skills. The student's journal, which is shared with the faculty member and often discussed during supervision time, enhances the faculty member's knowledge of the student's daily clinical experience.

Table 1 Sessions with clinical nurse specialists

Session	Content
1	Interpersonal techniques
	Nursing theory
2	Nursing conceptual frameworks
	Nursing diagnosis/pattern
3	Psychiatric diagnosis
	Nurse–patient relationship
4	Schizophrenia: a long-term perspective
	Therapeutic use of self
5	Role of the patient advocate and patient rights
	Anxiety
6	Student case presentation*
	Student case presentation*
7	Student case presentation*
	Altered thought process
	Hallucinations and delusions
8	Student case presentation*
	Student case presentation*
9	Student case presentation*
	Self-concept
10	Risk for harm to self or others
	Independent nursing interventions
11	Follow-up of case presentations
	Evaluation of nursing framework
12	Summary and evaluation

*Students' presentations have included application of the following nursing frameworks: King, Neuman, Orem, Orlando, Parse, Peplau, Reihl, Rogers, Roy and Travelbee.

The faculty member communicates with the clinical supervisor and the clinical nurse specialists on the student's progress and, in conjunction with the clinical supervisor, provides feedback to the student at midterm and final evaluations. The final grade for the clinical course is the responsibility of the faculty member.

Clinical nurse specialists

The students meet as a group with two clinical nurse specialists for a weekly 2-hour session to assist with the integration of theory into practice (see Table 1). The group session allows students to provide and receive support, solve problems, and learn from one another's experiences (Hughes 1985). The sharing of experiences in the group expands knowledge and understanding of the various services provided by the hospital.

Students integrate theory with practice from the beginning of their clinical experience. The introduction of theory-based practice begins by addressing the questions: What is a nursing conceptual framework? and What is its relevance to clinical practice? Students choose a nursing framework to use in developing a therapeutic relationship with a specific patient. Each student is responsible for a case presentation to the group based on the chosen framework and only that student is expected to know the framework well. The week prior to the scheduled presentation, the other students receive reading material which provides a basic knowledge and an overview of the framework.

Sessions are used to discuss research, concepts and issues specifically related to psychiatric—mental health nursing. Students are encouraged to bring both positive and negative experiences to the group sessions. Specific experiences are discussed to explore the dynamics involved, a process which enables the students to develop their analytical and problem-solving skills. Outcomes may include obtaining further information or attempting alternative strategies. Follow-up reports allow the students to evaluate the intervention or re-analyse the situation.

Evaluation

As with the rest of the placement, evaluations are completed collaboratively. Throughout the placement, students are encouraged to assess and evaluate their placement to ensure their learning needs are being met. If problems arise, the clinical supervisor, clinical nurse specialists, hospital educator and faculty member are resources to whom students can turn for assistance.

At the end of the placement, three evaluations take place: (a) the student is evaluated on clinical performance by the clinical supervisor and the faculty member; (b) students are requested to provide very specific feedback about various aspects of the placement on a form provided by the hospital educator; and (c) students, faculty, clinical supervisors, clinical nurse specialists and the hospital educator meet to evaluate the clinical experience and make recommendations for future placements. Minutes are taken and sent to all participants. The feedback is used to make revisions for the next term. For example, feedback has assisted in the preparation of resource packages for incoming students and in the alteration of clinical placements.

DISCUSSION

The collaborative model presented in this paper uses both clinical and courtesy appointments and clinical supervisors (preceptors) as vehicles for the clinical education of nursing students. Other agencies have reported that the use of joint appointees enhances student learning (Arpin 1979). However, joint appointments require both strong administrative and financial support. Although clinical appointments require a strong administrative commitment from both participating agencies, the absence of financial remuneration in these times of budgetary constraints may make this model easier to implement. Clinical appointments strengthen the links between the hospital and university. They are a source of professional growth and satisfaction for the clinical nurse specialists and for the hospital educator. The university benefits by increasing specialized teaching resources in the community.

Using this model, students receive varied placements and have access to more expert resources than in traditional models. The expectation that students will use theory-based practice has had positive outcomes for both students and nursing staff, including: knowledge and skill acquisition; development of a strong nursing perspective; peer support and collaboration; and the enhancement of nursing's image. The multidisciplinary teams have provided the nursing students with a unique experience in working with patients collaboratively with other disciplines. Due to the students' positive learning experience, they have begun to return to HPH for summer work programmes or for full-time employment after graduation.

Clinical supervisors

Clinical supervisors have indicated that their rewards stem from professional self-development and from their one-to-one relationship with a student, assisting the student to grow professionally. There are no monetary incentives. Recognition includes an acknowledgement and thank you in the hospital newsletter and a letter of appreciation on behalf of the School of Nursing.

This collaborative model has been beneficial to the faculty in the roles of educator and researcher. First, this model allows students to have more varied and individualized placements that cannot be given when one faculty member accompanies a group of students to a ward. Having students learn directly from clinical supervisors on the units has allowed the faculty member more time to provide consultation on teaching—learning principles to clinical supervisors, to provide educational sessions to hospital staff and to identify mutual research needs between the hospital and university.

When the education and service settings are separate, students often have difficulty making the links from theory to practice because they lack practitioner role models.

Table 2 Benefits and problems in the collaborative process

Benefits	Problems
Students	
Work with nurses (clinical supervisor) who have in-depth knowledge of the unit, the patients and the hospital	Dealing with many people
Work with clinical nurse specialists in the application of nursing theory into practice	Arranging appointments with various supervisors
Share experiences with other students	
Participate in evaluating experience	
Allows students to be more self-directed and develop problem-solving skills	
Faculty	
Increased research time	Dealing with many people
Variety of clinical experiences for students	Trusting the students will not 'learn' the 'wrong' things
Collaborate with staff nurses from various units	
Feedback regarding student performance	
Opportunity for research with hospital staff	
Clinical supervisor	
Expertise is recognized	Time constraints
Collaborative relationship with university faculty	
Exposure to various frameworks	
Development of teaching/supervising skills	
Clinical nurse specialists	
Collaborative relationship with faculty	Time constraints
Develops critical thinking about theory and practice	
Opportunity for research with faculty	
Hospital educator	
Stringent negotiating procedures assist in defining roles, clarifying expectations and identifying areas of responsibility	Time required in the negotiations with clinical programmes, departments, people, resources and outside agency
Provides a sound clinical experience which will encourage students to seek employment at hospital	
Encourages staff to participate in student education	

Students very often perceive faculty as theoreticians unable to practice nursing, and practitioners as technicians unable to relate theory to practice (Blazeck *et al.* 1982). When students discover faculty members and practitioners collaborating within this framework, they have the opportunity to view the worlds of education and practice as different but equal.

Conclusion

This collaborative approach has been advantageous to both the hospital and university (see Table 2). Practice/education and practitioner/educator links have been strengthened. The exchange of information between the university and practice setting has increased. Learning opportunities in the clinical setting have been enriched and staff nurses have developed skills in the clinical supervisor role. Although the process described in this paper is complex and time-consuming, the advantages far outweigh the problems. The working relationship which the authors and clinical supervisors have developed is one of mutual respect for the role that each plays in this collaborative process.

References

Arnswald L. (1987) Not fade away are psychiatric nurses an endangered species? *Journal of Psychosocial Nursing* **25**(5), 31–33.

Arpin K. (1979) Joint appointments: strengthening the clinical practice component in nursing education programmes. *Nursing Papers* **13**(2), 9–14.

Blazek A., Selekman J., Timpe M. & Wolfe Z.R. (1982) Unification: nursing education and nursing practice. *Nursing and Health Care* **3**(1), 18–24.

Byrne C., McKnight J., Roberts J. & Rankin J. (1989) Learning clinical teaching skills at the baccalaureate level. *Journal of Advanced Nursing* **14**, 678–685.

Christy T. (1980) Clinical practice as a function of nursing education: an historical analysis. *Nursing Outlook* **8**, 493–497.

Clark M. (1981) Staff nurses as clinical teachers. *American Journal of Nursing* **81**, 314–318.

Davis L. & Barham P. (1989) Get the most from your preceptorship program. *Nursing Outlook* **37**(4), 167–171.

Ford L.C. (1980) Unification of nursing practice, education and research. *International Nursing Review* **27**(6), 178–183, 192.

Fuenson L. & Conahan B. (1980) A clinical preceptor program: strategy for new graduate orientation. *Journal of Nursing Administration* **10**, 18–23.

Hughes C. (1985) Supervising clinical practice in psychosocial nursing. *Journal of Psychosocial Nursing* **23**(2), 27–32.

Johnson J. (1980) The education/service split. Who loses? *Nursing Outlook* **28**, 412–415.

MacPhail J. (1975) Promoting collaboration between education and service. *The Canadian Nurse* **71**, 32–34.

MacPhail J. (1988) Collaboration between nursing education and nursing practice for quality nursing care. In *Canadian Nursing Issues and Perspectives* (Kerr J. & MacPhail J. eds), McGraw-Hill Ryerson, Toronto, pp. 267–282.

Martin E.J. (1985) A speciality in decline? Psychiatric mental health nursing, past, present and future. *Journal of Professional Nursing* **1**(1), 48–53.

Noonan U.A. (1979) How to increase clinical learning opportunities in a psychiatric nursing setting. *Journal of Nursing Education* **18**(4), 5–15.

Wong J. & Wong S. (1987) Towards effective clinical teaching in nursing. *Journal of Advanced Nursing* **12**, 505–513.

SURGICAL EDUCATION

Influence of Clerkship Structure and Timing on Individual Student Performance

Frank A. Baciewicz, Jr., MD, Linda Arent, Michael Weaver, RN, MSN, Richard Yeastings, PhD,
Neil R. Thomford, MD, Toledo, Ohio

Student oral and written surgical clerkship performances may be related to the clerkship structure and the time of year the students rotate through the clerkship. The influence of calendar block, hospital site (university hospital, affiliated private tertiary-care hospital, and rural preceptor experience), and the mix of general surgical versus subspeciality rotations on oral and written student surgery clerkship scores was analyzed. Multivariate analysis of variance revealed significant differences in score for calendar block (p = 0.02) only; this difference resided in the written examination. The various combinations of rotations were not different from one another in terms of measured outcome.

At our institution, the surgical clerkship is a required part of the third-year medical school curriculum. Although it is a prerequisite for graduation, all students' experiences during the clerkship are not identical. The students take the clerkship at different times during their third year, matriculate at different hospitals, and are clerks on various general and subspecialty services. Each student's performance is rated by an oral examination and a national board-developed written examination given at the conclusion of the clerkship. The purpose of this study was to determine if the calendar block of the surgical clerkship, the hospital site (university hospital, affiliated private tertiary-care hospital, or rural preceptor experience), and the mix of general surgical and subspecialty rotations influenced the students' oral and written clerkship scores.

MATERIAL AND METHODS

One hundred thirty-nine third-year students rotated through the surgical clerkship from June 1985 to May 1986. Each surgical clerkship lasted 12 weeks and was divided into three 4-week rotations. There were four blocks during which students took the clerkship: June to August (29 students), September to November (34), December to February (36), and March to May (40).

From the Department of Surgery, Medical College of Ohio, Toledo, Ohio.

Requests for reprints should be addressed to Frank A. Baciewicz, Jr., MD, Division of Cardio-thoracic Surgery, Department of Surgery, C.S. 10008, Medical College of Ohio, Toledo, Ohio 43699.

Manuscript submitted July 18, 1988, revised April 7, 1989, and accepted April 21, 1989.

The 4-week rotations were taken at three combinations of locations: the tertiary-care university-care hospital, one of three private tertiary-care hospitals in the same metropolitan area affiliated in a teaching capacity with the medical school, or in a one-on-one preceptor teaching situation in one of three rural community settings. The students were required to take a minimum of 1 month but no more than 2 months at the university hospital. The possible combinations of hospital-based rotations included: (1) 1 month university hospital, 2 months private-care hospital; (2) 1 month university hospital, 1 month private-care hospital, 1 month rural preceptor; and (3) 2 months university hospital, 1 month private-care hospital. The sequence of 2 months university hospital, 1 month rural preceptor was experienced by only two students and was eliminated from statistical analysis.

The 4-week rotations were in general surgery, cardiovascular-thoracic surgery, and other subspecialties including orthopedics, urology, and plastic surgery. Neurosurgery and otolaryngology are separate departments and were not included in the third-year clerkships. Cardiothoracic and vascular rotations were considered separately from general surgery and the other subspecialties because they emphasize cardiorespiratory physiology. A minimum of 1 month of general surgery was required, and a maximum of 2 months of general surgery was assigned. Whether students received 1 or 2 months of general surgery depended on the subspecialties they requested and the availability of general and subspecialty slots.

The students' performances were assessed by oral and written examinations given on the last day of their 12-week rotations. Each student had two oral examinations based principally on the patients cared for and the required lecture series. The maximum score on each oral examination was 100, so the total maximum oral score was 200. A grade of 149 or lower resulted in failing the oral examination. The written examination was the standard national board-prepared surgery examination with a maximum score of 800.

Differences in preclinical preparation among the groups were identified as a potential explanation for any discrepancy in performance on oral and written scores. Each subject earned a percentile score for each basic science subject taken during the first two years of medical school. Each subject (anatomy, behavioral science, biochemistry, microbiology, pathology, pharmacology, and physiology) had a possible score from the 1st to the 99th percentile. Compilation of the seven scores gave a possible index ranging from 7 to 693 and was an indicator of overall preclinical performance.

As the average oral, written, and preclinical scores were intercorrelated, multivariate analysis of variance was applied to test for differences in these variables be-

TABLE I

Student Scores by Calendar Block (mean ± SD)*

	June–Aug	Sept–Nov	Dec–Feb	Mar–May
No. of students	29	34	35	39
Preclinical index (7–693)	355.3 ± 179.8	336.6 ± 167.5	346.6 ± 170.2	351.6 ± 169.6
Written score (200–800)	435.3 ± 108.4	468.1 ± 98.3	509.7 ± 92.4	504.1 ± 106.6
Oral score (0–200)	169.4 ± 12.8	170.0 ± 9.1	169.0 ± 9.5	171.8 ± 10.3

* Values in parentheses represent grading scales.

TABLE II

Student Scores by Site (mean ± SD)*

	Site Combination[†]		
	1	2	3
No. of students	13	77	47
Preclinical index (7–693)	364.1 ± 150.1	344.3 ± 170.9	347.8 ± 175.8
Written score (200–800)	495.4 ± 122.8	482.3 ± 100.9	478.0 ± 107.1
Oral score (0–200)	168.1 ± 12.7	170.1 ± 10.2	170.7 ± 10.1

* Values in parentheses represent grading scales.
† Combination 1 = 2 months university hospital, 1 month affiliated private tertiary-care hospital; combination 2 = 1 month university hospital, 2 months affiliated hospital; combination 3 = 1 month university hospital, 1 month affiliated hospital, 1 month rural preceptor experience.

TABLE III

Student Scores by Rotation Mix (mean ± SD)*

	Rotation[†]			
	1	2	3	4
No. of students	15	17	25	80
Preclinical index (7–693)	367.3 ± 180.3	329.1 ± 167.0	400.5 ± 164.7	330.9 ± 169.1
Written score (200–800)	462.7 ± 140.6	492.6 ± 84.4	508.2 ± 116.9	475.3 ± 96.7
Oral score (0–200)	166.3 ± 8.1	172.8 ± 11.0	170.5 ± 10.8	170.2 ± 10.5

* Values in parentheses represent grading scales.
† Rotation 1 = 2 months in general surgery, 1 month in cardiovascular-thoracic surgery; rotation 2 = 1 month in general surgery, 1 month in cardiovascular-thoracic surgery, and 1 month in other subspecialities; rotation 3 = 1 month in general surgery, 2 months in other subspecialities; rotation 4 = 2 months in general surgery, 1 month in other subspecialities.

tween the blocks, sites, and subspecialty rotations. Type III sums of squares were used in order to eliminate linear dependencies that might have resulted from the unequal cell sizes. Significant multivariate findings were followed up with univariate analyses of variance, with the studentized maximum modulus post-hoc test applied to significant univariate tests [1–3].

RESULTS

Tables I, II, and III give the average preclinical index and written and oral test scores for the students when compiled by block, combination of site, and rotation mix, respectively. These data were subjected to the statistical analysis described above.

Multivariate analysis of variance indicated no significant site ($p = 0.71$) or rotation ($p = 0.32$) effects, whereas the block effect was statistically significant ($p = 0.02$). Further univariate analyses demonstrated that this difference resided in the written score only ($p = 0.02$); there were no statistically significant differences in either oral or preclinical scores ($p = 0.71$ and $p = 0.89$, respectively). Post-hoc tests showed that December to February and March to May blocks had higher scores than the June to August block ($p = 0.05$).

COMMENTS

Previous studies in assessing student performance on the surgical clerkship have assumed that the students receive a homogenous experience. The difference in student performance has been attributed to the individual student's intelligence and aptitude for surgery [4–6] or to variance in educational format [7,8]. Consequently, studies have measured student performance as related to the pre-medical school performance on the Medical College Admissions Test and college grades [4–6]. Other investigators have pointed to difficult-to-quantitate student character traits [9,10] as significant reasons for differences in student performance. Other efforts have been aimed at studying various educational techniques to delineate a difference in student test results [11–15].

We observed that the student clerkship experience in surgery differed widely in our institution. The medical school class is approximately 150 students per year, and the university hospital is small at 300 beds. In order that all students have a 12-week surgical rotation in their third year, the student clerkship experience includes private tertiary-care hospitals in our community that have teaching services, one-on-one preceptor experience in rural community hospitals, and the university hospital services. This rural experience is called AHEC (Area Health Education Center) and is funded by the federal legislature. Our hypothesis was that the different combinations of teaching environments would be reflected in students' scores. In fact, our results demonstrate that any combination of university hospital, private-care hospital, and rural preceptor resulted in similar performances. This suggests that students at medical schools dependent on private-care institutions and individual instruction for surgical education may do as well as students at schools based entirely at a university hospital.

Calhoun et al [16] report that allocation of student time to rounds, the operating room, write-ups, laboratory work, and conferences is different at university, veterans administration, and affiliated tertiary-care hospitals. However, they demonstrated that patient care time and educational time were similar at all sites. If we assume that equal time was spent on education at all site combinations in the present study, it is not surprising that all site combinations had similar student oral and written scores.

In addition, whether the students matriculated for 4 or 8 weeks at the university hospital did not result in differences on oral or written scores. The second 4 weeks of university hospital experience did not have an additive effect on student performance. This similar performance for the 4- and 8-week university hospital experience may be unique to this medical school. Certainly, an experience in which students see different surgical delivery systems may be valuable in their career selection.

A second clerkship variable was the number of 4-week rotations that students spent on a general surgical rotation. All students spent at least 1 month on general surgery rotations, and 68% spent 2 months on general surgery. Our expectation was that students with 2 months of general surgery experience would perform better than those with only 1 month. Furthermore, we thought that 4 weeks spent on a cardiothoracic or vascular service that emphasizes cardiac, vascular, and respiratory physiology would favorably influence oral and written examination scores. The data shows that neither 2 months of general surgery nor an additional month of cardiovascular-thoracic surgery influenced student scores.

Although the students did have different site combinations and number of general surgery rotations, the students at all sites (with the exception of the outlying AHEC centers) were required to attend 3 hours of Friday afternoon lectures on core curriculum surgical topics. In addition, with the exception of students on rural preceptor rotations, their presence was mandatory at Saturday grand rounds. These common didactic sessions may have outweighed the effect of hospital site and number of general surgery rotations on student scores.

The timing of the calendar block, whether it was the students' first, second, third, or fourth clinical experience, was also assessed. Statistical analysis demonstrated a significant performance difference for the third and fourth calendar blocks compared to the first, with the difference residing in the written examination scores. Although not statistically significant, the mean written score in the second block was higher than that of the first but not as high as that in the third or fourth block. The perception that students should take a rotation they wish to excel at later in the clinical year appears accurate. Since the written examination is an assessment of medical knowledge, we would expect the students' performance to improve over the course of the academic year as their knowledge base increases. As pointed out by Calhoun et al [16], the percentage of time students spend on educational versus patient care activities increases as the academic year progresses. This increased educational time may be another explanation for the improved performance during the latter part of the academic year.

The fact that the student scores for their basic science courses did not vary among the groups makes it unlikely that inter-group difference was the reason for the difference in written scores. If their average basic science percentile scores were similar, our interpretation was that the students' entering those clinical rotations were comparable.

This study can help allay student fears that they will not score well on their examinations if they do not take a particular rotation at a specific hospital. The data do not implicate specific subspecialty rotations or specific type of teaching environments as affecting the students' oral and written test results. If students wish to improve their performances on the surgery clerkship, it may behoove them to take it later in their third clinical year.

In conclusion, student surgical clerkship written scores are significantly lower during the initial part of the clinical experience. Participating hospitals and the mix of surgical subspecialties have no effect on oral or written student surgical clerkship scores.

REFERENCES

1. Speed FM, Hocking RR, Hackney OP. Methods of analysis of linear models with unbalanced data. J Am Stat Assoc 1978; 73: 105–12.
2. Kendall M, Stuart A, Ord JK. The advanced theory of statistics. Vol. 3. London: Charles Griffin and Co., 1983.
3. Hochburg Y. Some conservative generalizations of the t-method in simultaneous inference. J Multivariate Anal 1974; 4: 224–34.
4. Cowles JT, Kubany AJ. Improving the measurement of clinical performance of medical students. J Clin Psych 1959; 15: 139–42.
5. McGuire FL. Fifteen years of predicting medical student performance. J Med Educ 1977; 52: 416–7.
6. Carline JD, Cullen TJ, Scott CS, Shannon NF, Schaad D. Predicting performance during clinical years from the new medical college admission test. J Med Educ 1983; 58: 18–25.
7. Linn BS, Cohen J, Wirch J, Pratt T, Zeppa R. The relationship of interest in surgery to learning styles, grades and residency choice. Soc Sci Med 1979; 13A: 597–600.

8. Patel VL, Dauphinee WD. The clinical learning environments in medicine, paediatrics and surgery clerkships. Med Educ 1985; 19: 54–60.

9. Turner EV, Helper MM, Kriska SD. Predictors of clinical performance. J Med Educ 1974; 49: 338–42.

10. Murden R, Galloway GM, Reid JC, Colwill JM. Academic and personal predictors of clinical success in medical school. J Med Educ 1978; 53: 711–9.

11. Laurence PF. Nelson EW, Cockayne TW. Assessment of medical student fund of knowledge in surgery. Surgery 1985; 97: 745–9.

12. Linn BS, Schimmel R, Wirch J, Pratt T, Zeppa R. Where national board exams pass and fail in evaluating knowledge of surgical clerk. J Surg Res 1979; 26: 97–100.

13. Stillman RM, Lane KM, Beeth S, Jaffe BM. Evaluation of student: Improving validity of the oral examination. Surgery 1983; 93: 439–42.

14. Stillman RM. Effect of prior clinical experience on students' knowledge and performance in surgery. Surgery 1986; 100: 77–82.

15. Zelenock GB, Calhoun JG, Hockman EM, et al. Oral examinations: actual and perceived contributions to surgery clerkship performance. Surgery 1985; 97: 747–3.

16. Calhoun J, Davis WK, Erlandson EE, Maxim BR. A multisite comparison of student activities in the surgery clerkship. Surgery 1982; 91: 662–7.

EDITORIAL COMMENT

Norman Snow, MD, Cleveland, Ohio

The preceding study by Baciewicz and co-workers proposes that the outcome of a basic surgical clerkship is independent of the rotation site utilized. The only difference noted among sites was that of the National Board of Medical Examiners (NBME) test score. Similar analyses in Miami (J Surg Res 1979; 26: 97–100) and at Case Western Reserve (personal communication) have concluded that the NBME examination is satisfactory for licensure but may be inadequate for internal review based on local curriculum content. The significance of the NBME score difference, therefore, is unclear relative to outcome, at least as locally defined. Rotation block time seemed

From the Department of Surgery, Case Western Reserve University, Cleveland, Ohio.

to influence NBME scores as well. Students are known to spend more educational time later in the academic year; therefore, factors extraneous to the curriculum may be responsible for this phenomenon, such as an upcoming NBME test, clinical maturation, and improvement in problem-solving ability.

I am personally bothered by the last sentence of the article, which seems to tempt students to "go for the grade" rather than the overall educational experience. The timing of clerkship rotations is multifactorial and includes administrative direction, prevalence of seasonal patient experiences, and personal preferences. All scores seem to rise as students learn the ropes and mature. It would seem more appropriate to adjust the curriculum content seasonally to reflect what we know about student behavior rather than to seduce

the matriculants by specialty preference.

Despite the problems with outcome measurement, the important conclusion of this study is that with careful attention to curricular development and with meticulous monitoring of its implementation, equally satisfactory, although not uniform, educational quality may be available at a wide variety of institutions other than the university hospital. Given the dissimilarities between hospitals, and despite disparate campus locations, one must emphasize fundamental general surgical principles within a uniform core curriculum. Little advantage was obtained in Toledo by manipulating the general surgery, cardiovascular, or specialty rotations, and I suspect that the core curriculum presented in a consistent fashion outweighed the hospital differences.

JAMES O. WOOLLISCROFT, M.D., and THOMAS L. SCHWENK, M.D.
Teaching and Learning in the Ambulatory Setting

Abstract—Changes in how and where health care is delivered have had an adverse effect on the traditional inpatient-based clinical education of medical students. Increasingly, medical educators are turning to ambulatory-based educational experiences as viable and useful adjuncts to the inpatient wards. However, when planning and developing an ambulatory clerkship, careful attention must be paid to the desired outcomes from the experience, the appropriate site, and instructional model to use to best meet the objectives. This report explores (1) the major differences between ambulatory and inpatient educational settings, (2) potential educational outcomes of clinical teaching in the ambulatory setting, (3) instructional models that can be used to meet educational objectives, (4) the potential barriers and critical issues that must be considered when implementing ambulatory educational experiences, and (5) evaluation strategies for measuring the educational outcome. *Acad. Med.* 64(1989):644–648.

The last great revolution in the education of physicians occurred in the late 1800s with the founding and development of teaching hospitals. The establishment of hospital-based clinical clerkships as integral components of the clinical education of medical students was part of this revolution.[1] Throughout the twentieth century, medical students have learned about the natural history and physiologic manifestations of disease, diagnostic and therapeutic rationales, and the nuances of physicianhood through interactions with patients in hospital wards. However, changes in how and where health care is delivered have affected, for the most part adversely, the traditional inpatient basis for students' clinical training. New financing arrangements and new medical technologies have caused inpatient lengths of stay to shorten, comprehensive evaluations to terminate prematurely (from an education perspective), and measures of severity of illness and intensity of service to increase. The modern teaching hospital has become a large intensive care unit where medical students have inadequate access to patients who represent only a small, albeit very ill, portion of the total spectrum of medical practice.[2] The suitability of using inpatient wards for the preponderance of students' clinical education is being questioned.

Education in the ambulatory setting has been advanced as a solution to this problem. Unfortunately, many medical educators may look to clinical teaching in an ambulatory setting as a panacea for the ills of the current medical education system. Similar to the way unproven medical technologies become adopted before appropriate rigorous clinical trials can be conducted, ambulatory medical education is being embraced before the educational consequences can be defined. Moreover, the phrase "ambulatory medical education" has almost as many meanings as there are medical educators. No physician educator would talk about the desirability of "inpatient education" without defining the type of inpatient experience; similarly, the spectrum of clinical experiences that a student can have in an ambulatory setting is tremendous. Even when the focus of ambulatory teaching is limited to primary care specialties such as family practice, internal medicine, and pediatrics, the possible educational experiences can differ as much as experiences in an inpatient neurosurgery ward differ from those in a labor and delivery unit.

Therefore, ambulatory-based teaching experiences must be devised to meet specific educational needs and be evaluated by specific and appropriate techniques to ensure that the desired outcomes are being achieved. Explicitly defining the desired outcomes for each experience will dictate the appropriate timing in the medical school curriculum and duration of the experience, the type of ambulatory setting, and the teachers' qualifications. For example, if the desired outcome is learning introductory interviewing skills, it is appropriate to begin such a program early in the basic science years. Finding a patient population that is willing to spend the requisite time and is capable of talking and acting as the resource base for such an experience is more difficult. Creative approaches have included programs in nursing homes and residential facilities for the elderly, where the residents act as "patients" for the students.[3] For such introductory interviewing courses, non-physicians can function superbly as teachers.

As another example, if the desired educational outcome is providing experience in continuity of care, this obviously cannot be achieved during a four-week block rotation. Rather, long-term experiences are needed with physicians who can be good role-models for the necessary clinical care behaviors. On the other hand, demonstrating "relevant" patient problems to reinforce basic science information can be done expeditiously in only one half-day of teaching in the ambulatory setting. A classic example is demonstrating the physical effects of the biochemical alterations of glucose

Dr. Woolliscroft is associate chairman for undergraduate medical programs, Department of Internal Medicine, and Dr. Schwenk is chairman, Department of Family Practice, University of Michigan Medical Center, Ann Arbor, Michigan

Correspondence and requests for reprints should be addressed to Dr. Woolliscroft, Department of Internal Medicine, University of Michigan Medical Center, 1500 E. Medical Center Drive, Ann Arbor, MI 48109-0368.

metabolism in a patient with diabetes mellitus. Having medical students rotate through the diabetes clinic, with its concentrated group of patients with this disease, is an efficient way to meet this educational objective.

We believe ambulatory-based medical teaching is indeed an "idea whose time has come,"[4] but uncritical acceptance does not mean that it will have strong or positive effects on students' education. In this paper we explore: (1) the major difference between the ambulatory and inpatient educational settings, (2) some of the potential educational outcomes of clinical teaching in the ambulatory setting, (3) some instructional models that can be used to meet these objectives, (4) potential barriers and critical issues that must be considered when implementing an ambulatory teaching experience, and (5) measurable educational objectives and evaluation strategies for different types of ambulatory settings.

We limit our discussion to medical student education. A considerable amount has been written about postgraduate ambulatory-based education, but little critical thought has gone into such training for students. In many ways, students' experiences are even more critical than residents' experiences because they are generally short and the impact of the experience, for better or worse, may be greater.

Ambulatory – Inpatient Differences

The major characteristic usually mentioned as the distinguishing feature between ambulatory and inpatient education is that patients in the ambulatory setting are not as ill as inpatients. Certainly this is true. The ambulatory setting is not the best site for learning the complexities of major organ-system failures and their amelioration by biomedical technologies. The ambulatory setting is a better, and perhaps the only, place to learn many of the skills and techniques required for daily patient care and the long-term management of chronic illness. However, the truly major difference between outpatient and inpatient teaching is that the "locus of control" of hospital care lies with the medical care system, and in ambulatory care it lies with the patient. This fundamental difference underlies all aspects of developing education programs, and it must be recognized and accommodated in ambulatory-based programs. The hospital has been organized for the efficiency and convenience of the system, its personnel, and technologies, while the ambulatory care system is generally organized for the convenience of the patient. Most educational issues flow from this basic difference, including those of appropriate and attainable educational objectives, effective instructional and evaluation methods, the effect of medical education on the patient and the patient's care, and the costs of teaching.

Potential Educational Outcomes

There are a multitude of possible educational goals for any ambulatory-based educational experience.[5] We discuss six goals that illustrate the potential spectrum. Each of these goals may be accomplished in an ambulatory setting. However, it would be an exceptional clerkship that accomplished all of them.

Observation of the Natural or Treated History

The outpatient setting allows the student to see the natural or treated history of an illness, rather than only the brief (albeit intense) episodes manifested in the hospital. Following patients through portions of or all phases of illness, from primary and secondary prevention through rehabilitation or death, provides a view of the impact of that disease upon a single patient that cannot be gained through other experiences. However, this "naturalistic" education generally requires a long-term experience rather than a four- to eight-week ambulatory clerkship if a single patient or small group of patients is intended as the focus for learning. A reasonable compromise is to have the student observe many patients with the same disease at different stages in its progression. The student then can synthesize an overall picture of the disease.

Developing Appropriate Professional Expectations and Attitudes about Chronic Illness

The ambulatory setting, compared with the inpatient ward, provides different opportunities for teaching students the realities of the impacts of diseases upon patients and their families. For example, when caring for patients with cancer, students may develop a skewed and negative attitude toward treating cancer patients because of their selective exposure to major complications, organ failure, and death.[6] Seeing active, functional patients being followed on a routine basis several years after their initial diagnosis and treatment provides a very different picture of oncological diseases. Similarly, treating elderly patients only in the inpatient setting may bias students against the elderly, as they often suffer from chronic debilitating diseases. Seeing elderly people function and live independently, as is often the case in ambulatory medical settings, may positively change the students' perceptions and professional attitudes.[3] Conversely, experiencing the impacts of diseases on patients who are seen on a continuing basis in their homes will usually make the long-term impact of catastrophic disease (and its biomedical treatment) more personal and immediately apparent. Having a student follow a man recently discharged with a major cerebrovascular event complicated by dense hemiplegia and aphasia, who cannot work and has significant family adjustment problems, is a far different emotional experience than writing discharge orders for the same man recovering from an apparent medical "success."

The mix of cases is as important in the ambulatory as in the inpatient setting in terms of the impact it has on students' attitudes and expectations. When planning ambulatory clerkships, program designers and directors must consciously consider what expectations and attitudes the student will be likely to develop.

Social, Financial, and Ethical Aspects of Medical Practice

Many issues that are not readily addressed in the inpatient setting are more naturally covered in the ambulatory setting. Examples include: office and practice management; the team approach to medical care, including developing collaborative relationships with medical personnel whose work may be more apparent in the ambulatory and community setting than in the hospital; the role of preventive medical care in the practice of modern medicine; financial and reimbursement issues, including the impacts of pharmaceutical, long-term care, and home-care costs on patients and their families; and ethical issues, which, of course, pervade all aspects of medical practice but are perhaps more subtle in ambulatory practice. An example is the ethical aspects of supervision or "gatekeeping" in managed care systems. These are problems that frequently confront practicing physicians but are rarely specifically addressed or taught in medical school curricula.

Patient Communication and Negotiation Skills

The ambulatory setting is especially suited for learning the skills of physician-patient communication necessary for managing patients long-term. Indeed, it may be the only setting where such skills can be learned. These skills, which differ markedly from the communication skills used in inpatient medical care, include negotiation and contracting skills, which figure prominently in a setting where patients have more autonomy. Since these communication and negotiation skills directly affect patient compliance and adherence,[7-9] the opportunity to learn contracting and negotiating skills is desirable. In general, the ambulatory setting, where patients have more control over their decisions and fate, highlights the critical importance of physicians' communication skills. Hence, students not only can develop their communication skills but also can see the im-

portance of communication to their future function as physicians.

Clinical Problem Solving

Clinical problem solving skills also differ in the ambulatory setting, where complex evaluations are rarely done simultaneously as they are, for efficiency, in the hospital. Ambulatory problem solving is usually stepwise and more deductive than that in the hospital, where students see patients who are admitted for specific sets of tests and procedures and are then discharged, to have the results obtained and interpreted at a later outpatient visit. However, once again, it must be recognized that critical thinking and problem solving skills are problem-specific and often site-specific and must be taught in a setting similar to that in which they will be applied. For example, the appropriate approach to a young woman who has a history compatible with multiple sclerosis will differ depending on the setting. In a tertiary care setting, it might include a nuclear magnetic resonance scan and follow-up in a neurology clinic, whereas in a remote rural clinic the appropriate approach might be careful clinical observation over time.

Often, the goal of teaching students to work up and treat common ambulatory problems well and efficiently is what is really meant by clinical problem solving in an ambulatory setting. As such, having the student see patients with the desired mix of diseases is important. However, if the objective is to teach or demonstrate how to formulate appropriate clinical questions and hypotheses, how to test them logically, and how to apply laboratory evaluations in a reasoned fashion, the physician-instructor is very important. But the choice of setting may be less important than when teaching other skills.

Faculty Role Models

Finally, ambulatory teaching offers opportunities for developing stronger teacher-learner relationships. This critical aspect of medical teaching

needs a great deal of improvement and attention,[10] yet using teams of residents, attending physicians, and consultants (as is done in inpatient settings) hampers such improvement. Unlike inpatient teaching, ambulatory teaching occurs mostly within a three-person relationship between one teacher, one learner, and one patient. This educational "intimacy" offers significant opportunity for identifying students' strengths and weaknesses, providing detailed feedback in a supportive environment, and having faculty serve as role models for appropriate professional skills and attitudes. This type of teaching may require a different educator than does inpatient teaching.[11] Teaching skills and expertise may be specific to particular sites or teaching formats, may not be transferable, and may require extensive faculty development efforts.

Instructional Models

Choosing the efficient and effective instructional model depends totally upon the desired educational objectives and the available clinical settings. For example, if the goal is to teach students to manage common ambulatory problems, a number of different models can be used. An experiential or apprenticeship model, in which students see patients who serve as the impetus and focus for learning, is one choice. However, the experience will vary considerably depending on the region, specialty, and time of year. A student in a rural family physician's office in February will be likely to see a spectrum of problems very different from those seen by a student in a suburban pediatrician's office in July. Indeed, there is likely to be a major difference in the types of acute infections a pediatrician's patients have in January as compared with July. Consequently, the student needs standardized materials such as teaching packets and computer-aided patient management problems for basic and supplemental information as each such problem is encountered.

If the desired goals are to develop

skills in clinical problem solving and in negotiating with patients, traditional faculty supervision in an outpatient teaching clinic may be best. This has been the de facto choice in many ambulatory education programs. Students see a patient and present the case to the faculty member, who then may perform a truncated history-taking and examination or simply expound on the case based upon the student's presentation. In a variation of this model, the faculty member and student use the chart to stimulate recall in a discussion. Often, this occurs during a formal presentation with the students during the clinic session. Other permutations of this model include decision analysis to lay out clearly the "decision tree" and then focus discussion upon the critical decision nodes, or the use of algorithms to demonstrate a consensus approach to the problem.

However, if the desired objectives are those of professional socialization or attention to the socioeconomic aspects of medical practice, using faculty role models may be the best approach. This is a more passive model. The faculty member demonstrates the role the student is to learn and, as a consequence, must see patients during the clinical time and involve students in his or her interactions with patients.

Problems, Pitfalls, and Barriers

The detailed nature of these objectives means programs must develop specific ambulatory experiences that are carefully planned and rigorously evaluated. A model for ambulatory teaching does not exist, although preliminary efforts are under way in a few centers.[12] Inpatient teaching has not been subjected to rigorous planning and evaluation, but the rich tradition of inpatient teaching implicitly defines the roles of the inpatient teacher and student and the expected educational outcomes. The present rapid shifts in medical care delivery and education will not allow 80 years for an ambulatory teaching tradition to develop in a similar fashion.

The most tangible barriers to ambulatory teaching are cost and patient acceptance. The negative impact of ambulatory teaching on faculty productivity, office staffing, and space is real.[13-15] A health maintenance organization has proposed special ambulatory teaching facilities,[16] but the experience of model family practice centers for residency training suggests that this idea has continuing as well as capital costs.[17] These financial disincentives exist regardless of the setting or model used for teaching.

Another barrier is the recruitment, development, and retention of qualified physician teachers. In university-based clinics, productivity pressures may make the faculty unwilling to participate in a teaching program that significantly reduces their efficiency.[13,14] Similarly, physicians in practice make significant sacrifices to be teachers; this must be recognized and appropriate compensation provided.[13,18] In addition, educational experiences in the ambulatory setting often entail far greater responsibility for the physician teacher. Unlike in inpatient clerkships, there are fewer house officers and fellows to share the teaching load. This concentration on the faculty physician may offer advantages to the student, but instructor "burnout" is a real problem that must be acknowledged and addressed. The best teachers may be the most conscientious and therefore most susceptible to this problem. Therefore, a larger number of instructors must be recruited and trained to ensure that "rest periods" without students are built into the program.

Finally, the patients' willingness to be part of educational programs will determine the success of new ambulatory teaching efforts. Medical education in general is characterized by the paradox of the students' need to learn by trial and error without the luxury and opportunity of making mistakes. Patients may have less enthusiasm for student involvement on their own "turf" than in the hospital, where they give up considerable autonomy. Even if student involvement is widely accepted by patients (and studies suggest that it may be under appro-

priate circumstances[12]), the presence of the student may alter the object of study, for example, the physician-patient relationship and its many ramifications. The version of the Heisenberg principle — the presence of a learner actually changes the medical care that the faculty member gives and that the student learns and emulates — may, like all laws of nature, be impossible to break. True learning in the ambulatory setting may not occur until the learner becomes the teacher.

Evaluation Strategies

Many evaluation strategies are appropriate, depending upon the educational objective. If the objective is to develop appropriate expectations and attitudes, change attributable to the ambulatory experience can be measured by any number of self-assessment instruments designed to measure such changes. If the objective is to develop an understanding of ambulatory care problems and models not readily addressed in inpatient settings, log books are useful in determining — and perhaps ensuring — that the student has the desired experiences. Skills in communicating and negotiating with patients can be assessed through interactions with standardized patients. The ability to assess common problems critically and logically can be assessed using computer or paper-and-pencil patient-management problems. Formal debriefings (ambulatory "oral exams") with the students to cover key points and objectives is a useful evaluation. These strategies allow the curriculum assessment needed to more closely match the training experience with the educational objectives.

As with potential objectives, models, and other aspects of ambulatory education, there is great diversity in the evaluation methods employed. The evaluation must be appropriate to the question asked, and the evaluation component must be planned from the outset of the program. Only through rigorous evaluation can programs determine whether their original intentions for the ambulatory-based experience are being met.

To summarize, education in the ambulatory setting is upon us, and the potential impact on medicine is enormous. Clearly, it may be looked upon as a momentous change similar to that which swept through this nation's system of medical education in the late 1800s. During that revolution, some established institutions were left behind and eventually closed, while innovative programs were developed in other existing schools. New schools, such as The Johns Hopkins Medical School, were developed based upon the "new" model. History may eventually record that we are in a similar era.

References

1. Ludmerer, K. M. *Learning to Heal*. New York: Basic Books, 1985.
2. Schroeder, S. A. Expanding the Site of Clinical Education. *J. Gen. Intern. Med.* 3(1988):S5–S14.
3. Woolliscroft, J. O., Calhoun, J. G., Maxim, B. R., and Wolf, F. M. Medical Education in Facilities for the Elderly: Impact on Medical Students, Facility Staff and Residents. *JAMA* 252(1984):3382–3385.
4. Perkoff, G. T. Teaching Clinical Medicine in the Ambulatory Setting. An Idea Whose Time May Have Finally Come. *N. Engl. J. Med.* 314(1986):27–31.
5. Lawrence, R. S. The Goals for Medical Education in the Ambulatory Setting. *J. Gen. Intern. Med.* 3(1988):S15–S25.
6. Chamberlain, R. M. Application of Cancer Prevention Knowledge: A Longitudinal Study of Medical Students. *J. Ca. Educ.* 2(1987):93–106.
7. Davis, M. S. Variations in Patients' Compliance with Doctor's Advice: An Empirical Analysis of Patterns of Communications. *Am. J. Public. Health* 58(1968):274–288.
8. Ware, J., and Snyder, M. Dimensions of Patient Attitudes Regarding Doctors and Medical Care Services. *Med. Care* 13(1975): 669–682.
9. Ley, P. Satisfaction, Compliance and Communication. *Br. J. Clin. Psychol.* 21(1982):241–254.
10. Muller, S. (Chairman). Physicians for the Twenty-First Century. Report of the Project Panel on the General Professional Education of the Physician and College Preparation for Medicine. *J. Med. Educ.* 59, Part 2 (November 1984).
11. Schwenk, T. L., and Whitman, N. A. *The Physician as Teacher*. Baltimore, Maryland: Williams and Wilkins, 1987.
12. Gravdal, J., and Glassar, M. The Integration of the Student into Ambulatory Primary Care: A Decade of Experience. *Fam. Med.* 19(1987):457–462.
13. Pawlson, L. G., Schroeder, S. A., and Donaldson, M. S. Medical Student Instructional Costs in a Primary Care Clerkship. *J. Med. Educ.* 54(1979):551–555.
14. Kirz, H. L., and Larsen, C. J. Costs and Benefits of Medical Student Training to an Independent HMO. *JAMA* 256(1986):734–739.
15. Isaacs, J. C., and Madoff, M. A. Undergraduate Medical Education in Prepaid Health Care Plan Settings. *J. Med. Educ.* 59(1984):615–624.
16. Kirz, H. L., and Larsen, C. J. An Independent HMO's Affiliation with a University. *HMO Practice* 2(1988):129–132.
17. Colwill, J. M., and Glenn, J. K. Patient Care Income and the Financing of Residency Education in Family Medicine. *J. Fam. Pract.* 13(1981):529–536.
18. Hale, F. A., Arnold, J. F., Salzman, J. New England Preceptors' Attitudes toward Teaching Compensation. *Fam. Med. Teacher* 12(1980, No. 5):1–4.

A Year-Long Clerkship in Ambulatory Care

Thomas J. Ruane, M.D.

Abstract—Decreased availability of hospitalized patients for medical student education, a changing clinical environment in both hospital and outpatient settings, and the need for teaching the specific skills of primary ambulatory care mandate the development of outpatient-based clinical clerkships. A required third-year clerkship at Michigan State University College of Human Medicine combines a long-term structure and a defined curriculum with a wealth of clinical encounters. New approaches to the basic clinical education of medical students are needed to connect clinical resources, specialty expertise, and the special knowledge and skills needed for primary care. The clerkship described in the present paper represents a model for such clinical education.

Although medical education in ambulatory care settings has been called an idea whose time has come (1), it has not entered the mainstream of the undergraduate curriculum. Education in ambulatory settings is often shunned or derided by proponents of traditional educational experiences based in the teaching hospital.

Since academic year 1983–84, all students entering their clinical curriculum at Michigan State University College of Human Medicine have taken a required third-year long-term clerkship based in a variety of ambulatory primary-care settings. The author's purpose in this report is to give data and reflections on clinical education that have grown out of this clerkship. These data suggest clinical education that incorporates both the traditional objectives of hospital-based rotations and those unique to outpatient practice into an ambulatory clerkship.

Rationale

Most arguments for increased ambulatory education are based on changes that have occurred in the teaching hospital over the past 20 years. First, decreased overall utilization and shortened hospital stays have markedly affected both the quantity and quality of patient contact for medical students. Peabody's (2) classic advice to medical students to take advantage of their opportunities to spend unhurried time with patients to learn clinical medicine is hardly applicable in a situation in which, as one surgery clerkship coordinator put it, " the patient meets the student as he is going under anesthesia and goes home throwing up." A second reason for increasing ambulatory-based education is that a variety of topics of evident importance such as health promotion, disease prevention, patient education, and the management of chronic

Dr. Ruane is associate professor of family practice and director of the ambulatory care clerkship, Michigan State University College of Human Medicine, East Lansing.

pain and chronic illness do not lend themselves well to being taught in a brief hospital-based clerkship. Third, a markedly increased proportion of acute and chronic medical problems that previously were evaluated and treated in the hospital are now managed entirely in the office setting.

A final and less discussed reason for looking to the ambulatory setting for medical education is the extent to which advances in knowledge and technology have altered the experience of caring for the hospitalized patient. Even as recently as 20 years ago the traditional clinico-pathologic conference served as an effective model for hospital-based medical education. Patients with multiple and complex symptoms and physical findings found their way to a university hospital often after weeks of mismanagement by the local physicians and staffs of community hospitals. A painstakingly complete history and physical examination supplemented by basic laboratory and X-ray studies provided the basis for a discussion by the professor, whose broad knowledge and clinical experience and acumen were applied to a discussion of the differential diagnosis of the disease. In such discussions, fine points of the medical history ("Had the patient recently travelled to Martha's Vineyard?") and physical examination frequently tipped the balance between one and another often obscure diagnostic possibilities. As a denouement, the clinical pathologist presented the findings of the postmortem examination and compared them with the professor's diagnosis.

However, with today's array of specific biochemical and immunochemical assays, computed tomography and magnetic resonance imaging (MRI) scans, endoscopies, and angiograms, few maladies for which a specific diagnosis can be reached remain undiagnosed for long.

The availability of these procedures promotes their widespread application, with undoubtedly positive results. This development of modern diagnostic tests requires increased specialized knowledge and technical skill in the care of the hospitalized patient. It seems also that these developments have fundamentally altered the intellectual challenge of medical diagnosis and management and have, in fact, moved the arena of diagnostic challenge (which is related to the application of the clinical skills of the interview and physical examination) out of the teaching hospital and into the office of the primary care physician.

The shift in the focus of diagnosis has rapidly bypassed even the nonhospital-based specialist. Several years ago John Fry, a British general practitioner and World Health Organization consultant, observed: "We have come to view our specialist colleagues more as expert 'technicians' than as consultants" (3). Advancing technology and its application have made this observation increasingly apt. Referral of the patient with chest pain, abdominal pain, or headache to the subspecialist produces an almost automatic heart catheterization, endoscopy, or MRI scan, respectively. Wider availability of and experience with these techniques, fear of charges of negligence against the consultant, and more appropriate referral by today's well-trained primary-care physician can only accelerate this trend. The basic clinical skills of the medical interview and physical examination in the ambulatory setting will be increasingly important. Development and evaluation of teaching programs in these sites is a challenge for medical educators.

The contrast between the skills taught to medical students in their courses introducing clinical medicine and those skills required to manage critically ill hospitalized patients is symptomatic of a culture shock within medicine and medical education in which the skills and values promulgated in such courses have lagged perhaps 20 years behind those most needed in the high-technology environment of modern hospitals.

Ironically, these basic clinical skills have become increasingly critical in diagnosis and management of outpatients as a larger portion of clinical care has shifted to outpatients. In describing an introduction to an outpatient medical clinic for internal medicine residents, Howell and colleagues (4) commented that "most of the time, the inpatient model simply isn't relevant to outpatient practice... [In the outpatient setting] you'll have the chance to be more thoughtful and less technical, using skills in which internists have traditionally prided themselves. . . ."

Description

The College of Human Medicine is a young medical school (graduating its first class in 1972) with a tradition of educational innovation and a commitment to the education of primary care physicians. While the two preclinical years are taught at the campus of Michigan State University, clinical education occurs in five communities across the state. (A smaller, Upper Peninsula program will not be further discussed here.) Until the Ambulatory Care Clerkship (ACC) began in 1983-84, the clinical curriculum required rotations in medicine, pediatrics, surgery, obstetrics and gynecology, and psychiatry. A fourth year consists of clinical electives.

In 1978 the faculty mandated the development of a clerkship with the following characteristics: It should occur in the third year of medical school; it should consist of 36 half-days of instruction and extend over a minimum of 26 weeks; and

the clinical experience should be located in the office of a primary care physician (family practice, medicine, or pediatrics) and involve a continuing one-to-one relationship between student and preceptor. After pilot programs in two of the clinical campuses in 1981-82, and offering the ACC as an elective in all five clinical campuses in 1982-83, the clerkship was implemented in 1983-84 as a requirement for all students by the designation of one half-day each week as ACC day— the specific day differed by community. On this half-day, students leave other clerkships to attend the ACC.

The ACC began as a preceptorship without defined academic content or structure. The only specific requirements were to attend the office sessions and to record in a log book information about patients encountered. A specific curriculum was later developed for this clerkship. In addition to the office practice experience, which is supervised and evaluated by the preceptor, the ACC now has several other educational elements. A set of required readings consists of approximately 100 text pages. These readings, which are updated annually, consist of both relevant review articles and material developed for the ACC by the college's faculty. These are provided to all students. The topics dealt with include an overview of primary care, screening and prevention, practical economics of primary health care, low back pain, and several others. A final examination tests the students' mastery of this material.

Four half-days (16 hours) spread through the year are designated as lecture time. While the ACC coordinator at each community has wide latitude in choice of topics and speakers, the following topics are presented in each community: organization of office practice, common dermatologic and ear-nose-throat problems, sports injuries, chronic pain syndromes, screening and prevention, and economic influences on primary care. The remaining lecture topics differ by community and represent an array of topics selected in response to student interest and local expertise.

All students must write a paper entitled "Cost and Quality of Care" by midway through the clerkship. In this exercise students select, from among several available, a brief vignette describing a common clinical problem; perform a computer based search of the medical literature using Medlines, the National Library of Medicine's online bibliographic retrieval system; and from the articles located develop and defend a written clinical protocol for evaluation and management of the problem. Finally, from a list of common fees (provided to them), students calculate the cost of applying their protocol to a patient.

The final examination consists of a written case presentation, a written review of the literature on a clinical problem, and a content examination. The student selects, by the middle of the clerkship, a patient with an active medical problem on whom the case presentation will be done. In this paper, the student must demonstrate the accumulation of an appropriate data base for both the evaluation and management of the patient's problem and for appropriate screening and health maintenance for the patient. The paper must demonstrate attention to patient education and appropriate continuity of care (5) for the active problem and for health maintenance issues. The written literature review must be relevant to the patient problem in the case presentation and must contain specific references from the current medical literature. Finally, the student takes a written examination covering the material in the required readings.

This curriculum has several unusual characteristics. The first is that it provides the only opportunity for all students in a clinical campus to meet and discuss important curricular topics several times each year. These meetings allow a curriculum and evaluation based on the students' development through the first clinical year. The long-term nature of the clerkship allows for easy coordination of readings, lectures, clinical application exercises, and evaluations. For example, the topic of screening and prevention is covered in the required readings and a lecture, and the student is required to apply this information over time to a patient and is evaluated on it through the final examination.

An educational exercise involving the functional assessment of elderly patients in the home is being pilot tested in one community during 1988–89.

Experience

A good deal of data about the ambulatory care clerkship has been accumulated through a review of the student logbooks. From 1984–85 through 1986–87 (the second through fourth year the ACC was offered), the number of initial and repeat patient visits per student, types of procedures performed by students (including such things as well examining a child, prescribing contraception, and consultation or referral), the age and sex of patients, and the specialty of the preceptor physician have been entered into a computer data-base file. Overall, ACC students have contact with approximately five patients per week or 150 in the course of the clerkship. The ACC thus adds approximately 15,000 patient-student contacts to the clinical curriculum.

Information regarding the diagnoses recorded in the student logs was collated in one community for 1984–85 through 1986–87. Beginning with academic year

1987–88, diagnoses will be included in the data-base file for all students.

The conviction among some faculty members that existing clerkships could not possibly survive with students absent one half-day per week was encountered early in the development of the ACC. Administrators' support for the program and a recognition that in the third year of medical school educational programs must take precedence over students' service commitments overcame this early resistance.

Students experience serious conflict only rarely between the ACC and other, block clerkships. After only two years of requirement of this clerkship students came to view their shared time as ordinary medical school scheduling. Many express surprise when told that the ACC curriculum is innovative. When conflicts occasionally occur, the structure of the ACC usually allows students to miss a session and complete it later in the year. In the past two years, ACC students report experiencing this conflict as generally good-natured teasing from residents and faculty members in surgical specialties about the great experiences that they are missing in going to the office of their ACC preceptor. This teasing is similar to the old joke, "The only thing wrong with every-other-night call is that you miss half the good cases."

Preceptors must be recruited each year. Because the ACC coordinators for each community are generally affiliated with residency programs in family practice and familiar with practitioners in the community, this recruitment has proved to be a manageable task each year. Few preceptors drop out of the program, though many take an occasional year off. Preceptors are unpaid clinical faculty members of the college, and their work in the ACC is evaluated both by their student and the community coordinator. Their basic educational role is similar to that of a community-based physician who admits and follows patients in a teaching hospital. Preceptors open their offices and practices to the ACC students and teach them about the practical aspects of patient care. Although virtually all preceptors go well beyond this basic role and provide a great deal of teaching about specific topics, the presentation and administration of the core curriculum is viewed as the responsibility of the full-time clerkship faculty and occurs in parallel with, but separate from, the clinical experience. Full-time faculty members provide the final evaluation of student performance in the ACC in all but the office practice experience.

Mechanisms have been developed to deal with poor performance by students but have had to be applied only rarely. Students meet and review their logbooks periodically with community coordinators. Problems with attendance and recording of data are thus detected early and dealt with appropriately. Unacceptable performance in required projects must be remedied by appropriately revising the report or project. Written papers and oral examinations can be used to offset poor performance on the content examination.

Planned Changes

Two further developments are planned: the first is internal development of the ACC, and the second relates to applying the lessons learned from this clerkship to other areas of general medical education. In the first area, two projects have priority. One is periodic evaluation of each student's clinical skills in data collection, problem-solving, and patient education. The evaluation method will be a variation of the clinical simulation technique reported from the University of Ottawa (6), in which the physician-evaluator simulates a patient and periodically halts the simulation to give students feedback about performance. Such a system will allow for periodic evaluations and an end-of-year final evaluation of third-year students in essential clinical skills.

A second area for internal development is implementing a system for collecting and coding the diagnoses for patients the students encounter.

Implications

The ACC has a curriculum focused on several important topics and principles of outpatient medical care and on common and chronic medical problems. This curriculum requires students to search the medical literature through computer data bases and to incorporate current knowledge into planning for continuing patient care. Repeated patient contact over time in a setting where they take responsibility for continuing primary care allows students to apply this knowledge immediately.

The faculty must develop new ways in which the clinical expertise of specialty faculty members can be combined with the clinical resources and long-term structure of the ACC to develop better ways of teaching many topics. For example, hypertension and hypercholesterolemia are chronic problems encountered frequently by all students in the ACC. Well-child care, contraception, detection and evaluation of breast masses, and anxiety and depression are all topics commonly encountered in primary care in settings, and these topics can be more easily taught in those settings than in teaching hospitals. Coordinating readings, lectures, papers and projects, and study questions with long-term patient care allows the development of clinical application exercises that can provide new and effective opportunities for clinical education. If specialty and primary care faculty members can work and teach alongside one another in primary-care ambulatory environments, the full potential of the clerkship described here can be realized.

References

1. PERKOFF, G. T. Teaching Clinical Medicine in the Ambulatory Setting: An Idea Whose Time May Have Finally Come. *N. Engl. J. Med.*, 314:27–31, 1986.
2. PEABODY, F. W. The Care of the Patient. *J.A.M.A.*, 88:877–882, 1927.
3. FRY, J. Hospital Referrals, Must They Go Up? Changing Patterns Over Twenty Years. *Lancet*, 148, July 17, 1971.
4. HOWELL, J. D., LURIE, N., and WOOLLISCROFT, J. O. Worlds Apart: Some Thoughts to be Delivered to House Officers on the First Day of Clinic. *J.A.M.A.*, 258:502–503, 1987.
5. RUANE, T. J., and BRODY, H. Understanding and Teaching Continuity of Care. *J. Med. Educ.*, 62:969–974, 1987.
6. ROSSER, W. W., and CROCCO, D. An Evaluation System for an Undergraduate Clerkship in Family Medicine. *J. Fam. Pract.*, 9:1049–1055, 1979.

132   February 1991

Family Medicine

A Profile of Required Third-Year Family Medicine Clerkships

Barbara G. Ferrell, PhD, Barbara L. Thompson, MD

ABSTRACT

A survey was conducted of programs which reported requiring a third-year clerkship in family medicine in the 1988-89 AAMC Curriculum Directory to determine the characteristics of these 36 programs. The program characteristics were compared to those outlined by the STFM Task Force on Predoctoral Education in the 1981 monograph, Predoctoral Education in Family Medicine. *Only one third of schools nationwide had a required family medicine clerkship; for 36 schools it was scheduled in the third year. Based on the information provided by the 25 (72%) of these 36 programs which responded, the third-year clerkship was likely to be a stand-alone, decentralized six- or eight-week rotation. The curricula were based on a set of "common problems" and emphasized those areas which separate family practice from other specialties. Students were most likely to be graded by faculty rating and a multiple choice examination. The curricula of the programs reviewed did reflect the recommendations of the Task Force, but there was great variability across programs.*

(Fam Med 1991; 23:132-6)

In 1981 the Task Force on Predoctoral Education of the Society of Teachers of Family Medicine produced a monograph on undergraduate education in family medicine.[1] In that document, two types of clinical educational strategies were outlined--the clerkship and the preceptorship. The Task Force recommended that "with adequate resources a family medicine clerkship should be required." It was felt that the clerkship provided "an opportunity to achieve more family medicine goals than any other single teaching strategy."

A clerkship was further defined by the Task Force as a more structured educational experience than a preceptorship. Clerkships typically take place in residency training inpatient facilities, usually affiliated with a university.[2] Evaluation of the student in a clerkship is both objective and subjective, rather than the purely subjective form used in most preceptorships.[1]

From the Department of Family Medicine. University of Texas Medical Branch. Galveston.

Address correspondence to Dr. Ferrell. Department of Family Medicine. 214 Family Medicine Unit D. University of Texas Medical Branch. Galveston, TX 77550.

The third year was thought to be the best time for the family medicine clerkship, during what has been called the "precision" phase of medical education.[3] Yet when the Task Force report was written, only 36 schools offered a clinical clerkship of any kind in family medicine, and very few schools had a third-year required clerkship in family medicine.[1]

Nearly a decade after the Task Force made its recommendations, 36 US medical schools in the *1988-89 AAMC Curriculum Directory*[4] listed a required clerkship in family medicine during the third academic year. This study addressed two questions: How well do these clerkships reflect the experience as outlined by the STFM Task Force 10 years ago? What do these clerkships look like?

Method

To obtain information about required third-year family medicine clerkships in the United States, it was first necessary to determine which schools offered such an experience. Data from the 124 allopathic schools of medicine listed in the *1988-89 AAMC Curriculum Directory* were summarized. Information regarding the curricula was used to determine the frequency of placement of a family medicine requirement in the clinical portion of a student's training and to characterize the experience in terms of time. Schools which indicated that they had a required clerkship in either family medicine or family practice in the core clinical years were included in the tabulation. Schools which listed a primary care clerkship were not included. A summary of the placement of required clerkships throughout the curriculum is found in Figure 1.

A letter was sent to the directors of all 36 programs which listed a required clerkship in family medicine during the junior year, requesting information about the program. The purpose of the request was to gather information about these programs that would assist in developing a required third-year clerkship, which had been mandated by state law. No guidelines as to the type of information to be sent were given to the schools; any information which they were willing to share was welcome. The materials which schools sent in response to the survey varied widely; all except one provided a copy of the materials given to students at the beginning of the clerkship. The qualitative method of content analysis was chosen to summarize the data from the student materials. Content analysis is a methodology that enables a researcher to make valid inferences from text.[5]

Figure 1

Placement of Clerkship in Clinical Years

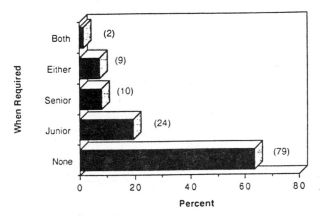

This graph is based on data summarized from the *1988-89 AAMC Curriculum Directory*. The total number of medical schools is 124, and the number of clerkships is in parentheses.

Table 2

STFM Goals and Objectives

Goals	Objectives
Teach the Knowledge Skills, and Attitudes of Family Medicine	I. Common, Undifferentiated Problems II. Patient as Whole, Emphasis on Wellness III. Family Medicine Problem Solving IV. Communication Skills V. Data Collection and Record Keeping VI. Family As a Unit VII. Consultation, Referral, and Continuity of Care VIII. Diagnostic and Therapeutic Modalities IX. Community Orientation
Student Self-Understanding and Development	X. Life-Long Learning XI. Self Understanding and Personal Growth
Other Aspects of Family Medicine	XII. Family Medicine As a Career XIII. Management and Cost-Effectiveness XIV. Family Medicine Research XV. Health Care Teams

Table 2

Twenty Problems Most Frequently Listed*

Problem	Number of Schools
Hypertension	14
Diabetes	13
UTI/cystitis/dysuria	13
Otitis media	12
Low-back pain	11
Headache	11
Abdominal pain	10
Arthritis	9
Depression	9
Vaginitis	9
Obesity	9
Anxiety	9
Pharyngitis	9
Bronchitis	8
Asthma	7
COPD	7
Diarrhea	7
Dermatitis	7
Pneumonia	6
Sexually transmitted diseases	6

*Based on 16 clerkships which listed common problems.

Results

Timing and Duration of the Clerkships

While the Task Force recommended a required clerkship, no recommendations were given regarding its placement in the curriculum or its duration. Based on data summarized from the *AAMC Curriculum Directory*, required family medicine clerkships varied a great deal in both length and placement, and third-year clerkships differed from those offered to fourth-year students. The length of the clerkships ranged from two to eight weeks; the average length of all clerkships was 5.2 weeks. Junior clerkships were longer on average (5.6 weeks) than senior clerkships (4.8 weeks). Four-, six-, and eight-week clerkships were most common, with 51% of the schools offering a four-week clerkship. In the third year, however, the six-week clerkship was most common (33%), and one fourth of the third-year experiences were eight weeks in length.

Twenty-one of the 36 (58%) programs that responded to the initial request sent some type of information about the clerkship. To increase the sample size, a follow-up letter was sent to those programs which had not responded. Data from an additional five programs were received, making the total number of programs responding 26 (72%).

To determine the generalizability of the data collected, the schools with required clerkships which responded were compared to the total listed in the *AAMC Directory*. The schools which sent information about third-year clerkships were similar to the national profile in terms of clerkship placement and length. The average length of clerkship for schools responding was 5.3 weeks. Again, four-, six-, and eight-week clerkships were most common. Eleven schools (44%) reported requiring a four-week clerkship. Just over two thirds required that the clerkship be taken in the junior year, while almost one third offered students an option of taking it in the junior or senior year. One school required the clerkship in the senior year and was deleted from further analysis. Thus, the total number of schools on which the description is based is 25.

Structure of Clerkships

Clinical clerkships have been described as inpatient based, usually taking place in tertiary care facilities, often associ-

Figure 2

STFM Objectives Included in Clerkships

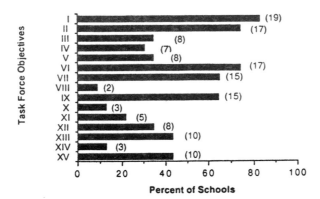

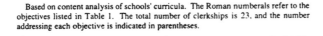

Based on content analysis of schools' curricula. The Roman numberals refer to the objectives listed in Table 1. The total number of clerkships is 23. and the number addressing each objective is indicated in parentheses.

Figure 3

Percent of Clerskhips Using Each Type of Evaluation

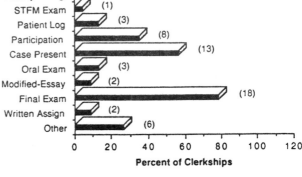

Based on content analysis of schools' curricula. The total number of clerkships is 23; the number using each form of evaluation is included in parentheses.

ated with academic medical centers.[6,7] Changes in the length of hospital stay and case mix have created a move toward clinical teaching in an ambulatory setting.[8] A family medicine experience, by its nature, is oriented toward ambulatory care. A survey of family medicine undergraduate education revealed that only 40% of the clerkships took place in hospital based teaching settings.[9]

All of the programs reporting a required clerkship had a stand-alone experience in which a block of time was set aside for the clerkship. None of the programs were based on a longitudinal continuity model, in which students' family medicine experience took place once a week over the entire clinical year.

Several models appear to have been generated for the third-year family medicine clerkship. One was a university based family practice clinic with a residency training program. Only four of the clerkships studied (16%) were housed entirely within such a university based residency training program. Almost half (44%) were decentralized, with students sent to physicians either in solo or group private practices away from the university setting, often in rural areas. In such clerkships there are no residents or full-time faculty on site; the practicing physician takes sole responsibility for teaching the student and for the core of required instruction of the clerkship.[10]

The remainder of the clerkships (40%) were a combination of the above models. Some students were accommodated at the residency training facility, others were sent to private physicians. Often, these clerkships were termed "decentralized," even though they used university based facilities.

Curriculum

The Task Force outlined three broad goals with 15 objectives for predoctoral training in family medicine (Table 1). The goals were: 1) teach, demonstrate, and facilitate practice in the knowledge, skills, and attitudes of family medicine; 2) foster student self-understanding and development; and 3) introduce other aspects of family medicine.[1] Of the schools included in the current study, 23 provided enough information to determine the extent to which their curricula matched these goals and objectives.

The first Task Force goal included the objective of teaching the diagnosis and management of "common, undifferentiated problems in ambulatory and community settings."[1] This theme of common problems in family medicine was evident in the curricular focus of the programs.

While most of the schools (78%) based their curricula on a set of common problems, there was considerable diversity in the number and type of problems comprising the set. Five schools required the student to generate a list of problems by logging the patients seen during the clerkship. For other schools, the number of problems in the list ranged from as few as 10 to as many as 32, with an average of 22. The origin of the common problems list was not specified for most programs. One school cited a reference for the list of problems, and another based the list on a local survey of the types of cases seen by physicians in the area. Table 2 shows the most frequently listed problems.

Six of the schools had a skills list, comprised of procedures that students were expected to learn during the clerkship. The average number of skills on the list was 15, but several schools had smaller lists.

In general, the schools had clerkship objectives similar to those presented in the STFM Task Force monograph (Figure 2). Two of the schools, in fact, had these objectives as the basis for their curricula. Objectives such as "approach to patient as whole person, with emphasis on wellness and health promotion" and "care of family as a unit," which reflected the uniqueness of family medicine as a discipline, were especially in evidence. Most schools also addressed "consultation, referral, and continuity of care" (65%) and "community-oriented skills and attitudes" (57%).

Fewer of the schools included objectives from Goals II and III (Objectives X-XV) in their curricula. Family medicine research was addressed in only one school, which did not base its curriculum on the STFM objectives. Family practice as a career, although implied in several programs, was specifically addressed in only one third of the curricula.

Evaluation

Evaluation of students in a clerkship should be both objective and subjective.[1,11] The types of scales used to rate students, which are typically completed by physicians at the end of a clinical rotation, are usually thought of as subjective measures, while standardized examinations and departmental multiple choice or modified essay tests are considered objective.

Most of the schools studied used a variety of methods to evaluate students (Figure 3). All of the schools which provided information about student evaluation used a physician or faculty rating to determine the student's grade, but the importance of this rating varied a great deal. At one school this rating was the sole determinant of the grade, while at other schools the weight of this factor varied from 40% to 80%. This rating constituted at least one half of the grade in 82% of the clerkships.

The second most frequent type of evaluation was a departmental test, in either a multiple choice (78%) or modified essay (9%) format. Only one school reported using the standardized examination developed by the STFM, and that school did not report the proportion of the student's grade for which it counted. The final examination or modified essay exam generally counted for between 20% and 30% of a student's clerkship grade.

A formal case presentation was used for student evaluation by half of the schools reporting. This tool typically counted for less of the student's grade, however, averaging 15%.

For approximately one third of the clerkships, a student's grade was determined at least in part by participation in some program activity or by completing a required assignment. While almost one half of the schools (45%) reported that some kind of patient log was required, only three incorporated these into their grading systems.

At most of the schools, students provided feedback about the program upon completion. Fully 70% of the programs had a clerkship rating form which the student completed at the end of the rotation. Almost one half of the programs (45%) had an additional form used by students to rate the physician, faculty, or resident with whom they worked. None of the programs reported the use of a clinical competency examination.

Clerkship Faculty

There was little information in the materials received about the method of selecting physicians to work with students in the clerkship; neither was there information regarding the type of training these individuals received in order to work with students. Some schools indicated that their "preceptors" were paid for their time. One school paid the preceptors $1,200 per student-month experience. Most schools indicated that some type of recognition or reward was provided these individuals in the form of a dinner or ceremony at least once a year.

Discussion

As stated above, nearly a decade after the STFM Task Force's recommendations were published, only one third of the medical schools in the US had a required family medicine clerkship. The third-year clerkship in family medicine is most often a decentralized six- or eight-week rotation, and generally, the objectives of required family medicine clerkships are consistent with those recommended by the Task Force.

While it might appear that schools which offer a clerkship are following the recommendations of the Task Force, there is a great deal of variability in the programs, and the students' experiences across programs may be quite different. While some schools call the experience a clerkship, many of the experiences do not meet the criteria for a clinical clerkship--a structured curriculum and objective methods of evaluation. Some programs listed as clerkships in the AAMC Directory appear to be no more than preceptorships occurring during the third year.

These findings are limited by the absence of information about 28% of the required third-year clerkships. In addition, information provided by the responding programs was not uniform; data pertaining to some important policies and practices were missing from some clerkship materials. The use of a structured questionnaire may have yielded more uniform information but may have missed relevant dimensions of the clerkship experiences that emerged through the content analysis of course materials. A combination of focused questions and open-ended queries may be the most effective method of obtaining a comprehensive profile of these clerkships.

It is somewhat discouraging that almost 10 years after the Task Force report, only one third of the medical schools in the country had a required clerkship. This, coupled with the short duration of the clerkships relative to other required clinical rotations, indicates the difficulty involved in establishing meaningful family practice training in the curricula of many schools. Obviously, much remains to be accomplished in this crucial area.

REFERENCES

1. Society of Teachers of Family Medicine Task Force on Predoctoral Education. Predoctoral education in family medicine. Kansas City: Society of Teachers of Family Medicine, 1981.
2. Rabinowitz HK. Student clinical experiences in family medicine: a comparison of clerkships and preceptorships. Fam Pract Res J 1989; 8:92-9.

3. Rabinowitz HK. The precision phase: seven years experience with a required family medicine clerkship for third-year medical students. Fam Med 1983; 15:168-72.

4. 1988-1989 AAMC curriculum directory. Washington, D.C.: American Association of Medical Colleges, 1988.

5. Weber RP. Basic content analysis. Beverly Hills, Calif.: Sage Publications, 1985.

6. Beasley JW. Using private practice settings for academically intensive family practice clerkships. J Fam Pract 1983; 17:877-82.

7. Parkerson GR, Muhlbaier LH, Falcone JC. A comparison of students' clinical experience in family medicine and traditional clerkships. J Med Educ 1984; 59:124-30.

8. Perkoff GT. Teaching clinical medicine in the ambulatory setting: an idea whose time may have finally come. N Engl J Med 1986; 314:27-31.

9. Taylor RB, Camp L, Rogers JM, Updike J, Lyle C. A third-year family medicine clerkship based in an academic family practice center. J Med Educ 1984; 59:39-44.

10. Hobbs J, Mongan PF, Tollison JW, Miller MD, Wilson OR. A decentralized clerkship: strategies for standardizing content and instruction. Fam Med 1987; 19:133-6.

11. Rabinowitz HK. The relationship between medical student career choice and a required third-year family practice clerkship. Fam Med 1988; 20:18-21.

A Model for Designing Clinical Education

JAN F. PERRY, MA

This paper presents a circular process of curriculum design combined with a matrix of clinical education activities and levels of student functioning. The result is a model for a process to improve the quality of clinical education by attending to the design of the learning experiences.

Key Words: *Clinical education, Physical therapy.*

The clinical phase of an educational program in the health professions is of critical importance to the students' development. The purpose of this paper is to present a model that will aid in the development of high quality clinical education experiences for the student in the health professions. The literature is cited only as it directly pertains to the subject—an extensive review of the literature is not intended.

Although the clinical education portion of the overall curricula is seldom viewed as a curriculum by itself, the literature on curriculum design offers some guidance in educational design. Tyler[1] and Taba,[2] in classics of their field, list the steps of curriculum design: select objectives, select learning experiences, organize learning experiences, and plan the evaluation of the curriculum.

In breaking those steps down to describe a plan which is more specific, the following process evolves: 1) determine the objectives of the clinical experience, 2) determine the evaluation of the objectives that were selected, 3) select learning experiences, 4) organize learning experiences, 5) develop learning experiences that do not already exist, 6) implement the learning experiences, 7) evaluate the student, the program, and the experiences, and 8) revise as necessary (Fig. 1).

In the following section these steps are expanded upon from the viewpoint of a clinical education facility. The examples are taken from the field of physical therapy, although the process is applicable to any field using clinical education experiences.

DETERMINE OBJECTIVES

The first step in clinical education design is to determine the objectives. This is currently done in a variety of ways. Some educators select clinical experiences as convenience dictates with little concern for objectives. Others use the Standards for Basic Education in Physical Therapy as a base for developing objectives.[3] Some attempt to meet the student's needs.[4] Still others depend on the objectives supplied by the clinical education center staff.[5] Most of these methods involve thoughtful planning, but few who use them look at the student's preparation (both didactic and clinical) for the experience and how that experience fits into the total picture of the student's clinical education.

Historically, the Academic Coordinator of Clinical Education (ACCE) has been responsible for designing the clinical education program. The ACCE determined the objectives of an experience and then distributed those objectives to all clinical facilities. Happily, this trend is now changing. More and more the staffs of clinical education sites are contributing to the development of objectives for clinical education programs. The ACCE outlines the types of experiences and broad goals for various levels of students,

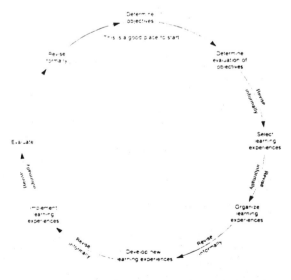

Fig. 1. *Process of learning experience design.*

Mrs. Perry is Assistant Professor, Department of Physical Therapy, Medical College of Georgia, Augusta, GA 30912 (USA).

The work on which this article is based was sponsored by Allied Health Special Project Grant #5-D12-AH00904-02.

This article was submitted March 27, 1980, and accepted March 31, 1981.

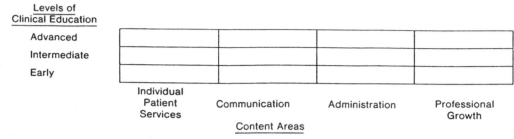

Levels of
Clinical Education

Advanced

Intermediate

Early

| Individual Patient Services | Communication | Administration | Professional Growth |

Content Areas

Fig. 2. Matrix for examining clinical education objectives. (Topics taken from Handbook of Information Concerning the Accreditation Process for Physical Therapy Education Programs: Revised 9/76.[6])

and then the Center Coordinator of Clinical Education (CCCE) and Clinical Instructor (CI) apply those general objectives to their facility. The need for input from both those in the educational program and in the clinical center cannot be stressed too much. The ACCE has an overview of the entire clinical education program; the CCCE and CI have the details. Working together they can produce a well-integrated program, but each will need to listen and learn from the other.

Matrix for Developing Objectives

The clinical staff should consider several items to gain a broader perspective of the clinical education experience. First, the objectives of the educational program sending the student must be examined. These can be examined as individual clinical education courses or as a series of courses that develop sequentially, or both. When examining the objectives of a program in this manner, a matrix can be developed (Fig. 2). The horizontal axis of the matrix indicates content areas, and the vertical axis indicates levels of clinical education experiences. This matrix

can be used throughout the planning process to examine completeness and sequence.

An early step in determining objectives for the clinical phase is a review of the coursework completed by the student. In addition, the unique aspects of the clinical facility should be reviewed. Both the coursework the student has had (eg, anatomy, physiology, kinesiology) and areas of specific interest offered at a center (pulmonary therapy, rehabilitation techniques, specific therapeutic exercise techniques) must be examined together. The student's coursework preparation can be assessed as it relates to each cell in the matrix (Fig. 3). If the clinical faculty members determine, after reviewing the matrix, that they want the student to have an experience for which he is not academically prepared, they will realize that they must present this to the student as new information.

The resources available at the center must also be examined. If there are objectives for which a center has few or no resources, these can and should be discarded. Objectives that could be met especially well by the center should be included and perhaps be made mandatory for the student to meet; objectives for which resources fall somewhere in the middle might be considered optional. After the educational program's objectives, the student's coursework to date, and the resources of the center are examined, the objectives specific to a certain level of student can be identified.

A typical review might reveal the following information:

Educational program objectives: The student will become skilled in evaluation techniques.
Pertinent coursework to date: Pulmonary function, goniometric, and manual muscle testing.
Clinical education site: Rehabilitation center with many experiences available for goniometric and manual muscle testing.

A general objective of the clinical education program for that site might become: "The student will acquire skill in the completion of goniometric assessment and manual muscle testing." The center staff has decided not to invent an experience in pulmonary

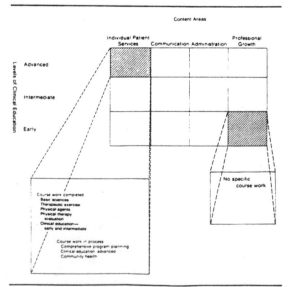

Fig. 3. Matrix applied to review of student preparation.

function assessment. The center staff are doing what they do best while working within the educational program objectives.

DETERMINE EVALUATION OF OBJECTIVES

The second step in the model is to select the method by which the objectives that were developed will be evaluated. The means of evaluation are closely tied to the way something is taught; therefore, the planning of evaluation must occur early in the process. To carry my previous example through this step, if the student will be judged on his goniometric assessment by a paper-and-pencil test, the actual experience offered to the student may simply be one of observation and, possibly, reading. If, however, the evaluation of the objectives will be through the actual completion of a test and comparison of the student's measurements with the instructor's measurements, the learning experience would, of necessity, include practice.

The method of evaluation is often outlined by criteria, which are related to each objective. As an example, examine the center's objective mentioned earlier: "The student will acquire skill in the completion of goniometric assessment. . . ." By further defining what is meant by "acquire skill" the clinical faculty will be adding criteria to the objective. For an advanced student, an appropriate level of skill may include criteria dealing with the completeness, speed, and accuracy of the examination. With the criteria, the objective might read: "The student will complete three goniometric assessments of patients' hips. Measurements should be within 5 degrees of the CI's measurement 90 percent of the time; all instances of abnormal range should be identified; the third goniometric evaluation should be accomplished within 30 minutes."

When the evaluation of an objective is spelled out to this extent, the activities necessary to accomplish the objective become much clearer. The necessity for determining the method of evaluation early in the process also becomes obvious.

The matrix, again, can be helpful in this process. In examining methods of evaluation as they evolve "up" the vertical component of the matrix (Fig. 2), a check is provided to make sure that the criteria are demanding higher-level performance by the student. The matrix also provides a review mechanism to help ensure that objectives are developed for all content areas.

SELECT LEARNING EXPERIENCES

In the selection of learning experiences, the resources of the center, the objectives developed by the center, and the manner in which the objectives will be evaluated are reviewed. The experiences selected are those that will enable the student to meet the objectives as described by the evaluation criteria. The importance of criteria in this process cannot be over-estimated.

After all factors are considered, the experiences that have been identified should be reviewed as to their efficiency and effectiveness. The use of media other than an instructor should be considered in some circumstances. For instance, if an orientation program is necessary and must be repeated numerous times throughout the year for new students, the CI or the CCCE might develop a media program (eg, slides plus narration) that would orient the students to the center. This could save time for both the CI and student and increase the consistency of the information that is presented.

ORGANIZE LEARNING EXPERIENCES

Once the learning experiences have been identified and possible areas appropriate for the use of instructional media have been identified, the organization of learning experiences must begin. This organization can remain loose because much depends on the types of patients available at various times.

Some basic principles of organization that apply are 1) simple activities should precede complex ones, 2) the whole picture should be presented before the specific skills, techniques, or knowledge needed to complete that "picture" are presented, and 3) observational periods should precede participatory experiences.

The student's activities should be written out for the purpose of designing lesson plans, media programs, handout materials, and lectures. An experience outline should include the student's activities, the instructor's activities, and their sequence. A lesson plan for goniometry might include the following items.

Before the activity: The instructor selects a patient and assures the availability of necessary equipment; the student reviews goniometric techniques and becomes familiar with the patient's problem.

During the experience: The student locates the goniometer and the appropriate recording form, carries out the assessment, and records the results. The instructor is available but is not present during this phase.

After the experience: The instructor repeats the measurements in order to assess the student's accuracy. The instructor and the student discuss the experience for both to receive feedback.

DEVELOP NEW LEARNING EXPERIENCES

When the objectives are determined and learning activities are selected and organized, the clinical fac-

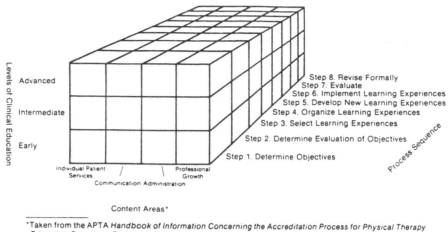

*Taken from the APTA *Handbook of Information Concerning the Accreditation Process for Physical Therapy Education Programs* (Revised 9/76).[6]

Fig. 4. Model for designing clinical education.

ulty may determine that the most effective means of presenting a topic has not been developed. The planning that has taken place to this point makes this an ideal time to design a new experience. A specific need has been identified, the objectives and how they will be evaluated are known, and the place of this activity in the sequence of the student's clinical experience has been determined. With these items known, the actual development is much easier.

IMPLEMENT LEARNING EXPERIENCES

The next step is to implement the learning experience. This occurs when the student arrives for the clinical education experience and should be the culmination of the five steps that have preceded it.

In addition to well-stated objectives, specific criteria, and pertinent and appropriately ordered learning experiences, the CI must bear in mind many other factors. The time frame of an experience, where it will be accomplished, where and when the CI and student can talk privately with each other, and the materials needed for an experience must all be, if not prearranged, at least considered. In reviewing necessary materials the CI should be aware of equipment needs (eg, audiovisual, therapeutic, or evaluative), supply needs (eg, paper and pencil, slides, linens, forms), and resource needs (eg, reference books, pictures, models, experts).

When the student arrives, the interpersonal skills of the CI can virtually make or break the experience.

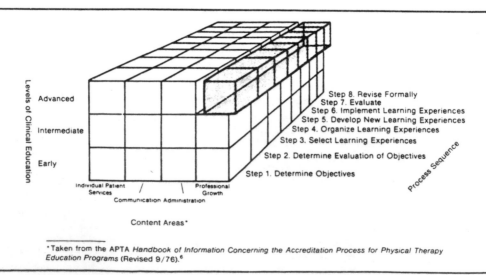

*Taken from the APTA *Handbook of Information Concerning the Accreditation Process for Physical Therapy Education Programs* (Revised 9/76).[6]

Fig. 5. Developing one content area through the complete process at the advanced level.

If a CI is brusque and uncaring, all of the careful earlier planning will not make this a pleasant experience. The student may learn, but the aftertaste of the experience may be bitter enough to undermine the objectives. The reverse is also true; the exuberance and caring of a CI can make a clinical experience a superior learning experience even though little planning has occurred. The latter is always to be welcomed, enjoyed, and capitalized upon; however, it should not be relied upon. The careful planning that has preceded an experience should be implemented by CIs who possess adequate interpersonal skills to motivate students, are skilled in appropriate subject matter, can coach and provide feedback to students in a constructive manner, and care about the students as growing individuals.

EVALUATE

After an experience is completed, evaluation can occur at several levels. Student performance (attainment of objectives) is assessed, preferably by the methods already identified. Additionally, the program through which the student has gone is assessed for 1) its ability to assist the student in attaining the objectives, 2) efficient use of student and instructor time, 3) the perpetuation of good patient care, and 4) the appropriateness of the objectives to the level of student functioning (ie, was the student asked to function at a higher/lower level than that for which he was prepared?). The performance of the instructor is also to be reviewed. The interpersonal concerns already mentioned can be considered as well as planning, subject matter expertise, coaching, and feedback skills. Obviously, evaluation in clinical education is

more than a comment on the student's performance. The purpose of these activities is to provide information for program revision and staff development.

REVISE FORMALLY

Based on evaluations, the program can be revised if necessary. If the objectives appear to be inadequate, they need revision: the selection, organization, and development of learning experiences can be revised if the evaluation procedures indicate problem areas. This is a circular process (Fig. 1) that should have no end; however, the pace of activity usually slows markedly after the first revisions are completed.

USE OF THE MATRIX

The matrix (Fig. 2) can be used through all steps of this process to examine any area of the development process. When the circular process described in Figure 1 and the matrix described in Figure 2 are combined, a complete model of clinical education design emerges (Fig. 4). By using this new model, the educational planner can have an overview of all levels and types of student activity as well as a clear view of each step of the design process.

An advantage of this model is that it allows the educational planner to look at the clinical experiences in a variety of ways. First, one content area at one level can be reviewed from the objective-setting stage through evaluation and revision (Fig. 5). Next, for each step in the planning process the different levels of clinical education can be compared (ie, objectives related to goniometry can be compared for early, intermediate, and advanced students) (Fig. 6). Fi-

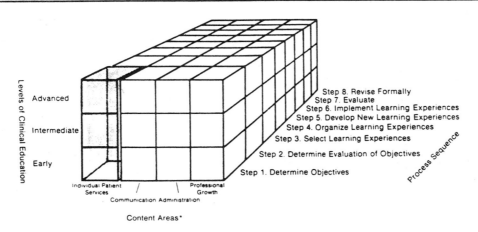

*Taken from the APTA *Handbook of Information Concerning the Accreditation Process for Physical Therapy Education Programs* (Revised 9/76).[6]

Fig. 6. *Examining the sequence of learning experiences in one content area from an early level of clinical education to an advanced level.*

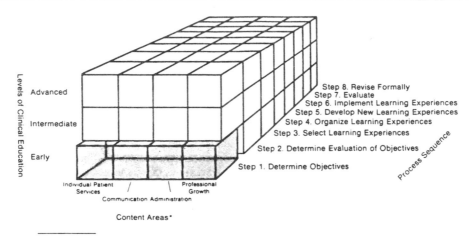

Fig. 7. *Examining clinical education at an early level.*

nally, the entire experience can be viewed at any point in the planning process (Fig. 7).

The new model can be used for multiple purposes and by different people. The CCCE can use it to design the clinical education program specifically for his facility, while the ACCE can use it for designing the entire clinical education program, which would be carried out in a variety of clinical facilities. The objective setting and the selection, organization, and development of learning activities would be done in detail by the CCCE and CI; whereas, the ACCE would be involved in the more general aspects of objectives development and the overall content and organization of learning experiences. All three would be involved in the evaluation and revision steps.

Another use of this model of great interest to all clinical faculty members (ACCEs, CCCEs, and CIs) is as a basis for clinical faculty development. The model outlines areas in which clinical faculty should be competent and, therefore, areas of potential continuing education activities.

ADAPTATIONS OF MODEL

The process of educational planning (setting objectives; planning the evaluation of the objectives; and selecting, organizing, developing, implementing, and evaluating the learning experiences) can enrich clinical education programs. One of the primary purposes for presenting the process described in this paper is to encourage adaptations of the model to meet individual needs. Some adaptations might include the following: The four experiential content areas (individual patient services, communication, administration,

professional growth) can be changed to fit the program of a given institution. The number and levels of clinical education experiences will vary from one place to another. A center that has students at only one level, but from many educational programs, could use the vertical axis of the model to indicate the different programs with which they affiliate. This process would allow them to identify components of their clinical education program common to all, as well as components that differ between institutions sending them students.

The presentation of this model is only the first step. The worth of the model will be determined by its usefulness to clinical educators and by the adaptations, modifications, and revisions that it stimulates.

Acknowledgment. I would like to thank E. Shepley Nourse for her editorial and design consultation as well as for her encouragement.

REFERENCES

1. Tyler RW: Basic Principles of Curriculum and Instruction. Chicago, IL, University of Chicago Press, 1950, p 1
2. Taba H: Curriculum Development: Theory and Practice. New York, NY, Harcourt, Brace, and World, 1962, p 12
3. Pinkston D, Hochhauser SL, Gardner-O'Loughlin K: Standards for basic education in physical therapy: A tool for planning clinical education. Phys Ther 55:841–849, 1975
4. Wightman ML, Wellock LM: A method of developing and evaluating a clinical performance program for physical therapy interns. Phys Ther 56:1125–1128, 1976
5. Hertz CG, Williams H, Hutchins EB: Designing a curriculum in a clinical setting: An iterative process. J Med Educ 51: 844–849, 1976
6. American Physical Therapy Association: Handbook of Information Concerning the Accreditation Process for Physical Therapy Education Programs, revised ed. Washington, DC, Americal Physical Therapy Association, 1974

Developing a Clinical Education Program from the Clinician's Perspective

PATRICIA A. WINDOM

As the number of physical therapy programs increases, more physical therapy departments will be developing clinical education programs. A guide for clinicians who are developing clinical education programs is presented. Suggestions are made for developing a philosophy of clinical education and for structuring the program. Topics discussed include guidelines for clinical instructors and students, learning contracts, negotiable time, and program evaluation. Examples adapted from the clinical education materials developed at Massachusetts Rehabilitation Hospital are included.

Key Words: *Affiliations, clinical; Education, clinical; Program development.*

To be effective, education for students in disciplines that emphasize direct patient care must include supervised practice in the clinical environment. While the physical therapy student is functioning in the practice setting, he is usually supervised by a clinician in an apprentice-like relationship.[1] As the number of physical therapy programs increases and the practice of physical therapy expands into nontraditional settings, such as public schools, private practice, home care, and industry, more clinical affiliations will be needed and programs will be needed in settings not previously used.[2,3 (chap 3:1)] Many physical therapy services that have not participated in the clinical education of physical therapy students will be developing affiliation programs. In addition, facilities currently affiliated with physical therapy schools may be redesigning their programs to become more effective in the planning and implementation of clinical education.[2,3 (chap 2:6, 3:1)]

Clinical education in physical therapy involves a cooperative effort between the faculty of an academic program and the staff of a clinical facility.[4] The individual on the faculty at the physical therapy school who is responsible for coordinating the clinical education of the students in the program is called the academic coordinator of clinical education (ACCE).[3 (chap 4:1)] The person from the clinical affiliation site who is designated to coordinate the clinical education program at that facility is called the center coordinator of clinical education (CCCE).[3 (chap 4:1)] The therapists who supervise the students during their clinical education program are called clinical instruc-

tors (CIs).[3 (chap 4:2)] The CCCEs and the CIs are often referred to as the clinical faculty.

The ACCEs usually supply the clinical faculty with curriculum descriptions, learning objectives, and student evaluation forms. However, the clinicians who work with the students in the clinical setting are primarily responsible for designing and implementing learning experiences for the affiliating students.[3 (chap 4:6, 8, 12)] The major responsibility for the quality of the clinical education program, therefore, rests with the CIs and the CCCEs. Although several guides have been developed to assist the academic faculty in planning clinical education,[4-6] little has been written specifically to help clinicians plan clinical affiliation programs for their facilities.

The purpose of this paper is to present information that may be of assistance to physical therapy clinicians who are developing or revising clinical affiliation programs. The materials and the examples presented in this article were adapted from those used by the Department of Physical Therapy at Massachusetts Rehabilitation Hospital in revising the clinical affiliation program for physical therapy students. Similar materials can be developed for clinical affiliation programs for physical therapist assistants.

DEVELOPING A PHILOSOPHY OF CLINICAL EDUCATION

Before planning a clinical affiliation program, the physical therapists at the affiliation site should formulate a philosophy of clinical education. The philosophy should combine what the therapists believe to be important in clinical education with what is feasible in their clinical environment.

The first step in developing a philosophy of clinical education is to identify and discuss important issues

Ms. Windom is Assistant Professor, Program in Physical Therapy, Old Dominion University, Norfolk, VA 23508 (USA).

This article was submitted July 10, 1981, and accepted June 4, 1982.

in clinical education: supervision and evaluation of students, structure versus flexibility in the program, and planned versus spontaneous learning. Many questions, including the following, need to be answered. Should the student be supervised by more than one CI? Who should evaluate the student? How structured should the program be? Who is responsible if a problem arises? The answers to these and similar questions depend on the staffing pattern of the clinical facility, the individual philosophies of the clinical faculty members, and the requirements of the academic programs. Through discussion, the clinical staff can identify and agree on those characteristics of clinical education they value and desire their program to have. Therapists who are developing clinical affiliation programs for the first time should attend clinical education workshops, consult references, and talk with others more experienced in clinical education for assistance in making decisions concerning these important issues.

The next step in developing a philosophy of clinical education is to make a critical analysis of the clinical site to determine its strengths and limitations. By making an analysis of the facility and staff, those developing the program will be able to decide what the facility has to offer students, at what educational level(s) students should affiliate at the facility, and how many students the facility could support. After assessing the strengths and weaknesses of the facility, the staff members may even decide that their facility should not serve as a clinical site.

All aspects of the department need to be explored. Locate educational resources, such as books and periodicals, that are available to students. Identify rounds and clinics that students can attend. Note special opportunities to be offered to students (eg, visiting the brace shops, observing surgery, using special equipment, working with staff members who have special skills). Analyze the staffing patterns of the department to determine the number of staff members available for supervising students. Determine the necessary patient:staff ratio. Identify the types of patients treated and the method of assigning patients to therapists. These and similar data will help determine the type and the scope of clinical education the department can support.

As a final step, the developers of the program should use what they have identified as important characteristics of clinical education and the profile of the department to determine the format of the clinical education program. Compromises may have to be made between what the staff would like to include and what the facility will allow. What should result is an outline for a program that takes maximum advantage of the strengths of the facility and reflects the philosophy of the department. In narrative form,

---

Figure 1. Excerpt from "Guidelines for the Center Coordinator of Clinical Education."

The center coordinator of education is responsible for

1. Overseeing the clinical education program.
2. Serving as a liaison between affiliating schools and the physical therapy department.
3. Presenting clinical instructors with pertinent information about the student and the school at least two weeks in advance of the student's arrival.
4. Preparing the physical therapy staff to participate in clinical education.
5. Updating the clinical education program yearly.

---

this becomes a statement of the philosophy of clinical education (Appendix).

All individuals who make decisions concerning clinical education have a philosophy governing those decisions. Developing a formal, departmental philosophy encourages staff members to agree on what is important in clinical education and improves compliance with policies and procedures that are developed from the statement of philosophy. In addition, a written statement of philosophy permits the staff, the academic faculty, and the students to know what can be expected from the clinical education program. As new clinical education plans are developed, they

---

Figure 2. Excerpt from "Guidelines for Clinical Instructors of Full-time Students."

The clinical instructor is responsible for

1. Supervising and evaluating the student in a manner that promotes the student's achievement of his own objectives and the objectives outlined by the school, the physical therapy department, and the clinical instructor.
2. Developing a contract with the full-time student during the first week of the affiliation.
3. Planning meaningful learning experiences for negotiable time.
4. Meeting with the center coordinator of clinical education at least twice during the affiliation and as needed.
5. Being available to the student for daily discussion of such topics as patients, problems, observations, and questions.

Figure 3. Excerpt from "Guidelines for Full-time Students."

The full-time affiliate is responsible for
1. Developing a contract with the clinical instructor.
2. Meeting all general objectives for the full-time student and those specific objectives outlined by the clinical instructor.
3. Preparing and presenting an in-service program or other project to the physical therapy department.
4. Supervising the care of at least one patient who is being treated by a physical therapist assistant and one who is being treated by an aide.
5. Communicating any dissatisfactions with the clinical education program to the clinical instructor or the center coordinator of clinical education.

---

should be evaluated for consistency with the stated philosophy, and as new staff members come to the department, the written philosophy must be reevaluated for consistency with all the staff members' philosophies.

STRUCTURING THE PROGRAM

When completed, the philosophy of clinical education can be used as a guide for organizing the affiliation program. The amount of structure should be adapted to the specific needs of the department. A highly structured program can save administrative time while assuring a baseline quality experience for all students. Methods that may be used to structure the program include providing guidelines for participants in the program, developing learning objectives for the program, using learning contracts to individualize instruction, and providing negotiable time for learning experiences.

Guidelines

Guidelines can be developed to specify the responsibilities of the CCCE (Fig. 1), the CI (Fig. 2), and the student (Fig. 3). Adopting guidelines for evaluating and supervising students is a way of structuring quality clinical teaching into the program. Guidelines for the student clarify what the CI expects of him, including any special projects the student must com-

plete. The guidelines may be used to orient students and new clinical instructors to the clinical education program. In addition, copies of the guidelines for the CI and CCCE can be given to the students to use as standards for evaluating the program.

Learning Objectives

"A learning objective is a description of the behavior expected of a learner after instruction."[7] Objectives developed as part of the clinical education program describe behavior expected of a student as a result of the clinical education program. Objectives can be written for the program in general (Fig. 4), for specific patient care assignments (Fig. 5), and for individually planned learning experiences. Learning objectives can be used by the student and the CI to plan and evaluate learning experiences; by the student and staff to direct independent study; to orient new staff members; and to guide the selection of educational resource materials for the department.

Learning Contracts

A learning contract is " . . . a mechanism for agreement between a teacher and a student . . . for the purpose of individualized learning . . . ."[8] The student and his CI outline their program objectives separately and combine them through discussion and negotiation into a learning contract. The contract then serves

---

Figure 4. Excerpt from "General Objectives for All Full-time Students."

1. By the end of the affiliation, the student will be able to independently perform an accurate patient evaluation using the appropriate patient evaluation form.
2. Upon completion of a patient evaluation, the student, with minimal assistance, will be able to establish realistic short-term and long-term goals and estimate a realistic time period for achieving them.
3. Upon establishment of short- and long-term goals, the student will be able to independently design and defend a treatment program to address these goals.
4. By the completion of the affiliation, the student will be able to independently perform the treatment program as planned, changing the program as necessary to meet the needs of the patient.

---

as a basis for communication, planning, negotiation, and feedback throughout the affiliation. When composing his portion of the contract, the student identifies objectives in three areas: strengths and weaknesses, supervision, and special interests (Fig. 6).

Strengths and weaknesses. In this portion of the contract, the student assesses his own strengths and weaknesses and identifies areas of insufficient practice or exposure. To formulate his objectives for the affiliation, he uses feedback he has received from other clinical and classroom instructors as well as his own judgment. Many students, particularly those on their first full-time affiliation assignment, need help in making their objectives concise and discriminating. Because of the independent nature of physical therapy practice and the need to stay abreast of changes in the field, therapists need to be able to assess their own abilities, limitations, and need for further skills development.[9] The learning contract provides students with the opportunity to practice these skills.

Supervision. The student is asked to outline the type of supervision he would prefer during his affiliation. Would he like to be left alone with the patient, or would he prefer close supervision? Does he want the type of supervision he receives to change as he becomes more skilled? This exercise is particularly helpful for the student who has had a negative past experience in his relationships with clinical instructors. It allows the CI to anticipate problems that might occur because of conflicting teaching-learning styles. The student learns to be open about his feelings, and problems are often avoided.

Special interests. In this section of the contract, the student lists the types of patients he would like to treat, the clinics and departments he would like to visit, and the special learning experiences he would like to have.

Figure 5. Excerpt from "Specific Objectives for Cardiac Rotation."

1. The student will work with at least three patients having one or more of the following: myocardial infarction, congestive heart failure, bundle branch block, atrial fibrillation, coronary artery bypass graft, valve replacement, pacemaker.
2. The student will be able to determine when to stop physical therapy because of poor patient tolerance as indicated by premature ventricular contractions, angina, dyspnea, confusion, hypotension, severe change in pulse.
3. The student will be able to recognize the following arrhythmias on EKG: premature ventricular contraction, atrial fibrillation, premature atrial contraction.
4. For each patient assigned to him, the student will be able to describe the pathological cardiac condition of the patient and relate it to the normal anatomy and physiology of the heart.

The CI's contribution to the contract can be partly standardized with the use of general and specific learning objectives and guidelines for students and CIs. Experience at a facility where the CI developed expectations for each student revealed that many of those expectations varied little from student to student and could be standardized for all students affiliating with the department. Clinical instructors are free to alter the objectives and guidelines to meet the needs of individual students and can contribute additional objectives to the contract. Copies of previously written

---

Figure 6. Excerpt from a Contract Written by a Student.

Weaknesses
1. Chest physical therapy and auscultation.
2. Interpretation of evaluative findings.
3. Receiving criticism.
4. Gait analysis.
5. Assessing abnormal tone.

Supervision
1. I would like to have close supervision during the first week of the affiliation and then increasingly less for the remainder of my time here.
2. I like to discuss thoroughly what I plan to do and why before going in to see the patient.
3. I need to be reminded to slow down and think about what I am doing when I get nervous.

What I Would Like to Do and See
1. Attend amputee and hand clinics.
2. Discuss common gait deviations and their causes.
3. Practice chest physical therapy and auscultation.
4. Evaluate and treat a hemiplegic patient.
5. Observe occupational therapist do a Kenny evaluation on a patient.

Figure 7. Excerpt from "Form for Student Evaluation of the Affiliation."

1. Comment on your supervisor's interest in your learning experiences; include the amount of help you were given with planning and with specific weaknesses.
2. Were you allowed to pursue your individual interests in the practice of physical therapy?
3. Did you have what you considered adequate input into the student program?
4. Do you believe your evaluation was a fair representation of your performance? Comment on how the evaluation was delivered. Were there criticisms of which you had previously been unaware?
5. Did you receive what you considered adequate constructive criticism at what you considered appropriate times? Were you given positive feedback when you believe it was indicated?

The student is responsible for managing his own negotiable time. To facilitate constructive use of the time, self-instructional and resource materials should be made available to the student. A file of resource people can be developed to identify staff members and their areas of expertise. When the student identifies a specific educational need, he can be given assistance in locating resources; however, most of the responsibility for managing the negotiable time should remain his.

The concept of negotiable time offers many advantages to the student and the CI. It gives the student the opportunity to take advantage of the many learning experiences available in the clinical setting. It adds flexibility to the program and gives the student some control over his schedule. It facilitates evaluation of affective behaviors such as "professional growth" and "constructive use of time" because it gives all students equal access to learning resources and time. But most importantly, negotiable time teaches the student how to learn on his own, a skill not emphasized enough in most educational settings.[10]

contracts can be made available to CIs and students as examples to follow.

In the final stages of negotiation, the CI can help the student set priorities for achieving the objectives of the affiliation. The amount of control the student is permitted to have over his program may vary with the needs of the student and the philosophy of the clinical faculty. Significantly, the strength of the contract lies not so much in its content as in the process of developing it.

Negotiable Time

No matter how interested the clinical staff is in providing clinical education, the primary responsibility of the clinical staff is direct patient care. In a busy clinic, both the student and the CI tend to fill their schedules with patient-care activities. As a result, the student is often unable to accomplish the other activities outlined in his contract. Opportunities for observation of treatments, visits to special clinics, and participation in special projects are often missed because they cannot be fit into busy schedules.

To remedy this problem, a specified block of time (eg, one hour) can be reserved daily for the student to use as negotiable time, that is, time reserved for planned learning experiences, self-instruction, observation, meetings between the CI or the CCCE and student, or other learner-centered activities. No routine patient care activities are scheduled during this period. Although having a consistent schedule for negotiable time is preferable, the schedule can be changed as necessary to accommodate the needs of the learner.

Evaluation of the Program

The clinical education program needs to be evaluated periodically to see that it is accomplishing what it was designed to do. One important source of feedback is the student. Most academic programs are designed to have students evaluate their clinical affiliations, but the clinical faculty does not always have access to that information. An evaluation form designed by the clinicians allows them to receive feedback specifically related to their clinical education program. Seeking input from students and new graduates when developing the evaluation form is a good idea because they are most cognizant of issues that concern affiliating students. In addition to providing clinical faculty with feedback on the clinical education program, student evaluations allow students to contribute to the program and offer students some insight into the difficulties of evaluation. Figure 7 illustrates some of the questions that can be used in student evaluations of the affiliation.

As a final check, the clinical education program should be evaluated for consistency with the philosophy of clinical education. Every statement in the philosophy should be reflected in the structure of the program.

SUMMARY

Suggestions for clinicians who are planning and developing a clinical education program have been presented. Not all aspects of clinical education have been addressed, however, and the reader is encouraged to consult other resources on clinical education for further assistance.[3, 11-13] The examples used in the figures were developed to meet the needs of one particular department and may not be suitable for every facility. Developing a planned clinical education program can be time-consuming initially, but the feedback from staff, students, and academic faculty indicates that it is well worth the effort.

Acknowledgments. The author wishes to acknowledge Jean Peteet, former director of physical therapy, and the physical therapy staff at Massachusetts Rehabilitation Hospital who helped develop the materials used in this article.

REFERENCES

1. Seaton JD: Clinical faculty issues. In Ford C (ed): Clinical Education for the Allied Health Professions. St. Louis, MO, The CV Mosby Co, 1978, p 158
2. Evans P: Future trends in clinical education. American Physical Therapy Association Section for Education Newsletter 14:1, Winter 1978
3. Moore ML, Perry JF: Clinical Education in Physical Therapy: Present Status/Future Needs. Washington, DC, Section for Education, American Physical Therapy Association, 1976
4. Moore ML, Parker MM, Nourse ES: Form and Function of Written Agreements in the Clinical Education of Health Professionals. Thorofare, NJ, Charles B Slack Inc, 1972, p 16
5. Ford CE (ed): Clinical Education for the Allied Health Professions. St. Louis, MO, The CV Mosby Co, 1978
6. Pascasio A: Selection, evaluation and utilization of clinical resources. In McTernan EJ, Hawkins RO Jr (eds): Educating Personnel for the Allied Health Professions and Services. St. Louis, MO, The CV Mosby Co, 1972, pp 35–42
7. Davis RH, Alexander LT, Yelon SL: Learning System Design: An Approach to the Improvement of Instruction. New York, NY, McGraw-Hill Book Co, 1974, p 29
8. Duley J: Out-of-class contract learning at Justin Morrill. In Berte N (ed): Individualizing Education by Learning Contracts. Lon Hefferlin JB (gen ed): New Directions for Higher Education, no. 10. Washington, DC, Jossey-Bass Inc, Publisher, 1975, p 54
9. Fuhrmann BS, Weissburg MJ: Self-assessment. In Morgan M, Irby D (eds): Evaluating Clinical Competence in the Health Professions. St. Louis, MO, The CV Mosby Co, 1978, p 139
10. Brunner J: Learning and thinking. In Hamachek D (ed): Human Dynamics in Psychology and Education. Boston, MA, Allyn & Bacon Inc, 1972, pp 12–21
11. Dickinson R, Freeman A, Peteet J: What's the Connection? Goals—Learning Activities—and Back Again. Washington, DC, National Institutes of Health, Public Health Service, US Department of Health, Education and Welfare, 1973
12. Pinkston D, Hochhauser SL, Gardner-O'Loughlin K: Standards for basic education in physical therapy: A tool for planning clinical education. Phys Ther 55: 841–849, 1975

APPENDIX

Physical Therapy Department Philosophy of Clinical Education

The physical therapists at this hospital recognize that clinical instruction is an integral part of physical therapy education. We seek to contribute to the education of physical therapists and physical therapist assistants by maintaining a student affiliation program committed to providing quality learning experiences. Affiliating with many different academic programs within and outside of the state provides us with exposure to varied approaches to physical therapy education and theories of patient care.

Because of the uniqueness of our staffing pattern and the complexity of the patient problems we treat, we believe our facility is best suited for the student who is already knowledgeable in the theories of therapeutic exercise and rehabilitation and who possesses beginning skills in evaluation and treatment. We believe our rehabilitation setting is an ideal place for a senior student to integrate information previously learned; it is not the best place for an entry-level student to practice basic physical therapy skills.

The physical therapists at this hospital believe clinical experiences should be planned, organized, and based on well-defined clinical objectives. Students should be actively involved in planning and evaluating their clinical experiences. They should be encouraged to pursue their individual, professional interests as much as possible within the framework of general physical therapy education.

The members of our department believe that continuity of supervision is important for developing student-supervisor rapport, for maintaining open communication, and for accurately assessing student performance. Because therapists are assigned to patient care areas where patients are grouped according to diagnosis, limiting the number of clinical instructors per student often results in limiting the variety of patient problems available to the student for management. However, we attempt to provide the student with the challenge of patients with various pathological conditions within the limitations of the rotation to which the student is assigned. In addition, time is made available for the student to seek experiences not provided by his particular affiliation assignment. When alternatives for student placement are available, the center coordinator of clinical education attempts to match the student to the patient care area most suited to the student's clinical needs.

Student evaluation should be immediate, on-going, and constructive. Feedback should be designed to help the student know how he is performing and how he can increase his strengths and improve his weaknesses. The clinical affiliation program needs to be evaluated also. We encourage the student to give us feedback on how the program is or is not meeting his needs and expectations. Several channels of communication are available to the student for giving and receiving formal and informal feedback. Because the purpose of evaluation should be to provide direction for planned behavioral change, nothing crucial to the outcome of the affiliation should wait until the final evaluation (of the student or of the affiliation) to be discussed.

While we as therapists recognize and accept the responsibilities inherent in providing quality clinical education, we believe that our first responsibility is to provide quality patient care to the community we serve and that all student-related activities must occur within that context.

Mock Clinic

Mock Clinic

An Approach to Clinical Education

BARBARA R. SANDERS, MS,
and JANE F. RUVOLO, MS

This paper presents a new clinical education experience initiated at the University of Wisconsin-La Crosse. A Mock Clinic was developed that simulates a real-life physical therapy department: students adopt roles of both physical therapist and patient. Each student is student-therapist and student-patient at least once each session. At the beginning of each session, the student-therapist selects a patient treatment card (containing instructions submitted by academic and clinical faculty members) and a faculty supervisor discusses the role of the patient with the student-patient to assist him in accurately displaying signs and symptoms. The student-therapist also meets with the faculty supervisor to review the patient and the approach. The student-therapist then "evaluates" and "treats" the student-patient. A group discussion concludes each session. Mock Clinic is a role-playing experience that provides the opportunity for students to see themselves in clinical situations and enables them to learn without involving real clients. Strengths and weaknesses of Mock Clinic identified by all participants are discussed.

Key Words: *Education, Clinical competence, Physical therapy.*

In the fall of 1978, the University of Wisconsin-La Crosse initiated a new clinical education experience. Mock Clinic simulates a real-life physical therapy department. It is a role-playing experience that provides the opportunity for students to see themselves in clinical situations, enabling them to learn without involving real clients who may be disturbed by an "inexperienced physical therapist."[1] The purpose of this paper is to present the planning and implementing of our Mock Clinic.

Mock Clinic was originally intended to serve as a remedial experience for a small number of students. Because of the success of this approach, Mock Clinic has now developed into an additional clinical experience for all physical therapy students. This approach would be useful in any physical therapy setting because it allows students to practice clinical techniques, thus decreasing the gap between thinking and doing.

The concept for Mock Clinic evolved through the joint efforts of the academic faculty members and several of the adjunct clinical faculty members to facilitate practical learning situations and to create a better understanding among students concerning clinical techniques. Implementation was then planned and coordinated by the Academic Coordinator of Clinical Education (ACCE).

The major objectives of the Mock Clinic were
1) to provide an additional site for clinical practice,
2) to provide a channel for working on specific problems of individual students,
3) to provide a more controlled environment than is available in a real-life clinical setting, and
4) to give the academic faculty the opportunity to work with the students and gain more information about each student's clinical skills.

BACKGROUND INFORMATION

The use of simulations and role playing in clinical education and evaluating clinical performance is increasing. Learning experiences using simulations and

Ms. Sanders is Academic Coordinator of Clinical Education, Physical Therapy Department, University of Wisconsin-La Crosse, La Crosse, WI 54601 (USA).

Ms. Ruvolo was a graduate student in the Adult Fitness/Cardiac Rehabilitation Program, University of Wisconsin-La Crosse, La Crosse, WI, when this manuscript was submitted. She is now Assistant Chief Physical Therapist, Lorain Community Hospital, Lorain, OH 44052.

This paper was a poster presentation at the Fifty-sixth Annual Conference of the American Physical Therapy Association, Phoenix, AZ, June 1980.

This article was submitted April 21, 1980, and accepted February 9, 1981.

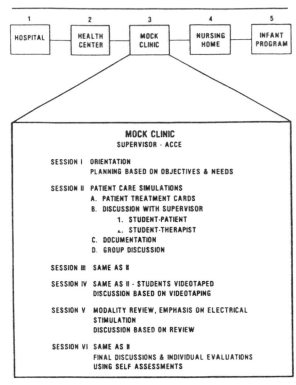

Fig. 1. *Format of Mock Clinic.*

role playing provide students with the opportunity to test skills and judgment in the context of reality, to get prompt and specific feedback on performance without risk to patients, to try a variety of approaches, to work on one part of a complex problem at a time, and to experience more flexibility than real-life situations allow.[2] Role playing provides an opportunity for the students to see themselves in situations and to learn from errors without involving real patients. These activities can be used in any context.[1]

Simulations and role playing as methods of instruction have numerous advantages over other methods. The first advantage is the low risk to the students and the patients. There is no discomfort for patients, and the student can practice over and over again. Another important advantage is the relevancy: simulations allow early clinical contact in which newly acquired skills and knowledge can be practiced and student motivation and interest maintained at a high level. A third advantage of simulations is the transfer to real-world situations: skills practiced with role-playing patients are the same skills that will be used with real patients in other clinical settings.[3] The student's performance in simulations and role playing can be assumed to parallel closely their performance in real life.[4]

The benefits to the learner and instructor are numerous. The student is an active participant, rather than a passive recipient of information in the class-

room. The student is required to apply knowledge and facts learned from the classroom and from other clinical settings. Appropriate information must be collected and integrated to formulate solutions for each situation. Successful completion of the clinical experiences can provide positive reinforcement by giving the student the opportunity to experience the success of accomplishment. A final benefit includes the ability to learn future roles that may not be currently available and for which the student must be prepared. An example might be the participation in a health team planning conference.[3,5] Through role playing the students can develop a measure of personal, emotional, and intellectual involvement in a wide range of clinical experiences.[1]

In addition to the benefits to the student, simulations can help increase the effectiveness of the clinical instructor. The instructor must decide what is to be learned and practiced and how to give the students feedback about what they have done. Another benefit is the control the instructor has over complex learning; very complex skills can be broken down and learned as basic skills, and more complex components can be introduced gradually as the student masters each skill. The use of simulations also allows control over distractions found in the real world. For example, instruction can be one-to-one and not complicated by the presence of visitors, other patients, and health care professionals who may be found in busy clinics. Simulations and role-playing experiences allow the instructor, in addition to the learner, to benefit from a wide range of clinical experiences that may not be available at any other time during the clinical education period.[3]

Disadvantages have also been identified. For example, simulations can be costly when obtained commercially or time-consuming when originally developed, the acquisition of facts may be more efficiently obtained through other methods, and the instructor may be placed in an unfamiliar teaching role.[2,3]

IMPLEMENTATION

To attain the objectives, a situation was designed that would parallel the real-life clinics, would be more structured than the usual laboratory practice sessions, and would provide experience in which patients could not be affected adversely. The development of Mock Clinic was based on three states of clinical education—laboratory experiences, limited clinical experiences, and internship experiences. The simulation experience enhanced the limited clinical experiences and was integrated with class work.

The concurrent format of clinical education allowed the scheduling of Mock Clinic as another clinical assignment to augment the existing sites (two general hospitals, three nursing homes, an infant developmental program, two school systems, a private practice, and a university health center). This format places the students in a clinical assignment two afternoons a week for three weeks in the second, third, and fourth semesters of the physical therapy program. During any semester, each student is scheduled for Mock Clinic in addition to four other clinical assignments. At least four students are scheduled at any one time.

Mock Clinic is supervised by the ACCE. Other academic faculty members and graduate assistants are also available to assist in Mock Clinic. An advantage of having more than one person involved in the supervision is that diversified role models are provided for the students. This also allows the ACCE time to visit, supervise, and evaluate students scheduled in the other clinics.

Each rotation through Mock Clinic includes an orientation and planning session in which individual objectives are shared and discussed and specific planning for that rotation is done[6] (Fig. 1). The students are asked to request any special attention they feel they may need, such as reviewing positioning for manual muscle testing of an upper extremity. In addition to direct patient care activities, the students may request a review of the use of a particular modality, help in solving an administration problem, or a general discussion of a topic. The schedule for the rest of Mock Clinic is then formulated around these decisions.

Mock Clinic is structured so that students simulate the roles of both a therapist and a patient. Each student is a student-therapist and a student-patient at least once each session.

At the beginning of each session, the student-therapist selects a patient treatment card (Fig. 2). The faculty supervisor then discusses the role of the patient with the student-patient to assist him in accurately displaying signs, symptoms, and any other manifestations of the problem or treatment. The student-therapist also meets briefly with the faculty supervisor to review his patient and his approach. The student-therapist is then expected to evaluate and treat the student-patient.

The patient treatment cards are submitted by academic and clinical faculty members. The instructions may be brief or detailed, may describe acute or chronic problems, and may have erroneous information. The faculty supervisor is free to instruct student-patients to respond in any way. If a student-therapist has had trouble in other clinics with overly emotional patients, the supervisor may want to instruct the student-patient to cry throughout the treatment; this would allow the supervisor to observe and intervene if necessary in order to help resolve the situation.

The student-therapists are required to record their evaluations and write progress notes, home programs,

or staffing reports when indicated. Written communication follows the Problem-Oriented Medical Records format and is critiqued by the supervisor.

Emergency situations and professional communication are programed by the supervisor: a cardiac arrest might occur, a patient might fall, or an angry health care professional might approach the student-therapist. All students are expected to respond appropriately.

A group discussion of the session's activities concludes each session. The patient types, individual student performances, feelings, and documentations are discussed. It is an open discussion and many subject areas may be covered. The group discussion period has stimulated the interchange of ideas and experiences between the students and supervisor.

Each student is videotaped at least once a semester. The students and the supervisor review the videotape. This review allows the videotaped student-therapist to do a self-assessment, the other students to do a peer review, and the faculty to critique the individual student. The peer review encourages the students to observe the student-therapist closely and to think about that student's approach. Through this experience the students sharpen their observation skills and learn to provide constructive feedback to their classmate. We have found that the students seem to be more critical of the students than the supervisor is. Areas of strengths and weaknesses for each student are then identified and future planning for meeting the individual's needs can be done.[7]

The self-assessments encourage the student to examine his own performance carefully. Self-assessment is a necessary skill for clinicians and is often not purposefully taught. The data collected can be valid and meaningful and can contribute to healthy function and competent performance.[7] When compared with the supervisor's assessment, the student's self-assessments tend to be similar, which contributes to the student's increased self-confidence. Guidelines for self-assessment include professional conduct; student-

---

Mrs. Hall is a 62 y.o. female outpatient with sudden onset of facial paralysis 2 days PTA. History is non-presenting. She has a referral from her physician for evaluation and treatment.

Mrs. Treader is a 65 y.o. school teacher. Her present complaint is of pain for several months' duration in her R shoulder. Her physician has diagnosed bursitis, referring her to you for evaluation and treatment.

Fig. 2. Examples of treatment cards.

patient relations; recognition, understanding, and use of factors involving patient behavior; sense of responsibility; communication; attitude; knowledge; and skills.

DISCUSSION

The merits of Mock Clinic are determined by written evaluations of students submitted by adjunct clinical faculty members before and after the student participation in Mock Clinic. The evaluations indicate that students who have participated in Mock Clinic exhibit more self-confidence in skills, enhanced individual clinical techniques, and better overall clinical performance. Mock Clinic provides the faculty and students with an educative experience wherein the cognitive and practical processes of physical therapy are developed and enhanced.

Strengths and weaknesses of Mock Clinic have been identified by academic and clinical faculty members and by students through written subjective evaluations and formal discussion group meetings.

Mock Clinic does provide an additional site for student placement and is included in each student's clinical schedule. Students have stated that they look forward to that assignment because of the stimulating experience they have had in previous semesters.

The students have the opportunity to select specific areas to review and practice. In addition, the faculty members can select a specific area for a particular student or group of students to focus on. This has been particularly beneficial when an adjunct faculty member has previously rated a student who needs help in a particular area or when a new subject has been introduced in a class and students wish to practice a skill before trying the skill with a real patient.

We have been able to simulate a real-life clinical setting while providing a more controlled environment. More direct supervision is possible because the supervisor has only the responsibility of the students and not the additional concerns of patients, colleagues, and support staff or other distractions found in many clinical settings. This direct supervision allows continuous and immediate feedback to the students, both during and after the performance of evaluation, treatment, and written documentation. Positive feedback and constructive criticism can be given immediately when the task is performed. The atmosphere and the availability of time prompt the students to ask questions and receive timely responses. Thus, the students feel more comfortable in asking questions without feeling that they should have known the answers. Ideas and questions can be shared and discussed with the other students and the supervisor. The informality and flexibility encourage the students to try new techniques without having the anxiety of harming the patient or endangering themselves, thus encouraging more creative thinking.

The academic faculty is now much more aware of the students' clinical competencies and of each clinical facility's contribution to the students' education. This has helped to improve communication between the academic faculty and clinical faculty. Prior to the implementation of Mock Clinic, the academic faculty did not have the opportunity to observe critically each student's clinical skills. The students were observed only briefly during routine visits to the clinical facilities. With the advent of this new approach, each student can be observed intermittently during his clinical development. His professional growth can be seen and shared. The feedback to the academic faculty is important because it often serves as a "pat on the back for a job well done" or as a reminder to continue to stress a certain area in a course.

The group discussion period following each session has been an unexpected advantage. These discussions have been instrumental in increasing the students' and faculty's awareness of the variety of approaches to patient care.

We feel that our original objectives have been accomplished. Other advantages have been identified and further objectives have been set as well. The project has not been without disadvantages, which we have also identified and tried to correct.

The students have stated in their written evaluations of Mock Clinic that they are expected to look at the "total patient." This expectation includes referral, initial evaluation, treatment plan and progression, and follow-up programs for discharge, referral, or home programs. Consequently, the problems of each patient can be identified and ideas for treatment programs can be discussed, along with possible alternatives and the inclusion of other health care personnel in the care of the patient. Such responsibility—to look at the total patient—is what is expected in any clinical setting; however, it is not always possible to carry out when students spend only two half-days a week in a health care setting.

The self-assessment through videotaping encourages the students to develop a format and habit of evaluating themselves that they can carry with them throughout their career. In Mock Clinic, the students have time to review the videotapes, evaluate their actions, discuss their evaluations with the supervisor, and determine any necessary actions based on these self-evaluations. The students then have the opportunity to refine their techniques or to try new methods. This experience helps them improve their clinical skills and develop self-confidence.

Through the role playing, the students gain clinical experience from the perspective of the therapist and the patient. As the patient, the student begins to develop an understanding of the patient's feelings and perspectives of his health care and an enhanced awareness of his patients and colleagues. The experience of portraying this situation from the patient's side is often very enlightening for the student.

Several weaknesses of Mock Clinic have been observed by the academic and clinical faculty members. One problem is that the students find the role playing difficult initially because of the lack of realism and their lack of confidence. However, with time and practice they appear to become more comfortable and competent in role playing. After their first or second attempt, and with increased coaching from the supervisor, they tend to lose their self-consciousness. We have also found that the students actually enjoy being the patient when they are more familiar with the diagnosis, signs, and symptoms of the patient they role play. To familiarize themselves with the patient's problems, they are encouraged to keep notes about patients they see in other facilities, talk with supervising therapists, and research the patients' problems.

A second disadvantage is that the clinic is time-consuming for academic faculty. At least one faculty member is required to provide supervision, guidance, and instruction. This becomes even more time-consuming when both junior and senior students are scheduled for clinical rotations.

Third, the availability of adequate facilities can be a problem. We use a teaching laboratory that closely resembles a therapeutic exercise gymnasium and treatment area of many physical therapy departments. It is set up to allow several treatment cubicles around the periphery of the gymnasium, with the necessary equipment and modalities available. Other uses for this classroom are scheduled around the Mock Clinic.

Unlimited modifications of Mock Clinic are possible. Our present plans include structuring the three semesters toward a more realistic situation. The first semester experience will remain as described. In semester two, the student-therapist would see the student-patient for an initial evaluation and several follow-up treatments, giving the students the opportunity to role play patient treatment progression or regression and to write progress notes. During the third semester, the student-therapist will be responsible for scheduling patients, supervising supportive personnel, and working with other health care personnel. There would be only one student-therapist each session, with the remaining students composing the patient load and the supportive staff. Mock Clinic provides an ideal setting for working on interpersonal communication skills that fall in the last semester. The students can have confrontations with physicians, nurses, patients and families, and supervisors with whom they can learn to interact.

There is a need for the simulated clinic to require the student to demonstrate more than patient care skills, that is, to include administrative skills such as supervision of personnel, care of the physical plant and equipment, time management such as scheduling in-service training, and other skills. Mock Clinic has served this purpose. Also, the Mock Clinic has reinforced didactic instruction given in the classroom and facilitated the transition into the clinic. It has provided the students with the opportunity to test skills and judgment in the context of reality, to get prompt and specific feedback on their performance without risk to patients, to try a variety of approaches, to work on one part of a complex problem at a time, and to experience more flexibility than most real-life situations allow.[2] This experience has also helped the students to be better prepared for other clinical assignments and to be more self-confident in their skills. The students have developed more individual competencies and better overall clinical performance than the students did prior to the implementation of Mock Clinic. We believe the experience assists the development of professional attitudes and values and promotes independent, creative physical therapists.

REFERENCES

1. Cross SP (ed): Interviewing and Communication in Social Work. Boston, MA, Routledge & Kegan Paul, 1974, pp 150–152
2. Ford CW, Morgan MK: Teaching in the Health Professions. St. Louis, MO, C. V. Mosby Co, 1976, pp 219–220
3. Ford CW (ed): Clinical Education for the Allied Health Professions. St. Louis, MO, C. V. Mosby Co, 1978, pp 150–152
4. Barrows HS: Simulated Patients: The Development and Use of a New Technique in Medical Education. Springfield, IL, Charles C Thomas, Publisher, 1971, pp 2–15
5. Gershen JA, Handleman SL: Role-playing as an educational technique in dentistry. J Dent Educ 38:451–455, 1974
6. Chesler M, Fox R: Role-playing Methods in the Classroom. Chicago, IL, Science Research Associates, Inc, 1966, pp 20–22
7. Morgan MK, Irby DM (eds): Evaluating Clinical Competence in the Health Professions. St. Louis, MO, C. V. Mosby Co, 1978, pp 140–145

Mock Clinic: One Program's Experience

Elizabeth M Strickler

ABSTRACT: *The Program in Physical Therapy at Grand Valley State University (GVSU) has used a Mock Clinic as the first component of the clinical education curriculum since 1984. This article discusses the reasons for using Mock Clinic at GVSU, describes the design of our Mock Clinic, which differs from that described by Sanders and Ruvulo in 1981, and reports on student, faculty, and clinician responses to Mock Clinic. Objective and subjective data regarding Mock Clinic were collected from students, faculty, and clinicians and were reviewed and discussed. The response to Mock Clinic in our curriculum has been overwhelmingly positive. Students and faculty believe that Mock Clinic effectively enhances student preparedness for clinical affiliations and is a valuable commitment of curriculum time. Strengths and weaknesses of Mock Clinic are identified.*

The Mock Clinic approach to clinical education in physical therapy was first described by Sanders and Ruvulo in 1981.[1] The purposes of this article are 1) to discuss reasons for using Mock Clinic at Grand Valley State University (GVSU) and to describe a modification of Mock Clinic for use as the earliest clinical experience in a physical therapy curriculum and 2) to report on student, faculty, and clinician responses to Mock Clinic.

BACKGROUND INFORMATION

A common problem in physical therapy clinical education is the placement of beginning-level students in clinical sites. Early clinical experiences for physical therapy students typically are viewed as essen-tial to the process of professional socialization and as an important step in the development of patient-care skills. Supervision of students during early clinical experiences, however, can be demanding and time consuming; this often limits the acceptance of students by affiliating sites for early clinical experiences. Additionally, recent changes in health care funding have affected the types and numbers of clinical sites available for early experiences. General hospital physical therapy departments that have traditionally served as early clinical affiliation sites now serve an increasingly acutely ill patient population, have staff numbers that are diminishing as more services are provided outside of the hospital setting, and face external and internal pressures to be very productive and expedient in patient management. These changes are forcing many physical therapy department staffs to reexamine their ability to accept beginning-level affiliate students. The expanding number of clinical sites where physical therapy services are offered outside of hospitals could provide alternative placement options for beginning-level students, but many of these sites have traditionally only accepted advanced-level affiliates and have served as speciality affiliations. Some of the staff in such sites are, therefore, hesitant to accept the beginning-level affiliate.

The Program in Physical Therapy at GVSU admitted its first class into the professional portion of the curriculum (junior and senior years) in 1983. As a new program in a part of the state where many clinical education sites had yet to be developed, limited acceptance of beginning-level students was seen as a potential problem, despite strong support for the program from the state and local professional community. To address this problem and also to improve student performance during initial clinical affiliations, a Mock Clinic, using physical therapist and patient role-playing experiences, was instituted at GVSU as the first clinical education experience for students.

Many authors have discussed the advantages and disadvantages of simulations and role-playing as a clinical teaching and evaluation tool.[1-6] The faculty at GVSU believed that the Mock Clinic approach to clinical education would be an ideal mechanism for developing and enhancing clinical problem-solving and self-assessment skills in students. May and Newman wrote that "effective problem solving skills are best learned in an environment in which the student is free to test skills, explore alternatives, and discover solutions that may or may not match the instructor's solution."[7] Problem solving can be a lengthy and risky process for physical therapy students completing early clinical affiliations. Because of time factors and other constraints in the clinic, this process may not always be cultivated. We believed it was important to cultivate problem solving first in the academic setting, where we could ensure that subject matter essential to arriving at solutions was provided and where we could foster the willingness to take a chance and develop the self-confidence that is so essential to the problem-solving process, especially during solution development and implementation.[7,8] In Mock Clinic, instructors have time to allow the problem-solving process to occur and the opportunity to observe the cognitive, affective, and psychomotor behaviors that comprise the process of problem solving. In-depth knowledge of previous and concurrent course content also allows instructors to design clinical cases for Mock Clinic that require immediate use of didactic material, thereby increasing the relevancy of information for students and enhancing retention.

Self-evaluation skills have been described as "a necessity for competent independent judgments by clinicians."[6] Fuhrmann and Weissburg point out that although specific components of self-evaluation have been identified, few clinicians are ever taught self-evaluation skills.[6] Our faculty saw Mock Clinic as the ideal situation in which to teach the process of self-evaluation and to allow students to practice and refine those skills, just as they would practice other clinical management skills.

Ms Strickler is Academic Coordinator of Clinical Education and Assistant Professor, Program in Physical Therapy, Grand Valley State University, Allendale, MI 49401. She is a doctoral student, School of Health Education, Human Performance, and Counseling Psychology, Michigan State University, East Lansing, MI. This paper was presented in poster format at the Combined Sections Meeting of the American Physical Therapy Association, Atlanta, GA, February 12–15, 1987.

First-year Professional Curriculum, Grand Valley State University Program in Physical Therapy

First Semester	Second (Orthopedic) Semester
Regional Human Anatomy	Anatomy of Joints
Applied Human Physiology	Clinical Biomechanics
Pathophysiology	Clinical Medicine I (radiology, orthopedics, rheumatology)
Human Physical Development	Orthopedic Evaluation and Treatment
Introduction to Physical Therapy	P.T. Procedures II (therapeutic exercise, traction, mobilization)
P.T. Procedures I (basic patient management skills: transfers, gait, training, thermal agents, patient interviewing, medical records)	Clinical Education I (Mock Clinic)

Many academic programs use part-time clinical affiliations (ie, half days or a few days a week) as the earliest clinical experience for students. At GVSU, Mock Clinic is used as an alternative to early part-time clinical affiliations. The location of the university provided a limited number of clinical sites within an hour's drive. Several sites within that area had a small staff or were new to clinical education, making it difficult for them to accommodate more than one student at a time. Larger local facilities with experienced clinical educators already had active affiliate programs that limited their capacity for additional student placements. The faculty also wanted to avoid student fatigue and adjustment problems as a result of split clinical and academic days and other problems associated with part-time clinical affiliations described by Kondela and Darnell.[9] Based on past experience, we also believed that part-time affiliations can become largely observational experiences for the student and can produce a fragmentation of patient care, limiting benefits to the student, clinical instructor, facility, and patient. Additionally, the curriculum design encouraged initial full-time (versus part-time)

clinical affiliations focusing on specific patient populations and allowing students to participate in all aspects of patient care with those populations (Fig. 1).

DESCRIPTION OF MOCK CLINIC

Mock Clinic is offered as a 60-hour course, Clinical Education I, for second-semester junior students in the first year of the professional curriculum. Figure 1 outlines the first-year professional curriculum, shows where Mock Clinic fits into the curriculum, and provides brief descriptions of course content where necessary. Mock Clinic is offered during the orthopedic semester, which is followed immediately by a three-week, full-time orthopedic affiliation, Clinical Education II.

The original design of Mock Clinic, as described by Sanders and Ruvulo, was concurrent with part-time affiliations during the second, third, and fourth semesters of the professional curriculum and provided an alternate clinical assignment for students.[1] There were a total of six Mock Clinic sessions, including four patient-care simulations, with a minimum of four students scheduled in Mock Clinic at any time.[1]

The design of Mock Clinic used in our curriculum is shown in Figure 2. As a preface to clinic sessions, initial class periods are devoted to instruction in problem solving and self-evaluation processes. Students are divided into two groups that alternate roles as patient or physical therapist. Each student has the opportunity to assume the role of a physical therapist at least nine times during the semester. Clinic sessions are similar to those described by Sanders and Ruvulo.[1] Student physical therapists are provided with case information similar to the example shown in Figure 3. They spend approximately 15 minutes preparing their treatment area, planning their evaluation, and gathering necessary equipment. Meanwhile, student patients are provided with background information on their case. An example of this information is shown in Figure 4. Students review the information, provide missing data (when necessary), and discuss the case briefly with an instructor to ensure accuracy and consistency of presentation. For the first two to four clinic sessions, only one case is presented per clinic; thereafter, two cases are presented per clinic so that each student assumes both the role of physical therapist and patient during a clinic session. This allows from 1 hour to 1 hour and 15 minutes for the student physical therapist to complete an initial evaluation and design and implement a treatment program on new patients or reevaluate and continue treatment on previously seen patients. All sessions conclude with a brief question-and-discussion period where students can share ideas on the management of their patients. When time permits, students are given the opportunity to begin documentation of their case in SOAP (subjective, objective, assessment, plan) note format. All students must write notes on their patients and include home programs when appropriate. All notes for the semester are kept in a notebook and are intermittently reviewed by the instructor with written and verbal feedback provided.

The academic coordinator of clinical education (ACCE) coordinates Mock Clinic, serves as the primary instructor, and is assisted by one other faculty member during clinic sessions. The ACCE must be aware of course objectives, content, and schedules for previously taught and concurrent courses so that cases used in Mock Clinic will require students to use recently presented didactic material. For instance, when lectures and laboratories on radiology, rheumatology, goniometry, and certain elements of therapeutic exercise are completed, cases might include diagnoses of rheumatoid ar-

Figure 2
Design of Mock Clinic Used at Grand Valley State University

Time Allotment	Clinic Sessions	Participants
Three hours	Student-patient/student-physical therapist preparation Patient evaluation and treatment (videotaped) Questions/discussion Documentation	16 Students (8 physical therapist-patient pairs) 2 Instructors
One hour	Group discussion and videotape reviews	32 students
	Four hours per week per student	

Figure 3
Mock Clinic Sample Case Information Provided to Student Physical Therapists

Mr./Ms. Leonard is a 26 y o factory worker who sustained a fracture of the distal ⅓ of the femur 4 months ago. He/she was immobilized in a long leg cast until 1 week ago when it was determined that the fracture was adequately healed to begin rehabilitation and allow PWB ambulation. At the time of removal of the cast it was discovered that the patient had a compression neuropathy of the common peroneal nerve. The patient is referred by Dr. James, his orthopedist, for evaluation, gait training PWB, and other treatment as indicated.

thritis or related disorders. Likewise, cases involving various problems of the shoulder would follow course material that focused on the dissection and biomechanics of the shoulder joint, clinical medicine lectures on shoulder conditions, and instruction in all evaluation and treatment procedures for that joint. Academic and clinical faculty members assist the ACCE in development or modification of cases as appropriate throughout the course. Consistent with principles of organization of learning experiences,[10] cases presented in Mock Clinic progress from simple to complex. Cases become more complex by providing less diagnostic information and open referrals, presenting patients with multiple medical or surgical problems, or inserting significant psychosocial or vocational concerns. Toward the end of the semester, student patients research and develop their own case presentations.

Videotaping of students during Mock Clinic is initiated about the fourth week of clinic sessions. Every student is videotaped at least once in his or her role as physical therapist. All students are given the opportunity to review their tape individually, and then, based on their consent, parts of the videotape are used for class videotape review and discussion sessions. During these sessions, the student physical therapist is given the first opportunity to critique his or her performance, followed by peer and instructor feedback.

At the midpoint and end of Mock Clinic, each student completes a self-assessment form identifying his or her strengths and weaknesses in several broad categories, including interaction skills, evaluation and interpretation, treatment planning and application, problem solving, flexibility and judgment, and self-assessment. The criteria by which the students judge their performance in these areas are the course objectives, which closely parallel subsequent clinical education performance objectives and evaluation criteria. Based on their self-assessment at midterm, students develop individualized objectives for the remainder of the course.

Figure 4
Mock Clinic Sample Case Information Provided to Student Patients

You are Mr./Mrs Leonard, a 26 y o factory worker. 4 months ago you were involved in a MVA which resulted in numerous contusions, lacerations, and a Fx of the distal R femur. You were hospitalized for 2 weeks and discharged in a LLC. You have been ambulating on crutches since then. One week ago the cast was removed and it was discovered that you had a compression neuropathy of the common peroneal nerve. While you were casted you had noticed some tingling along the lateral and anterior aspects of your lower leg and dorsal aspect of your foot. However, you were unaware that the area had subsequently become anaesthetic. You are unmarried and live alone in a ground floor apartment. You have a stick shift car and are unable to drive presently because of stiffness and weakness in your leg. A friend brought you to PT today.

Your physical presentation is as follows:

1) Inability to flex knee past 50, with pain at end range; full knee extension.
2) Ankle dorsiflexion to neutral with knee flexed or extended
3) Anaesthesia in the distributions of the lateral cutaneous n. of the calf and the superficial and deep peroneal nn.
4) Strength in the following R LE mm in the P + to F − range: _____
5) Strength in the quadriceps and hamstrings in the F + range
6) Gait _____

Mock Clinic is a required course in the professional curriculum and is offered as a credit or no-credit course. Credit is based on timely and accurate completion of all written assignments and participation in both Mock Clinic and discussion.

EVALUATION OF MOCK CLINIC

Because Mock Clinic was an innovative and time-consuming addition to the professional curriculum, we believed it was important to evaluate students' responses to Mock Clinic. Specifically, we wanted to know 1) whether students believed Mock Clinic met stated objectives for the course and 2) whether they believed it would, and did, affect subsequent clinical performance. Additionally, feedback from clinicians regarding student performance during early clinical affiliations was monitored, and informal feedback from faculty members regarding Mock Clinic was collected.

METHOD

From 1984 to 1986, all students enrolled in Mock Clinic completed a 21-item course-evaluation form (Appendix). The design and content of Mock Clinic during these years did not change significantly. The evaluation form was completed by students after they had completed Mock Clinic and before a three-week, full-time orthopedic affiliation and again immediately after the affiliation. Minor editorial changes were made in items 14 and 15 of the evaluation form to reflect the intervening time and affiliation. A Likert scale was used to rate responses to each item. Frequency distributions of responses to items were tabulated, and percentages of students responding in each category were calculated.

Evaluations of students' performance during their orthopedic affiliation were reviewed. The evaluation tool used was the Competency Assessment Report (CAR).[11] This report asks clinical instructors to rate students' performance as unsatisfactory, marginal (performing below expectations), satisfactory (performing as expected), or superior (performing above expectations) at the conclusion of the affiliation.[11] We believed that student performance on initial clinical affiliations, as measured by the CAR, could be one indicator of the effectiveness of Mock Clinic, although we recognized that many factors, and not Mock Clinic alone, contributed to students' performance during their first clinical affiliation.

Feedback from faculty regarding Mock Clinic was gathered through informal interviews and discussions.

Table

Percentages of Students' Responses on Mock Clinic Evaluation Form Before and After Clinical Affiliation

Item	Strongly Agree		Agree		Indifferent		Disagree		Strongly Disagree	
	Pre[a]	Post[b]	Pre	Post	Pre	Post	Pre	Post	Pre	Post
1 Increased understanding of basic problem-solving processes.	64	56	34	39	2	5				
2 Improved clinical problem-solving skills.	52	46	48	47	0	7				
3 Improved verbal/nonverbal patient communication skills.	47	43	46	40	7	14	0	3		
4 Improved understanding of SOAP note format.	75	61	22	37	3	1	0	1		
5 Improved SOAP note writing.	66	50	31	47	3	1	0	2		
6 Improved performance of clinical evaluation skills.	62	59	37	39	1	2				
7 Improved interpretation of information from patient evaluations.	47	42	49	50	4	7	0	1		
8 Improved treatment planning and design skills.	47	38	42	52	11	9	0	1		
9 Improved treatment skills in the following areas:										
a. application of modalities	17	40	49	38	27	19	7	3		
b. therapeutic exercise	34	25	60	53	5	19	1	3		
c. transfer training	20	20	56	51	20	26	4	2	0	1
d. gait training	21	30	67	48	11	21	1	1		
e. use of body mechanics	45	40	48	48	6	10	1	2		
f. preparation of treatment area	57	55	38	36	4	8	1	1		
g. preparation of patient for treatment	58	58	35	34	5	8	2	0		
10 Improved ability to adjust to changes in the environment or patient status.	21	21	53	49	26	26	0	4		
11 Improved ability to constructively assess peer performance.	31	41	55	50	14	9				
12 Improved ability to assess own performance.	51	58	45	36	4	6				
13 Improved understanding of the patient in the health care system.	45	26	40	50	11	23	4	1		
14 Will have (did have) a positive impact on clinical performance in Clinical Education II.	89	86	11	14						
15 Will *not* (did not) affect performance in Clinical Education II.					1	2	11	14	88	44

[a] Preaffiliation.
[b] Postaffiliation.

SUBJECTS

Ninety-two students completed the course-evaluation form during the three years it was administered. Seventy-eight percent of the students were female (n = 72), and 22% of the students were male (n = 20). The age range of the students was from 19 to 44 years, with a mean age of 23.6 years.

RESULTS

Percentages of student responses on the Mock Clinic evaluation before and after the orthopedic affiliation are shown in the Table. Response to Mock Clinic was consistently positive during the three years studied, with 100% of the students agreeing or strongly agreeing that Mock Clinic would, and did, have a positive impact on their clinical performance. Ninety-eight percent of the students preaffiliation and 95% of the students postaffiliation believed that Mock Clinic had increased their understanding of basic clinical problem-solving processes. Ninety-seven percent of the students preaffiliation and 98% of the students postaffiliation believed that Mock Clinic improved their understanding of the SOAP note format, and 97% of the students both preaffiliation and postaffiliation agreed that Mock Clinic had improved their actual SOAP note writing. Ninety-nine percent of the students preaffiliation and 98% of the students postaffiliation believed that their clinical evaluation skills had improved as a result of Mock Clinic. Ninety-six percent of the students preaffiliation and 94% of the students postaffiliation agreed or strongly agreed that their ability to assess their own performance had improved, and 86% of the students preaffiliation and 91% of the students postaffiliation believed that their ability to constructively assess the performance of their peers had improved as a result of Mock Clinic. For all evaluation items, with one exception, 70% or more of the students agreed or strongly agreed that Mock Clinic had met stated objectives for the course both before and after a clinical affiliation. When asked if Mock Clinic had improved their treatment skills in the application of modalities, 27% of the students preaffiliation were indifferent and 7% disagreed; 19% of the students postaffiliation were indifferent and 3% disagreed.

The evaluation form also asked students to list the two cases or activities from which they learned the most. In response to this question, students consistently listed the more complex or challenging cases presented, cases where evaluation and treatment had to be limited or modified because of surgical or medical contraindications, or cases that they had researched themselves.

Subjective and objective feedback and evaluation from clinical instructors indicated that our students performed at or above the instructors' level of expectation for junior-year students completing a first affiliation. All 92 students participating in this study received satisfactory or superior overall performance ratings during their first affiliations. Although numerous factors obviously contributed to the students' clinical performance, Mock Clinic was one of those factors for our students. Some of the areas that were consistently identified as strong areas for our students during their first clinical affiliation included note writing and documentation, evaluation skills, and self-assessment skills.

Because the program in physical therapy at GVSU has included Mock Clinic in the curriculum since the beginning of the program, we cannot evaluate or compare the early clinical performance of students who participated in Mock Clinic with that of students who did not participate in Mock Clinic. This could be a question for future study.

Informal interviews of the faculty members of the GVSU Program in Physical Therapy indicate that they believe that Mock Clinic is a valuable commitment of curricular time and that it offers the following benefits:

1. Provides a viable alternative to early part-time or shorter full-time clinical affiliations.
2. Helps students integrate, apply, and retain didactic material.
3. Gives faculty the opportunity to observe affective, cognitive, and psychomotor skills of students simultaneously, allowing early identification and management of potential clinical problems.
4. Enhances student preparedness for, and performance during, initial clinical affiliations.

Based on the success of the orthopedic Mock Clinic, the faculty decided to integrate Mock Clinic experiences into laboratories of other appropriate courses in the curriculum, and with the implementation of the master's degree entry-level curriculum, we plan to offer an additional neurologic Mock Clinic course.

DISCUSSION

Students' evaluations of Mock Clinic before and after their first clinical affiliation indicated a very positive response to the Mock Clinic experience in general. From the students' perspective, the strongest areas of gain from Mock Clinic were problem-solving skills, evaluation skills and interpretation, and self-assessment and peer-evaluation skills. Although the great majority of students reported that Mock Clinic had improved their performance in all areas addressed in the evaluation, less improvement was noted in treatment planning and application, adjusting to changes in patient status or environment, and understanding the patient in the health care system. Several reasons for these perceptions can be proposed. As constraints were placed on students in Mock Clinic to complete evaluations and treatments in more clinically realistic time frames, the treatment component of patient care sometimes suffered. Although student physical therapists may have completed their evaluation and designed a treatment program for a patient, they may have had only 10 to 15 minutes to then carry out their treatment program in some cases. As student evaluation skills improved, this became less of a problem. Because cases progressed from simple to complex, it was not until the latter part of the semester that students were presented with significant changes in patient status during treatment (eg, angina, stumbling during gait training) to which they had to adjust. The relatively small exposure to these kinds of situations probably diminished the students' feeling of significant improvement in this area. It may be beneficial to introduce complex cases slightly earlier in Mock Clinic. Perhaps the lack of past experience with actual patients limited students' perception of how well they understood the patient in the health care system. Nonetheless, student patient preparation and role-playing in Mock Clinic became a valued learning experience for the instructor and the students. It served as a time to review a variety of materials. For example, in the case depicted in Figure 4, the student patients needed to 1) know the muscles innervated by the common peroneal nerve, 2) mimic their actions and manual muscle testing grades, and 3) describe and mimic the type of gait pattern that might be seen in such a patient.

The overall small variability between percentages of student responses to each questionnaire item preaffiliation and postaffiliation is interesting, given the emphasis often placed on clinical affiliations as the "final integrator" by students, clinicians, and faculty. Because of this emphasis, I expected postaffiliation responses to be much less positive than preaffiliation responses to questions regarding Mock Clinic. Even though the trend was toward slightly less-positive postaffiliation responses on most items, I interpreted the relatively small variability between preaffiliation and postaffiliation scores as another indication of the effectiveness of Mock Clinic in preparing students for clinical affiliations.

Many of the strengths and weaknesses of Mock Clinic identified and described by Sanders and Ruvulo remained in our program even with the modified design.[1] Particular strengths are 1) the relatively low-risk environment (ie, a credit-no credit course, no potential harm to patients as a result of a misjudgment) that fosters questioning, problem solving, and creativity; 2) the group discussions reviewing a variety of patient care approaches to the same patient; and 3) the developing and fostering of self-assessment skills through instruction and videotaping. Previously described weaknesses, such as students' difficulty with role-playing and the faculty time commitment, also existed with our Mock Clinic.[1] We addressed the problems with role-playing by requiring the student physical therapists to wear clinical attire (eg, laboratory jackets) with surprisingly positive results. Role-playing also improved significantly when students researched their own cases and came to Mock Clinic prepared and with appropriate props. Although Mock Clinic was originally described with fewer students participating at any time,[1] we found clinic sessions to be satisfactory with up to eight student pairs and a faculty-to-student ratio of one to eight (or one faculty member to four student pairs). Our laboratory space easily allows this number of students to participate and is similar to many physical therapy departments. The time commitment of the course coordinator, however, is 98 hours of actual classroom time and approximately 40 hours of preparation and videotape-reviewing time for the semester. The second laboratory instructor must spend 66 hours in the classroom during clinics and approximately 20 hours of preparation time for the semester.

The primary advantages of Mock Clinic as perceived by the faculty are discussed in the Results section. Our Mock Clinic experience and perceptions mirror the perceptions of the faculty members at the University of Wisconsin-La Crosse regarding their Mock Clinic experience.[1] Several other advantages of Mock Clinic as a component of clinical education in the program have been identified. First, because of the curriculum design and the use of Mock Clinic, performance objectives for students on their first clinical affiliation (working with defined populations) can be set at higher levels than might normally be set for a junior-year student completing an initial clinical experience. For example, we expect students during the orthopedic affiliation to manage adult or pediatric patients with orthopedic or rheumatologic disorders. This includes completing evaluations, planning and implementing all components of treatment programs, referring patients to other services or professionals, discharging patients when appropriate, and documenting all aspects of patient care. Student preparation for clinical affiliations and these higher-level performance objectives have increased and improved the acceptance of first-rotation students by clinical facilities. We believe that our curriculum design and Mock Clinic have enabled us to continue placing first-rotation students in traditional early clinical affiliation settings (eg, acute-care general hospitals) but has also allowed us to use other nontraditional sites (eg, specialty private practice or outpatient offices, industrial clinics, home health agencies) for early clinical affiliations. Clinical faculty in the latter sites (previously considered advanced level or specialty experiences) are willing to accept our students based on a review of the curriculum (including Mock Clinic). These clinicians have been satisfied with students' performance even at the beginning level.

CONCLUSION

In summary, response to the use of Mock Clinic in our curriculum by students, faculty, and clinicians has been overwhelmingly positive. As the students complete senior-level affiliations and provide feedback on the strengths and weaknesses of their academic preparation, they continue to consistently identify Mock Clinic as a strength of the GVSU Program in Physical Therapy. The faculty members strongly believe that Mock Clinic offers a curricular alternative for enhancing student preparedness for clinical affiliations and is an extremely valuable commitment of faculty time and curricular hours.

ACKNOWLEDGMENT

I thank Barbara Sanders, MS, for her advice and consultation when Mock Clinic was first being developed at GVSU.

REFERENCES

1. Sanders BR, Ruvulo J: Mock clinic: An approach to clinical education. Phys Ther 61:1163–1167, 1981

2. Ford CW, Morgan MK: Teaching in the Health Professions. St. Louis, MO, C V Mosby Co, 1976, pp 219–220

3. Ford CW (ed): Clinical Education for the Allied Health Professions. St. Louis, MO, C V Mosby Co, 1978, pp 145–152

4. Barrows HS: Simulated Patients—The Development and Use of a New Technique in Medical Education. Springfield, IL, Charles C Thomas, Publisher, 1971, pp 2–15

5. Maatsch JL, Gordon M: Assessment through simulations. In Morgan MK, Ford CW (eds): Evaluating Clinical Competence in the Health Professions. St. Louis, MO, C V Mosby Co, 1978, pp 123–131

6. Fuhrmann BS, Weissburg M: Self-assessment. In Morgan MK, Ford CW (eds): Evaluating Clinical Competence in the Health Professions. St. Louis, MO, C V Mosby Co, 1978, pp 137–140

7. May BJ, Newman J: Developing competence in problem solving—A Behavioral Model. Phys Ther 60:1140–1145, 1980

8. Sanford TL: The therapist of the 21st century—Medical science curriculum. Phys Ther Education, 1984, vol 29, pp 8–11

9. Kondela PM, Darnell RE: Receptivity to full-time early clinical education experience. Phys Ther 61:1168–1172, 1981

10. Perry JF: A model for designing clinical education. Phys Ther 61:1427–1432, 1981

11. Competency Assessment Report. Detroit, MI, Detroit Area Clinical Educators Forum, 1982

Appendix
Mock Clinic Course Evaluation Form

Course Evaluation
P.T. 321
Clinical Education I—Mock Clinic

Please rate the following statements relating to mock clinic on the following scale:
1 = strongly agree, 2 = agree, 3 = indifferent, 4 = disagree, 5 = strongly disagree

CHECK ONE:

Mock Clinic:

	1	2	3	4	5
1) Increased my understanding of basic clinical problem solving processes.					
2) Improved my skills in clinical problem solving.					
3) Improved my verbal and non-verbal patient communication skills.					
4) Improved my understanding of the SOAP note format.					
5) Improved my SOAP note writing.					
6) Improved my performance of clinical evaluation skills.					
7) Improved my interpretation of the information gained through patient evaluation.					
8) Improved my treatment *planning* and design skills.					
9) Improved my treatment skills in the following areas:					
a) Application of modalities					
b) Therapeutic exercise					
c) Transfer training					
d) Gait training					
e) Use of body mechanics					
f) Preparation of treatment area					
g) Preparation of patient for treatment					
10) Improved my ability to adjust to changes in the environment or patient status.					
11) Improved my ability to constructively assess the performance of my peers.					
12) Improved my ability to assess my own performance.					
13) Improved my understanding of the *patient* in the health care system.					
14) Will have a positive impact on my clinical performance in Clinical Education II.					
15) Will *not* affect my performance in Clinical Education II.					

Of all the experiences in mock clinic please list the 2 cases or activities from which you feel you learned the most:

Evaluation and Research

"Research is a high-hat word that scares a lot of people. It needn't. It is nothing but a state of mind—a friendly, welcoming attitude toward change. It is the problem-solving mind as contrasted with the let-well-enough-alone mind. It is the composer mind instead of a fiddler mind. It is the tomorrow mind instead of the yesterday mind."

Charles Franklin Kettering

Methods of
Evaluation
of Student
Competence

Physical Therapy Competencies in Clinical Education

JOAN C. NETHERY, MA

General principles for using the physical therapy competencies in clinical education are presented. Several systems for using the competencies in a physical therapy internship curriculum are described.

Key Words: *Clinical education, Physical therapy.*

Uses of the physical therapy competencies have been discussed in several publications.[1-3] The physical therapy staff at University Hospitals of Cleveland has used the competencies in various aspects of education and evaluation during the past three years. The greatest use of the competencies has been in our clinical education curriculum for physical therapy internship.

PRINCIPLES

In order to use the competencies in clinical education effectively, the clinical instructor must have a basic understanding of the competencies. The clinical instructor also must be familiar with general principles for application of the competencies.

The physical therapy competencies are designed to describe the work activities of the profession and the specific standards of performance that must be met. The use of the competencies for education in the clinical setting—the site of professional practice—is, therefore, logical.

Figure 1 depicts a competency box diagram. All competencies have several levels of tasks as represented by boxes. The competency is stated in the single box at the top of the diagram. The boxes directly beneath the top box are called the Task Level 1 boxes. These Task Level 1 boxes identify the component skills and knowledge required to achieve the competency. Boxes beneath these component boxes contain a further breakdown of the prerequisite knowledge and skills required to perform each task. The upper level boxes of the competency, especially the Task Level 1 component boxes, contain information that is important in clinical education. These upper level boxes specify knowledge and skills directly related to clinical practice. The lower level boxes specify knowledge and skills learned prior to participating in clinical education or practice.

Each competency statement is a performance objective with standards of performance represented. Each competency statement can also be an educational objective with the standards of performance serving as behavioral criteria. As with all educational objectives, the competencies and their standards must be shared with the student to let him know what performance responses are expected.

Clinical instructors can use the competencies for planning learning experiences and for assessing the student's performance. In planning learning experiences, the clinical instructor must determine the starting level for each student. Once the student's starting level is determined for a competency, the clinical instructor can plan experiences to enable the student to progress upward in the diagram toward achieving a total clinical performance, as represented by the top box. Knowledge and skills on the competency diagram are developed from bottom to top and from left to right, and therefore, the competency statements provide guidance regarding content and sequence of learning experiences. The competencies also provide standards regarding evaluation of the various clinical performances. In some cases, the standards need to be further defined. Clinical educators can expand the definitions of the standards based on the needs, requirements, and resources of their facilities. In evaluating the student's performance, the clinical instructor starts at the top box. If the student is able to meet the standards of the competency statement, no further evaluation is necessary. If the student is unable to meet the standards of the competency statement, the instructor must analyze each component, working down and from right to left through the boxes to identify areas of deficiency. Identified areas of deficiency then become the foci for subsequent learning experiences.

Miss Nethery is Assistant Director, Department of Physical Therapy, University Hospitals of Cleveland, Cleveland, OH 44106 (USA).

This article is adapted from a paper presented at the APTA Reconvened Meeting, HI, 1978, and from presentations at clinical faculty seminars at Cleveland State University, Cleveland, OH, and the University of Wisconsin, Madison, WI.

This article was submitted January 28, 1980, and accepted March 17, 1981.

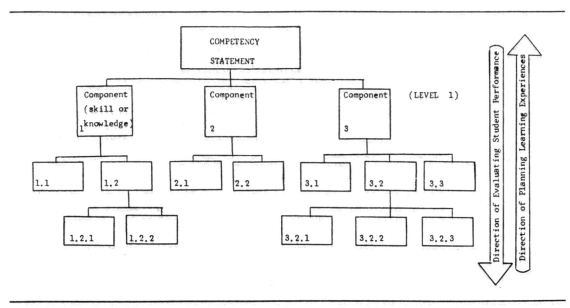

Fig. 1. Competency box diagram.

In other words, when the competencies are used in clinical education, the clinical educators have a system for planning learning experiences based on student needs, the student knows what is expected of him, and the student is evaluated on his ability to meet specified criteria in a standardized manner.

APPLICATION

Background

The physical therapy internship curriculum at University Hospitals of Cleveland was developed in 1971. Internship at our facility is full-time clinical education following successful completion of all academic coursework required for entry level. Interns spend an average of 12 weeks at our facility. Ten weeks is the minimum period of internship; there is no maximum. Within a given framework, interns select the physical therapy divisions in which they desire to have clinical education experience as well as the amount of time they will spend in each of the five divisions (pediatrics, chronic illness, respiratory, general medicine and surgery, and outpatient). Interns are evaluated formally three times during each rotation: during the first three days for the initial evaluation, at the midpoint of a rotation, and at the end of the rotation. A final composite narrative report is sent to the academic program faculty. School forms are not used for recording evaluations or submitting reports to the school, but the forms are reviewed to identify content areas; this is done to ensure that schools receive the information they need. Our curriculum includes a set of 25 departmental education objectives with criteria.

The objectives are used for evaluating intern performance throughout the division rotations. Baseline, initial evaluation data are used to determine the intern's starting level and to plan pertinent learning experiences. Midpoint and final evaluations are performed to redefine the level of the intern and plan additional learning experiences and to identify areas of improved performance. Informal evaluations with timely feedback are performed regularly. Interns play an active role in determining the content and sequence of their learning experiences including selecting the educational objectives on which they wish to focus. Prior to incorporating the competencies into our clinical education program, interns were required to develop independence in 10 particular objectives that were specified as "basic" to the curriculum. Improved performance was required on other objectives selected. A rating system was developed to define the intern's quality of performance on the objectives and their criteria. In brief, the performance ratings are

0   Intern is unable to perform or prefers not to perform.

I   Intern performs satisfactorily with assistance.

II   Intern performs satisfactorily with guidance or supervision.

III   Intern performs independently.

The competency text, *Competencies in Physical Therapy: An Analysis of Practice*,[1] provided a new resource related to clinical practice. Although we were satisfied with our existing curriculum and our strategy for teaching and evaluating interns, this new resource enabled us to develop a more clearly defined and objective means for evaluating performance.

Initial Evaluation
Competency 2.1.1. Conduct a Gross Evaluation

I

1/ II	2/ II	3/ I	4/ I	5/ II	6/ II	7/ II	8/II
1.1/II	2.1/II	3.1/I	4.1/I	5.1/II	6.1/NA	7.1/II	
1.2/II	2.2/II	3.2/II	4.2/I	5.2/II	6.2/II	7.2/II	
			4.3/II	5.3/II	6.3/II	7.3/NA	
			4.4/III	5.4/II	6.4/II	7.4/NA	
				5.5/II			
				5.6/II			

Midterm Evaluation
Competency 2.1.1. Conduct a Gross Evaluation

II

1/ III	2/ III	3/ II	4/ III	5/ III	6/ III	7/ III	8/III
1.1/II	2.1/III	3.1/II	4.1/III	5.1/III	6.1/NA	7.1/III	
1.2/III	2.2/III	3.2/III	4.2/III	5.2/III	6.2/III	7.2/III	
			4.3/III	5.3/III	6.3/III	7.3/III	
			4.4/III	5.4/III	6.4/II	7.4/NA	
				5.5/III			
				5.6/III			

Fig. 2. *Physical therapist intern evaluation—General medicine and surgery division.*

Competencies in Physical Therapy, commonly referred to as the "Red Book," was purchased for our department in 1977. At a continuing education session, the staff was introduced to the competencies and the use of the "Red Book." Following the educational session, the physical therapists of each treatment division were asked to review and revise the systems for determining satisfactory performance of interns in their division. Use of the competency statements was encouraged.

Since entry level remains undefined for the competencies, it was not to be assumed that competence at entry level would require independent performance, according to the standards, for each competency statement. It was necessary to determine: 1) which competency statements are relevant to clinical practice at our facility, 2) which competency statements appear pertinent to entry level practice, and 3) what performance rating (ie, independent, supervised, assisted) should be required for satisfactory intern performance.

Each of the five physical therapy divisions developed new systems: all of the systems function within our previously established clinical education curriculum for internship, and all use the described rating system to evaluate intern performance.

The Systems

The pediatric and respiratory divisions chose to develop systems requiring interns to achieve specified

performance ratings on various departmental educational objectives and their criteria. The "Red Book" competency statements are not a required part of the system. They supplement the system and are an optional resource when dealing with problem areas. For example, if an intern has difficulty with the departmental basic educational objective, "Planning an effective treatment program," the "Red Book" competency statement, "Designing a physical therapy plan of care," can be used to help identify problems. The evaluation results, from both the departmental objective and the competency statement, can be used to plan learning experiences that help resolve identified problems. Having the competency statements for a reference aids in communication, facilitates problem resolution, and increases objectivity.

The general medicine and surgery (GM&S) division developed a system using 11 of the "Red Book" competencies. The departmental educational objectives are used to supplement the competencies. Interns selecting a GM&S division rotation must achieve a designated performance rating on each of the 11 competencies in order to pass. Interns are introduced to the competencies and perform self assessment on their performance at midpoint and final evaluation times. During the formal evaluation sessions for midpoint and final evaluations, the self assessment and the instructor assessment of intern performance are compared and discussed. Forms developed from the "Red Book" Self-Assessment Recording Sheets are used or the evaluations are handwritten in diagram fashion. Figure 2 presents a sample portion of a physical therapy intern evaluation from the GM&S division. The competency 2.1.1., "Conduct a gross evaluation," is demonstrated. The number at the top of the diagram indicates the overall performance rating for the competency. The remainder of the diagram pertains to the two upper levels of boxes for the competency. The Task Level 1 boxes are identified by the single number to the left of the diagonal slash. The Task Level 2 boxes, breakdown boxes of the Task Level 1 component boxes, are identified by two numbers to the left of the diagonal slash. The Roman numerals to the right of the diagonal slashes indicate the intern performance ratings for each of the labeled boxes. The figure describes that the intern initially performed competency 2.1.1. with assistance (performance rating I) and progressed by midpoint evaluation to independent performance (rating III) except for component box 3. Specific areas of improvement are easily identified as are areas needing additional improvement. The midpoint rotation difficulty in component box 3 can be immediately related to box 3.1, thus providing the focus for subsequent learning experiences.

The system developed for the outpatient and chronic illness divisions is represented by Figure 3, a sample portion of a physical therapist intern evaluation form from the outpatient division. The division staff studied the "Red Book" competencies and selected those pertinent to their divisions. The staff then determined that many of the competencies could be combined or condensed for use in their system. For example, "Red Book" competencies 2.2.1., "Design a physical therapy plan of care," and 2.2.2., "Modify physical therapy goals or plan," were combined to become outpatient/chronic illness physical therapy division competency 1.2.: Treatment design, planning, and modification with subareas 1.2.1.: Design and 1.2.2.: Modify. The staff from the outpatient and chronic illness divisions agreed that they could effectively evaluate the intern's performance in these areas

by focusing on certain content areas of the "Red Book" competency statements rather than the competencies in their entirety. Specific content areas were identified (each considered to be critical to satisfactory performance) and standards were defined.

In this system, as in the others, interns were evaluated using the department performance rating scale of 0 to III. To pass an outpatient division or a chronic illness division rotation, interns must have performed with a specified rating for each competency within the division system. Figure 3 illustrates the progress made by a physical therapy intern during his outpatient division rotation. During that rotation, the information from the evaluations was used to identify the intern's areas of need or improvement and to plan relevant learning experiences.

With both the GM&S division and the outpatient/chronic illness division systems, departmental objectives must be incorporated to give the intern documented feedback in areas not dealt with specifically in the "Red Book." Areas requiring regular use of the departmental objectives include communication skills, effective use of time, personal integrity, and appreciation of the coordinated efforts of health professionals.

DISCUSSION

The systems described demonstrate several ways of using the "Red Book" competencies in clinical education. These systems are distinctly different although they have similarities and incorporate common factors such as the departmental educational objectives and the performance rating scale. When the systems were implemented, we were concerned that interns and staff might have difficulty accepting and working with the different systems. Surprisingly, interns had no complaints and reported no problems. Their descriptions of the systems were positive and included words such as "helpful," "objective," and "comfortable." They also expressed appreciation for exposure

1.2. Treatment Design, Planning and Modification

			Levels of Intern Performance		
			Initial	Mid	Final
1.2.1.	Design				
	criterion 1.		II	III	III
	criterion 2.		II	II	III
	criterion 3.		I	III	III
	criterion 4.		II	III	III
	criterion 5.		II	III	III
1.2.2.	Modify				
	criterion 1.		0	II	III
	criterion 2.		0	I	II
	criterion 3.		0	III	III

Fig. 3. Physical therapist intern evaluation—Outpatient division.

to and experience in use of the competencies. Physical therapists serving as clinical instructors felt that the systems using the competencies required more time to document performance than systems not using the competencies, but that the information obtained was more specific.

Physical therapists must recognize that each clinical educator has a responsibility to the community and to the profession to prepare competent individuals to enter physical therapy practice. This is especially critical while competency-based testing is not used as part of the licensure procedure. Each clinical educator is placed in the position of preparing students to enter

practice and determining their competence in this capacity. The use of the physical therapy competencies for planning clinical education learning experiences and evaluating physical therapy student performance is one means to achieve this goal.

REFERENCES

1. Competencies in Physical Therapy: An Analysis of Practice, ed 1. San Diego, CA, Courseware, Inc, 1977
2. Davis CM, Anderson MJ, Jagger D: Competency: The what, why, and how of it. Phys Ther 59:1088–1094, 1979
3. Nethery JC: Physical therapy competencies: An overview. The Pyramid 9:1–6, 1979

Competency Based Evaluation of Student Performance

Bella J. May, Ed.D.

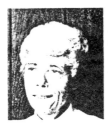

Bella J. May is Professor and Chairperson, Department of Physical Therapy, School of Allied Health Sciences, Medical College of Georgia, Augusta, Georgia 30901.

Abstract: Criterion referenced evaluation instruments are used to determine student achievement in a competency based educational system. The general concepts underlying competency based education and evaluation are described and the method used to implement these concepts in the Department of Physical Therapy of the Medical College of Georgia are outlined. Student performance is evaluated against external criteria and not against each other. A variety of instruments are used to determine if students meet entry level requirements for practice.

Competency based education has been a popular topic in recent years, but little has been said about the evaluation of student achievement in a competency based program. Traditionally, curricula have been organized around the subject matter concepts to be acquired and tasks

Adapted from a paper presented at the Tenth Annual Meeting of the American Society of Allied Health Professions, November 1977.

to be performed. Faculty have been concerned with covering the material and achievement has been measured through subject matter oriented normative evaluations, where student scores are compared to each other. In a normative system, class averages are computed and grades are assigned along the normal distribution curve. Graduates of many programs are evaluated for purposes of licensure in a similar subject matter oriented normative manner. The results of such evaluations indicate only how any one student's score compares to the score of other students who take the same examination at a similar time. The score does not indicate how competent a student may be in relation to the demands of the profession. Such examinations also do not indicate whether or not a student can utilize the subject matter concepts that have been retained.

In the Department of Physical Therapy of the Medical College of Georgia we have been involved in competency based education and evaluation since 1971. We currently have a baccalaureate program to prepare individuals to meet entry level competencies as physical therapists and an associate degree program to prepare individuals to meet entry level competencies as physical therapist assistants. Program objectives reflect terminal entry level competencies; unit and course objectives reflect the enabling competencies necessary to reach the terminal competencies. Student performance is evaluated through criterion referenced examinations where performance is measured against the stated standard or criteria to be achieved.[1]

GENERAL CONCEPTS

The concepts underlying competency based education and criterion referenced measurement can be simple or complex, depending on one's approach to educational theory and practice. In this paper a flexible and pragmatic approach to criterion referenced measurement used in two allied health educational programs will be described. It should be recognized at the outset that there is more flexibility in the application of educational theory to student evaluation in individual educational curriculum as compared to its application to the licensing of practitioners. While the competency based educational programs themselves will not be described, it is important to simply note that competency based education is a system of education based on the specification of what constitutes competency in a given profession. The emphasis is on achievement of desired competencies, and the psychological viewpoint is that learning is enhanced if the student is actively involved in the learning experiences. The goal of the educational endeavor is to have at least 90% of the students achieve 90% of the competencies 90% of the time, and the learning experiences are designed to that end.[2]

In planning and implementing instructional events, it is important to delineate between competencies and tasks. While the differentiation may become hazy at times, competency statements reflect the total performance, including the cognitive, affective and psychomotor aspects applicable, while a task statement usually reflects only one part of the performance.

In a competency based system, criterion referenced evaluation instruments are used to determine student achievement. Mager stated: "The measurement of instructional success is accomplished mainly through the development of situations or test items that precisely match each objective in scope and intent."[3] Criterion referenced evaluation instruments are developed from the stated competencies to be attained. External criteria for acceptable performance are established, and student performance is evaluated against such external criteria, not in comparison to the performance of other students. Criteria are based on minimally acceptable levels of performance; this seems appropriate in programs where selective admission procedures are used to determine who will be allowed to enroll.

DEVELOPING TERMINAL AND ENABLING COMPETENCIES

The first step in the establishment of a competency based educational program is the development of the terminal competencies. The process is both difficult and time consuming. Each educational program should determine for itself the competencies it wants its graduates to exhibit at the completion of the program.

Very broadly, at the Medical College of Georgia, we believe that the physical therapist should be able to analyze and solve problems in a wide range of areas, treat many different patients, administer a department, teach patients and families, understand the results of research in the field and communicate effectively with others. Physical therapist assistants should be able to apply selected procedures, communicate effectively, assist the physical therapist in many different situations and communicate effectively. Our terminal competencies were derived following careful study of available materials, conferences with clinical instructors and review of accreditation requirements. Competencies do not only reflect current practice, but anticipate future practice. In fast changing allied health fields, it is our belief that the educational program must be ahead of practice if graduates are to be contributors to improvement in health care.

In developing our terminal competencies for each program, we did not rely on the minimal requirements of state licensure, since the purpose of licensing is to identify individuals who are not competent to practice. Rather, we prepare our graduates for the highest possible competency level, confident that in this manner, they will meet the minimal levels established in different states.

While there is always some question regarding what constitutes entry level for a profession, the judgment of both the didactic and clinical faculty is a reliable source for this determination. In establishing terminal competencies, care must be taken not to make them so specific that the job of planning instructional events becomes restricted. Terminal competencies may be stated in the form of terminal program objectives which represent all areas of function. In our department they are reviewed regularly to insure continued relevancy.

After the terminal competencies in the form of terminal behavioral objectives are specified, the enabling competencies or steps to the attainment of the final objectives must be identified. These are usually the unit or course objectives for the different learning experiences in the curriculum and are the parts that eventually compose a terminal competency. For example, a terminal objective in our baccalaureate program specifies that the physical therapist should be able to select and apply appropriate physical therapy evaluation procedures for any patient referred for treatment. The steps to the attainment of this competency might include:

1. Define the function of specified evaluation procedures.
2. Define the effect on human function of a disease process.
3. Apply specified evaluation procedures on a fellow student in a safe and effective manner.
4. Apply specified evaluation procedures on a specified patient.
5. Differentiate between the functional effects of different disease processes.
6. Compare and contrast the validity of a number of evaluation procedures to determine the physical therapy needs of patients with specified disability.
7. Exhibit an awareness of the varying reactions of patients of different ages to the physical therapy evaluation.
8. Analyze the value and limitations of specified evaluation procedures in determining the physical therapy needs of patients with a wide variety of disabilities.
9. Exhibit the ability to communicate the purpose of different evaluation procedures.

The list is only illustrative and not exhaustive of all enabling objectives necessary for the attainment of the terminal competency. One could make a more detailed list, but this would only be necessary if such details were helpful guides for the instructor in the development of the learning experiences. In our department, we have developed behavioral objectives from the cognitive, affective and psychomotor domain for each course and integrated unit in our curricula. The objectives become the guides from which the instructors develop the learning experiences and the evaluation instruments.

ESTABLISHING PERFORMANCE LEVELS

Before designing a criterion referenced evaluation instrument one must establish the minimal acceptable level of performance. This may be the most difficult part of the process, for there are few guidelines to follow. In our program we decided not to adopt the generally accepted level of 90%, since we did not believe it was appropriate in a setting where the student could not be given all the time necessary to achieve at that level. Traditional competency based education provides the student as much time as necessary to attain the desired competencies. Under these conditions, a 90% achievement level is realistic. However, such a system is not always financially feasible and would not be possible in a department with limited resources and faculty.

After much discussion and examination of alternatives, we established a 75% performance level for all nondirect patient care units and courses such as anatomy, physiology and administration, and an 80% performance level for all other units. Students must make either 75 or 80% correct responses in all evaluations.

Since both of our curricula are developed in a sequential pattern of integrated problem solving units, each student must meet the minimal acceptable level of performance in one unit before being allowed to progress to the next.[4] Students who do not meet minimal acceptable levels of performance in any one evaluation are given remedial work and retested. If a student does not achieve mastery level in a total unit, he may be given remedial work or may repeat the total unit the following year.

Since we use a selective admission process, it is our intent to graduate all we admit. If a student cannot achieve mastery at the pace of the curriculum, we develop an individualized program at a slower pace to the extent possible. The goal is to have each student function at the minimally acceptable level, and within reason, the length of time it takes can be modified.

In some instances, we have been able to allow students to work through the units designed for nondirect patient care competencies separately from those related to direct patient care activities. The design of our curriculum allows for this degree of flexibility.[4] While not ideal, it does ease the burden on the student who cannot achieve at the pace of the rest of the class. To date, we have had three students who have taken three years to complete the last two years of the baccalaureate curriculum and only three students have been dropped for academic reasons. Some students have required additional help between units to reach mastery level. The design of the unit system assists with this activity. All evaluation instruments are criterion referenced and developed from the objectives that specify the competencies to be achieved.

SELECTING AND DESIGNING EVALUATION INSTRUMENTS

Evaluation instruments in a criterion referenced system may be of the same type as any other instrument and include paper and pencil tests, practical performance evaluations, simulations, orals or a combination. Criterion refer-

enced evaluations must be valid, internally consistent and clearly delineated. Criterion referenced tests gather their meaning from connection to the external criteria, therefore, variability is immaterial. One may gather useful information from item analysis if it is used judiciously. A non-discriminating item may be a good item if it reflects an important aspect of the criterion. Positively discriminating items indicate to the instructor where instructional event needs to be improved, while negatively discriminating items usually reflect a flaw in the item itself or in the learning activities.[5]

The difference between criterion referenced tests and other tests lies in the outlook of the tester, the relation of the test items to the objectives and the scoring. Items in criterion referenced tests are developed directly from the stated outcomes of the learning activities, and each student's score reflects the extent to which that student's performance matches the desired performance. There is no need to compare student scores or compute class averages. The instructional event can be assumed to be successful if all or most of the students exceed the minimal acceptable level of performance. If more than 10% of the students fail to achieve the desired level, then the faculty needs to review the learning activities.

The following general guidelines may be helpful in developing criterion referenced examinations:

1. "The test items should call for the same principal performance specified in the objectives."[6] Asking a student to list muscle attachment does not indicate if that student can solve a biomechanical motion problem.
2. "The indicator behavior called for in the test items should be congruent with the ability of the learner."[6] Questions should be asked in a simple straightforward manner.
3. "Any condition of performance implicitly or explicitly specified in the objective should be incor-

porated in the test item."[6] If your objective calls for the student to select the appropriate modality for a patient with a learning disability, don't evaluate him with an adult hemiplegic.

4. "Test items should cover the complete class of behaviors specified in the objectives."[6] This may require both performance and paper and pencil tests if the objectives for a particular unit call for the student to perform a task, describe a phenomenon, analyze a problem and exhibit an appreciation of different points of view.

A number of evaluative instruments may be used in any course or unit. Some examinations may cover only a few of the objectives. However, students should be evaluated on all objectives when all examinations for a unit are considered; comprehensive final examinations may serve that purpose. Each item is developed in relation to the relative weight of each objective in both importance and time spent in the instructional events. It is not necessary to write an individual item for each objective; some items may reflect the behaviors required in several objectives.

A variety of paper and pencil instruments are available to the creative test writer. To determine if students can select appropriate evaluative instruments to determine the needs of a particular patient, one can develop a simulated patient situation and simply ask the student what evaluative instruments would be used in this instance. The student's thinking processes can be explored if the student is asked to justify the selection of the evaluative tools rather than just list them.

Affective objectives are more difficult to evaluate. However, a series of questions asking the student to respond to patient comments may provide some data to determine if the student can interpret the emotional state of a given patient.

In addition to the paper and pencil tests, practical examinations are a useful tool in allied health and are an effective method of determining achievement of performance objectives. Practical examinations may be used to evaluate attainment of objectives from the cognitive and affective as well as the psychomotor domain by structuring the problem to be solved by the student. Videotaping practical examinations provides an added dimension as the student can evaluate his own performance and the tape can be used as a learning tool.

Criterion referenced examinations are not limited to the more traditional methods. In one of our courses, an objective specified that the student should be able to plan, implement and evaluate an inservice education session. Achievement of that objective is assessed by having the student plan, implement and evaluate an inservice education session for a local clinical facility.

In one of our interdisciplinary courses on the health care environment an objective states: "The student should be able to function as a collaborative member of a team according to the criteria established by the group." In this unit the students themselves establish the criteria by which they will determine if the individual group member has met the competency. At the end of the unit they evaluate themselves and each other, and the results of this evaluation are used in determining the unit grade. In this same course, students are expected to learn about the health care system in a case study method. Their attainment of the competencies is evaluated through a group presentation of their case study. As long as definitive criteria for performance are outlined, the method of evaluation can be as creative as necessary.

ASSIGNING GRADES

The final step is to assign a grade to the student at the completion of the unit. Ideally, in a competency based educational program, there should be no grades, only a determination of achievement of competencies. In our university this is allowed only for clinical education, and we must assign letter grades for each course in the curriculum. To meet the demands of our university, we have developed a rather arbitrary system of assigning grades to our students. In those units where students must achieve a 75% level, grades are assigned as follows: A = 100 to 92%; B = 91 to 83%; C = 82 to 75%; and below 75% is failing. For those units where students must achieve an 80% mastery level, the bottom of the C range is raised and the rest of the scale remains the same: A = 100 to 92%; B = 91 to 83%; C = 82 to 80%; and below 80% is failing. We do not give the grade of D.

In this system it is possible for all students to earn the grade of A. Since we are interested in the achievement of competencies based on external standards, we would be happy to have all students perform above 91%.

DISCUSSION AND SUMMARY

It is our belief that competency based educational programs with achievement measured through criterion referenced evaluations are most appropriate for allied health education at all levels. It has been our experience that the system encourages the development of relevant learning experiences aimed at helping the student acquire the necessary competencies for practice. The evaluations reflect the degree to which the student has achieved the competencies and whether or not he meets entry level standards for practice. The system tends to actively involve the student in the learning experiences, since objectives are shared prior to the start of a unit. The system also tends to diminish competition between students and foster team work, since students are no longer competing for grades. Motivation becomes internalized as the student knows where performance must be improved.

In a competency based educational program, the individual is variable to the extent that one can individualize instruction; time is variable to the degree that one can give each student as much time as necessary to attain the competencies; and the instructional process is variable to the extent that one can manipulate the educational activities. But, the product is constant in that the minimal acceptable level of performance is specified.

The system has been in operation in our department for the past six years, and we have found it to be a clear and relevant method of determining student achievement and if our graduates do indeed meet the desired competencies for practice.

REFERENCES

1. May BJ: Evaluation in a competency based educational system. Phys Ther 57:28-33, 1977.
2. Sanders JR, Murray SL: Alternatives for achievement testing. Educ Tech, March 1976, pp 17-23.
3. Mager RF: Measuring Instructional Intent. Belmont, California, Fearon Publishers, 1973.
4. May BJ: An integrated problem solving curriculum design for physical therapy education. Phys Ther 57:807-813, 1977.
5. Popham WJ: Criterion Referenced Measurement. Englewood Cliffs, New Jersey, Educational Technology Publications, 1971.
6. Woodley KK: Matching Test Items to Behavioral Objectives, handout, Educational Technology Conference Workshop on Competency Based Evaluation, New York, 1973.

A Method of Developing and Evaluating a Clinical Performance Program for Physical Therapy Interns

MARCIA L. WIGHTMAN, BS,
and **LOIS M. WELLOCK, PhD**

A method used by interns and supervisors in developing and evaluating a clinical performance program during a 6-week internship in the Division of Physical Therapy at the University of Michigan Medical Center is presented. This method required a statement of educational resources available, establishment of criteria for judging acceptable performance, statement by the intern of his educational objectives, negotiation of a written contract, and maintenance of a log. The 32 participants thought that this was a rational and acceptable program and stated that they would, if given a choice, elect to follow the same procedure again.

A method of developing and evaluating a clinical performance program with physical therapy interns was designed to establish a system for clinical education in keeping with sound learning principles. Learning experiences are too often those of convenience. The intern may be assigned to a physical therapist on the medical or chest service and is expected to show great enthusiasm in his work and to develop proficiency in the treatment of such patients. Maybe the intern's interests are elsewhere, and his main concern is to please the supervisor, achieve a satisfactory performance report, and to be assigned to that part of physical therapy which is of real interest to him. Such experiences are frustrating to all concerned—the student, the supervisor, the academic faculty, and the patient.

If the internship is to have maximum meaning to the intern, he must view the learning experience as realistic, achievable, and useful. The learning will be effective not in terms of how the supervisor views the experience offered but in terms of how the intern perceives the situation. By the time the full-time internship is available, the intern has preconceived ideas of what his needs are in order to acquire the knowledge and skill necessary to become an effective physical therapist. Learning "initiated by need and purpose is likely to be motivated by its own incompleteness."[1] Because learning is dependent to a great extent upon motivation, the more intrinsic motivation the learner can bring to the situation the better the chance for meaningful learning. Extrinsic motivation may still be necessary and can be offered in a manner acceptable to the learner when criteria for acceptable performance have been established by the intern and the supervisor before the learning experience takes place.

This method was developed in 1974 in response to the concerns of the interns, the clinical coordinator and supervisors, and the academic faculty associated with the clinical education program for physical therapy interns at the University of Michigan Medical Center. Twenty-one interns and 11 supervisors participated in this program the first year. Some of the expressed concerns which indicated a need for change in the then pres-

Ms. Wightman is Assistant Director, Division of Physical Therapy, Department of Physical Medicine and Rehabilitation, University Hospital, Ann Arbor, MI 48109.

Dr. Wellock is Assistant Professor of Physical Therapy, Department of Physical Medicine and Rehabilitation, University of Michigan, Ann Arbor, MI 48109.

ent system were very real to those involved. The interns were concerned that they had "no say" in planning their clinical internship. They were anxious because they did not know what the supervisors expected of them in terms of performance. The interns asked for more feedback from the supervisors. The clinical coordinator and supervisors and the academic faculty were dissatisfied with the written performance evaluation for each intern and identified a need for more objectivity and documentation.

DEVELOPMENT OF THE METHOD

Educational Resources

This method required the physical therapists at the facility to list the educational resources available at the facility. These resources included such items as diagnoses frequently seen, conditions treated, evaluation procedures and physical agents used, and therapeutic exercises frequently employed. The availability of conferences, rounds, clinics, and specialty rotations such as assignment on the burn unit or the chest service were also included.

Criteria for Acceptable Performance

Criteria for judging acceptable performance of a physical therapist in specific physical therapy procedures were written by the clinical coordinator of the facility and reviewed and accepted by the staff at the facility. Criteria were written for chart reading, muscle testing, measurement of joint range of motion, body mechanics, note writing, patient safety, ambulation training, conduct, verbal communication, instruction for home programs, modalities, sterile technique, and burn and chest physical therapy. Criteria were also written for acceptable performance in participation in rounds, clinics, and conferences.

Selection of Objectives

Before arriving at the physical therapy department, the intern received information on the educational resources available at the facility. He was asked to compile a list of educa-

tional objectives in keeping with his own needs and the resources available. Upon arrival at the facility, the intern and the supervisor discussed the intern's objectives for the 6-week internship in relation to the intern's needs and previous experience in a clinic. Mutually acceptable goals were then outlined.

The Contract

A written contract was then negotiated by the intern and the supervisor. The contract included the goals to be accomplished, the criteria by which acceptable performance would be judged, and an outline of the student's and the supervisor's responsibilities. Also written into the contract were statements concerning daily meeting time and place, type of supervision to be given the intern, and any other information which would promote better communication. The primary responsibility of the intern was to fulfill the educational objectives upon which he and the supervisor had mutually agreed. The supervisor was responsible for stating the criteria for acceptable performance for each of the objectives and for offering the environment in which the objective could realistically be met. A typical section in the contract might read:

Given a patient with muscle weakness, the intern will gain skill in manual muscle testing by testing the patient three times during a 3-week period. The supervisor will observe the initial test and one reevaluation. Evaluations of the intern's skill in manual muscle testing will be based on the criteria for acceptable performance for this procedure at this facility which are:
1. Rationale of test was explained to patient.
2. Commands were clear and in terms to which the patient could respond.
3. Patient was draped, with part to be tested exposed.
4. Patient was positioned so therapist's body mechanics were maximized.
5. Tests were organized by position.
6. Appropriate stabilization was applied to obtain accurate test.
7. Substitutions were minimized by positioning and by verbal commands.
8. Muscle, when possible, was palpated during testing.
9. Test was completed efficiently, one to two minutes per muscle was average time.

TABLE
Log, 1974 Summer Internship

Objective: Given patients with neurologic diagnoses, the intern will increase his proficiency in muscle testing by performing at least three muscle tests.

Student's Comments	Supervisor's Comments
3/19/74 Performed initial muscle test on patient with a C7 lesion (left upper extremity, only). Took 45 minutes. Supervisor observed and assisted me as I had difficulty with muscles of the hand. My grades for shoulder and elbow agreed with my supervisor's grades. I did not remove the shirt and did not palpate muscle bellies until reminded to do so by my supervisor.	**3/19/74** Jane's test today showed she needed to organize her testing positions to avoid moving the patient so often. She realized she should have removed the patient's shirt when testing the shoulder. She was reminded to palpate muscles during the test. All other requirements met for a good muscle test as outlined in criteria for acceptable performance.
3/21/74 Performed muscle test on a patient with MS, without supervisor's observation. Had test organized so it took only 35 minutes to do complete test. Found strength to be G- except for ankles bilaterally which were Poor.	
3/28/74 Reevaluated patient with MS and found strength remained the same. Supervisor observed this test but offered no assistance. Took 25 minutes.	**3/28/74** Good testing. No comments for improving this test.
3/30/74 Performed muscle test on patient with peripheral neuropathy. Radial and median nerve deficit found. Performed muscle test of hand with only minimal assistance while supervisor observed.	**3/30/74** Jane did well and does excellent muscle test— fulfilled objective to my satisfaction.
4/4/74 Could not retest patient with neuropathy because he was discharged from the hospital.	

10. Test was executed accurately (80 percent of intern's grades agreed with the supervisor's).
11. Test results were recorded accurately and on proper form.

Minimum requirements for a contract were established by the supervisors of the facility in order to eliminate contracts that had little educational value and to emphasize that which, according to the supervisor's judgment, was important to the intern's experience. The contract stated that the intern would participate in certain minimal experiences during the 6-week period. These were:

1. Treatment of six patients per day
2. Performance of muscle testing, goniometry, sterile technique; instructing a patient in a program to be continued after discharge; activity involving the family or an allied health professional in the treatment procedures for at least one patient
3. Attendance at a minimum of two conferences or clinics
4. A one-half hour educational presentation to aides, staff, or other allied health professionals

Evaluation of Performance

A log was kept by the intern and the supervisor. The intern described what was done to meet a stated objective and noted any comments necessary to clarify the procedure. The supervisor noted the degree to which she judged the intern had achieved the criteria for acceptable performance and entered specific suggestions for improvement. An example of an entry from a 1974 log is given in the Table.

Summaries of the performance, as described in the log, were compiled separately by the intern and the supervisor. Each summary expressed the degree to which the intern had achieved the educational objectives stated in the contract and identified the intern's strengths and weaknesses as indicated by the information in the log. Information from these summaries was used by the clinical supervisor in completing evaluation forms from the intern's school when requested.

EVALUATION OF THE METHOD

The interns and supervisors were interviewed weekly during the internship by the clinical coordinator of the facility. Interns and supervisors completed a questionnaire at the end of the internship covering overall impressions of this method of developing and evaluating the clinical performance. The interns stated that they appreciated the high degree of responsibility placed upon them for establishing their own objectives and evaluating their own performance. They mentioned that writing in the log forced them to analyze what they were doing and to evaluate themselves. They appreciated the structure and direction the contract offered and said the criteria provided a guide of what was expected by supervisors for successful completion of the internship. They also stated that the establishment of criteria for the judging of acceptable performance provided consistency in their supervision and evaluation.

The less experienced supervisors stated that the establishment of criteria for acceptable performance aided them in establishing what to look for when observing the intern. Experienced supervisors expressed the opinion that the learning environment, when using this method, was more relaxed and conducive to learning than some other systems in which they had functioned. Both interns and supervisors expressed satisfaction with the use of the log. They stated they could often write more accurately concerning observations, attitudes, and opinions than they could express themselves when verbally discussing such topics. The supervisors stated conferences enhanced the learning experience when the student was aware of the items to be discussed and had done some preparation

for the discussion. A conference based on known expectancy was less traumatizing for both participants. The clinical coordinator at the facility was able, through use of the log entries, to evaluate the quality and amount of supervision each intern received and to use this information in counseling the supervisors. The 32 participants stated that they would, if given a choice, elect to follow the same procedure again.

SUMMARY

Everyone likes to know "how am I doing?" Through a method of cooperative planning and evaluating, this question can be discussed in a rational and objective manner. Acceptable behavior can be reinforced and suggestions for improvement can be made through the log entries. While this method was developed primarily to lessen the anxiety and uncertainty of the intern, confusion and uncertainty on the part of physical therapists supervising interns for the first time were also lessened.

The concerns of the interns, the clinical coordinator and supervisors, and the academic faculty were reduced. The interns realized they had a "say" in the planning of their clinical experience. They knew what was expected of them and the manner in which they would be evaluated. They had immediate feedback through the log entries. The clinical coordinator and supervisors and the academic faculty had objective documentation of the interns' performances.

Burton says, "The learning products achieved by the learner are those which satisfy a need, are useful and meaningful to the learner, and are so perceived by him. The realness of the condition under which learning takes place and the readiness of the learner contribute to integration."[1] From the responses of the interns and supervisors who participated in this method of developing and evaluating the clinical performance program, we conclude that the environment was conducive to learning.

REFERENCE

1. Burton WH: The Guidance of Learning Activities. New York, Appleton-Century-Crofts Inc, 1962

Use of the Rasch Model in the Development of a Clinical Competence Scale

Wendy Rheault, PhD, PT
Elizabeth Coulson, MBA, PT

ABSTRACT: This article illustrates the use of the Rasch model in the development and implementation of a student clinical competence scale. The short instrument described was used by the academic coordinator of clinical education to assess the clinical competence of 47 physical therapy students. The Rasch analysis converted scores from an ordinal scale to student scores on an interval scale. It also provided us with a ranking of item difficulties on an interval scale. The items, ranked from easiest to hardest, were as follows: exhibits professionalism, exhibits effective communication skills, performs effective treatment skills, performs safe treatment skills, can problem-solve, and works from an adequate knowledge base. More research is needed on this scale to ascertain whether the item difficulties remain constant across time, academic settings, and raters. If this can be demonstrated, then students can be compared from one year to the next and across educational programs.

INTRODUCTION

One of the difficulties faced by educators is the development of adequate ways to measure student clinical competence. Because of the nature of clinical competence, educators may measure clinical competence with ordinal rating scales such as 0=poor, 1=fair, and 2=good. The problems associated with using scores from an ordinal level of measurement are well known.[1] Because there is not equal distance between the numbers on ordinal scales, meaningful and accurate comparisons of scores for the same student between different clinical rotations or between different students cannot be made. Additionally, some statistical procedures cannot be used with data from an ordinal level of measurement.

Dr Rheault is Chairman and Professor, Department of Physical Therapy, The University of Health Sciences/ Chicago Medical School, 3333 Green Bay Rd, North Chicago, IL 60064. Ms Coulson is Assistant Chairman and Associate Professor, Department of Physical Therapy, The University of Health Sciences/Chicago Medical School.

The Rasch model, as described by Wright and associates, was developed to solve some of the inherent problems associated with ordinal level measurement.[2] Wright and Linacre[3] explained their approach in the November 1989 issue of *Archives of Physical Medicine and Rehabilitation.* The Rasch model is a mathematical model used to convert nominal or ordinal scores to measures on an interval scale with equal distance between the numbers. The new measures thus enable the educator to make correct inferences about the rate of student change and allow the educator to make more accurate comparisons among students. The original Rasch model was developed for two response categories.[4] Wright and associates[5] have expanded the model to include multiple response categories (eg, 0=incompetent, 1=minimally competent, and 2=fully competent).

The purpose of this article is to demonstrate the use of the Rasch model in the analysis of a scale to measure student clinical competence.

PROBLEMS WITH USING NONLINEAR SCORES

A person's score on a test will depend on the difficulty of the items. By simply taking a count of the number of right answers, however, the particular difficulties of the items are not taken into account. To illustrate the problems with using nonlinear scores, the following example is presented in the text and in the Figure. This example assumes that each student has a "true" level of clinical competence. The "true" score is imperfectly represented by a score on an ordinal scale. The Figure shows the clinical competence (C) of two students, student "n" and student "m." We can see that for all three cases, the "true" clinical competence of each student remains the same; it is positioned at the same point on the line for the three scenarios. Student m is clearly more competent than student n. The small hatched lines indicate the item difficulties for five items on a hypothetical clinical competence scale. By simply

taking a count of the items that students pass, we see that in the first case, student m gets all five items correct, while student n is unable to get any of the items correct. Therefore, the difference in their clinical ability is 5. In the second scenario, four of the items are too easy for both students and one is too difficult. In this case, we would conclude that there was no difference between the clinical competence of our two students. The third scenario gives us yet another possible conclusion. What do we believe? Is there a drastic difference in clinical competence between the students, as the first case suggests, or is there no difference, as the second scenario demonstrates? Remember that students m and n are positioned at the same point on our line for all three cases, indicating that their clinical ability has not changed. This points to the extreme hazard of making comparisons when the scores are nonlinear. The Rasch model will take the item difficulties into account when estimating the clinical competence of the student. Therefore, in the example given, after Rasch analysis student m and student n will receive their "true" ability scores irrespective of which clinical competence "test" they took. That is, their scores will not be dependent on the particular items taken. For each scenario, the difference between student abilities will be the same.

THE RASCH MODEL

The item-response models developed by Rasch and Wright specify that a person's response to a test item is related to two parameters—the person's ability (in our case, an overall measure of clinical competence) and the difficulty of the particular item.[2] Rasch believes that items on a scale form a hierarchy from easiest to hardest. From each student's particular response pattern to the items, we can estimate his or her ability. It should be noted that as a result of Rasch analysis, both item difficulty and person ability are located on a linear scale.

The procedure for item calibration and person measurement is called *unconditional*

Reprinted with permission from the Section for Education, APTA

maximum likelihood estimation (UCON). When items and people meet on a test, the result is a data matrix that records how people responded to particular items and how the items were responded to by the students. See Table 1 for part of the data matrix for this scale. Based on the data matrix, maximum likelihood estimation seeks the set of item difficulties and student abilities that maximizes the probability of the observed matrix. The computer progressively tries to calculate the best item difficulties and student abilities that fit the data from the matrix. Each UCON iteration is an attempt to bring item and student measures closer to that aim. See Wright and Stone[2] and Wright and Masters[5] for the specific mathematics involved in the Rasch model.

DEVELOPMENT OF CLINICAL COMPETENCE SCALE

Many of the clinical competence scales now in use are lengthy instruments that are difficult to interpret. The lengthy evaluation tools may give us rich information about individual students and the techniques they have mastered; however, it is often difficult to derive an overall rating or standing for the student, and the overall rating may not be meaningful. Another problem typically encountered is that scores are derived from different clinicians at various clinical sites, making comparisons of students impossible. We developed an instrument designed to address these problems. We specified two criteria: 1) the instrument should be a short and very general measure of clinical competence, and 2) ratings could be made by the academic clinical coordinator of education (ACCE) who visited all students and discussed the student's progress with the center clinical coordinator.

APPENDIX
Clinical Competence Scale

The purpose of this questionnaire is to assess the physical therapy student's clinical competence. Please rate the student on each item.

The student:
1. Works from an adequate knowledge base.

	low	high	
poorly	average	average	good
0	1	2	3

2. Exhibits effective communication skills.

	low	high	
poorly	average	average	good
0	1	2	3

3. Performs safe treatment techniques.

	low	high	
poorly	average	average	good
0	1	2	3

4. Performs effective treatment techniques.

	low	high	
poorly	average	average	good
0	1	2	3

5. Can problem-solve in the clinical setting.

	low	high	
poorly	average	average	good
0	1	2	3

6. Exhibits professionalism befitting of a health professional.

	low	high	
poorly	average	average	good
0	1	2	3

The items on the instrument were adapted from research conducted by Kubany and Cowles.[6] Kubany and Cowles interviewed 12 experienced faculty members in medicine and asked them to outline the most important characteristics needed for competent performance as a medical student. Kubany and Cowles then made a reduced list of eight characteristics based on the commonalities in the experts' list. From the list, we further limited the items to the six items that we believed were most important for clinical competence in physical therapy. See the Appendix for the complete instrument.

METHOD

The ACCE used the instrument for 47 students from the University of Health Sciences/The Chicago Medical School following their final full-time clinical experience and based on information from all sources. These sources included the ACCE's own visits (at least three during the professional phase of the program) and telephone contacts with the various clinical instructors (at least three phone calls). The information was entered into the computer, and the computer program MSCALE[7] was used to calculate the item difficulties and student abilities. MSCALE is the program used for Rasch analysis.

The Rasch analysis calculates student abilities and item difficulties that are located on an interval scale and that share a common unit. The units used are *logits* or *log odds units*. The student's position on the clinical competence scale reflects his or her "true" ability. Thus, the analysis produces 1) a linear representation of the order of difficulty of the individual items based on the data matrix, and 2) the student's overall level of clinical competence on a linear scale.

RESULTS

Table 2 lists the items from easiest to hardest with their associated difficulties (in logits) and the standard error. The most

Table 1
Partial Data Matrix

	Items on Clinical Competence Scale					
Student	Item 1	Item 2	Item 3	Item 4	Item 5	Item 6
1	3	3	2	2	3	2
2	2	2	2	2	2	3
3	2	1	2	2	2	3
4	1	2	2	2	1	2
5	3	2	2	2	3	2
6	1	2	2	2	3	3
7	3	3	2	2	2	2
8	2	2	2	2	2	2
9	1	2	2	1	1	2
10	3	3	3	3	3	3

Table 2

Hierarchy of Items on Clinical Competence Scale Determined Through Rasch Analysis

Item	Difficulty (in Logits)	Standard Error (in Logits)
Difficult item		
Knowledge	.71	.36
Problem-solving	.63	.31
Safe treatment technique	.46	.45
Effective treatment technique	.46	.42
Communication	−.89	.37
Professionalism	−1.39	.32
Easy item		

difficult items were knowledge and problem-solving. The least difficult items (the items that more students received a "3" for) were professionalism and communication. This gives the educator a ranking of the relative difficulty of the various clinical skills.

Likewise each of the 47 students received an ability measure with the associated standard error. Table 3 summarizes the students' abilities. Recall that Rasch analysis produces the model of item difficulties and student scores that best fits the collected data from the students. There may be students, however, who do not fit the calculated model; they may not possess the modeled response to items and have a different item difficulty hierarchy. Their scores are thus termed *misfits*. Only two of the 47 students misfit the constructed model. In both cases, the students did better than expected on the problem-solving item; that is, they found problem-solving easier than rendering safe and effective treatment skills. This is an interesting finding because clinical educators often observe students who are average clinicians (can treat appropriately) but who particularly excel at problem-solving. The analysis was able to distinguish this small subset of students who score differently from the rest of the students.

DISCUSSION

The purpose of this article was to demonstrate the use of the Rasch measurement model for a clinical competence scale. The student abilities derived from the Rasch analysis can now be used to track student progress from one rotation to the next or to compare students for the purposes of making scholarship or other important decisions. Parametric statistics can also be used on the data because the data are on an interval scale.

Lengthy inventories that specify the specific skills and techniques the student has mastered have their use in physical therapy education. The longer inventories are very useful as formative measuring instruments,

informing students of their progress toward mastery of the material. The tool described in this article is more appropriate as a summative measuring tool that documents overall final performance. This may be important in the future as accrediting agencies and others ask educators to demonstrate the overall competence of students in an objective and accountable manner. Both types of instruments are, therefore, appropriate for documenting student competence.

None of the items from the clinical competence scale misfit the model produced by Rasch analysis. If an item had misfit, it would have indicated that it was not a relevant item for the variable of "clinical competence." Thus, the Rasch analysis is extremely useful for test development and editing.

It is essential that any scale be valid and reliable. Wright and Masters[5] explained how the traditional concepts of validity and reliability fit into the Rasch model. For example, the standard error associated with each student score and each item difficulty reflects measurement error. The MSCALE standard error is preferable to the traditional standard error statistic because the Rasch model includes modeled test error variance that is not

an average of the whole test but is particular to the test score.[5] Wright and Masters[5] explained that content and construct validity are verified by examining the item difficulty hierarchy to see whether it makes sense. The item difficulties should be compared with the intentions of the item writer to ascertain whether the scale conforms to the writer's theory or expectations concerning item difficulties. They term this *item order validity*. The fit of the items to the model also provides information about content and construct validity. The reader is referred to Wright and Masters[5] for more specific information on validity and reliability.

Not all educators may have access to the software needed to change raw scores to measures on a linear scale. Conversion charts for specific instruments can be developed. Table 3 can be used to convert a raw score on the clinical competence scale to a measure that is on an interval scale. For example, a student with a raw score of 10 on the clinical competence scale would have a converted score of .65 logits. A student may receive a raw score of 10 by a number of different response patterns. One student may exhibit the following responses to the six items: 1,2,1,2,1,3; while another student may possess a different pattern: 2,2,1,2,1,2. In both cases we would assign the student a converted score of .65 logits. This score assignment is justified because we have found an overall fit of students to the model as calculated by the Rasch analysis. The standard error becomes important because it indicates the amount of measurement error that we might expect for that particular converted score.

Table 3 is based on the data from our institution. The next step in this line of research is to collect data from different

Table 3

Summary of Clinical Competence Values for 47 Students

Raw Score	Number of Students with Score	Measure (Logits)	Standard Error
17	2	5.43	1.16
16	3	4.60	1.04
15	6	3.90	1.01
14	2	3.22	1.58
13	4	2.55	1.62
12	3	1.89	1.99
10	4	.65	1.29
9	5	.04	1.41
8	7	−.59	1.67
7	3	−1.24	1.65
6	3	−1.91	2.03
5	1	−2.57	.91
3	1	−3.87	1.10
1	3	−5.46	1.53

institutions and to determine whether the item difficulties remain the same. If we find that the item difficulties remain the same across academic settings, then we have a universal tool that can be used to measure student clinical competence from different settings. A conversion chart can be developed to transform scores to an interval scale, and appropriate inferences can be made based on the measures.

Linacre[7] has recently expanded the Rasch model to take into account the difficulty of the raters (in our case, the ACCE). The data matrix would then have a third dimension for rater difficulty. Student clinical competence and item difficulty would then be calculated taking into account rater difficulty. Thus reliability among raters is taken into account.

CONCLUSION

This article illustrates the use of the Rasch model in test development and implementation. When first developing a measuring scale, the test developer selects the items and the scaling method. Our items were selected based on work by Kubany and Cowles.[6] After item development, data were collected from 47 students. The student responses were analyzed using the Rasch model. Rasch analysis provided student measures that took into account item difficulty. Therefore we were given 1) student clinical competence scores and 2) item difficulties, both of which were on a linear scale with equal distance between units. The new student competence measures could now allow meaningful and valid analyses among and within subjects. Because a *model* was constructed through Rasch analysis, it was possible that particular students or items would not fit the model. Only two students misfit the model, and no items were misfits. If any items had misfit, it would have indicated that the item did not fit the definition of the variable of "clinical competence." These items would have been deleted. If the spacing between item difficul-

Figure

Illustration of problems with nonlinear scores. (Small hatched lines indicate difficulty position of item. Cn=clinical competence of student n; Cm=clinical competence of student m.)

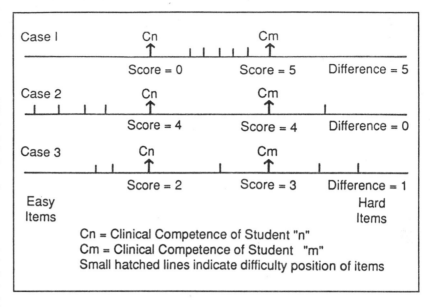

ties had been inappropriate, this would have indicated another problem. That is, if all the items had bunched together (been of the same difficulty), then this would have shown us that items at a different difficulty needed to be written. Therefore, Rasch analysis can provide the researcher or clinician with useful information about test development and possible revision.

The Rasch model appears to be a very useful tool for the physical therapist. This mathematical model has much potential for research in both physical therapy and physical therapy education. It can be used for any rating scale. For example, the clinician or researcher can utilize the Rasch model for analyzing pain scales, pediatric assessment tools, and functional scales. Physical therapists are urged to explore the possibility of

using the Rasch measurement model for many different variables.

REFERENCES

1. Merbitz C, Morris J, Grip JC: Ordinal scales and foundations of misinference. Arch Phys Med Rehabil 70:308–312, 1989
2. Wright BD, Stone MH: Best Test Design. Chicago, IL, MESA Press, 1979
3. Wright BD, Linacre JM: Observations are always ordinal; measurements, however, must be interval. Arch Phys Med Rehabil 70:857–860, 1989
4. Rasch G: Probabilistic Models for Some Intelligence and Attainment Tests. Copenhagen, Danish Institute for Educational Research, 1960, and Chicago, University of Chicago Press, 1980.
5. Wright BD, Masters GN: Rating Scale Analysis. Chicago, IL, MESA Press, 1982
6. Kubany AJ, Cowles JT: Improving the measurement of clinical performance of medical students. Journal of Clinical Psychology 15:139–142, 1959
7. Linacre JM: Many-Faceted Rasch Measurement. Chicago, IL, MESA Press, 1989

Development
of Evaluation
Instruments

Group Development of a Clinical Education Instrument

Bonnie Teschendorf
Pamela Gramet
Louise Heubusch

ABSTRACT: *Academic coordinators of clinical education and center coordinators of clinical education formed a special interest group in New York State. The group cooperatively developed an evaluation instrument for use in the clinical training of students. The background, theory, and philosophy of the group is reflected in the discussion and in the content of the evaluation instrument. Major components of the instrument are presented.*

INTRODUCTION

Academic coordinators of clinical education* often work in isolation from each other, developing and redeveloping separate student evaluations for each program and dealing independently with frustrating student problems. As the number of physical therapy programs in New York State grew, it became apparent that improved communication and sharing would benefit each program. As a result of this need for closer communication and cooperation, the New York State Physical Therapy Academic Clinical Coordinators group was formed. There are currently 11 physical therapy programs in New York State: seven are located in the downstate New York area and four are in the upstate New York area.

---

* Academic Coordinator of Clinical Education (ACCE): An individual, employed by the educational institution, whose primary concern is relating the students' clinical education to the curriculum. This coordinator administers the total clinical education program and, in association with the academic and clinical faculty, plans and coordinates the individual student's clinical experience with academic preparation and evaluates the students' progress (Moore ML, Perry JF: Clinical Education In Physical Therapy: Present Status/Future Needs. Washington, DC, Section for Education, American Physical Therapy Association, 1976).

Ms Teschendorf is Associate Director, Assistant Professor, Program in Physical Therapy, College of Physicians and Surgeons, Columbia University, New York, NY 10032. Ms Gramet is Assistant Professor, Program in Physical Therapy, College of Health Related Professions, SUNY Health Science Center at Syracuse, Syracuse, NY 13210. Ms Heubusch is Director of Clinical Education, Clinical Assistant Professor, Department of Physical Therapy and Exercise Science, State University of New York at Buffalo, Buffalo, NY 14214.

The purpose of this article is to describe the development of a uniform tool for evaluation of students in the clinical education settings used by all of the programs. The evaluation instrument developed by the group was the product of the cooperative efforts of this ACCE group.

HISTORY OF THE NEW YORK STATE ACCE GROUP

In 1982, five academic coordinators of clinical education (ACCEs) from the downstate New York physical therapy programs met with the goal of developing an agenda for the first New York State ACCE meeting. Later that year, ACCEs from 10 of the 11 physical therapy programs in New York State met in Queens.

Initially the group spent time becoming acquainted and comparing philosophies and experiences regarding clinical education. Mutual frustrations and problems were identified through extensive discussion. Topics emerged as mutual concerns, including the difficulty of scheduling clinical rotations, performing clinical visits, the development and retention of clinical education sites, and most importantly the lack of a common, standardized evaluation instrument.

The meeting concluded with a commitment to continue participation as related to the following objectives:

1. Designing a uniform clinical evaluation instrument for all New York State programs of physical therapy.

2. Obtaining grant funding to support workshops with clinical instructors.

3. Organizing a meeting of both ACCEs and center coordinators of clinical education (CCCEs) at the New York State Chapter APTA annual conference in 1983.

4. Planning a one-day workshop with clinical instructors to be held in the downstate New York area.

5. Maintaining the enthusiasm to continue group efforts.

Based on these objectives, committees were organized to deal with evaluation forms, grant proposals, and education workshops. A chairperson was selected from the group to serve for the first year. A letter was sent to 468 CCCEs affiliated with the academic programs to inform them of the formation and objectives of the group and to invite them to participate. The input of clinicians was viewed as essential to the success of future programs.

EVALUATION INSTRUMENT DEVELOPMENT

The first major project the group tackled was the development of a standardized evaluation tool for clinical education. The emphasis of the clinical education phase of training has in recent years moved toward a competency-based system. That is, specific standards for student performance (minimal competence) are identified in professional practice and must be met prior to the completion of the clinical experience. The use of various evaluation tools by the member programs with their open interpretation and diversified format challenged us to design a uniform instrument to measure competence based on standards. Common problems with the evaluation process that the group identified included the difficulty of identifying an appropriate standard of practice, the lack of reliability and validity in rating scales, and the uncertainty concerning the intended specific goals and objectives of clinical instructors. Prior to the development of a form, it proved helpful to refer to current literature regarding evaluation in clinical education.

In 1977 the "Red Book" of Competencies in Physical Therapy was endorsed by APTA, and facilities and schools began using it as a reference.[1,2] This book discussed the basic competencies of the physical therapy profession. A short time thereafter, in 1979, the Texas Consortium for Physical Therapy Clinical Education developed a tool called the Blue MACS (Mastery and Assessment of Clinical Skills).[3] The Blue MACS represents a comprehensive listing of professional competencies and their subskills. Despite the disadvantage of being a time-consuming task, as reported by clinical instructors, the use of the instrument has been widespread. The provision of specific standards for mastery is a helpful guide in planning and evaluating student clinical experiences.

A publication in 1973[4] described an evaluation instrument developed for use by programs of physical therapy in New York State. This instrument was intended to generate narrative reporting of student progress related to specific categories. Standards for student achievement were not listed, nor was a grading procedure indicated.

PROBLEMS TO BE RESOLVED

Problems of evaluating students in all categories of clinical performance are well described in the literature. One problem the group shared was the identification and acceptance of appropriate entry-level standards of practice for physical therapy. Because some standards are subject to change and all could be subject to interpretation, it is difficult to assure uniformity in assessment of skill acquisition. The student may be evaluated variably from setting to setting, as well as from supervisor to supervisor within a setting.[5] The radiology profession is able to equate competence with standards by using outcome measures.[6] Consideration of outcome measures may be unique to radiology, for a product is produced with fewer variables to measure as compared to physical therapy.

A second problem the group addressed was the issue of reliability and validity in rating scales devised for the assessment of students. Studies of evaluation tools have described a low interrater consistency, and difficulties were presented when using observational assessment. Squier concluded that "studies of the reliability and validity of rating scales for the assessment of clinical progress are disappointing." He also stated, "Ratings given to the students proved to be unreliable and lacking in validity. Repeated modification of the rating scales and careful preparation of raters failed to improve significantly the interrater consistency obtained."[7]

One factor contributing to the lack of validity is a "halo" effect, or tendency for the rater to use a global mind set when rating all categories. This effect may be diminished if the student reports to several clinical instructors during one clinical rotation. This enables the multiple instructors to write a composite evaluation of overall performance, which may then result in a more objective assessment. A problem with multiple instructors, however, is variable expectations regarding student performance.

The problem from the students' perspective is uncertainty concerning the intended specific goals and objectives of clinical instructors. Through development of specific objectives, discussion of the student's responsibilities prior to the affiliation, use of a negotiated contract, and use of continuous verbal feedback, this problem may be reduced.[8,9] Clear channels of communication as well as thorough discussion and agreed-upon objectives make it easier to assess the student throughout the clinical experience and reassure him or her that performance is meeting expectations.

EVALUATION PROCESS AND PURPOSE

The process of evaluation is intended to be a description of change or of current status compared to a previous status. The reasons for evaluating the student in the clinical setting are to make informed decisions regarding student progress and to provide feedback about the academic program of training. The evaluation tool may be helpful in identifying inadequacies consistent among students. This, in turn, should provide an impetus for modifications in program content or method of presentation.[10]

The most important purpose in the use of evaluation is to provide the student with a permanent record of progress toward professional competence. Assisting a student in the identification of tasks that have been mastered versus those that require continued attention is an important function of the evaluation tool. The student may use this feedback to improve future clinical performance and develop learning objectives. Such documentation may also assist the academic clinical coordinator in planning appropriate remedial assignments for the student who falls behind the expectations expressed in the standards.

The evaluation also reinforces the student's personal image as a developing professional. A sense of competence, skill, self-esteem, and perceived ability to function in the clinical environment is an important foundation for professional life. The student can be encouraged to use the evaluation tool as part of a self-assessment process. This realistic self-critique learned in the student role may contribute to future ability to plan continuing education and use newly learned skills in practice.

In summary, the literature supports our impression that clinical evaluations are subjective regardless of the use of rating scales or narrative reporting. The purpose of recording change in behavior, however, if utilized as a mechanism to assist the student toward higher levels of clinical competence, continues to offer sound rationale for use of the process. Our group believes that students should be provided with written standards and procedures for evaluation. All students should be treated equally, negative situations should be recorded with documentation in a timely fashion, and evaluations should be discussed openly with the opportunity to refute the assessment of performance. Providing ongoing oral feedback, in addition to written evaluations, allows students to incorporate feedback into future behavior.

THE EVALUATION INSTRUMENT

Concepts derived from the literature and from group experiences reinforced the need to develop a competency-based instrument for student assessment. Group convictions regarding clearly stated objectives and opportunities for feedback required the incorporation of these components into the structure of the form.

In order to actually implement the process, the group was divided into subcommittees that were assigned separate parts of the evaluation form. The subcommittees worked for the next year to develop the individual sections. Each subcommittee studied forms shared by other schools and clinics. When materials were completed, the total group met to draft the form. By 1984 the first draft of the form was presented to 39 clinical coordinators and instructors at the New York State Chapter APTA annual conference in Buffalo. A workshop held several weeks later in the New York metropolitan area repeated the presentation for another 37 clinical instructors. Feedback solicited from both groups resulted in revision of the form. Several schools began to utilize the form with students in the fall of 1984. In 1985 clinics using the form were randomly surveyed for opinions and further suggested changes.

The final format of the clinical performance evaluation instrument consists of ten sections. Each section specifically identifies terminal behaviors expected of students. The sections are entitled:

  I. Professional Behavior and Attitude

  II. Safety

  III. Communication and Interpersonal Relationship Skills

  IV. Evaluation

  V. Integration of Academic Knowledge

VI. Program Planning
VII. Treatment Implementation
VIII. Management
IX. Teaching
X. Data Retrieval and Data Analysis

The final page of the form provides a space to describe strengths, areas needing change, and areas improved during the affiliation period. This format is used at mid-term and final evaluation periods. In addition to this specific narrative summary, there is space in each of the ten sections for narrative comments.

Grading is based on a scale of 1 to 3. Students are expected to receive an overall grade of 3, which indicates competence in each category. The individual physical therapy programs have the liberty of specifying the competencies to be achieved during the early part-time clinical experiences.

Feedback from clinical instructors surveyed after using the form for one year indicated a high level of satisfaction with the form. They also were pleased to eliminate the multiple evaluation forms previously required by affiliated programs. The form continues to be evaluated; a study currently underway will assess the validity and reliability of the instrument.*

_____

* Authors will make copies of the form available upon request.

CONCLUSIONS

The group was successful in achieving its primary goal: development of the New York State Performance Evaluation Instrument. The tool has been widely accepted by the clinical sites affiliating with New York State programs. Several nonmember programs also are using the form.

An unanticipated benefit of the group's formation was the network of cohesive support developed within the group. Members have enjoyed the camaraderie and shared enthusiasm experienced as active participants. The success with the first project has been a motivating factor in generating new ideas. Future projects are approached with renewed conviction to strive for excellence in clinical education.

ACKNOWLEDGMENTS

Group contributors included the following: Jill Auster-Liebhaber, Susan Bennett, Melanie Gillar, Barbara Goldberg, Pamela Gramet, Louis Heubusch, Millee Jorge, Linda Krasilovsky, Wen Ling, Pat Marino, Marie Nardone, Eileen Nathanson, Dee Dee Perneti, Elaine Rosen, Barbara Silvestri, Ann-Marie Sirois, Mardi Steppacher, Bonnie Teschendorf, and Karen Tunney.

REFERENCES

1. American Physical Therapy Association: Competencies in Physical Therapy: An Analysis of Practice. San Diego, CA, Courseware Inc, 1977
2. Nethery JC: Physical therapy competencies in clinical education. Phys Ther 61:1442-1446, 1981
3. The Blue MACS: Mastery and Assessment of Clinical Skills, ed 3. Galveston, TX, Texas Consortium for Physical Therapy Education, 1981
4. Dickinson R, DiMarino J, Pfitzenmaier J: A common evaluation instrument. Phys Ther 53:1075-1080, 1973
5. Wysocki R: Evaluation of student clinical performance. Aust Nur J 10:42–43, 1980
6. Guidelines and Forms for Measurement of Clinical Competence for Radiography Students. Ottawa, Ontario, Canada, Canadian Association of Medical Radiation Technologists, Radiographic Section, Council on Education, 1978
7. Squier, RW: The reliability and validity of rating scales in assessing the clinical progress of psychiatric nursing students. Int J Nurs Stud 18:157–169, 1981
8. Wightman ML, Wellock LM: A method of developing and evaluating a clinical performance program for physical therapy interns. Phys Ther 56:1125–1128, 1976
9. Windom PA: Developing a clinical education program from the clinician's perspective. Phys Ther 62:1604–1609, 1982
10. Ramsborg GC: Evaluation of clinical performance: Part I. JAA Nurs Anesth, February 1983, pp 55-62

education

The Development and Use of an Evaluation Instrument for Clinical Education

BARBARA P. KERN, M.A.,
and JOHN M. MICKELSON, Ed.D.

The development and use of an evaluation instrument for clinical education is described. The objectives contained within the instrument are stated in behavioral terms, that is, the visible activities the student is expected to display. The rating scale is based on levels of supervision required in order for the student to meet the objectives. After a three-year trial, the instrument has yielded data about the strengths and weaknesses of students, clinical programs, and the didactic curriculum.

The objective evaluation of clinical experience is always a matter of difficulty whatever the profession, and physical therapy is no exception. Supervisors of clinical experience have long felt the need for an evaluative procedure which is valid, reliable, practical to administer, and yields data which permit the evaluation of the student and the professional program designed to prepare him.

The first class of students to enter Temple University's Department of Physical Therapy enrolled in September 1967. At that time, a program had been planned, initial classes organized, and preparations were underway to provide for clinical education to begin the following semester. The last included developing working arrangements with clinics, orientation of personnel in treatment facilities, and developing means of evaluation.

Initially, those persons involved in the development of the evaluation instrument for clinical experience included the coordinator of the Clinical Education Program, a curriculum consultant from Temple University's College of Education, and the faculty of the Department of Physical Therapy. Later this group was augmented by the clinical supervisors.

IDENTIFYING BEHAVIORAL OBJECTIVES

Evaluation has been defined as the process of determining the extent to which educational objectives are achieved; therefore, the first step in preparing for the construction of the

Miss Kern is Assistant Professor and Clinical Coordinator, Department of Physical Therapy, College of Allied Health Professions, Temple University, 3525 Germantown Avenue, Philadelphia, Pennsylvania 19140.

Dr. Mickelson is Professor of Curriculum Instruction, College of Education, Temple University, Philadelphia, Pennsylvania 19140.

evaluation instrument was the identification of the objectives for clinical education.[1] The members of the faculty agreed to state the objectives in behavioral terms, that is, the *overt* activity the student is expected to display. Terms such as *to know, understand,* or *appreciate* were avoided. Such terms are not explicit enough to be useful; what is meaningful and measurable is what the student is *doing* when demonstrating that he understands or appreciates.[2] Also, objectives relating to knowledge and understanding are emphasized within the didactic portion of the curriculum; by the time the student is assigned to clinical work he should already have achieved in the classroom the basic cognitive objectives necessary for that phase of clinical education. In the clinic, the prime concern should be the behaviors resulting from the cognition the student has developed or is developing.

The members of the faculty in physical therapy were asked to submit, on index cards, statements of the behaviors which the students should be capable of performing upon the completion of their professional curriculum. Each faculty member was encouraged to list as many terminal behaviors as possible without concern for duplication. These ranged from specific or limited behaviors to those which were more general.

The behavior cards were shuffled to break up any existing patterns and then grouped, letting the categories develop naturally as similar behavior cards were placed together. There were no predetermined categories. From these natural groupings terminal behavioral hierarchies developed which, in turn, became the behavioral objectives for clinical education.

The procedure just described was then repeated with a group of clinical supervisors. The repetition was one phase of the plan for involving clinical supervisors in program development. It also served to ensure that coverage was complete and to provide a check on the validity of the tentative list of terminal behavioral objectives. The value of this procedure was evident when an analysis of the behavior cards secured from the clinicians revealed that essential supervisory and administrative behaviors had been overlooked in developing the first list of objectives.

After additional refinement, a list of ten terminal behavioral objectives were identified for clinical education. Component behaviors, derived from the objectives submitted, were identified for each of the ten. These were the behaviors the student must perform to achieve the objective.

CONSTRUCTING THE INSTRUMENT

Check lists and rating scales are instruments commonly used to objectify the evaluation of

PROFESSIONAL PRACTICES

	Satis-factory	Unsatis-factory
The student presents a professional appearance.		
Grooms himself properly	☐	☐
Wears clean uniform and shoes	☐	☐
Practices personal hygiene	☐	☐
The student conducts himself in a professional manner.		
Accepts responsibility	☐	☐
Assists and cooperates willingly with co-workers	☐	☐
Cleans treatment area after use	☐	☐
Responds favorably to criticism and suggestions	☐	☐
Follows chain of command	☐	☐
Respects confidential material	☐	☐
Abides by regulations of facility	☐	☐
Uses free clinic time to advantage	☐	☐
The student maintains appropriate interpersonal relationships.		
Reacts appropriately to the moods of others	☐	☐
Masks emotional reactions in presence of others	☐	☐
Contributes to a friendly but professional atmosphere	☐	☐
The student prepares appropriate reports.		
Records results of treatments	☐	☐
Submits reports when indicated	☐	☐
Expresses ideas logically and understandably	☐	☐
Adapts communication to the comprehension of each individual	☐	☐
Uses appropriate medical terminology	☐	☐

COMMENTS:

Fig. 1. Student behaviors for evaluating professional practices.

procedures. The first is the more appropriate for an "either-or" situation (the student wears a clean uniform, or he does not wear a clean uniform), while the scale is the instrument of choice when the behavior to be rated exists on a continuum, and variations in the quality of performance are to be expected.[3] The present instrument is a combined check list-rating scale.

For convenience, the terminal behavioral objectives and their component behaviors were grouped into three general categories: professional practices, treatment skills, and administrative and supervisory practices. Later a fourth category, specific techniques, was added to complement the category of treatment skills. The category of professional practices (Fig. 1) is designed as a check list; the other categories (Figs. 2, 3, and 4) are designed as rating scales. The sequence of Figures 1, 2, 3, and 4 represent the sequential organization in the total instrument.

With the basic format of the instrument completed, the next step was the development of performance criteria for the rating scale. Performance on the check list was indicated simply as satisfactory or unsatisfactory.

Callahan's work on levels of proficiency provides useful clues for a solution to the problem of ambiguity in rating scales. She outlined sequences of development through which a student must progress to achieve the highest level of competency. The first three sequences deal primarily with understanding the treatment, experiencing it, and applying it to "normal" classmates. The last five sequences relate to psychomotor skills; a student observes the treatment, assists in the treatment, applies treatment while being closely supervised, applies treatment without direct supervision, and has his results checked in order to evaluate the mastery of his skill.[4]

TREATMENT SKILLS

Please rate according to student's most typical and frequent manner of performance.

    5. Student demonstrates skill when fulfilling objective with only guidance.
    4. Student demonstrates skill when fulfilling objective, but requires occasional supervision.
    3. Student requires supervision and occasional assistance when fulfilling objective.
    2. Student is unable to fulfill objective without assistance.
    1. Student fails to meet objective.
N/O No opportunity to observe.

TREATMENT ORGANIZATION

The student evaluates the patient.
____ Obtains necessary preliminary information
____ Assesses level of disability
____ Assesses appropriateness of patient's appliances, devices and/or equipment
____ Measures patient's potential for appliances, devices and/or equipment
____ Analyzes results of evaluation
____ Requests change in treatment when indicated
____ Reports findings to appropriate personnel

The student plans treatment programs.
____ Identifies long and short term goals
____ Selects procedures appropriate to long/short term goals
____ Progresses patient in logical sequence
____ Provides for assessment of procedure
____ Suggests referrals to other health services when indicated

COMMENTS:

TREATMENT TECHNIQUES

The student prepares for each treatment.
____ Reviews patient's medical chart
____ Reviews techniques of selected physical agents if necessary
____ Prepares area prior to treatment
____ Checks equipment prior to use
____ Drapes patient properly

The student applies treatment techniques.
____ Instructs patient as to method and purpose of treatment procedure
____ Instructs patient in proper use of assistive devices
____ Adapts procedure to patient's needs
____ Practices principles of body mechanics
____ Notes any adverse reactions in the patient
____ Treats patient within limits of tolerance (fatigue/pain)
____ Uses and adjusts equipment properly

Fig. 2. Student behaviors for evaluating treatment skills.

SPECIFIC TECHNIQUES

Please rate according to student's most typical and frequent manner of performance.

5. Student consistently demonstrates skill when performing technique with only guidance.
4. Student is skilled in performance of technique, but requires occasional supervision.
3. Student requires supervision and occasional assistance when performing technique.
2. Student is unable to perform technique without assistance.
1. Student is unable to perform technique.

N/O No opportunity to observe.

MODALITIES
———— Massage
———— Infrared
———— Diathermy
———— Microthermy
———— Ultrasound
———— Ultraviolet
———— Electrical stimulation
———— Ion therapy
———— Cervical traction
———— Others

HYDROTHERAPY
———— Whirlpool
———— Hubbard tank
———— Paraffin
———— Therapeutic pool
———— Hydrocollator packs
———— Others

COMMENTS:

THERAPEUTIC EXERCISES
———— Passive and/or stretching
———— Active, active assistive
———— Progressive resistive
———— Isolated muscle reeducation
———— Coordination
———— Posture training
———— Neuromuscular facilitation
           techniques
———— Pulmonary exercises
———— Others

PROSTHETIC TRAINING
———— Stump care
———— Stump bandaging
———— Preprosthetic training
———— Prosthetic training
———— Others

TESTING PROCEDURES
———— Manual muscle test
———— Goniometry
———— ADL evaluation
———— Functional muscle test
———— R.D. test
———— Chronaxy
———— Strength-duration curves
———— Others

FUNCTIONAL ACTIVITIES
———— Bed activities
———— Lead-up activities
———— Dressing
———— Wheelchair management
———— Wheelchair transfers
———— Others

AMBULATION TRAINING
———— Stand/sit activities
———— Elevations
———— Gait training

Fig. 3. *Student behaviors for evaluating specific techniques of treatment.*

ADMINISTRATIVE AND SUPERVISORY PRACTICES

Please rate according to student's most typical and frequent manner of performance.

5. Student demonstrates skill in fulfilling objective with only guidance.
4. Student demonstrates skill when fulfilling objective, but requires occasional supervision.
3. Student requires supervision and occasional assistance when fulfilling objective.
2. Student is unable to fulfill objective without assistance.
1. Student fails to meet objective.

N/O No opportunity to observe.

The student assists in supervision of a physical therapy department.

———— Supervises supportive physical therapy personnel
———— Schedules patients for treatment
———— Analyzes patient load served
———— Coordinates patient's treatment times with other therapies

The student assists in the administration of a physical therapy program.

———— Suggests areas for staff in-service training programs
———— Instructs other health professionals in principles of physical therapy
———— Interprets the role of the physical therapist to other health professionals

COMMENTS:

Fig. 4. *Student behaviors for evaluating administrative and supervisory practices.*

An analysis of these last five sequences suggested that the degree of direction required from the supervisors was an important component in evaluating clinical performance. This led to the definition of three levels of required direction.

1. Guidance. The student seeks suggestions, approval, or both, from the supervisor prior to fulfillment of the objective. This does not necessitate the presence of the supervisor in the immediate treatment vicinity. The student is able to meet the objective independently.

2. Supervision. The presence of the supervisor is required in the immediate vicinity in order for the student to meet the objective.

3. Assistance. Actual physical assistance must be offered by the supervisor in order for the student to meet the objective.

With the foregoing as guidelines, new performance criteria were created.

> 5. Student demonstrates skill when fulfilling objective with only guidance.
> 4. Student demonstrates skill when fulfilling objective, but requires occasional supervision.
> 3. Student requires supervision and occasional assistance when fulfilling the objective.
> 2. Student is unable to fulfill objective without assistance.
> 1. Student fails to meet the objective.
> N.O. No opportunity to observe.

These criteria are used in judging the students' performance in the areas of treatment skills, specific techniques, and administrative and supervisory practices.

METHOD OF DETERMINING A GRADE

Once an evaluation has been made and the form returned to the college, a final grade is reached through a predetermined scale which takes into account the student's previous experiences. As a student progresses through all the phases of clinical education, the criteria for grades also progress. For example, if a student receives ratings of 3 at his first rehabilitation affiliation, this would be the equivalent of an A; if he receives the same rating (3) at his fourth or last affiliation in a rehabilitation center then he would receive a D. This grading scale is predetermined on the basis of minimal acceptable standards established by the faculty for performance in each phase of clinical education.

USING THE INSTRUMENT

The primary function of an evaluation form for clinical education is to provide a reliable means of assessing student performance in the clinical setting. In addition to providing information regarding student performance, the present instrument has been designed to provide feedback concerning the effectiveness of clinical programs and the professional curriculum.

Since the objectives on the evaluation form are written in the form of terminal objectives, the total instrument is not always applicable for all phases of clinical education, especially early assignments. At Temple University, the instrument is used as follows for junior and senior students.

The objectives of clinical education for junior students are concerned mainly with developing positive attitudes and proficiencies in the application of basic modalities; thus, the categories of professional practices and specific techniques comprise the basic instrument to be utilized in the evaluation of students at this level.

The senior students should be capable of applying treatment procedures. In addition, they should be able to assess the patient's level of disability and then plan and organize treatment programs to meet the patient's specific needs; therefore, the category of treatment skills is added to the instrument. As the seniors progress to full-time clinical assignments, they are expected to demonstrate beginning skills in administrative and supervisory activities. This completes the total evaluation instrument as used for students in their final phase of clinical education.

Assessing the Student

Prior to his assignment to a clinic, each student receives a copy of the evaluation form and a copy of the objectives for that specific phase of clinical education. In this way, the student has in writing exactly what he is expected to achieve during his assignments in the clinic. Similarly, the clinical supervisors are provided with the objectives for each phase of clinical education.

By virtue of the performance criteria specified in the rating scale, the possibility of a conflict over the evaluation of clinical performance is averted, with rare exceptions.

The rater's attention is directed to the criteria listed; his judgments are focused. A student who requires constant supervision and occasional assistance in attempting to meet the objectives knows he is performing at a 3 level. Most students can evaluate themselves with a remarkable amount of candor. They have a clear notion of their own competencies and needs.

Assessing the Clinical Program

The clinics and the college have immediate feedback available on each phase of clinical education. The appropriateness of objectives and the effectiveness of learning experiences can be assessed by reviewing both the number of ratings completed and the categories in which the ratings occurred. Specific techniques is the one area which yields the most feedback of this type; such feedback provides an excellent basis for reviewing the total clinical programs.

After the first class of seniors at the College of Allied Health Professions had completed all the clinical work required for the first and second semesters, the number of ratings administered by the clinics for each modality were plotted on a graph. The results of this study were enlightening and interesting both to the clinical supervisors and to the faculty of the college. One could see quickly the areas where students were or were not receiving clinical experience throughout a full year of clinical education. The data obtained from the graph were further broken down into an analysis of the ratings offered by each clinic. These findings were then utilized as bases for discussions between clinical supervisors and the coordinator of clinical education from the college. The relevancy of college preparation to clinical experience was readily apparent, while at the same time inadequacies in the clinical programs were identified.

Assessing the Curriculum

By again reviewing the category of specific techniques, this time for the quality of ratings received from the clinical supervisors rather than categories in which ratings occurred, strengths and weaknesses in the college program could be pinpointed and necessary corrective action could be planned. For instance, the fact that the majority of students received relatively low ratings in manual muscle testing would be cause to investigate the instruction provided at the college in this course. Perhaps concepts were not thoroughly understood, perhaps instruction was too superficial or insufficient time was provided. What ever the cause, the college has been alerted to search for it.

SUMMARY AND CONCLUSIONS

An evaluation instrument has been presented which, after a trial run of three years, has yielded highly useful data about the strengths and weaknesses of the students, clinical programs, and the didactic curriculum.

Problems still exist but all seem resolvable. The major problem is training clinical personnel in the proper use of the instrument.

The instrument is primarily a diagnostic tool and, only secondarily, a means of determining grades. The clinical supervisors are asked to rate the student on his performance in terms of the criteria in the rating scale. The tendency to interpret the rating scale in terms of grades $5 = A = $ Excellent, rather than in terms of the criteria, is occasionally apparent. As the supervisors become more familiar and comfortable with this concept, the tendency to "grade" decreases.

A particularly satisfying result of the approach used in the development of this instrument is its adaptability to other health professions. At the College of Allied Health Professions, two departments other than physical therapy have recognized the value and advantages of such an approach and are using it in developing their own clinical evaluation instruments.

A formal study to evaluate the reliability and validity of this instrument will be carried out when sufficient data are available.

REFERENCES

1. Gronlund NE: Measurement and Evaluation in Teaching. New York, The MacMillan Company, 1965
2. Mager RF: Preparing Objectives for Programmed Instruction. San Francisco, Fearon Publishers, 1962
3. American Physical Therapy Association. Handbook for Physical Therapy Teachers. New York, American Physical Therapy Association, 1967
4. Callahan ME, Dickinson R, Scully R: Cooperative Planning for Clinical Experience in Physical Therapy. Washington, D.C., Office of Vocational Rehabilitation, U.S. Department of Health, Education, and Welfare

the authors _____

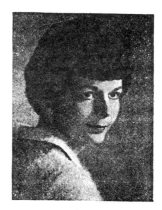

Barbara P. Kern is assistant professor of physical therapy at the College of Allied Health Professions of Temple University. She has been coordinator of clinical education in the Department of Physical Therapy at Temple University since the professional curriculum was initiated in 1967. Prior to her present role, she was assistant director of physical therapy at New York State Rehabilitation Hospital, West Haverstraw, where she was actively involved in student programs as a clinician. Miss Kern attended the 1965 and 1967 annual educational programs for physical therapy teachers, sponsored by the American Physical Therapy Association and Vocational Rehabilitation Administration.

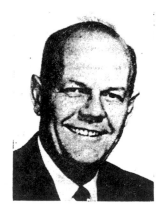

John M. Mickelson, Ed.D., has specialized in curriculum development for many years and formerly taught tests and measurements. He is now professor of Curriculum and Instruction at the College of Education, Temple University. Dr. Mickelson has been curriculum consultant for the College of Allied Health Professions, and has worked with other professional schools and educational laboratories. He has published in the curriculum field.

education_____

Reliability of a Method of Evaluating the Clinical Performance of a Physical Therapy Student

MARY JO MAYS, M.S.

Forty-three physical therapists participated in a study to determine the reliability of evaluations completed on thirty senior physical therapy students during their two six-week affiliations. The results indicated that the evaluation form could be considerably shorter and yield more reliable results. A proposed shorter form was constructed and is presented to show what types of objectives were statistically evaluated to be reliable and to present the way in which a student's performance can be graded on items which require a gradation of ability.

Methods used by physical therapy clinical instructors to evaluate physical therapy students during clinical affiliations contain discrepancies which are well known to the educators in our profession. Evaluation forms used to record the clinical performance of students have been criticized for being too long and too subjective. Variability in the health status of patients appears to add to the difficulty of evaluating the clinical performance of a student. The length of the affiliation period has been criticized for being too short to allow the clinical educator to make and provide valid evaluations.

Miss Mays is Assistant Professor in Physical Therapy, Division of Physical Therapy, University of Nebraska College of Medicine, Omaha, NB 68105.

This study was done in partial fulfillment of a master's degree at the Medical College of Virginia, Richmond, VA 23219.

RELATED STUDIES

The evaluation of students' clinical performance has been the subject of several studies. Hinz stated that a method of evaluation should apply to actual working situations. He believed that multiple observations of a large number of individual students by multiple observers were needed and that, to observe and assess students with validity and reliability, the perception and skill of faculties and other raters needed to be improved.[1]

In oral examinations, some examiners have been accused of grading extroverted students higher than introverted students, although the introverted students were more knowledgeable.[2] Bull suspected factors related to personality may have played a major role in determining clinical grades and that factual knowledge played only a minor role.[3,4] The biases of the evaluator have also affected evaluation. Some examiners press for a preconceived response; other examiners do not encourage students who are not doing well; and still others interrupt students while they are replying to questions.[5]

Although some investigators have found that seniority does not reduce observer variation,[6] some have found that less experienced examiners are less objective,[7] and some have found that the less experienced are unable to avoid personal bias when assessing students.[8] Evaluators generally agree that, unless the raters apply essentially the same standard in rating items under study, the pooling of ratings is not appropriate.[5,9,10]

Vigliano and Gaitonde found that the good student in medicine expressed genuine concern for his patients, empathized with his patients' feelings, carefully observed both the patient and himself, and, when alerted to his own reactions to a patient, was successful in managing those reactions. He was also reliable and had the ability to use his theoretical learning in the clinical care of patients.[9]

In the following study, the reliability of the information received on an evaluation form used by one school of physical therapy was investigated. The following hypotheses were proposed: 1) the raters will agree significantly about ranking of the objectives in order of importance, 2) certain objectives will be ranked significantly higher in importance than other objectives, and these higher ranked objectives will correlate significantly with the student's overall grade, and 3) certain criteria for a specific objective will be rated significantly higher in importance than other criteria for the same objective.

METHOD

Form and Subjects

The evaluation form used for this study has been used at the Medical College of Virginia since 1966 for the evaluation of senior physical therapy students during their full-time clinical affiliations. This final phase of the baccalaureate degree program consists of two different affiliations of six weeks each.

Thirty senior students, three men and twenty-seven women, aged from twenty-two to thirty-eight years, participated in this study during the summer of 1970. These students had generally similar learning experiences during the first two years of college, although they came from different colleges and universities. All had been enrolled for two years at the Medical College of Virginia for their physical therapy education.

The experience of the raters (n = 43) in physical therapy ranged from less than one year to twenty-five years. Their experience as clinical educators ranged from less than one to eighteen years; however, some had never used the evaluation form and some had used it as many as twenty times. Each clinical educator received the same detailed written directions for evaluation of student performance and the same interpretations of the form. Each was a graduate from an accredited curriculum in physical therapy. Although these variables are broad, they are common in physical therapy clinical education.

Each student was evaluated by two different raters, one for each six-week affiliation period. In some instances, the rater was assisted by other physical therapists in evaluating the student.

Ranking Objectives

Each rater was sent a data form which contained eleven objectives, each with two or more criteria (Tab. 1). These were the same objectives and criteria which were used in the form for evaluation of the students. The raters were asked to rank the objectives from 1 through 11 with none being given the same rank. Number 1 was assigned to the objective deemed most important; number 2 to the next most important; and so on through 11. Ranks 1, 2, 3, and 4 were grouped as the top-ranked objectives; ranks 5, 6, and 7 were grouped as the medium-ranked objectives; and 8, 9, 10, and 11 ranks were grouped as the least important objectives.

Rating Criteria

The raters were also asked to rate each of the criteria as high, medium, or low for each objective. For example, if an objective contained six criteria, a rater may have rated them

TABLE 1
Objectives and Criteria Which Appeared on Both the Evaluation and Data Forms

OBJECTIVE 1: Oral and Written Communication
Criteria:
a. Follows standard procedures of department
b. Expresses self in understandable and grammatically correct manner (and legibly when writing)
c. Reports in a manner which is objective, pertinent, reliable, inclusive, concise, organized
d. Respects confidential information
e. Uses accurate medical terminology
f. Exhibits tact and discretion
g. Completes progress notes and final summaries

OBJECTIVE 2: Application and Teaching of Physical Therapy Procedures
Criteria:
a. Understands goals of treatment
b. Prepares for treatment by reading chart and planning treatment procedures or teaching method
c. Organizes area and equipment for treatment
d. Prepares patient by proper positioning and draping
e. Explains and demonstrates treatment procedures to the patient
f. Performs procedures with manual skill in timing and efficiency

OBJECTIVE 3: Location and Recognition of Information
Criteria:
a. Seeks information from appropriate sources
b. Contributes to patient review sessions
c. Draws conclusions and makes recommendations regarding treatment, when appropriate

OBJECTIVE 4: Needs of Patient
Criteria:
a. Provides for physical needs in regard to comfort
b. Provides for physical needs in regard to medical conditions
c. Relieves apprehension and instills confidence
d. Establishes appropriate treatment atmosphere to achieve realistic goals
e. Initiates discussion with instructor regarding referrals to other services within hospital and community to meet patient's social and vocational needs

OBJECTIVE 5: Safety Procedures
Criteria:
a. Checks equipment before and after use regarding function, designated temperatures, repair, and placement
b. Provides supervision and protection of patients
c. Utilizes isolation and aseptic techniques
d. Checks patient's physical condition before, during, and after treatment
e. Guards own safety and health

OBJECTIVE 6: Application of Basic Knowledge to Physical Therapy Procedures
Criteria:
a. Sets realistic goals and plans treatment programs in a logical sequence
b. Compares patient's physical and physiological status with normal function and structure
c. Explains the rationale for choice of modality or procedure

OBJECTIVE 7: Organization and Utilization of Time
Criteria:
a. Uses unscheduled time for self-education, departmental maintenance, case presentation, or other assignments
b. Adheres to schedule
c. Prepares for patients by planning daily schedule
d. Utilizes nonprofessional personnel to advantage

OBJECTIVE 8: Interpersonal Relationships
Criteria:
a. Adjusts approach and level of communication to individual's age, education, and understanding
b. Contributes to the maintenance of a friendly and professional atmosphere

TABLE 1—*continued*

---

c. Understands and adjusts to mood and behavioral changes in self and others
d. Responds to criticisms and suggestions
e. Explains and gives instructions in treatment procedures to patient, his family, and others
f. Communicates with medical and paramedical personnel regarding the patient and physical therapy procedures

OBJECTIVE 9: Appraisal of His Own Performance and Behavior
  Criteria:
    a. Identifies his own weaknesses and strengths
    b. Analyzes and discusses his own performance with clinical instructor
    c. Seeks necessary information and assistance when carrying out treatment
    d. Demonstrates his understanding of the professional code of ethics

OBJECTIVE 10: Observation
  Criteria:
    a. Asks questions about what he has observed
    b. Indicates change in patient's status in oral and written comments
    c. Notes and responds to patient's clinical signs
    d. Observes patient's responses and analyzes performance
    e. Recognizes need for assistance and offers his help to patients and staff
    f. Recognizes signs of patient's apprehension
    g. Evaluates patient's total response following treatment
    h. Provides for progression of treatment on basis of analysis

OBJECTIVE 11: Maintenance of Physical Facilities, Including the Care of Equipment
  Criteria:
    a. Cleans up treatment area and equipment after use
    b. Reports need for equipment repair and need of supplies

---

so that three of the criteria were high, two were medium, and one was low. In addition to the data provided by the clinical raters, the grades which the students received on the objectives and the overall grade were collected.

Statistical Method

The grading scale of the form used to evaluate student performance contained terms such as unsatisfactory, satisfactory, highly satisfactory, and outstanding. The investigator used nonparametric statistics to indicate relative position of objectives and of criteria. The n value for raters (43) was considered a large value, statistically.

Interpretation of the reliability of the data was achieved by the Kendall coefficient of concordance. Differences in frequency rankings were compared by the Kolmogorov-Smirnov Goodness of Fit test. The comparison was made in terms of proportions and was unaffected by the size of the sample. If an objective were ranked in the high grouping (1, 2, 3, and 4)

twenty times out of thirty and if another objective were ranked in this grouping only five times out of thirty, the difference (D) would be .667 minus .167, or the D value would equal .500. The statistical significance of the Kendall coefficient value and the Kolmogorov-Smirnov Goodness of Fit test values was determined by chi-square. Furthermore, the grades which the students received on each objective were compared with the overall grades received by the students by using the Spearman rank correlation coefficient, sometimes called the rho correlation coefficient.

RESULTS

Interrater reliability was statistically significant at the .001 level (Kendall coefficient, .604); thus, the significant agreement among the raters in the rankings of the objectives could occur by chance only one in one thousand times. Although the Kendall coefficient is significant at the .001 level, it is not a high correlation value, showing that a strong

TABLE 2

Total Number of Times Each Objective Was Ranked "High," "Medium," or "Low," and the Kolmogorov-Smirnov (KS) Values[a]

Objectives	"High" Rank (1-4)	KS_H	"Medium" Rank (5-7)	KS_M	"Low" Rank (8-11)	KS_L
1. Oral and written communication	12	−.095	22	.265	9	−.170
2. Application and teaching of physical therapy procedures	37	.544	6	−.144	0	−.400
3. Location and recognition of information	4	−.300	12	.009	27	.291
4. Needs of patient	30	.365	13	.035	0	−.400
5. Safety procedures	10	−.147	17	.137	16	.009
6. Application of basic knowledge to physical therapy procedures	40	.621	2	−.247	1	−.374
7. Organization and utilization of time	0	−.402	10	−.042	33	.444
8. Interpersonal relationships	21	.135	13	.035	9	−.170
9. Appraisal of his own performance and behavior	3	−.326	10	−.042	30	.368
10. Observation	16	.007	23	.291	4	−.298
11. Maintenance of physical facilities, including the care of equipment	0	−.402	0	−.298	43	.700

[a] KS values were determined by a one-tailed test for each objective within a rank.

factor (or factors) exists which limits the agreement among the raters.

The objectives judged to be significantly more important than other objectives (by the Kolmogorov-Smirnov test) were "application of basic knowledge to physical therapy procedures," "application and teaching of physical therapy procedures," "needs of patient," and "observation" (Tab. 2). These results were significant at the .01 level.

The grades for the top four objectives had high correlation values with the overall grades received by the thirty students; however, other objectives had correlation values which were as high or higher. For example, the grade for "location and recognition of information" in both six-week affiliation periods had a high correlation with the overall grade which tends to suggest a halo effect since this objective was considered less important than the top four objectives. A comparison of correlations between grades on objectives and the overall grades for the first six-week affiliation period with the correlations derived from the second six-week affiliation period shows the latter to be higher (Tab. 3).

The most significantly rated criteria for the four objectives judged to be the most important by the raters are shown in Table 4. Each objective contained at least one criterion rated significantly high, one rated significantly medium, and one rated significantly low, except "application of basic knowledge to physical therapy procedures." This objective contained three criteria of which one was rated significantly higher than the other two; the remaining two showed no significant differences in ratings.

A shorter evaluation form was developed which consisted of the top four objectives and the criteria rated significantly high for each objective (Tab. 5). The criteria were arranged, as were the objectives, so that the first was the most important and the last was the least important.

Forty-three raters ranked the objectives and thirteen made at least one error in rating the criteria. Errors included failure to rate one of the criteria and rating all of the criteria of an objective as medium and low, and none as high. Errors were seldom the same; only three criteria contained more than one error. These errors were determined to be of no consequence to the results (Kolmogorov-Smirnov test).

DISCUSSION

The clinical education in health professions curricula is necessary and important; therefore, a valid and reliable method for evaluating the students' performances in the clinics is a high priority of our educational programs. Although this study did not achieve a method of evaluation which is completely valid and totally reliable, it has identified objectives and criteria agreed upon by the clinical educators who used this particular evaluation form.

Of the four objectives which were ranked as the most important, the two relating to knowledge and skills may be evaluated on specific observable behavior. One objective, "needs of patient," is in the affective domain and illustrates some of the "good student" qualities described by Vigliano and Gaitonde; i.e., if a student appears concerned about patients and shows respect and understanding, the rater has a tendency to say that the student is good.[9] Also, since the raters' observations were always face-to-face, personality factors such as considering another's needs may have been a determining factor in a rater's evaluation of a student's performance. This conclusion is supported by Holloway.[2]

The objective which was selected as fourth in importance by the raters was "observation." The author believes that in order for the student to fulfill the other objectives which were ranked of higher importance than this objective, the student must first be capable of making astute observations. Interestingly, the raters ranked this objective as fifth in importance during the first of the two full-time affiliation periods, and first in the second affiliation period (Tab. 3).

Table 3 suggests that during the first affiliation period the raters were more concerned about the student's basic knowledge and his abilities to locate information and to write acceptable progress notes. By the second affiliation period, the raters apparently assumed that the student knew the procedures of therapy and had communication skills, and they then expected the student to begin to recognize the patient's needs, to improve his observation skills which would enable him to evaluate the patient's condition and the results of therapeutic procedures, and to establish

TABLE 3
Objectives, Ranks, and RHO Correlations between Grades on each of the Eleven Objectives and the Overall Evaluation Grades Received by the Students (n = 30)

Objective	Rank	Rho First 6 Weeks	Rho Second 6 Weeks
1. Oral and written communication	6	.84	.83
2. Application and teaching of physical therapy procedures[a]	2	.79	.90
3. Location and recognition of information	8	.91	.90
4. Needs of patient[a]	3	.69	.88
5. Safety procedures	7	.61	.77
6. Application of basic knowledge to physical therapy procedures[a]	1	.85	.88
7. Organization and utilization of time	10	.73	.75
8. Interpersonal relationships	5	.67	.86
9. Appraisal of his own performance and behavior	9	.61	.77
10. Observation[a]	4	.76	.95
11. Maintenance of physical facilities, including the care of equipment	11	.56	.61

With an n of 30, a rho coefficient of .364 is significant at the .05 level, while a value of .478 is significant at the .01 level.

[a] These objectives were considered the four most important.

acceptable standards of interpersonal relations.

The agreement of the raters on the criteria which they ranked as significantly high may have resulted from the fact that those particular criteria expressed achievement of the more elementary criteria for the stated objective. For example, in Table 4, the criterion of objective 2 which was ranked significantly high was "understands goals of treatment." In order to meet this criterion, the student must first meet the more elementary criteria listed for the objective which were "organizes area and equipment for treatment" and "prepares for treatment by

TABLE 4
Kolmogorov-Smirnov Test Values and the Chi-Square Values of the Most Significantly Ranked Criteria for the Four Significantly "High" Ranked Objectives

Objectives and Criteria	Kolmogorov-Smirnov Value	Chi-Square Value
6. Application of Basic Knowledge to Physical Therapy Procedures		
Sets realistic goals and plans treatment programs in a logical sequence	.651	48.34
2. Application and Teaching of Physical Therapy Procedures		
Understands goals of treatment	.492	34.61
Prepares for treatment by reading chart and planning treatment procedures or teaching method	.336	16.16
Prepares patient by proper positioning and draping	.604	21.19
Organizes area and equipment for treatment	.663	62.78
4. Needs of Patient		
Provides for physical needs in regard to medical conditions	.442	26.83
Relieves apprehension and instills confidence	.268	9.91
Provides for physical needs in regard to comfort	.256	9.08[a]
Initiates discussion with instructor regarding referrals to other services within hospital and community to meet patient's social and vocational needs	.465	29.72
10. Observation		
Provides for progression of treatment on basis of analysis	.421	26.55
Notes and responds to patient's clinical signs	.315	14.85
Recognizes signs of patient's apprehension	.338	17.10
Asks questions about what he has observed	.307	13.50

[a] Chi-square value significant at the .05 level. All others significant at the .01 level.

reading chart and planning treatment procedures or teaching method."

CONCLUSION

Caution must be taken when interpreting the results of this study. Although each of the statistical levels of significance was at the .01 level, except for one of the criteria in Table 5, one can state only relationships of the results obtained in this study, not absolute truths, as many unknown variables are present. At this time, information is insufficient to make a conclusive statement about any of the objectives or criteria as they relate to the thoughts of the raters at the time they evaluated the students and at the time they documented the information for this study. Several investigators have stated that evaluators can distinguish only one or two components such as skill and knowledge. Considering the results of this study, I suggest that the preferred evaluation form would be one which measures the skill and knowledge components and omits material such as the student's appearance or his inter-personal relationships. These last components are probably best evaluated in the classroom during the first months of the academic curriculum and not in the clinic where the students are seen for only four to eight weeks. The short form derived from this study contains those components of skill and knowledge which the raters considered most important. The remaining objectives and criteria could be omitted because the raters' rankings and ratings and the correlations with those in practice indicate that they are inconsistent and unstable.

By using the criteria ranked significantly high, medium, and low for each of the top objectives in the evaluation of student performance, unnecessary items can be omitted and student performance can be gradated. The latter provides information concerning the level at which the student is performing (high, medium, or low). The quality ratings currently being employed would continue to be used in order to indicate the level of performance as unsatisfactory, satisfactory, highly satisfactory, or outstanding.

TABLE 5
Proposed Short Form

	Unsatisfactory	Satisfactory	Highly Satisfactory	Outstanding
OBJECTIVE 1: Application of Basic Knowledge to Physical Therapy Procedures				
Sets realistic goals and plans treatment programs in a logical sequence	_____	_____	_____	_____

Overall Grade: 1   2   3   4   5   6   7   8

OBJECTIVE 2: Application and Teaching of Physical Therapy Procedures				
Understands goals of treatment	_____	_____	_____	_____
Prepares for treatment by reading chart and planning treatment procedures or teaching method	_____	_____	_____	_____
Prepares patient by proper positioning and draping	_____	_____	_____	_____
Organizes area and equipment for treatment	_____	_____	_____	_____

Overall Grade: 1   2   3   4   5   6   7   8

OBJECTIVE 3: Needs of Patient				
Provides for physical needs in regard to medical conditions	_____	_____	_____	_____
Relieves apprehension and instills confidence	_____	_____	_____	_____
Provides for physical needs in regard to comfort	_____	_____	_____	_____
Initiates discussion with instructor regarding referrals to other services within hospital and community to meet patient's social and vocational needs	_____	_____	_____	_____

Overall Grade: 1   2   3   4   5   6   7   8

OBJECTIVE 4: Observation				
Provides for progression of treatment on basis of analysis	_____	_____	_____	_____
Notes and responds to patient's clinical signs	_____	_____	_____	_____
Recognizes signs of patient's apprehension	_____	_____	_____	_____
Asks questions about what he has observed	_____	_____	_____	_____

Overall Grade: 1   2   3   4   5   6   7   8

Final Overall Grade: 1   2   3   4   5   6   7   8

Comments:

The short form is a means of improving interrater reliability by providing consistent results based on the student's level of ability. Since some forms used in other physical therapy programs are similar to the one used in this study, those forms might also be strengthened by revising the objectives into the components of skill and knowledge.

I also suggest that all raters receive instruction and practice to enable them to produce valid and reliable ratings. A form alone cannot provide an adequate evaluation. The evaluator's ability to observe and interpret his observations is crucial to providing information which determines whether a student passes or fails. This instruction should be provided by someone qualified to teach others to be teachers, and it should include teaching the rater what and how to teach students, how to observe students, and how to evaluate that which has been observed.

Students should have the opportunity to learn to treat patients in the clinical setting prior to being evaluated. Until more practical, supervised, clinical experience can be provided for the students during the academic portion of their physical therapy education, the problems inherent in entering full-time clinical education remain. The clinical evaluator must not base the student's evaluation on what he thinks the student should know as a result of classroom study; rather, he should evaluate the student on what he has been taught in the clinic as well as on the skills and knowledge he had at the beginning of the affiliation.

Observation and evaluation of student clinical performance is complex, and the patient, the rater, and student contribute to the variability present in this type of evaluation. To arrive at an accurate evaluation of student performance, the rater must be instructed carefully so that he can observe and interpret his observations in the clinical setting. More emphasis must be placed on correlation of information received in the didactic program. In addition, the student must be taught to apply his basic knowledge in the clinical situation.

Some unanswered questions which are considered important have resulted from this study. What criteria did the raters use to apply the term *important* at the time they ranked and rated the criteria? To what degree do the differences in the clinical and educational experiences of the raters affect interrater agreement? In order to answer these questions, further investigative studies need to be done. In addition to replicating this study, further studies should concentrate on areas such as the value of early clinical experiences for the student and the progression of abilities which one might expect. The results of such studies could yield a standard method of evaluating student clinical performance.

REFERENCES

1. Hinz CF: Direct observation as a means of teaching and evaluating clinical skills. J Med Educ 41:150-161, 1966
2. Holloway PJ, Collins CK, Start KB: Reliability of viva voce examinations. Br Dent J 125:211-214, 1968
3. Bull GM: An examination of the final examination in medicine. Lancet 2:368-372, 1956
4. Bull GM: Examinations. J Med Educ 34:1154-1158, 1959
5. Waugh D, Moyse CA: Medical education; part II, oral examinations: a videotape study of the reliability of grades in pathology. Can Med Assoc J 100:635-640, 1969
6. Wilson GM, Harden R, Lever R, et al: Examination of clinical examiners. Lancet 1:37-42, 1969
7. Salzman LF, Romano J: Grading clinical performance in psychiatry. J Med Educ 38:746-751, 1963
8. Oaks WW, Sebeinok PA, Justed FL: Objective evaluation of a method of assessing student performance in a clinical clerkship. J Med Educ 44:207-213, 1969
9. Vigliano A, Gaitonde M: Evaluation of a method of assessing student performances in a clinical clerkship. J Med Educ 40:205-213, 1965
10. Hammond RR, Kern F: Teaching Comprehensive Medical Care. Cambridge, Massachusetts, Harvard University Press, 1959
11. Clissold GK, Metz EA: Evaluation—a tangible process. Nurs Outlook 14:41-45, 1966
12. Medical College of Virginia School of Physical Therapy: An Investigative Study Concerning Clinical Education. Vocational Rehabilitation Training Program, grant OVR 30-61, Dept HEW, 1961-1966

THE AUTHOR

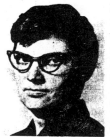

Mary Jo Mays is assistant professor of physical therapy, Division of Physical Therapy, University of Nebraska College of Medicine, Omaha, Nebraska. She received a certificate in physical therapy from the University of Colorado and a master's degree in physical therapy from the Medical College of Virginia. Before the latter degree was received, she worked for four years at the University of Minnesota Hospitals and spent three of those years as a clinical educator.

Evaluating Student Clinical Performance in the Affective Domain
CAROL M. DAVIS

Teaching students in the clinic setting can be a rewarding experience. Clinical instructors rarely experience difficulties teaching or evaluating students in cognitive or psychomotor domains. However, teaching and evaluating student performance in the affective domain can be a challenge. Affective behavior, or the appropriate attitudes, values and beliefs of a professional, exist in each person as constructs, or combinations of a variety of human processes including emotion. When evaluating affective behavior, we must do so indirectly. Because, behavior that is value-laden is never the value itself, rather it is an outward expression or reflection of an inner construct. For this reason it is necessary that clinical educators clearly describe those clinical behaviors they are looking for when evaluating affective behavior of students. For example, if we do not know what the behavior "displays initiative" looks like when we see it, how can we evaluate it? Therefore, barriers to successful clinical education evaluation of student affective behavior must be identified, and an approach to skillful evaluation of affective behaviors of students must be developed.

THE AFFECTIVE DOMAIN

Krathwohl and others[1] organized a taxonomy of affective learning into five stages (Figure 1). Each new student has a partly developed and regularly expanding set of attitudes, beliefs and values, most of which supported the choice of an allied health profession as a meaningful career. Attitudinal differences students display are more often due to individual priority of values than to actual value content. For example, some students will have career goals directed toward working in the areas of prevention and athletics while others will express a driving force to work with children or the elderly. This goal diversity is healthy and contributes to the wide range of interests that our professions can embrace and accept.

When evaluating the affective domain, the challenge is to identify appropriate clinical performances behaviors (and the accompanying attitudes, beliefs and values) as well as describing those behaviors that are inappropriate as professional ideals. However, when attempting to identify and describe these behaviors key questions arise. For example, what behaviors demonstrate the affective ideals of physical therapy? Where can we go to learn what we ought to value, what we want to identify and reinforce as professional values in our students? Perhaps even more important, where do we look to identify behaviors that clearly violate our profession's standards of excellence? Many physical therapists would quickly reply that the American Physical Therapy Association's Code of Ethics provides these guidelines. Professional Codes and their Standards of Conduct imply behavior that is acceptable and unacceptable in professional practice. Most Codes of Ethics enjoin professionals to do no harm, but do all one can for the patient.[2] These documents fail to guide clinicians in their daily patient care challenges. Specifically, these ethical codes do not provide much help in making those minor patient care choices that do not fall clearly within the Code of Ethics, but do clearly delineate an average clinical performance from one that is outstanding. This daily or formative evaluation process constitutes the very foundation of clinical education, and challenges our abilities to differentiate between student behaviors.

Major Category in the Affective Domain	Description of Major Category
1. Receiving	Willingness to attend to a stimulus
2. Responding	Active participation by the student
3. Valuing	Worth or value a student attaches to a particular object, phenomenon, or behavior.
4. Organization	Bringing together of different values, resolving conflict, and beginning the building of an internally consistent values system.
5. Characterization by a value or value complex	A value system so internalized that it has become a pattern of "life style". The behavior is consistent, pervasive, and predictable.

Figure 1.
Krathwohl's description of major categories in the taxonomy of the affective domain.

AN APPROACH TO CLARIFYING EXPECTATIONS OF AFFECTIVE PERFORMANCE

Before students report to a clinic, the supervisor of clinical education at that facility (usually the Center Coordinator of Clinical Education, CCCE) convenes the total patient care staff and distributes a copy of the evaluation form to be used with students. The evaluation instrument is reviewed and all unclear or vague terms are listed on a chalkboard for discussion. How to evaluate a student's professionalism is an example of the problems clinical instructors face when evaluating affective domain behavior. In spite of the absence of a widely accepted description of the value priorities in our profession, most performance evaluation instruments require clinical instructors to evaluate a student's professionalism. This type of clinical performance objective may be stated that: "The student must demonstrate professional behavior". Criteria to measure this objective could be as follows: a) Maintains patient confidentiality, b) Displays initiative, c) Maintains proper perspective between professional and personal affairs, d) Organizes time effectively, e) Arrives punctually and leaves according to standard hours.

Using this approach for clarifying affective performance, the CCCE first asks the staff: "Do you agree that these five criteria adequately describe what we mean by 'professional behavior' at this facility?". Staff members are invited to add, delete or change the given criteria for the objective.

Next the CCCE asks, "Which words seem vague or unclear to you?". Staff members may express difficulty describing the behaviors associated with criterion b, displays initiative. Some people may want to also clarify criterion c, maintaining a proper perspective. Criteria a, d and c, patient confidentiality, time organization, and punctuality describe behaviors that are easier to identify and evaluate.

In the third step of this process, the CCCE writes, "Displays initiative," on the chalkboard. The staff then collaborates to identify and describe examples of behavior that are representative of outstanding, acceptable and unacceptable performances. Figure 2 illustrates the beginning of this process. Results of this collaborative process are a clear description of expected behavior from students as well as a better understanding of what student behaviors look for on the part of physical therapy staff members. Having this information makes both the clinical instructors and the students aware of those activities that assure outstanding patient care.

Objective: Demonstrates professional behavior

Criterion b: Displays initiative

LEVELS OF PERFORMANCE

Unacceptable	Acceptable	Outstanding
Refuses to consult tests, articles; can think of no questions, even wants "the" answer spelled out. Never helps out with staff duties (clean up, weekend duty, etc.).	Looks answers up, asks good questions, willing to problem solve, helps out with staff duties.	Is willing to present continuing education without being asked. Questions reveal complex reasoning. Tolerates ambiguity well. Volunteers with staff duties without being asked.

Figure 2
Staff clarification of vague or unclear criteria in student evaluation.

In conclusion, clinical instructors are often confused and unclear about the nature of what is being evaluated when observing student behavior, especially in the area of evaluating affective performance. Attitudes, values and beliefs are elusive, inner constructs. Evaluating behavior that seems to point toward racial prejudice, for example, gets blurred by such things as a desire to please, peer group pressure, ambivalences from experiences in life, lack of self-awareness and inconsistency.[3] Clinical instructors can not use the same direct types of approaches for evaluating attitudes and values as they use to evaluate a student's knowledge and skills. When evaluating a student's affective performance, the clinical instructor should keep the following suggestions in mind. View patterns of the student's behavior rather than focusing on a one-time incidence. Gather specific indicators of a behavior on more than one occasion and on more than one activity. When questioning students about their behaviors, maintain a non-judgmental attitude. For example, saying: "Yesterday I noticed...", rather than, "Why did you...", gives a student the opportunity to respond nondefensively. Remember that students are just learning how to transpose life-long behaviors to professional patient care. Invite them to ponder the reasons behind

their choices in such a way that the behavior itself remains primary rather than the need to please instructors. A few behaviors are clearly not acceptable under any circumstance, for example, striking a patient and telling untruths for personal gain. The physical therapy staff should be responsible for identifying unacceptable student behaviors. Also, they must know what to do if a student should demonstrate such a behavior. Daily journals and logs or other self-report mechanisms done by students can yield rich descriptions of learning and development. But, to be used effectively as indicators of learning, self-reports need to be collected, read and discussed with students on a frequent basis.

Effective clinical education demands instruction in the values, beliefs and attitudes appropriate to the helping professions. If we are unwilling to respond to that challenge, we have to assume responsibility for the inappropriate, or worse, harmful actions of our graduates.

Dr. Davis is an Associate Professor in the Division of Physical Therapy, School of Medicine, University of Miami, 5801 Red Road, Coral Gables, FL, 33146.

REFERENCES

1. Krathwohl DK, Bloom BS, Masia BB: Taxonomy of Educational Objectives. New York, NY, David McKay, 1984.
2. Henderson ME, Morris LL, Fitz-Gibbons CT: How to Measure Attitudes. Beverly Hills, CA, Sage Publications, 1978.
3. Purtilo RB: Ethics in allied health education: State of the art. J of Allied Health 12(3):210-220, 1983.

Evaluation of Clinical Sites and Clinical Faculty

Evaluation of Clinical Education Centers in Physical Therapy

JEAN S. BARR,
JAN GWYER,
and ZIPPORA TALMOR

The purpose of this research was to test a set of 20 physical therapy clinical education standards and three related evaluation forms that were published in 1976 by Moore and Perry.[1] Mail questionnaires and telephone interviews with 134 Academic Coordinators of Clinical Education, 708 Center Coordinators of Clinical Education, 15 Clinical Instructors, and 52 students were used to collect data reported here. The resulting standards and evaluation forms were found to be practical, reliable, and valid for use by personnel of physical therapy and physical therapist assistant educational programs responsible for selecting clinical education centers for part-time and full-time students. We recommend that the standards and evaluation forms be used by personnel of physical therapy educational programs, clinical education centers, and selected committees of the American Physical Therapy Association because the standards and forms incorporate aspects of clinical education currently believed important to providing high-quality learning experiences in physical therapy practice.

Key Words: *Clinical education, Physical therapy.*

Physical therapy education comprises academic and clinical activities designed to assure students acquire the knowledge, attitudes, and skills required for physical therapy practice. To meet this objective, the content and skills learned in the classroom or laboratory must be applied, analyzed, synthesized, and evaluated in physical therapy clinical environments. For this reason, availability of high-quality clinical education centers is vital to the profession of physical therapy.

The physical therapy profession has had no widely accepted set of standards and forms for the evaluation and selection of clinical education centers. In the past,

Dr. Barr was Director, Project on Clinical Education, and Visiting Research Associate, Division of Physical Therapy, University of North Carolina at Chapel Hill, Chapel Hill, NC, when this study was performed. She is now a consultant in physical therapy education, Rt 8, Box 38, Chapel Hill, NC 27514 (USA).

Ms. Gwyer was Visiting Research Assistant. Division of Physical Therapy, University of North Carolina at Chapel Hill, when this study was performed. She is now a doctoral candidate, School of Education, University of North Carolina at Chapel Hill, Chapel Hill, NC 27514.

Mrs. Talmor was Visiting Research Assistant, Division of Physical Therapy, University of North Carolina at Chapel Hill, when this study was performed. She now resides at 1610 Frisch Rd, Madison, WI 53711.

Requests for further information about the project should be directed to Institute for Research in Social Science, Manning Hall, University of North Carolina at Chapel Hill, Chapel Hill, NC 27514.

This project was supported, in part, by Grant No. 1 D12 AH 90181 from the Public Health Service. Bureau of Health Manpower, US Department of Health, Education and Welfare.

This article was submitted September 29, 1980, and accepted January 4, 1982.

this void was filled by personnel of each educational program developing their own criteria and forms, which have not usually been tested for practicality, reliability, or validity. Additionally, some centers for clinical education were selected primarily on the basis of availability of "slots" for students; geographic proximity of the centers; and perceptions, beliefs, and values concerning learning, physical therapy, and clinical education believed held by the centers' staffs.[1]

A preliminary set of 20 clinical education standards and three related evaluation forms were published in 1976.[1] Neither the reliability and validity of those standards and evaluation forms nor their applicability to clinical education centers of varying sizes and types was tested. Our recent Project on Clinical Education (1980) focused on testing and revising the 1976 documents, and the results of that project are reported here.

This article introduces to physical therapy professionals a clinical education center evaluation process that has been demonstrated through nationwide testing to be 1) practical for use by Academic Coordinators of Clinical Education (ACCEs), Center Coordinators of Clinical Education (CCCEs), and students; 2) reliable in that there was a high degree of agreement among independent evaluations of centers when the evaluators had identical information to use in making their evaluations; and 3) valid in that the identical information with which the evaluators were provided conveyed the same meaning to them, enabled them to have similar interpretations of it, and led to a high degree of agreement in their independent evaluations of the centers. This process makes use of "Standards for a Clinical Education Center in Physical Therapy" and three evaluation forms: "Self Assessment of a Physical Therapy Clinical Education Center" (Self-Assessment form), "Profile of a Physical Therapy Clinical Education Center" (Profile form), and "Student's Evaluation of a Clinical Education Experience" (Student's form). This article 1) describes briefly how these products were derived, 2) reports the results of reliability and validity studies of the products, and 3) discusses the potential uses of the products by individuals and components of the professional physical therapy community.

METHOD

The project focused on the following research questions:

1. Are ACCEs and personnel of clinical education centers using the 1976 Standards and Evaluation Forms?
2. Are standards for selection of clinical education centers needed?
3. Is each 1976 Standard clear?
4. Is each 1976 Evaluation Form practical in terms of time and cost required to complete it?
5. Are the 1976 Evaluation Forms useful, clear, specific, consistent with the Standards, and of appropriate lengths?
6. Can the 1976 Standards and Evaluation Forms be used with all sizes and types of centers, during all stages and lengths of clinical education assignments, and by personnel of physical therapy and physical therapist assistant educational programs alike?
7. Should the 1976 Standards be grouped or combined into general categories pertaining to clinical education (eg, Administration, Resources)?
8. Do the 1976 Standards reflect the implicit standards that ACCEs report they use in evaluating clinical education centers?
9. How do ACCEs and CCCEs rank the importance and practicality of each 1976 Standard?
10. Are any of the 1976 Standards so essential that a center's lack of compliance would cause an ACCE either not to initiate an affiliation with that clinical education center or to cease affiliation with it?
11. Are the revised (1980) Self-Assessment, Profile, and Student's forms reliable?
12. Are the revised Self-Assessment and Student's forms valid?
13. Is the total evaluation process that is based on use of the revised standards and evaluation forms reliable and valid?

Several individual studies were designed to answer the above questions. Table 1 identifies each study by name and by numbers of the research questions it was designed to answer and outlines pertinent details of the study.

Mailed questionnaires alone or in combination with telephone interviews were used to obtain data about the practicality, reliability, or validity of standards and evaluation forms to be used in physical therapy clinical education programs. Altogether, 134 ACCEs, 708 CCCEs, 15 Clinical Instructors (CIs),

TABLE 1
Summary of Method for Each Project Study

Study Name	Research Question(s)[a]	Sample/Size	Method	Return Rate (%)
Status	1	ACCEs/134	Q[b]	79
Pretest	2–6	ACCEs/28	Q + I[c]	100
		CCCEs/28	Q + I	100
		Students/28	Q + I	100
Grouping	7	ACCEs/15	Q	87
Profile	8	ACCEs/89	Q	78
		CCCEs/128	Q	62
Weighting	2, 9, 10	ACCEs/71	Q	89
		CCCEs/400	Q	64
Interrater reliability	11, 12	CCCEs/5	SA[d] + P[e]	80
		CIs/20	SA + P	75
		Students/25	S[f]	76
Internal consistency	11	CCCEs/100	SA	50
Test	13	CCCEs/20	SA + P	85
		ACCEs/54	SA + P	80

[a] See text.
[b] Q = Mailed questionnaire.
[c] I = Telephone, semistructured interview.
[d] SA = Completed Self-Assessment form.
[e] P = Completed Profile form.
[f] S = Completed Student's form.

TABLE 2

Center Coordinators of Clinical Education Expressed Need for Standards by Size and Type of Center: Variables in Analyses of Variance

Center Size and Type Category	n	Mean Score[a]
General hospital > 400 beds	6	4.1
General hospital < 400 beds	4	4.3
Rehabilitation hospital	4	4.8
Other hospital (mental, children's)	3	4.7
Extended care facilities	4	4.5
Special outpatient with clinic setting (private practice, day care)	4	3.8
Community, public, or mental health without clinic setting	3	4.3

[a] Scale: 1 = strongly disagree; 5 = strongly agree.

and 52 physical therapy and physical therapist assistant students participated in this two-year, nationwide study. We have compiled a comprehensive description of the methods used during the project (unpublished data).

RESULTS

The 1976 and 1980 Standards are essentially alike. They address the same topics and contain nearly identical content in standard statements and interpretations. The differences are in the order in which the standards are listed and in the wording changes included in the 1980 set to clarify ambiguities identified in the earlier standards and interpretations. The 1976 Standards were used in the first five studies presented in Table 1.

Standards

Need for standards. All ACCE and CCCE participants in the Pretest study agreed that standards for clinical education in physical therapy are needed. An analysis of variance test was made of CCCE responses by seven categories based on size and type of center. The information analyzed is given in Table 2. No significant difference among the means in Table 2 was found, indicating that standards are needed regardless of the size and type of the center. Sixty-five percent of the Pretest respondents also stated that standards should be used as guidelines rather than as minimal requirements.

Content of the standards. Figure 1 lists the 20 1980 Standards thought by ACCEs and CCCEs to embody the basic characteristics of a center. These standards are specifically related to the quality of clinical education the center can provide. Data related to the content of the standards were collected during the Status, Weighting, Profile, and Grouping studies.

More than 60 percent of the ACCE respondents in the Status study indicated that, with the exception of the standard concerning "Professional Associations" (1980 Standard 15) mentioned by 50 percent of the ACCEs, all of the 1976 Standards are essential. (This

standard was also listed by 13 percent of the ACCEs and CCCEs participating in the Weighting study as one that could be dropped. Although the standard concerning "Professional Associations" appeared not to be essential to some ACCEs and CCCEs, it was essential to a large number of others. The data, when taken together, did not clearly mandate dropping this standard or any other from the 1976 list of 20.)

From 8 to 13 percent of the Weighting study participants, as indicated by the percentages listed below in parentheses, suggested that the following standards be dropped: "Consumer Satisfaction" (13%); "Support Services" (12%); "Affirmative Action" (11%); and "Internal Evaluation" (8%). Standards that the Weighting study participants suggested be added to the original 20 were found by the project staff to be already included or implied.

Respondents to the Grouping study did not believe that the 1976 Standards should be grouped into more general categories of interest in clinical education (eg, resources). Seventy-seven percent of the participants stated the standards were useful as they appear in Figure 1.

In the Profile study, ACCEs and CCCEs listed 38 characteristics of a "strong" (high-quality) clinical education center. Eighteen of these characteristics were paraphrases of 1976 Standards. "Consumer Satisfaction" and "Affirmative Action" were not mentioned. The project staff was able to match each of the remaining 20 characteristics with one of the 1976 Standards or interpretations. Table 3 lists these 20 characteristics and the key words of the standard or interpretation to which each was matched.

In summary, the data indicated that the 1976 Standards adequately represent the implicit standards that ACCEs and CCCEs report using to evaluate centers for physical therapy clinical education. These implicit standards also describe a high-quality clinical education center in physical therapy. Because of the small percentages of respondents who suggested deletions, none of the 1976 Standards were dropped.

Clarity of the standards. The ACCEs and CCCEs in the Pretest study reviewed and critiqued the clarity of each 1976 Standard with its interpretation. The data

Number	Text
1	The physical therapy service provides an active, stimulating environment appropriate for the learning needs of the student. (Learning environment)[a]
2	Clinical education programs for students are planned to meet specific objectives of the educational program, the physical therapy service, and the individual student. (Program planning)
3	The clinical center has a variety of learning experiences available to students. (Learning experiences)
4	The physical therapy staff practices ethically and legally. (Ethical standards)
5	The clinical center is committed to the principle of equal opportunity and affirmative action as required by federal legislation. (Affirmative action)
* * * * * * * * * * * * * *[b]	
6	The clinical center's philosophy and its objectives for patient care and clinical education are compatible with those of the educational institution. (Compatible philosophy and objectives)
7	The clinical center demonstrates administrative interest in and support of physical therapy clinical education. (Administrative support)
8	Communications within the clinical center are effective and positive. (Effective communications)
9	The physical therapy staff is adequate in number to provide a good educational program for students. (Staff number)
10	One physical therapist with specific qualifications is responsible for coordinating the assignments and activities of the students at the clinical center. (Center coordinators of clinical education)
11	Clinical instructors are selected based on specific criteria. (Clinical instructor selection)
12	Clinical instructors apply the basic principles of education—teaching and learning—to clinical education. (Principles of teaching and learning)
13	Special expertise of the various center staff members is shared with students. (Sharing special expertise)
14	There is an active staff development program for the clinical center. (Staff development)
15	The physical therapy staff is interested and active in professional associations related to physical therapy. (Professional associations)
16	The physical therapy service has an active and viable process of internal evaluation of its own affairs and is receptive to procedures of review and audit approved by appropriate external agencies. (Internal evaluation)
17	The various consumers are satisfied that their needs for physical therapy service have been met. (Consumer satisfaction)
18	Roles of the various types of physical therapy personnel at the clinical center are clearly defined and distinguished from one another. (Personnel roles)
19	Selected support services are available to students. (Support services)
20	Adequate space for study, conferences, and treating patients is available to students. (Adequate space)

[a] Key words in parentheses are used for identification purposes in this article.
[b] List of 20 standards is divided into two groups; a satisfactory level of compliance with 1–5 should be achieved before assigning or accepting students to a center.

Fig. 1. *1980 Standards for a clinical education center in physical therapy.*

TABLE 3

Selected Characteristics of a "Strong" Clinical Education Center in Physical Therapy Compared to "Standards for a Clinical Education Center"

Characteristic Key Words	Standard Key Words and Numbers	
Independent practice	Learning experiences	3
Evaluation of students	Principles of teach/learn	12
Variety of patients	Learning experiences	3
Equipment	Learning experiences	3
Balance in variety of experiences	Learning experiences	3
Orientation program	Program planning	2
Primary patient care	Learning experiences	3
Treatment techniques	Learning experiences	3
Students from several schools	Administrative support	7
Convenient geographical location	Program planning	2
Length of affiliation	Program planning	2
Written agreements	Administrative support	7
PTs from diverse schools	Learning environment	1
Methods	Learning experiences	3
Medical direction	Effective communications	8
Students to challenge staff	Learning environment	1
Community acceptance	Compatible phil/objs	6
Accredited institutions	Administrative support	7
PTAs on staff	Personnel roles	18
Staff accept PTA program	Learning environment	1

collected indicated that improvements were needed in the wordings of standards and interpretations on "Compatible Philosophy and Objectives" (1980 Standard 6) and "Staff Number" (1980 Standard 9). Additional changes were recommended in the interpretations of standards concerning "Learning Experiences" (1980 Standard 3); "Administrative Support" (1980 Standard 7); "Effective Communications" (1980 Standard 8); "Clinical Instructor Selection" (1980 Standard 11); "Principles of Teaching and Learning" (1980 Standard 12); "Staff Development" (1980 Standard 14); "Professional Associations (1980 Standard 15); "Internal Evaluation" (1980 Standard 16); and "Consumer Satisfaction" (1980 Standard 17). The interpretations of six standards were cited as overlapping. Two of these six interpretations, and three others, were found not to pertain to clinical education.

In summary, several 1976 Standards and interpretations were identified by Pretest study participants

TABLE 4

Composite Important, Practical, and Crucial Rankings of Standards by All Respondents

Standard Key Words[a]	Rank Order		
	Important	Practical	Crucial
Learning environment	1	1	3
Program planning	3	4	4
Learning experiences	4	3	7
Ethical standards	5	6	1
Affirmative action	17	12	8
Compatible philosophy and objectives	6	8	5
Administrative support	13	10	6
Effective communications	8	9	9
Staff number	2	2	2
Center clinical coordinator	7	5	10
Clinical instructor selection	11	14	11
Principles of teaching and learning	12	13	12
Sharing special expertise	9	7	19
Staff development	10	11	16
Professional associations	20	19	18
Internal evaluation	14	16	15
Consumer satisfaction	16	20	14
Personnel roles	19	15	17
Support services	18	18	20
Adequate space	15	17	13

[a] Standards with accompanying data are presented in their 1980 order.

STANDARD 2

CLINICAL EDUCATION PROGRAMS FOR STUDENTS ARE PLANNED TO MEET SPECIFIC OBJECTIVES OF THE EDUCATIONAL PROGRAM, THE PHYSICAL THERAPY SERVICE, AND THE INDIVIDUAL STUDENT.

Planning for students should take place in meetings among the Center Coordinator of Clinical Education (CCCE), the Clinical Instructors (CIs), and the Academic Coordinator of Clinical Education (ACCE). The clinical education objectives of the educational program and the physical therapy service should be used in planning student learning experiences. Students should participate in planning their learning experiences according to mutually agreed upon objectives. The staff in the clinical center should be prepared to modify particular learning experiences to meet individual student needs, objectives, and interests. A thorough orientation to the clinical education program and the personnel of the clinical center should be planned for the student. Evaluation of student performance is an integral part of the learning plan. Opportunities for discussion of and feedback about strengths and weaknesses should be scheduled on an ongoing basis.

	Yes	No
2.j. During the student's orientation, are the following objectives, policies, and procedures made available to students?		
1). clinical center's objectives?	___	___
2). physical therapy service objectives?	___	___
3). administrative procedures?	___	___
4). patient care procedures or ethical standards of practice?	___	___
5). procedure manual for clinical education?	___	___
6). accident report?	___	___
7). personnel policies?	___	___
8). patient care plans?	___	___
9). monthly and annual reports?	___	___
10). physical therapy service table of organization?	___	___
11). other? _____	___	___

Fig. 2. Format of Self-Assessment form.

as being unclear or redundant. The wordings of the 1980 Standards and interpretations are the results of revisions that were made based on these findings.

Order of the standards. The 1980 Standards shown in Figure 1 are in two groups: 1 through 5 and 6 through 20. They appear in these groups, and partially in a specific order within each group, based on data collected during the Weighting study.

With two exceptions, the standards in Figure 1 are ordered according to the data on crucial, important, and practical standards. "Staff Expertise" appeared in the 1976 Standards as a part of the standard concerning "Staff Number" (1980 Standard 9). Pretest study participants identified "Staff Expertise" as redundant with the interpretation of what is now Standard 1; therefore, data on this standard were ambiguous. The standard concerning "Affirmative Action" was moved into the top five because of the legal requirement that all federal facilities and all facilities receiving any federal support abide by the principles of affirmative action and equal opportunity.

The composite rank order of the standards with each descriptor—important, practical, or crucial—is presented in Table 4. All of the standards were found to be important and practical by the three groups of respondents. Of the five standards identified as most important and practical, four were also among the five most frequently mentioned crucial standards.

In summary, the order of the 1980 Standards was determined, in part, by results from the Weighting study. The standards appear grouped 1 through 5 and 6 through 20. Because the first four are considered by ACCEs and CCCEs to be most important and the fifth is a federal requirement, it is recommended that satisfactory compliance with these be achieved before students are accepted by or assigned to a center for clinical education.

Standard Key Words	Non-compliance	Questionable Compliance	Compliance
Learning environment			
Program planning			
Learning experiences			
Ethical standards			
Affirmative action			
Compatible philosophy and objectives			
Administrative support			
Effective communications			
Staff number			
Center clinical coordinator			
Clinical instructor selection			
Principles of teaching and learning			
Sharing special expertise			
Staff development			
Professional associations			
Internal evaluation			
Consumer satisfaction			
Personnel roles			
Support services			
Adequate space			

Fig. 3. Format of Profile form.

Evaluation Forms

Self-Assessment form. The 1980 Self-Assessment form[2] documents the characteristics of and the material and nonmaterial resources available at a particular center for clinical education of physical therapy and physical therapist assistant students. The 38-page form requires that seven documents from the center (eg, curriculum vitae of the CCCE and list of clinical education objectives) be attached and that 15 others be available for review upon request. One page from the Self-Assessment form appears in Figure 2 as an example of the general format of the form.

Data were collected during the Pretest study on the clarity and content validity of the 1976 Self-Assessment form. Center Coordinators of Clinical Education unanimously agreed that the instructions were clear and that the form was consistent with the standards. Twenty-four percent of its 226 items were identified by at least 10 percent of the participants as items to be revised, deleted, or placed elsewhere in the form. In analyzing these suggestions, we found it

obvious that many of the comments resulted from confusion about terminology that probably would not have arisen if the interpretation of each standard had appeared on the form along with the corresponding standard.

The content and construct validity of the 1976 Self-Assessment form were evaluated by the project staff as well. Three staff members and a consultant independently reviewed each item on the Self-Assessment form. Each item was coded as to whether it 1) was relevant to clinical education, 2) measured the standard, 3) best measured the standard, and 4) might predict high-quality clinical education. Coded responses from each of the four evaluators were tabulated per item. Any discrepancies in staff responses were discussed until a consensus about the evaluation for each item was reached. Those items thought to best measure the standard or to predict high-quality clinical education were included in the revised Self-Assessment form.

The reliability of the revised Self-Assessment form was tested in the Interrater Reliability and Internal

Consistency studies. The Interrater Reliability study was designed to provide data about the agreement of responses on the Self-Assessment forms completed independently by the CIs and the CCCEs of a particular center. When the proportion of items for each standard on which all raters or all but one of the raters agreed was tabulated, near perfect agreement was achieved 75 percent of the time. Perfect agreement among raters was reached on 51 percent of the items. (A table of these results is available upon request.) We concluded that *within* centers and among raters with different roles (ie, CCCE or CI), the Self-Assessment form was reliable.

Because the small sample used in the Interrater Reliability study precluded the use of internal consistency approaches to estimate reliability, a separate Internal Consistency study was designed. In this study the closed-ended responses from 50 CCCEs to the Self-Assessment form were collected. This sample, which focused on the perspective of one individual in the clinical education process (the CCCE), included a random sample of sizes and types of centers and analyzed responses across centers. The Reliability computer subprogram from the Statistical Package for the Social Sciences was used to analyze the data. Reliability was defined as the ratio of true-score variance to total variance over an indefinitely large number of independent, repeated trials[3] and expressed as Cronbach's alpha. Alpha (α) levels ranged from .372 to .909 for 16 of the 20 standards. Alpha levels of .6 or greater are acceptable levels of reliability.[4] Responses to items for the remaining four standards were the same for all respondents and therefore reliable by definition. We concluded that *across* centers of varying sizes and types and among raters with

the perspective of the CCCE, the Self-Assessment form was generally reliable.

In summary, the 1976 Self-Assessment form was revised based on data collected during the Pretest study and from the project staff, was tested in two later studies, and was found to be reliable. Revision of the form resulted in a decrease in the mean time required to complete it (from 6.00 hours to 3.75 hours), a decrease in the number of attachments requested (from 10 to 7), and a decrease in the total number of items (from 226 to 192) included in the form.

Profile form. The purpose of the Profile form[2] is to measure compliance of a center with the standards by using information from a completed Self-Assessment form. The Profile form is four pages in length and includes a section for graphic representation of the compliance of a center with each standard (Fig. 3) and a section for narrative comments about a center's strengths and weaknesses. This form was developed by the project staff and used in the Interrater Reliability study and the Test phase.

Analysis of the reliability within centers of the 20 objective items on the Profile form was conducted during the Interrater Reliability study. Alpha values ranged from .604 to .809 with an aggregated α of .892 across all four centers. (A table of these results is available upon request.) Because of the small sample size within any one center, analysis of the data across centers provides a closer estimate of the value of α for a larger sample. These data demonstrate that the objective graphic portion of the Profile form is reliable. The validity of the form was not tested except as it is a component of the evaluation process discussed below.

---

3. After your arrival at the center, were written objectives, policies, and procedures made available to you during your orientation?

	Yes	No
a. Clinical center's objectives	___	___
b. Physical therapy service objectives	___	___
c. Administrative procedures	___	___
d. Patient care procedures or ethical standards of practice	___	___
e. Procedure manual for clinical education	___	___
f. Accident report	___	___
g. Personnel policies	___	___
h. Patient care plans	___	___
i. Monthly and annual reports	___	___
j. Physical therapy service table of organization	___	___
k. Other _____		

Fig. 4. Format of Student's form.

Student's form. Responses on the Student's form[2] are meant to provide information about the strengths and weaknesses of the clinical education experience to the CCCE of the particular center and the ACCE of the affiliating educational program. The form is 10 pages long with both open- and closed-ended items. An example of its format is shown in Figure 4.

Student participants in the Pretest study generally agreed that the instructions for use of the 1976 Student's form were clearly written and that the form could be used with all sizes and types of centers, by part- and full-time students, and by physical therapy and physical therapist assistant students. Eleven of the 34 items on the form were identified by at least 10 percent of the students as items to be either revised for clarity or deleted. The specific suggestions for improving clarity guided revision of the form.

The reliability of the revised Student's form was tested in the Interrater Reliability study. Results of this study were analyzed in three ways: 1) the reliability of the whole form across centers, 2) the reliability of the whole form according to topics of common interest in the form (eg, orientation) across centers, and 3) the reliability of the form according to topics in the form within each center. Results support the reliability of the Student's form whether analyzed within or across centers. (A table of these results is available upon request.)

Twenty-five questions on the Self-Assessment and Student's forms are similar or identical as examples in Figures 2 and 4 demonstrate. In the Interrater Reliability study, the degree of agreement between CCCE or CI responses to these questions on the Self-Assessment form and student responses to the corresponding questions on the Student's form were analyzed. By comparing the responses from the two groups to these items, insight into the reliability and validity of the forms can be gained. If the responses of the two groups are in perfect agreement, it can be argued that the forms are both reliable and valid. If there is not perfect agreement, it may reflect random error (unreliability) on the part of one or both groups or disagreement between the two groups as to the meaning of the items (invalidity). The data show that for two-thirds (68%) of the corresponding items or questions on the two forms there was 75 percent agreement in responses and for 40 percent of the matching items there was perfect (100%) agreement. (A table of these results is available upon request.)

In summary, the 1976 Student's form was revised based on data collected during the Pretest study. It was later tested and found to be reliable and valid.

Evaluation Process

The proposed evaluation process for physical therapy clinical education centers is based on the use of the 1980 Standards and on the Self-Assessment, Profile, and Student's forms. Data from the studies already reported demonstrate the reliability of the evaluation forms and the validity of the standards and the Self-Assessment and Student's forms. The Test phase of the project was designed to establish the reliability and validity of the evaluation process.

Each CCCE participant in the Test phase evaluated his center by completing a Self-Assessment form. ACCE participants evaluated particular assigned centers on two variables, Strength and Compliance. A

TABLE 5
Description of Each Score Reported in the Test

Scores	Raters		Variables		Conditions	
	Staff	ACCE	Compliance[a]	Strength[b]	I. With Self-Assessment Information (No CCCE Identity)	II. No Self-Assessment Information[c] (With CCCE Identity)
Staff compliance score	X		X		X	
ACCE compliance score I		X	X		X	
ACCE compliance score II		X	X			X
Staff strength score	X			X	X	
ACCE strength score I		X		X	X	
ACCE strength score II		X		X		X

[a] Compliance with the standards.
[b] Overall strength of the clinical education center.
[c] ACCEs could use other written materials in their files about a center to be evaluated.

TABLE 6
Correlation Matrix of Test Results

	Staff compliance score	ACCE compliance score I	ACCE compliance score II	Staff strength score	ACCE strength score I	ACCE strength score II
Staff compliance score	...					
ACCE compliance score I	.83[a] a	...				
ACCE compliance score II	.67[a] b	.62[a] c	...			
Staff strength score	.96[a] d	.75[a] e	.54 f	...		
ACCE strength score I	.73[a] g	.83[a] h	.39 i	.71[a] j	...	
ACCE strength score II	.62[a] k	.48 l	.57 m	.63[a] n	.62[a] o	...

[a] Significant at $p \leq .003$; $\alpha = .05$ divided by 15 (the number of nonindependent comparisons). The letter in the bottom right corner of each cell is used to identify the particular cell being discussed or reported.

score representing the overall Strength of a center was obtained by rating that center on a scale of 1 to 20. The Compliance score was obtained by averaging the ratings on a completed Profile form. These evaluations were made under two conditions: 1) with Self-Assessment information, but no identity of the CCCE or center (Condition I) and 2) without Self-Assessment information, but with identity of the CCCE and center and use of any written materials available in the ACCE's personal files (Condition II). Three project staff members also rated each center under Condition I.

Six sets of scores were developed to express the results of these evaluations. As can be seen in Table 5, the sets of scores varied according to 1) raters used, 2) variables measured, and 3) conditions imposed. The scores were obtained by averaging all ACCE or staff ratings across all centers.

Data on the compliance variable collected under Condition I for one randomly chosen center were analyzed for interrater reliability among the three staff raters and between two ACCE raters. Correlation coefficients calculated from three pair-wise analyses of the staff scores were .71, .73, and .89, while those for the ACCEs were .69. All were significant at $p \leq .05$.

Table 6 summarizes the results of the correlation matrix for the Test phase. Each cell of the table represents the correlation of two scores and contains

the calculated r values. Each correlation has been assigned a lower-case letter, which appears in the lower right corner, to facilitate discussing and reporting correlations. For example, r_a, the correlation of ACCE Compliance Score I with Staff Compliance Score, is .83. Using a conservative approach to significance testing that set α at .05 divided by 15 (=.003) to allow for the simultaneous testing of 15 correlation coefficients, all but four of the correlations (r_f, r_i, r_l, r_m) are statistically significant.

Reliability of parallel measures of the same variable[5] is demonstrated in Table 6 by the correlations a, b, and c for Compliance and by j, n, and o for Strength. More consistency in ratings occurred when different raters reviewed information from a completed Self-Assessment form (Condition I) before rating a center ($r_a = .83$, $r_j = .71$). Less consistency in ratings occurred when the raters and conditions both varied ($r_b = .67$, $r_n = .63$) and when the ACCEs rated a center under two different conditions ($r_c = .62$, $r_o = .62$).

Based on the parallel-test model, correlations d through m, except j, pertain to validity in that they show relationships between the Compliance and Strength variables. These correlations were higher when the raters had information from completed Self-Assessment forms (Condition I) before rating a center ($r_d = .96$, $r_e = .75$, $r_g = .73$, $r_h = .83$). Means and variances of the six variables were examined to deter-

TABLE 7
Means and Variances of the Test Compliance and Strength Scores

Condition	Compliance[a]			Strength[b]		
	Score	X̄	Variance	Score	X̄	Variance
I	Staff compliance score	7.45	0.445	Staff strength score	13.588	7.854
II	ACCE compliance score I	7.62	0.578	ACCE strength score I	15.230	8.477
II	ACCE compliance score II	7.97	0.479	ACCE strength score II	16.509	4.255

[a] Scale: 0 = noncompliance; 9 = compliance.
[b] Scale: 1 = weak; 20 = strong.

mine the effect of using the Self-Assessment information to rate a center. We hypothesized that the mean score would be higher when the raters were evaluating centers under Condition II and the variance of the scores would be greater under Condition I. Table 7 presents the results of these analyses. The difference in means and variances were not statistically significant at $p \leq .05$ for either the Compliance or Strength scores; however, the direction of the differences was consistent with the hypotheses.

A more stringent test of the data is derived from the true-score model.[5] This analysis is based on the assumption that an error-free score (true score) exists and is known. In the Test phase, staff Compliance and Strength scores were assumed to be true scores and ACCE scores on the same variables were correlated with the true scores ($r_a = .83$, $r_b = .67$, $r_j = .71$, $r_n = .63$ in Table 6). The data show that the ACCE scores correlate with the true scores more highly when they have Self-Assessment information to guide their ratings than when under Condition II.

In summary, results of the Test phase of the project established the reliability and validity of the evaluation process based on use of the standards and Self-Assessment and Profile forms.

DISCUSSION

Physical therapists who participated in this project generally agreed that standards for clinical education in physical therapy are needed. They also generally agreed that the Self-Assessment and Profile forms are consistent with the 1980 Standards and are helpful in evaluating centers of all sizes and types. Physical therapy and physical therapist assistant student participants also agreed that the Student's form is clear and can be used to evaluate centers of all sizes and types. Use of these standards and evaluation forms by committee members and staff of the physical therapy profession is the next step in achieving the purpose of the Project on Clinical Education.

Currently, the CCCE is often asked by each educational institution with which the center affiliates to complete a form or forms detailing various characteristics about the center related to clinical education. Often these forms cannot be used for more than one educational program because of a few items peculiar to each. Completing a different set of evaluation forms for each educational program represents a duplication of effort for the CCCE whose center affiliates with two or more educational programs. This duplication of effort could be decreased by general acceptance of one set of reliable and valid evaluation forms and by the APTA encouraging the use of the forms among physical therapy clinical centers and educational programs.

Under such a plan, the clinical center would have one evaluation to complete on a regular basis and copies of it could be shared with any educational program desiring to affiliate with the center. In the process of completing a Self-Assessment form, the CCCE and center staff would have an opportunity to assess current and potential learning opportunities, inventory material and nonmaterial resources, identify staff-development programs needed, and suggest specific curricular changes to faculty of affiliating educational programs.

The ACCE would benefit by receiving 1) organized material to review prior to initially selecting or annually renewing affiliations and 2) reliable and valid forms for use in collecting such data. Information from a completed Self-Assessment form would permit the ACCE to select a clinical education center that could provide a specific type of learning experience for a particular student. The Profile form would provide a concise overview of, as well as references to, the strengths and weaknesses of a particular center or several centers.

CONCLUSIONS

As a result of this project, a reliable and valid set of evaluation forms consistent with "Standards for a

Clinical Education Center in Physical Therapy" have been established. These standards and evaluation forms are acceptable to ACCEs, CCCEs, and students. They can be used to evaluate and develop all sizes and types of clinical education centers in physical therapy. Use of such documents will benefit the center, the academic educational program, and the profession.

Acknowledgments. We wish to acknowledge the administrative assistance and subject-matter consultation of the principal investigators of the project, Margaret L. Moore, EdD, and Barry R. Howes; consultation about the overall design of the Project from Eugene Michels; consultation and assistance with data analysis from Richard T. Campbell, PhD; consultation about statistical tests and computer programming from Donna Hoffman, Kar Wang Lau, and Tom Novak; consultation about categories of centers from Richard T. Campbell, PhD, Priscilla Guild, and George Stiles; critiques of the manuscript by Suzann Campbell, PhD, Mary Clyde Singleton, PhD, and Irma Wilhelm; and preparation of the manuscript by Linda Barton, Ellen Willard, and Verna Taylor.

REFERENCES

1. Moore ML, Perry JF: Clinical Education in Physical Therapy: Current Status/Future Needs. Washington, DC, American Physical Therapy Association, 1976
2. Barr JS, Gwyer J, Talmor Z, et al: Standards for Clinical Education in Physical Therapy: A Manual for Evaluation and Selection of Clinical Education Centers. Washington, DC, American Physical Therapy Association, 1980
3. Nie NH, Hull CH, Jenkins JG, et al: Statistical Package for the Social Sciences: Update Manual. New York, NY, McGraw-Hill Book Co, March 1977, p 62
4. Robinson JP, Athanasion R, Head K: Measures of Occupational Attitudes and Occupational Characteristics. Ann Arbor, MI, The University of Michigan, Institute for Social Research, 1969, pp 62–64
5. Nunnally JD: Psychometric Theory, ed 2. New York, NY, McGraw-Hill Book Co, 1978, pp 200–203

Using Assessment Centers to Promote Clinical Faculty Development

Susan S Deusinger, PhD, PT
Suzy L Cornbleet, MA, PT
Jennifer S Stith, MS, PT

ABSTRACT: Development of a cadre of practitioners who can effectively guide the clinical learning of entry-level students is an essential concern for the physical therapy profession. Current systems for clinical faculty development are not systematic and rarely incorporate formal assessment of teaching abilities. This article describes a unique approach for assessing the knowledge and skills of clinical faculty. The approach facilitates individual analysis of teaching behaviors and promotes planning for further training or study to enhance existing ability. Reliance on self-assessment is emphasized as a responsibility for professional development.

INTRODUCTION

Designing and implementing effective clinical learning experiences are exceptionally challenging aspects of physical therapy education.[1] Numerous practitioners are recruited to serve as clinical faculty for the many entry-level physical therapy education programs in existence. To date, however, formalized training in the art and science of clinical teaching has been inconsistent and has not been paired with appropriate mechanisms to assess training outcomes. This article presents one approach for assessing the basic knowledge and skills needed for effective clinical teaching. Results of the assessment can then guide clinical faculty to develop a large repertoire of teaching strategies that foster student learning.

THE CHALLENGE OF CLINICAL FACULTY DEVELOPMENT

All curricula in physical therapy include both didactic and clinical components. These

Dr Deusinger is Director, Program in Physical Therapy, Washington University School of Medicine, 660 S Euclid Ave, St. Louis, MO 63110. Ms Cornbleet is Academic Coordinator of Clinical Education, Program in Physical Therapy, Washington University School of Medicine. Ms Stith is Associate Director for Entry Level Education, Program in Physical Therapy, Washington University School of Medicine. This article was adapted from a presentation for the Section for Education at the Combined Sections Meeting of the American Physical Therapy Association, Honolulu, Hawaii, February 1–4, 1989.

components are integrated in their intent to produce competent practitioners. Each component, however, poses unique challenges to the faculty member attempting to facilitate effective learning and performance. In the didactic component, educators assist students to gain background knowledge in the basic and clinical sciences and to develop skills and attitudes needed in the clinical setting.[2] In the clinical education component, instructors must promote the student's ability to synthesize and apply that background under many different and often complex clinical circumstances.[3] Clinical faculty serve as important role models and resources for professional development.[4]

To achieve these goals, clinical faculty are expected to design individualized learning experiences for students who have a wide range of abilities and backgrounds. This requires a broad-based appreciation of alternative learning strategies, knowledge of methods by which performance can be assessed, and skill in designing remedial activities for students who are having difficulty performing.[2,5] To succeed in the role of clinical instructor requires considerable attention to aspects of teaching that may not have been included in the clinical instructor's professional education. Training to meet these expectations, therefore, is essential to ensure quality clinical education.

A number of mechanisms are currently available to assist practitioners in becoming effective clinical teachers. Educational institutions,[6] consortia,[7] and individuals with expertise in clinical education[8] have all contributed to the training necessary for practitioners to become clinical instructors. Many clinical instructors, however, do not have access to these resources and have had to rely exclusively on trial and error and on-the-job training. The profession continues to lack a systematic method of assessing whether these training programs and experiences result in sufficient clinical teaching skill to facilitate the growth and competence of future practitioners.[9]

Feedback from students is a primary source of information for the clinical instructor who is seeking to develop or enhance his or her skill in clinical teaching. Feedback from peers, supervisors, and personnel from affiliating educational institutions may also be useful for these goals. Although feedback from these sources is invaluable, additional information is needed to provide a comprehensive picture of each individual's strengths and limitations as a clinical instructor. Dinham and Stritter noted that self-assessment is a method that contributes information valuable for developing skill in clinical teaching.[2] Rippey concluded that self-assessment is a necessary prerequisite for improving one's teaching because it allows the individual to recognize personal limitations and to internalize the need to change.[10] Thus, multiple sources of information are essential to facilitate development of clinical faculty and should be incorporated into any methods used to train clinical instructors.

Clinical faculty in physical therapy are challenged through their roles as clinical teachers to help ensure the next generation of competent practitioners. They are an extremely dedicated and conscientious group of professionals who are usually self-selected and often self-trained. The profession has clearly identified the need for more systematic training of clinical faculty[11] and, by extension, the need for a more formalized method of assessing the outcomes of this training. The next section will describe a model proposed to systematize training and assessment of clinical teaching in physical therapy education.

SYSTEMATIC DEVELOPMENT OF CLINICAL TEACHING SKILLS

The assessment center methodology has been suggested as an appropriate strategy with which to achieve the goals for clinical faculty development outlined above.[12] An assessment center traditionally uses a variety of methods to test skills essential to a job role. Centers are designed to simulate the actual work setting as closely as possible so that testing has the highest possible validity. In addition, numerous sources of input are required to make judgments about competence in the job setting.[13] Assessment centers have been promoted as potentially effective methods for physical therapy clinicians to identify directions for professional development[14] and to evaluate student performance in preparation for promotion within a curriculum or for graduation.[12] This section will describe the components and operation of an assessment center designed specifically to test the skills required for effective clinical teaching.

Development of the Center

Developing an assessment center requires careful preparation, adequate resource allocation, and collaboration of numerous individuals to ensure that the center operates smoothly. A clinical faculty assessment center was offered in 1988 at the Annual Clinical Instructor's Meeting sponsored by the Program in Physical Therapy at Washington University. Four factors were important in developing the center:

1. Personnel. A committee comprised of both clinical and academic faculty was formed to develop and implement the center. A consultant (Frank T. Stritter, PhD) was retained to ensure comprehensive attention to relevant principles of teaching, learning, and professional development. The committee's role was to identify the most salient directions for clinical faculty development in physical therapy and to select strategies to test the ability of clinical instructors to meet challenges in each direction.

2. Test content. The committee's first responsibility was to identify specific skills or knowledge essential for clinical teaching in physical therapy. This was accomplished by consulting the literature, acknowledging feedback from students and clinical faculty, and projecting teaching skills needed to work effectively with various levels of students. The content chosen for this assessment center emphasized skills and knowledge in interpersonal communications, administration, student performance evaluation, role modeling, and principles of the teaching and learning process. These aspects of teaching had been addressed in prior training programs and in educational materials distributed on a regular basis to clinical faculty.

3. Testing methods. Five methods were selected as appropriate for assessing the aspects of clinical teaching outlined above. These tests utilized a variety of formats including multiple choice and short answer, videotape analysis, role play, and in-basket. The committee recognized that no single testing method would ensure comprehensive assessment of the multiple dimensions of performance expected of each clinical teacher. The variety of methods selected for the center met an important criterion of useful assessment systems—having multiple and varied methods of testing.[15] A more detailed description of the actual tests will be provided later in this article.

4. Evaluation. Evaluation of the impact and outcomes of the center was an important consideration in its design. Measures of participant reaction and performance were used as indicators of the success of this center. Written and verbal feedback were solicited to assess the reaction of participants to the concepts and processes incorporated in the center. In addition, although performance in the assessment center was primarily judged by the participant himself, a computerized scoring system for each test was designed to provide each participant with a profile of his performance. The Figure illustrates the profile given to one participant. This normative information allowed each participant to identify his or her performance on individual tests and in the center as a whole. It also allowed participants to compare their performance with that of the entire group. Individuals were encouraged to combine these sources of information to construct an accurate picture of strengths and limitations in their own clinical teaching and to begin planning their future development as a clinical educator.

Developing an assessment center requires meticulous attention to detail, generous allowance of time for preparation, and allocation of numerous resources. The committee's central concerns were to provide sufficient personnel, operational space, and equipment so that the center could run smoothly. In addition, it was important to solicit sufficient input from students and faculty so that the center would be stimulating and relevant to the needs of clinical education. The entire process of development spanned six months.

Center Implementation

Representatives from all clinical sites affiliating with Washington University were invited to participate in the assessment center. Prior to the meeting, all sites were provided with a copy of the clinical instructor's training manual developed by our regional academic coordinator of clinical education (ACCE) consortium.[16] The participants were encouraged to review the manual prior to entering the assessment center. The effect of this review was later assessed to determine whether self-study of this reference affected performance in the center.

A total of 69 clinical instructors participated in the center. Demographic data were collected on all participants in an effort to ascertain whether certain characteristics, such as length of time in the profession, numbers of students supervised previously, or amount of prior training in clinical teaching, would have an impact on performance in the assessment center.

The total group of participants was divided so that half attended a two-hour seminar on clinical decision-making while the other half participated in two hours of testing. The schedule was then reversed so that all individuals eventually participated in both events. The split scheduling allowed efficient management of the large group of participants. It also allowed a test of whether formal instruction in the process and pitfalls of clinical decision making influences participants' performance.

The five testing methods were arranged in stations that were in physical proximity to each other. To facilitate the flow of testing, the two large groups were subdivided into six smaller groups, each scheduled to begin the testing at a different station. A sixth station was designated for breaks so that participants could rest or wait for rotation to another station. Because it was not projected that performance on one test would influence performance on other tests, the order of the tests was not controlled. The groups rotated every 20 minutes.

The specific components of the five tests were as follows:

1. Interpersonal communications (Test A). Effective communication is regarded by both students and faculty as an essential ingredient of the learning environment.[5,16] The participant's ability to communicate with a reticent student was tested using a role-play simulation. The test required the clinical instructor to give verbal feedback to a student about his or her clinical performance and to attempt to clarify the cause of a poorly defined set of performance problems. Actual students from our program, who had been trained by faculty, assumed the role of students in this simulation. The role play took place in a private faculty office to simulate the actual setting in which a clinical instructor might counsel a student. Criteria for the test included the ability to exhibit appropriate attending and listening skills, to balance complimentary and critical feedback, and to develop a collaborative relationship with the student in planning remedies for problems. Both self-assessment and ratings given by the student were used to evaluate the participant's performance during this test.

2. Administration (Test B). Implementing effective learning experiences in the clinical setting requires a considerable range of management and decision-making skills.[17] Administrative aspects of clinical teaching were tested using an in-basket test, a format that assesses an individual's ability to prioritize, delegate, and weigh decisions of importance in the work setting.[14] This two-part exercise required the participant to imagine holding the position of center coordinator of clinical education (CCCE). In the first part of the test, several concurrent messages were given to each participant. The task was to prioritize actions to be taken in response to typical clinical situations that could present themselves simultaneously (eg, evaluate new patients, treat existing patients, respond to student requests and complaints, and deal with employee absences). The second part of the test required the participant to evaluate whether a set of given responses to these situations was appropriate.

3. Student performance evaluation (Test C). Perhaps one of the most challenging aspects of clinical teaching is to accurately describe and document student behavior. In our current model of physical therapy education, the responsibility for evaluating student performance during clinical education rests almost entirely with the clinical faculty. The challenge for the clinical instructor is to conduct accurate performance evaluations and to provide meaningful feedback that guides further development.[12] The participant's ability to be both specific and objective in evaluating student performance was assessed by critiquing the documentation typically generated during student evaluations. Comments from actual student performance reports were first analyzed by participants for the qualities of objectivity and specificity. In the second part of the test, participants were then asked to use these standards to rewrite given evaluative comments in a way that would be more meaningful for the student and more informative in the evaluation process.

4. Role modeling (Test D). A clinician's professional behavior is strongly influenced by the role models encountered during clinical education.[4] In this station, participants viewed a videotape depicting the first meeting of a clinical instructor and a new (nervous) student. The scenario included examples of how a clinical instructor explains expectations, communicates professional values, interacts with colleagues, and manages

student anxiety. Participants were asked to critique the videotape by identifying both positive and negative examples of role modeling. This process allowed participants to identify how these essential characteristics of a clinical teacher affect the learning environment and to project the outcomes of clinical education when role modeling is ineffective.

5. Principles of the teaching/learning process (Test E). Background knowledge in educational principles relevant to clinical teaching is a necessary prerequisite for success as a clinical educator. Paper-and-pencil tests using multiple-choice or true-false formats are useful for assessment of such background knowledge.[15] For this station, a sample of principles presented in the clinical instructor's manual[16] was selected for testing. A written test using true-false and multiple-choice questions was given to assess participants' knowledge about writing behavioral objectives, planning learning experiences, defining remedies for student problems, and working in the legal context of clinical education. This test enabled participants to identify deficits in the knowledge base of educational methodology essential to being an effective clinical instructor.

Center Outcomes

The outcomes of the assessment center for clinical faculty were assessed by soliciting

feedback from faculty and students and by computing scores on each test to form a profile of performance. Both students and faculty agreed that the center offered a positive and challenging learning environment. Input from both groups assisted the committee to plan improvements in the operational structure of the center and to identify additional criteria of effective teaching that are important for the development of clinical education in physical therapy. Feedback indicated the need for more variety in the rotation schedule for testing and a desire for more opportunities for interactive participation during tests (eg, with students, colleagues, and media). The feedback also indicated the need to expand content areas tested in the center to include the ability to ask probing questions, to promote critical thinking, to challenge the exceptional learner, and to facilitate the development of professional values and attitudes.

Feedback from students strongly indicated the value of role play in preparing for various levels of clinical experiences. In response, our faculty have begun incorporating more simulations related to clinical teaching and learning in the curriculum. These simulations require students to assume various roles expected of clinical educators and to develop a

FIGURE

Percentage scores were generated from five tests in the assessment center for clinical faculty. The tests included Test A, a test of interpersonal communication skills; Test B, an in-basket test used to assess the administrative aspects of clinical teaching; Test C, an analysis of documentation relating to student performance in clinical education; Test D, a videotape critique of role-modeling behaviors during clinical instruction; and Test E, a written objective test of knowledge needed for effective clinical teaching. The group score reflects the mean percentage score for 69 participants. The total score (TOT) is a mean percentage score across all tests.

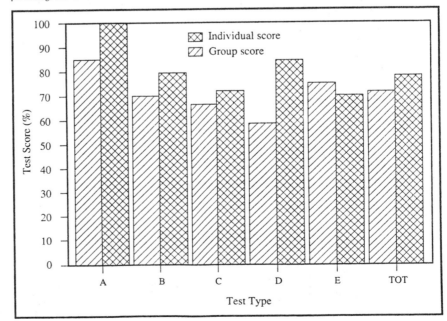

repertoire of interpersonal skills to be tapped during difficult encounters in clinical education. This is intended to promote a larger future cadre of individuals who can competently teach students in the clinic—as well as to assist our students in being effective learners during their own clinical training.

Review of the aggregate of scores for each test yielded little definitive evidence that performance on these tests was influenced by the demographic variables assessed (eg, length of career, amount of experience an individual has with students, or the type of facility in which one works). In addition, neither prior self-study of the clinical instructor's handbook nor placement of the decision-making seminar before or after the assessment center appeared to influence performance on these tests. Conclusions about the impact various individual differences make on performance in an assessment center would require a more thorough examination of potentially influential characteristics (eg, learning style, formal education, chronological age).

The group test scores (Figure) suggest that the documentation test may have been the most difficult for participants. Performance on any test such as this may reflect actual ability of participants, interest in the content area, characteristics of the test, or reaction to the testing conditions. To be maximally useful in clinical faculty development, tests should be constructed to enable participants to develop an accurate picture of their knowledge or skills in clinical teaching. Examination of the content, the testing process, and the standards applied to performance are important directions for the future if assessment centers are to be used for clinical faculty development.

Implementation of this clinical faculty assessment center was essentially a demonstration of the potential such testing systems may have in development of clinical faculty. Favorable reactions from participants, committee members, and students suggest that the goals of clinical education could be facilitated by using assessment centers to promote development of expertise in clinical teaching.

CONCLUSION

The enthusiasm shown by clinical faculty for the assessment center implemented in 1988 at Washington University confirmed the dedication of practitioners to excellence in clinical teaching. The assessment center methodology shows potential as a structure for training, a mechanism for self-assessment, and possibly a means for formalized assessment and credentialing of clinical instructors. Other options for assessing the outcomes of training for clinical instructors should be studied and compared with the assessment center methodology suggested in this article. These directions should enable the profession to develop a more systematic approach to clinical faculty development and to ensure and extend the quality of clinical education in physical therapy.

ACKNOWLEDGEMENT

Appreciation is extended to Frank T. Stritter, PhD, the University of North Carolina at Chapel Hill, for his assistance in developing the concepts and structure of the clinical faculty assessment center, and to Barbara J. Norton, MHS, PT, for her assistance in designing the computerized scoring system used in the center. Also appreciated are the efforts of committee members Elaine Angelo, Ann Marcolina, and Beth Slama, who assisted in developing and implementing the center.

REFERENCES

1. Watts NT: Handbook of Clinical Teaching—Exercises and Guidelines for Health Professionals Who Teach Patients, Train Staff and Supervise Students. New York, NY, Churchill Livingstone, Inc, 1990
2. Dinham SM, Stritter FT: Research on professional education. In: Handbook of Research on Teaching (ed 3). New York, NY, MacMillan Publishing Co, 1986, pp 952–970
3. Stritter FT, Flair MD: Effective Clinical Teaching. Bethesda, MD, US Department of Health Education and Welfare, Public Health Service, National Institutes of Health, National Library of Medicine, 1980
4. Jacobson B: Role modeling in physical therapy. Phys Ther 54:244–250, 1974
5. Emery MJ: Effectiveness of the clinical instructor: Student's perspective. Phys Ther 64:1079–1083, 1984
6. Phillips BU Jr, McPhail S, Roemer S: Role and functions of the academic coordinators of clinical education in physical therapy education: A survey. Phys Ther 66:981–985, 1986
7. Radtka S, Dragotta N, Needham S: Texas consortium for physical therapy clinical education: A model for interinstitutional consortium arrangements. Phys Ther 63:971–974, 1983
8. Curtis K: Creating Adult Learners by Clinical Teaching: A Clinical Instructor Training Program. Los Angeles, CA, Health Directions, Educational Services for the Health Professions, 1988
9. American Physical Therapy Association: Current patterns for providing clinical education in physical therapy education. Alexandria, VA, APTA, 1985
10. Rippey RM: The Evaluation of Teaching in Medical Schools. New York, NY, Springer Publishing Company, 1981
11. American Physical Therapy Association: Pivotal Issues in Clinical Education: Present Status/Future Needs. Alexandria, VA, Section for Education, Department of Education, APTA, 1988
12. Deusinger SS: Evaluation in clinical education. In: Pivotal Issues in Clinical Education: Present Status/Future Needs. Alexandria, VA, Section for Education, Department of Education, American Physical Therapy Association, 1988
13. Moses JL, Byhem WC (eds): Applying the Assessment Center Method. New York, NY, Pergamon Press, 1977
14. Deusinger SS, Sindelar BJ, Stritter FT: The assessment center—a model for professional development and growth. Phys Ther 66:1119–1123, 1986
15. Neufeld VR, Norman GR (eds): Assessing Clinical Competence. New York, NY, Springer Publishing Company, 1985
16. Regional ACCE Associates of Kansas, Oklahoma and Missouri: Clinical Instructor's Handbook. Printed by Regional ACCE Associates of Kansas, Oklahoma, and Missouri, 1987

Academic Resources

"Quality is never an accident; it is always the result of intelligent effort."

John Ruskin

Predictors of Student Clinical Performance

Relationship Between Academic Achievement and Clinical Performance in a Physical Therapy Education Program

WENDY RHEAULT
and ELIZABETH SHAFERNICH-COULSON

This study was performed to ascertain whether a relationship exists between physical therapy students' preprofessional academic achievement and their academic or clinical performance while attending professional school. A comparison was also made between professional academic achievement and clinical performance. The records of three classes of graduates (N = 65) were examined in relation to preprofessional grade point average, professional grade point average, and clinical performance. Pearson product-moment correlations showed no significant relationship between preprofessional and professional academic achievement or preprofessional academic achievement and clinical performance. The correlation between professional academic achievement and clinical performance was higher, but did not reach statistical significance. This study did find that preprofessional and professional grade point averages were related. The authors urge further study of current admission criteria and their relationship to clinical performance.

Key Words: *Achievement; Clinical performance; Education: physical therapist, admissions.*

Considerable competition exists among students for admission to physical therapy programs. The selection of well-qualified students is crucial for the growth of our profession into the 1990s. Gartland found that in the United States, prior academic performance was the primary admission criterion to physical therapy school.[1] Preprofessional grades have been demonstrated to correlate well with later academic achievement in a physical therapy education program; however, the importance of this factor in predicting clinical performance is less clear.[2–5]

Classroom educators assign grades to students based on their achievement in the nonclinical, or didactic, phase of the program. Because much of the classroom work in physical therapy programs involves laboratory and simulated patient care, students' grades may reflect how well they will perform ultimately in the clinic. If grades do indeed reflect clinical performance, then students who are in need of assistance for clinical skills can be identified early in their education, and remediation can be instituted.

The purpose of this study was to answer the following questions:

1. Does preprofessional academic achievement predict how well a student will do in the didactic phase of a physical therapy program?

2. Does preprofessional academic achievement predict how well a student will do in the clinical phase of a physical therapy program?

3. Does a relationship exist between achievement in the didactic phase of a physical therapy program and clinical performance?

REVIEW OF THE LITERATURE

Several studies in medical and allied health education have shown a positive relationship between previous and future academic performance.[6–8] Ronai et al point out, however, that very few studies have explored the relationship between early academic performance and subsequent clinical competence.[9] Indeed, some of the research indicates that the correlation between grades and clinical performance may be low.[10,11] McGinnis points out that a student's grade point average (GPA) may be a relevant predictor of future academic achievement because it represents past behavior that is similar to the predicted behavior.[12] Clinical competence probably involves an array of skills and attitudes, as well as academic knowledge.

Canadian researchers have studied the relationship between early academic achievement and clinical performance in physical therapy. Pickles reported a positive relationship between prior academic grades in the social sciences and clinical performance, although the correlation did not reach the 5% level of significance for all academic years studied.[3] Olney found a positive, but nonsignificant, relationship between early academic achievement and clinical performance.[4] Although Peat et al reported that the admission average was related significantly to clinical performance, only 9% of the variation in clinical performance could be explained by the

W. Rheault, MA, is Chairman and Associate Professor, Department of Physical Therapy, University of Health Sciences-The Chicago Medical School, North Chicago, IL 60064 (USA).

E. Shafernich-Coulson, MBA, is Academic Coordinator of Clinical Education and Assistant Professor, Department of Physical Therapy, University of Health Sciences-The Chicago Medical School.

This article was submitted July 8, 1986; was with the authors for revision 30 weeks; and was accepted June 9, 1987. Potential Conflict of Interest: 4.

admission average.[5] From their experience with a US physical therapy school, Tidd and Conine reported a correlation of .29 between clinical performance and preprofessional academic achievement ($p < .0001$).[2]

The relationship between didactic and clinical grades in the professional phase of a physical therapy program has been demonstrated to be high.[2,3] Pickles reported positive correlations ranging from .29 to .91 between didactic averages and clinical performance, with a variation between the academic years studied.[3] Because most of the information to date is based on Canadian physical therapy students or medical students and because few studies have been published on physical therapy students in the United States, a closer examination of the relationship between clinical performance and academic achievement in US physical therapy programs is needed.

METHOD

Subjects

The sample (51 women, 14 men) consisted of all prospective physical therapy graduates of the University of Health Sciences-The Chicago Medical School from 1983 to 1985. The mean age of the students was 22.7 years ($s = 2.1$ years). Table 1 shows the descriptive statistics of the sample.

Procedure

We examined all academic records of the students and determined their preprofessional academic achievement as their college GPA on admission to the professional phase of the physical therapy program. A preprofessional science GPA and an overall GPA were calculated on a four-point numeric scale (4 = A, 3 = B, 2 = C, 1 = D). Science GPA was included because it is a common admissions criterion for physical therapy schools in the United States.[1]

Academic achievement in the program was calculated based on all courses taken in our two-year program. Professional GPA was also expressed on a scale of 1 to 4. Clinical achievement was determined from the Illinois Consortium for Clinical Education's Physical Therapy Student Performance Report. This widely accepted measurement instrument is used by all physical therapy programs in Illinois. Originally developed in 1981 by a group of clinicians and educators, the so-called Illinois Consortium form underwent detailed revision in 1984. Although no formal studies on reliability and validity have been conducted, the form is considered a reliable and valid tool for assessing clinical performance. The Illinois Consortium form is competency-based; the student is expected to perform the listed behaviors in a safe, independent, and effective manner to receive a "yes" response. "No" responses indicate that by the end of the particular clinical education experience, the student's performance is not characterized by safe, independent, and effective practice.

The form is divided into two sections. The first section addresses the cognitive and affective domains, particularly the four major areas: professional qualities, communication skills, interpersonal relationships, and patient evaluation and program-planning abilities. The second section addresses the student's psychomotor performance. This part is divided into three subsections: evaluation procedures, treatment procedures, and physical agents. Each of the subsections is evaluated based on 12 to 14 performance criteria.

TABLE 1
Descriptive Statistics[a] for Variables

Variable	$\bar{X}$	s
Preprofessional science GPA (N = 65)	2.9	.34
Preprofessional overall GPA (N = 65)	3.1	.29
Professional GPA (N = 65)	3.2	.35
Clinical performance (N = 64)[b]	11[c]	15

[a] All values are grade point averages (GPAs) (on a four-point scale) except for clinical performance.
[b] One student did not complete all clinical work.
[c] Number of "no" responses on clinical performance evaluation form.

TABLE 2
Pearson Product-Moment Correlation Coefficients Between Variables

Variable	Professional GPA[a] (N = 65)	Clinical Performance (N = 64)[b]
Preprofessional science GPA	.25[c]	−.05
Preprofessional overall GPA	.23[c]	.04
Professional GPA		−.09

[a] GPA = grade point average.
[b] One student did not complete all clinical work.
[c] $p < .05$.

Grading of this form is based on the ratio of yes-no responses. Some of the items are deemed minimal for passing (ie, safety, basic communication, and implementing patient programs). The mean number of no responses received by the students on two of their three full-time senior affiliations (no specialty clinics included) constituted the measurement for clinical achievement.

Data Analysis

We used Pearson product-moment correlation coefficients to analyze the data. Hypothesis testing was performed to ascertain whether the correlations were significantly different from zero at the .05 alpha level.

RESULTS

The Pearson product-moment correlation coefficients revealed a significant relationship between preprofessional GPA and professional GPA (Tab. 2). A positive correlation of .25 was found between preprofessional science GPA and professional GPA, and a positive correlation of .23 existed between preprofessional overall GPA and professional GPA. Both correlations were significant at the .05 level. Nonsignificant correlations, however, were found between preprofessional academic achievement and clinical performance and between professional academic achievement and clinical performance ($p > .05$).

DISCUSSION

The results of this study indicate that a significant relationship exists between preprofessional GPA and professional GPA. Balogun et al found that preprofessional GPA was the best predictor of how well a student would perform academically in physical therapy school.[13] This finding supports the use of GPA in the selection process for physical therapy students.

Of particular interest to us was the finding that professional GPA and clinical competence were not significantly related. This finding contradicts Pickles' study; he found a high correlation between these two variables.[3] Because professional GPA included achievement in laboratory-based courses, we believed that a significant relationship might exist.

The absence of a significant relationship between preprofessional GPA and clinical performance is also noteworthy. It appears that other variables may be related to clinical ability. Perhaps problem-solving capabilities, manual dexterity, or personal attitudes are more closely related than preprofessional or professional academic achievement to clinical competence. Some studies have explored the use of personality predictors of clinical success. Further study is needed to delineate the important skills, attitudes, and areas of knowledge needed for success in the clinic.

In this study, clinical achievement was based on performance across two clinical rotations. Because other studies evaluated clinical achievement on only one rotation, our study may truly represent the student's clinical ability.

As with any other correlational study, a problem exists when studying a restricted sample. Because we evaluated only those students who were successful in being admitted to physical therapy school, we do not know how the rest of the applicant pool might have done in our program. The GPA is probably important in screening out those students who will be unsuccessful in physical therapy school.

CONCLUSION

This study was undertaken to ascertain the relationship between admission GPA and performance in a physical therapy program and to determine whether clinical and academic performance within a program were related. Our study supports earlier studies that found a relationship between preprofessional and professional academic achievement. No significant correlation existed between preprofessional academic achievement and clinical competence or between professional academic achievement and clinical competence. We urge educators to study other admission criteria and to delineate the variables that may be related to clinical competence.

REFERENCES

1. Gartland GJ: Synopsis of a study of admission criteria to physical therapy programs. Physiotherapy Canada 29:6–10, 1977
2. Tidd GS, Conine TA: Do better students perform better in the clinic? Relationship of academic grades to clinical ratings. Phys Ther 54:500–505, 1974
3. Pickles B: Correlations between matriculation entry requirements and performance in the diploma program in physical therapy at the University of Alberta. Physiotherapy Canada 29:249–253, 1977
4. Olney SJ: Prediction of clinical competence of students of physical therapy. Physiotherapy Canada 29:254–258, 1977
5. Peat M, Woodbury MG, Donner A: Admission average as a predictor of undergraduate academic and clinical performance. Physiotherapy Canada 34:211–214, 1982
6. Keck JW, Arnold L, Willoughby L, et al: Efficacy of cognitive-noncognitive measures in predicting resident-physician performance. J Med Educ 53:759–765, 1979
7. Mawhinney BS: The value of ordinary and advanced-level British school-leaving examination results in predicting medical students' academic performance. Med Educ 10:87–89, 1976
8. Turner EV, Helper MM, Krista SD: Predictors of clinical performance. J Med Educ 49:338–342, 1974
9. Ronai AK, Golmon M, Shanks CA: Relationship between past academic performance and results of specialty in-training examinations. J Med Educ 59:341–344, 1984
10. Hamburg RL, Swanson WC, Sohner CW: Perceptions and usage of predictive data for medical school admissions. J Med Educ 46:959–964, 1971
11. Schimfhauer FT, Broski DC: Predicting academic success in allied health curricula. J Allied Health 5(1):34–36, 1976
12. McGinnis ME: Admission predictors for pre-physical therapy majors. Phys Ther 64:55–58, 1984
13. Balogun JA, Karacoloff LA, Farina NT: Predictors of academic achievement in physical therapy. Phys Ther 66:976–980, 1986

Predictors of Academic and Clinical Performance in a Baccalaureate Physical Therapy Program

JOSEPH A. BALOGUN

The purpose of this retrospective study was to determine the best predictors of academic and clinical performance in a physical therapy undergraduate program. The records of 42 graduates of the program were reviewed to obtain data concerning 1) preadmission cumulative grade point averages (GPAs), 2) written composition scores, 3) interview ratings (INTVs), 4) preprofessional faculty ratings, 5) mean Allied Health Professions Admission Test (MAHPAT) scores, and 6) scores on the comprehensive examination administered at the end of the educational program. The results of the comprehensive written and oral-practical examination were used as a measure of the students' academic achievement and clinical performance. Multiple regression analyses revealed that both academic achievement and clinical performance can be predicted reliably ($p < .001$) from the preadmission requirements. The two viable predictors of academic achievement were GPA and MAHPAT. The GPA and MAHPAT accounted for 30.5% and 8.0%, respectively, of the total variance (40.6%) in academic achievement. The INTV and GPA were the two viable predictors of clinical performance. They accounted for 34.6% and 7.5%, respectively, of the total variance (44.8%) in clinical performance.

Key Words: *Education: physical therapist, admissions; Educational measurement.*

The number of physical therapy education programs has increased steadily over the years, and staffing demands are projected to remain high.[1] Because of the large numbers of qualified candidates competing for limited openings, physical therapy educators increasingly are demanded to document the criteria by which student selection decisions are made. One of the responsibilities of an admission committee is to design an efficient means of identifying candidates who will complete the educational program and become successful physical therapists. Currently, a paucity of literature exists on the admission process of physical therapy education programs.[2]

In 1976, French and Rezler commented on the "inadequate and poorly validated criteria" used in selecting students into allied health professions programs. They suggested that "the best combination of predictors should be locally established and may even vary from year to year, depending on local differences in curriculum, grading methods and the climate of learning."[3] Clinical skill is the "backbone" of physical therapy practice; therefore, determining the preadmission requirement that is the most viable predictor of clinical performance is important.

LITERATURE REVIEW

Previous academic achievement generally is assumed to be a fair and reliable indicator of the ability of students to succeed in any educational program. As such, cumulative grade point average (GPA) and standardized (aptitude) test scores are common criteria used in the selection of students into medical and allied health professions education programs.[2-5] Other criteria used include personal interview ratings, personality or interest inventory scores, written composition (ESSAY) scores, letters of recommendation, motor dexterity test scores, and biographical information. Previous investigations have shown consistently that academic course work is the best predictor of scholastic (cognitive) achievement at the end of the professional education.[2,6-11] Many studies indicate, however, that academic course work shows much lower or no correlation with clinical grades or performance on the job.[3,4]

Studies in nursing,[12] occupational therapy,[13] and medical programs[14-16] have revealed weak correlations between academic (preprofessional and professional) course work and clinical performance. On the contrary, studies in physical therapy have shown significant correlation between academic achievement (in preprofessional and professional courses) and clinical performance.[6,8,10] The best predictor of clinical performance currently is unclear.

Researchers who have investigated the relationship between academic requirements and academic and clinical performance have used the overall GPA in professional courses, grades in clinical internship, or ratings of job performance by employers as the criterion variable.[6-16] The use of GPA, clinical grades, and job rating scales as a measure of success, however, has a major psychometric weakness. Because the variables have a narrow range, they may not discriminate adequately among the usually homogeneous pool of candidates for admission to professional programs.[3,4]

Statement of the Problem

In 1983, Richardson advocated the need for physical therapy education programs to evaluate the proficiency of their graduates.[17] In the fall of 1984, we introduced a policy in our

J. Balogun, PhD, is Lecturer 1, Department of Medical Rehabilitation, Faculty of Health Sciences, Obafemi Awolowo University, Ile-Ife, Oyo State, Nigeria, West Africa. He was Assistant Professor, Department of Physical Therapy, Russell Sage College, Troy, NY 12180, at the time this study was completed.

This article was submitted March 24, 1986; was with the author for revision 35 weeks; and was accepted April 7, 1987. Potential Conflict of Interest: 4.

program that requires all physical therapy students to take a comprehensive written and an oral-practical examination at the end of their professional education program. The graduating class of 1985 was the first to take the comprehensive examination. The written component of the comprehensive examination was designed to test the students' theoretical knowledge of the basic and clinical sciences and physical therapy procedures. The oral-practical component of the comprehensive examination was designed to evaluate the students' communication, interpersonal, patient examination, and therapeutic intervention skills. In a recent study, my colleagues and I investigated the best predictor of academic achievement in our program, but we did not evaluate clinical performance at the end of the professional education program.[11]

The purpose of this retrospective study was to determine the best predictors of academic and clinical performance in our educational program. I hypothesized that the preprofessional GPA would be the most viable predictor of academic achievement and clinical performance in physical therapy.

METHOD

Subjects

The subjects for this study consisted of 42 recent graduates of a four-year baccalaureate program in physical therapy. All subjects were admitted into the professional program during the "screening" in the fall term of their sophomore year and began the professional program in the fall of their junior year. The research protocol was approved by the Institution Review Board on the Protection of the Rights of Human Subjects.

Procedure

Each student's file was reviewed for information used during the screening: 1) overall preprofessional GPAs, 2) ESSAY scores, 3) interview ratings (INTVs), 4) preprofessional faculty ratings (FACEVs), and 5) mean Allied Health Professions Admission Test (MAHPAT) scores. The student's score on the comprehensive written and oral-practical examination also was recorded. The scores on the components of the comprehensive examination were widely distributed, thus, differentiating the students better than the restricted GPA and clinical internship grades.

The preprofessional GPA was the mean of the grades for all courses taken in the first two years. The ESSAY was the student's score in a composition examination administered in the sophomore year. The INTV was the average of the ratings in a semi-structured interview. The FACEV was the mean of the ratings provided by two instructors from humanities and basic science departments. The MAHPAT was the average score for the five subsections (verbal ability, quantitative ability, biology, chemistry, and reading comprehension) of the Allied Health Professions Admission Test (AHPAT). The mean score, rather than the subscores of the test, was used because previous investigations showed that the MAHPAT is correlated most highly with academic achievement.[11,18]

The results of the comprehensive examination were used as a measure of the students' academic achievement and clinical competence at the end of their professional education program. The written component of the comprehensive examination consisted of two parts: 1) a basic-applied sciences section and 2) a clinical application section. The scores on both parts were averaged to represent the students' academic

achievement. The case studies presented during the oral-practical component of the comprehensive examination were limited to musculoskeletal, neurological, and cardiopulmonary content areas. A separate evaluation sheet was used for the three content areas. All evaluation sheets contained a list of specific behaviors to be assessed during the examination (Appendix). Each behavior, when correctly demonstrated or stated, was checked and later converted to numerical scores to reflect the weightings previously assigned to that particular behavior. To avoid bias, experienced clinical physical therapists administered the oral-practical component of the comprehensive examination, and students were assigned randomly to each case study. To control for interrater error, the same examiner evaluated all students assigned to each case study. I used the average of the scores of the different sections of the oral-practical component of the comprehensive examination (physical evaluation, problem and goal definition, therapeutic skills, and communication skills) to represent the students' clinical performance.

Data Analysis

In this investigation, the criterion (dependent) variable was defined as the performance on the comprehensive written and oral-practical examination administered at the end of the professional education program. Pearson product-moment correlation coefficients were computed to determine the relationship between the criterion variable and the predictor variables (preprofessional GPA, ESSAY, INTV, FACEV, and MAHPAT). The data were analyzed using multiple and stepwise regression models; both clinical and academic performances were used as dependent variables. The stepwise regression procedure selects the predictor variables in the order of their relative strength in predicting the criterion variable.[19] The tolerance was set at an F ratio of 4.00 and at a probability level of .01.

RESULTS

The MAHPAT score for the subjects in this study was 58.2 ($s = 17.5$). This value is slightly higher than the normative MAHPAT score of 57.0 for female physical therapy students (J. R. Silvestro, unpublished data, 1983–1984).

Presented in Table 1 are the Pearson product-moment correlation coefficients for the relationships between the criterion (academic and clinical performance) variables and independent (predictor) variables. Significant correlations were noted between academic performance and MAHPAT ($r = .50$, $p < .01$) and preprofessional GPA ($r = .55$, $p < .01$). Clinical performance was significantly related to preprofessional GPA ($r = .34$, $p < .05$) and INTV ($r = .59$, $p < .01$).

The results of the multiple regression analyses for academic and clinical performance are presented in Tables 2 and 3, respectively. The analyses revealed that the predictor variables (ie, admission requirements) can be used reliably ($p < .01$) to forecast the academic and clinical performance at the end of the professional program.

A summary of the stepwise regression analysis for academic performance is presented in Table 4. The results of the analysis revealed that preprofessional GPA is the best predictor of academic performance at the end of the professional program. It accounted for 30.5% of the total variability. The MAHPAT score is also a significant predictor ($F = 5.38$, $p < .01$) of academic performance. When MAHPAT was entered into the regression equation containing preprofessional GPA, they both accounted for 38.5% of the total variability. The findings suggest that 8.0% of the variance in academic performance was explained by MAHPAT. All predictor variables combined accounted for 40.6% of the total variability. The findings suggest that FACEV, INTV, and ESSAY have minimal predictive utility. The three variables accounted for only 2.1% of the variance in predicting academic performance (Tab. 4).

Presented in Table 5 is the summary of the stepwise regression analysis for clinical performance. The results of the analysis revealed that INTV and preprofessional GPA were the two viable predictors of clinical performance. Both variables accounted for 42.1% of the total variability. The INTV and preprofessional GPA accounted for 34.6% and 7.5%, respectively, of the variance of predicting clinical performance. All predictor variables combined accounted for 44.8% of the total variability. The findings suggest that ESSAY, MAHPAT, and FACEV accounted for only 2.7% of the increase in the ability to predict clinical performance in an equation containing INTV and preprofessional GPA.

DISCUSSION

The results of this study revealed that academic performance was significantly related to preprofessional GPA and MAHPAT (Tab. 1). This finding supported the results of a previous investigation by Balogun and colleagues.[11] They found significant ($p < .01$) correlations between academic achievement in the professional courses and preprofessional GPA ($r = .63$), ESSAY ($r = .31$), and MAHPAT ($r = .28$). In this study, however, the relationship between academic achievement and ESSAY ($r = .08$) was not statistically significant. The correlational findings of this study suggest that preprofessional GPA and MAHPAT may be viable predictors of academic achievement in our program (Tab. 1). The results of the stepwise regression analysis supported this speculation (Tab. 4). The analysis revealed that the most significant predictor of academic achievement was preprofessional GPA. The findings supported the research hypothesis and are consistent with the findings in previous research.[2,6-11] The MAHPAT is a viable ($p < .01$) predictor of academic achievement, but it accounted for less than 8% of the total variance (40.6%). From a practical perspective, the contribution of MAHPAT toward predicting academic achievement is minimal. The MAHPAT is not a viable predictor of clinical performance (Tab. 5).

The relationship between preadmission criteria and clinical performance (eg, internship grades, on-the-job ratings) has been a subject of considerable interest in the litera-ture.[6,8,10,12-16] Contrary to previous findings,[12-16] the results in this study revealed significant correlations between cognitive admission requirements and clinical performance. Preprofessional GPA and INTV were significantly related to clinical performance (Tab. 1). The results of the multiple regression analysis revealed that clinical performance can be predicted reliably from the admission requirements considered in this study (Tab. 3).

One of the primary objectives of this investigation was to determine the best predictor of clinical performance in our

TABLE 1

Correlation (r) Between Academic and Clinical Performance and the Predictor Variables (N = 42)

Predictor Variable	Criterion Variable	
	Academic Performance	Clinical Performance
Mean Allied Health Professions Admission Test	.50[a]	.03
Preprofessional grade point average	.55[a]	.34[b]
Written composition scores	.08	.08
Preprofessional faculty evaluation	.28[c]	.02
Interview ratings	.11	.59[a]

[a] r value significant at the .01 level of confidence.
[b] r value significant at the .05 level of confidence.
[c] r value significant at the .10 level of confidence.

TABLE 2

Analysis of Variance for the Multiple Regression Equation for Academic Performance

Source	df	SS	MS	F	p
Regression	5	616.3	123.3	4.92	.002
Residual	36	902.2	25.1		

TABLE 3

Analysis of Variance for the Multiple Regression Equation for Clinical Performance

Source	df	SS	MS	F	p
Regression	5	2083.3	416.7	5.84	.0005
Residual	36	2569.0	71.4		

TABLE 4

Summary of the Stepwise Regression Analysis for Academic Performance Showing Changes in Zero-Order (r) and Multiple Regression (R) Correlation Coefficients with Addition of Different Variables

Predictor Variable	R[a]	R²	R² Change (%)	F	df	p
Preprofessional grade point average (GPA)	.55	.31	30.52	17.57	1,40	.001
GPA + Mean Allied Health Profession Admission Test (MAHPAT)	.62	.39	7.96	12.19	2,39	.001
GPA + MAHPAT + FACEV[b] + INTV[c] + ESSAY[d]	.64	.41	2.11	4.92	5,36	.001

[a] R = r when only one predictor variable is being considered.
[b] FACEV = preprofessional faculty evaluation.
[c] INTV = interview ratings.
[d] ESSAY = written composition scores.

TABLE 5
Summary of the Stepwise Regression Analysis for Clinical Performance Showing Changes in Zero-Order (r)
and Multiple Regression (R) Correlation Coefficients with Addition of Different Variables

Predictor Variable	R^a	R^2	R^2 Change (%)	F	df	p
Interview ratings (INTV)	.59	.35	34.62	21.18	1,40	.001
INTV + preprofessional grade point average (GPA)	.65	.42	7.46	14.17	2,39	.001
INTV + GPA + ESSAY[b] + MAH-PAT[c] + FACEV[d]	.67	.45	2.70	5.84	5,36	.001

[a] $R = r$ when only one predictor variable is being considered.
[b] ESSAY = written composition scores.
[c] MAHPAT = mean Allied Health Professions Admission Test.
[d] FACEV = preprofessional faculty evaluation.

program. The results in Table 5 showed that the most viable predictor of clinical performance was INTV. This finding did not support the research hypothesis and is inconsistent with the previous reports in physical therapy.[6,8,20] Wiesseman found that preprofessional GPA and age were the strongest predictors of success in the professional board examination in physical therapy.[20] The GPA and age accounted for 35% of the total variance (49%) found in Wiesseman's study. Peat et al found preprofessional GPA as the most viable predictor of clinical performance.[8] It accounted for 9% of the total variance (12%) found in their study. Tidd and Conine reported the strongest correlation ($r = .43$) between clinical performance and GPA in physical therapy courses.[6] Clinical performance also was significantly ($p < .001$) related to overall GPA ($r = .39$), preprofessional GPA ($r = .29$), GPA in biological and physical sciences ($r = .28$), and GPA in behavorial sciences ($r = .23$). The previous studies[6,8,20] did not consider the same predictor variables in their design; thus, their findings cannot be compared objectively.

Educational Implications

College grades in preprofessional and professional courses and standardized aptitude test (AHPAT) scores, which are representative of cognitive measures, have been considered in previous studies in physical therapy.[6-11,20] In this study, a noncognitive measure (INTV) was the most reliable predictor of clinical performance. It accounted for 34.6% of the variance in clinical performance. Cognitive knowledge (preprofessional GPA) accounted for 7.5% of the total variability ($p < .01$). This finding suggests that noncognitive characteristics and previous academic achievement have relevance as predictors of clinical performance. During the clinical practicum, students were expected to demonstrate knowledge in all three behavioral (cognitive, psychomotor, and affective) domains. The cognitive domain includes theoretical knowledge and problem-solving skills. The psychomotor domain deals with the student's manipulative and performance skills during "patient" evaluation and therapeutic procedures. The affective domain evaluates the student's attitudes and rapport with the patient (Appendix). In the current changing health care system, physical therapists are required to perform, in addition to the "traditional" clinical functions, more diverse activities such as organizing in-service training, staff supervision, and health promotion. The inclusion of the three behavioral domains in any instrument designed to evaluate clinical competency in physical therapy, therefore, is crucial.

The five independent variables considered in this study accounted for 40.6% and 44.8% of the variance in predicting academic and clinical performance, respectively. The unexplained variance (59.4% and 55.2% for academic and clinical performance, respectively) may be attributable to other cognitive admission criteria (high school grades and aptitude test scores) and noncognitive admission criteria (motor skills, motivation, attitude, and personality) not considered in this study. Because physical therapy is both a "science" (academic knowledge base) and an "art" (techniques of clinical practice), considering both cognitive and noncognitive measures is important when admitting students into physical therapy education programs.

The predictive power of the subjective variables (ESSAY, INTV, and FACEV) can be improved by refining the measurement instruments.[3,4,21,22] We recently standardized the method of administration of the INTV and revised the FACEV questionnaire. We shortened the INTV and FACEV rating scales by removing the items we considered ambiguous and increased the spread (range of continuum) of the Likert scales. We also modified our criteria for grading the ESSAY. The changes made in the measurement instruments were based on the findings of previous research by Balogun and colleagues[11] and Balogun.[23] We recently used the modified measurement instruments to test candidates for admission to our program and obtained interrater reliability coefficients of .49 ($p < .01$) and .84 ($p < .001$) for ESSAY and INTV, respectively. The r value for ESSAY is low, probably because some of the items included in the grading criteria are ambiguous and difficult to decipher and quantify. It is plausible that the refinement of our measurement instruments would improve the contribution of the subjective variables in predicting academic and clinical performance in our program. A follow-up study is needed to support this speculation.

Limitations of the Study

The findings of this study should be applied with caution because of the small sample size. The high unexplained variance in predicting academic achievement (59.4%) and clinical performance (55.2%) limits the generalization of the results of this study. Additional research is warranted before more conclusive recommendations as to the best predictor of success in physical therapy can be made.

The reliability and validity of the instruments used in evaluating the proficiency of our graduates have not been determined. The test questions for the written component of the comprehensive examination were similar to those published by Hershey and Seibert[24] and Hershey[25] and cover all aspects of physical therapy; however, empirical documentation of its content validity is needed.

Implications for Future Research

To date, few research studies relating to the prediction of academic and clinical performance in physical therapy have been published. In view of the increasing costs in graduate education[17] and the desire of the profession to raise the entry-level requirement to postbaccalaureate degree, additional research to determine the best predictors of academic and clinical performance in physical therapy is crucial to inspire the trust of both the public and the college administration. Results of such studies will be helpful in admitting the next generation of students into physical therapy education programs.

Further studies are needed to determine the interrater and intrarater reliability and validity of the instrument used in our program for grading the oral-practical component of the comprehensive practical examination. Results of such studies may strengthen the validity of the findings in this study. Further interrater reliability studies are also needed after the interview forms are revised.

These findings suggest that academic achievement at the time of graduation may be a viable predictor of future clinical competence; however, follow-up research is needed to determine the relationship between students' academic achievement and performance in actual practice. The contribution of biographical information and noncognitive factors (such as motivation, personality, and motor skills) toward predicting success was not evaluated in this study. This area might form the basis of further research.

CONCLUSION

A significant correlation exists between academic achievement and MAHPAT, preprofessional GPA, and FACEV. Clinical performance was significantly related to FACEV and INTV.

The strongest predictors of academic achievement and clinical performance in the program studied were preprofessional GPA and INTV, respectively. The findings suggest that prediction of success in physical therapy may be enhanced by considering cognitive and noncognitive measures.

Acknowledgments. I express my appreciation to Dean Ursula Sybille Colby for providing the funds for computer analysis and a search of the literature. I give special thanks to John R. Silvestro, PhD, of The Psychological Corporation for providing literature on the reliability and validity of the AHPAT. Finally, I thank Fran Delaney for her contribution in the development of the oral-practical evaluation sheet and the multiple choice questions of the comprehensive examination.

APPENDIX
Summary of Criteria for Grading Oral-Practical Examination*

Lower Quarter Screening
  History and interview, initial observation, active and passive lumbar spine movements, neurological tests, specific tests (straight leg raising, neck flexion, Ely's test), provocation tests for sacroiliac joint
Specific Joint Evaluation
  Active and passive resisted movement tests, anthropometric measurements, special tests (stress, Apley's distraction and compression, Draws', McMurray's, Grind's, Tinel's sign)
Patient Problem List and Therapeutic Goals
  Assessment for appropriateness, specificity to problem, logical progression, and comprehensiveness
Treatment and Home Program Activities
  Assessment for appropriateness, specificity to problem, logical progression, comprehensiveness, and precautionary measures observed during treatment
Communication Skills and Affective Behaviors
  Assessment for patient setup and instruction, body mechanics, and professional presentation

* The format of the evaluation sheet has been changed to facilitate reproduction. Interested readers can write to the author for an original copy of the evaluation sheet.

REFERENCES

1. Johnson GR: Twentieth Mary McMillan lecture: Great expectations—A force in growth and change. Phys Ther 65:1690–1695, 1985
2. McGinnis ME: Admission predictors for pre-physical therapy majors. Phys Ther 64:55–58, 1984
3. French RM, Rezler AG: Student selection in four-year programs. In Ford CW, Morgan MK (eds): Teaching in the Health Professions. St. Louis, MO, C V Mosby Co, 1976, pp 94–110
4. Chaisson GM: Student selection: Logic or lottery. J Allied Health 5:7–16, 1976
5. Gartland GJ: Synopsis of a study of admissions criteria for physical therapy programs. Physiotherapy Canada 29:6–10, 1977
6. Tidd GS, Conine TA: Do better students perform better in the clinic? Relationship of academic grades to clinical ratings. Phys Ther 54:500–505, 1974
7. Pickles B: Correlations between matriculation entry requirements and performance in the diploma program in physical therapy at the University of Alberta. Physiotherapy Canada 29:249–253, 1977
8. Peat M, Woodbury MG, Donner A: Admission average as a predictor of undergraduate academic and clinical performance. Physiotherapy Canada 34:211–244, 1982
9. Kerr KM: Pre-entry requirements and academic performance in primary degree courses in physiotherapy at the Ulster Polytechnic. Physiotherapy 71:468–472, 1985
10. Olney SJ: Prediction of clinical competence of students of physiotherapy. Physiotherapy Canada 29:254–258, 1977
11. Balogun JA, Karacoloff LA, Farina NT: Predictors of academic achievement in physical therapy. Phys Ther 66:976–980, 1986
12. Taylor CW, Nahm H, Loy L, et al: Selection and Recruitment of Nurses and Nursing Students: Review of Research Students and Practices. Salt Lake City, UT, University of Utah Press, 1986
13. Anderson HE, Jantzen AC: A prediction of clinical performance. Am J Occup Ther 19:76–78, 1965
14. Benor DE, Hobfoll SE: Prediction of clinical performance: The role of prior experience. J Med Educ 56:653–658, 1981
15. Hobfoll SE, Benor DE: Prediction of student clinical performance. Med Educ 15:231–236, 1981
16. Hobfoll SE, Anson O, Antonovsky A: Personality factors as predictors of medical student performance. Med Educ 16:251–285, 1982
17. Richardson RW: Thinking for tomorrow. Phys Ther 63:1795–1801, 1983
18. Adams JR, Skinner DM: Can the AHPAT help evaluate comparable GPA from various academic institutions? Laboratory Medicine 11:258–264, 1980
19. Kim J, Kohout FJ: Multiple regression analysis. In Nie NH, et al (eds): Statistical Package for the Social Sciences, ed 2. New York, NY, McGraw-Hill Book Co, 1975, p 340
20. Wiesseman J: Does the AHPAT Add Enough Predictive Ability to the College GPA to Justify Its Use? Cleveland, OH, The Psychological Corporation (a subsidiary of Harcourt Brace Jovanovich Inc), 1984
21. Shepard KF: Use of small group interviews for selection into allied health educational programs. J Allied Health 9:85–94, 1980
22. Dietrich MC: Putting objectivity in the allied health student selection process. J Allied Health 10:226–239, 1981
23. Balogun JA: Predictive validity of the Allied Health Professions Admission Test. Physiotherapy Canada 39:39–42, 1987
24. Hershey RA, Seibert HK: Physical Therapy Examination Review Book: Basic Sciences, ed 4. New Hyde Park, NY, Medical Examination Publishing Co Inc, vol 1, 1984
25. Hershey RA: Physical Therapy Examination Review Book: Clinical Application, ed 2. New Hyde Park, NY, Medical Examination Publishing Co Inc, vol 2, 1973

Significance of Prior Experience on Students' Clinical Performance

Mary Ann Dettmann
Marcia T Linder

ABSTRACT: *This study was designed to determine if prior clinical experience is related to clinic success, and to substantiate the use of prior programs. Seventy-five percent of entry-level physical therapy educational programs use prior experience as an admission criterion. Sixty-one senior physical therapy students were ranked according to 1) the amount of prior clinical exposure they had; 2) clinical success, as measured by their rating on eleven Blue MACS skills and the subjective rating of their clinical instructor; 3) cumulative grade point average; and 4) their scores on the State-Trait Anxiety Inventory. Students with more prior experience were rated more highly by their clinical instructors and had lower anxiety levels.*

INTRODUCTION

Many physical therapy educational programs use prior experience as an admission criterion. This requirement apparently is based on the premise that such experience is beneficial. There is a lack of published data to substantiate the use of prior clinical experience as a criterion for admission.

To ascertain how many physical therapy schools require prior experience, a letter and a return postcard were sent to the directors of 105 entry-level physical therapy educational programs in August 1985. The letter requested information about whether the school used prior clinical experience as an admission criterion and, if so, how much was required. Seventy-five percent of the entry-level physical therapy school directors responded that prior experience was used as an admission criterion. A 1977 report by Gartland found that 47% of the United States physical therapy educators who responded to a survey emphasized work experience.[1] This apparent increase in the importance placed on prior experience is

Mrs Dettman is Associate Professor, Program in Physical Therapy, Marquette University, Walter Schroeder Complex, Room 346, Milwaukee, WI 53233. Mrs Linder is a physical therapist at St Elizabeth's Hospital, Appleton, WI. At the time of this study, she was Assistant Adjunct Professor, Program in Physical Therapy, Marquette University.

not accompanied by studies supporting its purpose.

Does prior clinical experience improve students' clinical performance? Several investigators studied the relationship between academic achievement and clinical performance and found small but significant relationships.[2-5] Grade point average was found by Peat et al to be the only reliable predictor of clinical performance.[2] May, investigating the relationship between group grade point means of academic and clinical courses, age, and type of work experience, found that no significant differences existed.[3] Pickles found a lack of consistency in the correlation between academic grades and clinical performance.[6]

Some of the advantages of prior experience are evident. Students may be able to make a more informed career choice when they have a better understanding of physical therapy, which can be gained through practical experience. The experience can provide role models and expand the students' understanding of the profession. The student who enrolls in a physical therapy program without being well informed, and who later drops out because he or she is disillusioned with the practice of physical therapy, has used a space that could have been used by another applicant. This is an important consideration in physical therapy education because enrollment is limited and programs have more qualified applicants than can be accommodated.[7,8]

A disadvantage of obtaining prior clinical experience is that it is time-consuming for the student, especially when a large number of hours are required. Because jobs that fulfill requirements are often reimbursed at near-minimum wage, the student may earn less money than at other employment. Students who are unable to get a physical therapy job must volunteer to meet the requirements. Experience requirements may therefore be a financial burden for some students.

Schools that require many hours of clinical experience have little control over the quality of that experience. Students can

develop bad habits. Clinical experience as a volunteer or aide puts the student in a subservient role that can be difficult to change when he or she must be "in charge" of patient care in the clinic. Conversely, students employed as aides have reported "treating" patients even before they have learned appropriate techniques and rationale for them. When prior experience consists primarily of repeated routine tasks, students may not view physical therapists as problem solvers.

Clinics located near physical therapy schools may be inundated with requests for experience. This problem can be more acute when the facility is already being utilized by the school for clinical experience of their students. Some clinics, however, may appreciate the opportunity to have volunteers or employees who can be recruited following graduation.

We decided to limit the scope of this study to exploring the relationship between performance in the initial clinical experience and the amount of prior experience. An experiment was designed to determine if performance in the first clinical experience for senior students was related to their previous clinical background. Because the literature reported both an inconsistent and a low but significant relationship between academic achievement and clinical performance, academic achievement in the form of grade point average (GPA) was added to the analysis. Similarly, an anxiety inventory was administered to all students because of the high levels of anxiety frequently observed as students anticipate their first clinical experience.

METHOD

Sixty-one students beginning their senior year (last professional year) were surveyed about their clinical experience and grouped according to whether they had experience in physical therapy. Clinical experience was defined as clinical exposure to date, excluding that which was part of junior coursework. Points ranging from 1 to 12 were assigned to the amount of experience. A

TABLE 1

Prior Experience Requirements for Admission to Physical Therapy Programs (Fall 1985)

Type of Program	n	Prior Experience Required		$\bar{X}$ in Hours	Range
		No	Yes		
Bachelor's Degree					
Freshman Admission	14	4	10	60	(8–100)
Junior Admission	69	18	51	129	(8–1,000)
Certificate	9	3	6	275	(100–600)
Entry-Level Master's	13	3	10	65	(40–100)
TOTAL	105	28	77	128	(8–1,000)

"1" indicated no experience and a "12" indicated 640 or more hours (about 16 weeks) of experience in a physical therapy department.

The senior physical therapy students had a two-week practicum (80 hours) which was their initial full-time clinical experience. We requested that the clinical instructors (CIs) evaluate the students based on 11 preselected skills from the Blue MACS assessment form.[9] The skills selected were basic skills, such as manual muscle testing, range of motion, goal setting, and patient rapport. The CIs had been trained in the use of the Blue MACS and had experience using the instrument. Several key indicators are listed for each of the 11 skills. Each student was evaluated on approximately 25 to 30 of these performance statements. A total numerical value was obtained by assigning positive points to "checks" (which indicate satisfactory performance) and negative points to "Ns" (which denote need for improvement). No points were assigned to question marks (insufficient observation) or if the key criterion was not addressed.

At the end of the two-week clinical experience, the CIs were asked to rate the students subjectively on a continuum ranging from "incompetent" to "consistently superior." Subsequently a numerical value was assigned to points along the continuum to obtain a quantitative assessment. Students' GPAs based on their first three years of college were included in statistical analysis as another measure of success.

A month before the clinical experience, all students took the Trait portion of the State-Trait Anxiety Inventory.[10] The Trait portion is an indication of general anxiety. On the morning of the first day of the clinical experience, students took the State portion of the Inventory which indicated anxiety at that moment. Five students were not given the State portion of the Inventory on the first day, and therefore some of our data report the results of 56 of the 61 students.

Data were subjected to analysis by chi square, Pearson correlation coefficient, and regression analysis.

RESULTS

Ninety-five of the 105 entry-level physical therapy program directors (90%) responded to the survey regarding prior clinical experience. The entry-level programs were divided into four categories: freshman admission bachelor's degree, junior admission bachelor's degree, certificate program, and entry-level master's degree. A majority of programs in all categories used prior experience as an admission requirement (Table 1).

The average amount of required experience was 128 (range 8–1,000) hours. Not all respondents indicated the exact number of hours, although most did. In some instances the student with many hours got more points than did the student with few hours. It is interesting to note that the certificate programs required the highest number of hours of prior experience (275) and the entry-level master's programs had a low hourly average (65). It should be noted, however, that the number of respondents in both of these categories was small.

There was no significant correlation, using Pearson correlation coefficient, between the amount of clinical experience and the Blue MACS rating. Although clinical experience did not correlate with the Blue MACS, the Blue MACS rating had a significant relationship with the CI's rating and was the strongest Pearson correlation obtained (Table 2). The state of anxiety correlated with the trait of anxiety, as one would expect. Both anxiety scores also correlated significantly with the CIs' ratings and the amount of clinical experience. Grade point average did not correlate with any of the variables.

Students' prior physical therapy experience was compared to the CIs' subjective rating using chi square analysis. Students were put into groups of no experience, 20 to 160 hours of physical therapy experience, and more than 160 hours of experience. Clinical instructors' subjective ratings were divided into low, medium, and high. There was a statistically significant relationship between the CIs' subjective rating of the student and the amount of clinical experience (Table 2). This suggests that the student with more prior clinical experience will receive a higher rating from his or her CI. Chi square was also significant between the CIs' rating and the Blue MACS rating. Blue MACS scores were divided into low, medium, and high. A student whose performance was rated high by the CI also tended to receive more "checks" and fewer "Ns" on the Blue MACS.

The only variable that had any predictive value, as demonstrated by multiple regression analysis, was the relationship between trait anxiety and the subjective CIs' rating. No other factors were predictive and, therefore, multiple regression analysis yielded no significant findings.

DISCUSSION

Prior clinical experience is probably one of the better ways for a student to learn about the profession and to make an informed career decision. There is limited space in entry-level curricula, and those

TABLE 2

Relationship Between Prior Experience, Clinical Performance Evaluations, and Student Anxiety

Correlations	r^a	P	X^2	df	P
Blue MACS Rating with CI Rating	.424	.001	12.89	4	.05
Prior Experience with CI Rating	.185	NS	10.68	4	.05
State of Anxiety with Trait of Anxiety	.389	.002			
State of Anxiety with CI Rating	−.299	.01			
State of Anxiety with Prior Experience	−.249	.03			
Trait of Anxiety with CI Rating	−.361	.003			
Trait of Anxiety with Prior Experience	−.304	.01			

aPearson correlation coefficients.

spaces should be given to the student who has made an effort to be informed about physical therapy.

There is an indication from this study that prior experience reduces anxiety levels in students. Students with low anxiety levels were rated higher by the CIs during their first clinical experience. Students with prior experience may have learned to be more comfortable with professionals and more at ease with patients.

Students with more prior experience tended to be rated higher on their performance by their clinical instructors. Familiarity with a clinic, equipment, and some disabilities and diseases may also facilitate learning and influence clinic behavior.

Grade point average did not show any correlation with the other variables in this study. Studies of the relationship between academic grades and clinical performance continue to be inconclusive.

The relationship between the CIs' scoring of the Blue MACS skills and their subjective rating of the student was the only variable that was significant on both the Pearson correlation coefficients and chi square. This tends to support the reliability of scoring of the 11 Blue MACS skills to represent the opinion of the CI concerning the performance of the student. The Blue MACS, however, like any clinical rating tool, is limited by subjectivity.

The value and usefulness of prior clinical experience as an admission criterion is not clear. More studies are needed to assess the impact of prior clinic experience on clinical performance. If there is a difference in the clinical performance of students with prior experience, does that difference still exist when students have satisfactorily completed the clinical segment of their education? If prior experience proves to be advantageous, then we need to know how much and what type of experience is both efficient and effective in assuring future success as a physical therapist.

REFERENCES

1. Gartland GJ: Synopsis of a study of admissions for physical therapy programs. Physiotherapy Canada 29:6–10, 1977
2. Peat M, Woodbury MG, Donner A: Admission average as a predictor of undergraduate academic and clinical performance. Physiotherapy Canada 34:211–214, 1982
3. May BJ: Academic achievement in physical therapy: Related to factors of age and work experience. Phys Ther 47:26–34, 1967
4. Tidd GS, Conine TA: Do better students perform better in the clinic? Relationship of academic grades to clinical ratings. Phys Ther 54:500–505, 1974
5. Olney SJ: Prediction of clinical competence of students of physical therapy. Physiotherapy Canada 29:254–258, 1977
6. Pickles B: Correlations between matriculation entry requirements and performance in the diploma program in physical therapy at the University of Alberta. Physiotherapy Canada 29:249–253, 1977
7. Position paper in support of physical therapist entry-level at postbaccalaureate degree level. In: House of Delegates Handbook. Washington, DC, American Physical Therapy Association, 1979
8. Physical Therapy Entry-Level Programs, Alexandria, VA, American Physical Therapy Association, Department of Education, 1986
9. The Blue MACS: Mastery and Assessment of Clinical Skills, ed 3. Galveston, TX, Texas Consortium for Physical Therapy Clinical Education
10. Spielberger CD, Gorsuch RL, Lushene RE: State-Trait Anxiety-Inventory Manual. Palo Alto, CA, Consulting Psychologists Press, Inc, September 1970

education

Do Better Students Perform Better in the Clinic?

Relationship of Academic Grades to Clinical Ratings

GRETCHEN S. TIDD, M.S.,
and TALI A. CONINE, H.S.D.

Grade point average data were obtained from the records of 285 physical therapy alumni of Indiana University. Based on correlation coefficients, answers to two broad questions were sought: Are academic grades significantly related to successful performance of students in the clinic? Are some specific aspects of the learning experiences better predictors than others of clinical ratings of students? The conclusions relating to each question were affirmative.

Have you ever heard a colleague say that "better students do not necessarily become better clinicians"? This belief implies that academic achievement is not a predictor of on-the-job performance in physical therapy. More specifically, it means that the learning experiences being provided in college courses are not critically related to successful performance in the clinic. The establishment of evidence that substantial relationships between academic achievement and clinical performance exist or do not exist would be of significance in selection of criteria for admission of physical therapy students, in decisions on emphasis to

be placed in an academic program, and in employers' choice of appointments to physical therapy positions. In fact, without conclusive research evidence, 1) physical therapy programs in general have used past academic performance as one important criterion for admission,[1] 2) the basic curricular requirements and emphasis in physical therapy have not been changed or revalidated since 1955,[2] and 3) at least in one major institution, the Veterans Administration hospitals, the beginning salary of physical therapists is based on scholastic standing of the applicants.

In 1972, a study was designed at Indiana University to investigate the relationship of academic achievement to clinical performance of students in physical therapy. The answers to two broad questions were sought:

1. Are academic grades significantly related to successful performance in the clinic by the students?

Miss Tidd is Assistant Professor of Allied Health Sciences at Indiana University and serves on the staff of Home Care Agency of Greater Indianapolis, 3190 North Meridian, Indianapolis, IN 46208.

Dr. Conine is Professor of Education and Physical Therapy and Chairperson of Allied Health Sciences Education at Indiana University, Indianapolis, IN 46202.

2. Are some specific aspects of the learning experiences better predictors than others of clinical performance of students?

REVIEW OF RELATED LITERATURE

Investigators in the past have sought to find and validate test batteries in such areas as intelligence, personality, interest, temperament, attitude, and biographical data to be used for student selection in physical therapy.[3-6] Published research related to academic predictors of clinical performance in the field is scarce, however, as compared with nursing, dentistry, medicine, and occupational therapy.[7-14]

Nearly twenty years ago, Gobetz published the results of a national survey in physical therapy in which didactic average, clinical practice evaluations, and job performance ratings were compared.[3] He reported positive coefficients of correlations between didactic grade average and clinical practice ratings for men (.34, .19) and women (.49, .38) students entering the professional program in 1950 and 1951.* He concluded that "generally speaking, the better students make the better therapists . . ." but noted that the men were less consistent and had lower correlations than the women.

In 1959, Stockmeyer reported a coefficient of .45 between academic average and clinical performance grades of one hundred physical therapy students at Stanford University.[15] She also found coefficients ranging from .15 to .45 between selected courses at the University and the clinical performance ratings. She observed that, although the correlations were not high enough to be of predictive value, the relationship between academic and clinical performance varied in the positive direction. In another unpublished study, a similar conclusion was drawn by Everett, who, in 1962, investigated the interrelationships among groups of University of Connecticut courses and an overall level of achievement rating of eighty-six students in that school.

_____

* Coefficients, designated by the letter r, essentially may be thought of as a *ratio*, which in this case expressed the extent to which the didactic grades are accompanied by changes in the clinical ratings. In a perfect positive relationship r = 1.00 but only rarely, if ever, will a coefficient be that high.

Research findings cited above have been somewhat inconclusive and limited. The coefficients of correlation obtained between grades and clinical ratings were low, although consistently in the positive direction. The areas of educational experiences or academic achievement investigated were not always clearly defined. In two studies, results were generally confined to performance of students in single courses in a given institution rather than representing achievement in broad educational constructs.[15,16] Furthermore, results might have been contaminated by extraneous variables since the grades of certificate and baccalaureate level students were not studied separately and a wide range of experiential backgrounds existed among the subjects.

DESIGN

The following null hypotheses were proposed and tested at the 5 percent level of significance to guide the objective investigation of the two questions underlying the study:

1. No significant relationship exists between a student's academic achievement and his clinical performance.
2. No significant relationship exists between a student's preprofessional performance and his clinical performance.
3. No significant relationship exists between a student's performance in physical and biological science courses and his performance in the clinic.
4. No significant relationship exists between a student's performance in behavioral science courses and his performance in the clinic.
5. No significant relationship exists between a student's performance in physical therapy courses and his performance in the clinic.

Two main assumptions were made. First, a student's performance can be measured and expressed in grades. The subject of grades has received considerable attention in the literature. Grades may lack reliability and validity, but a fairly accurate estimate of a student's capacity is obtained when a grade represents several estimates from more than one teacher.[17] No attempt was made in this study to test the reliability or validity of the grades. The grades used in the testing of the hypotheses, however, were based on several estimates in given areas of performance. The second assumption was that the student's clinical grade was predictive of his subsequent on-the-job performance. Gobetz noted only a slight difference in the magnitude of the correlations when comparing didactic average to clinical performance ratings and employer ratings after one year of the subject's employment.[3]

The sources of data were the records of all graduates of the physical therapy program of Indiana University between 1960 and 1972. The program is a four-year baccalaureate degree curriculum; the final two years make up the professional education which is offered at the Medical Center Campus in Indianapolis. The preprofessional course work may be completed at the university or at another accredited institution. During the professional education period, the students receive two grades for their clinical performance. The more intensive clinical practicum takes place at the end of academic studies in the senior year. The clinical ratings are based on composite evaluations by clinical instructors pertaining to students' ability to evaluate, plan, and implement a patient care program, use effective verbal and nonverbal communication, participate in administrative activities of a unit, and support and augment professional activities.

From the alumni files of the physical therapy department, the following information was selected: the total college grade point average (GPA) of the graduates, excluding the clinical grades; and the sub-GPA for the clinical practicums, the preprofessional courses, behavioral science courses, biological and physical science courses, and physical therapy courses. The *Essentials of an Acceptable School of*

Physical Therapy[2] and the criteria used by the university provided the definition of the last three subcategories as listed in Table 1.

The Indiana University grading scale was used to quantify any letter grade for which no mark was recorded on a 0 to 100 point scale (Tab. 2). The clinical grades, and grades transferred from other institutions, formed the major portion of this category. The median values in each range of 0 to 100 points were used for the conversion of letter grades (Tab. 2). This conversion was necessary for statistical analyses of correlations. All grades were weighted according to the number of credit hours they represented before averaging. The grade for each course was grouped in its appropriate category, whether it was a required or an elective experience. The data were not separated according to the sex of the subjects because only a very small percentage (5.26%) of the graduates were men and no skewness of the distribution was detected.

The Product Moment Correlation was used to measure the extent of association (coefficients, or r) between the various grade-point averages. The Chi square procedure was used to analyze the frequency of data in their qualitative values of A, B, C, D, or F grades and to determine if the procedure of quantifying the grades may have introduced errors in measuring the extent of association by the Product Moment Correlation.

RESULTS

Complete information was available for 285 (96%) of the 297 graduates of the Indiana University program between 1960 and 1972. The data not included in the study related to 8

TABLE 1
Groupings Used for the Calculation of Sub-GPA Categories

Categories	Courses	Semester Hours Credit
Biological and physical sciences	Anatomy, botany, chemistry, microbiology, physics, and physiology	27-57
Behavioral sciences	Anthropology, economics, geography, linguistics, political science, psychology, and sociology	7-26
Physical therapy	Tests and measurements, therapeutic exercise and assistive devices, and physical agents	16-18

TABLE 2
Indiana University Grading Scale

Descriptions	Grade	Points	Percentages	Medians
Unusual degree of academic performance	A	4	93-100	96.5
Above average achievement	B	3	85-92	88.5
Average achievement	C	2	78-84	81.0
Passing work but below standards	D	1	70-77	74.5
Failure in a course or failure to complete a course without authorized withdrawal	F	0	Below 70	—

graduates who had incomplete preprofessional grades (3) or professional records (1), had satisfactory-unsatisfactory type reports instead of A to F or 0 to 100 scaled grades (3), or did not have the minimum required semester hours in the behavioral sciences (1).

The correlation coefficients shown in Table 3 related GPA in clinical performance, academic achievement, preprofessional college achievement, achievement in biological and physical sciences, achievement in behavioral sciences, and achievement in physical therapy courses. All coefficients, ranging from .23 to .88 were found to be significant at or beyond the .001 level (P < .001).

The Chi square tests, not reported in this article, also indicated that the null hypotheses should be rejected. Thus, relative to the first question of this study, a significant relationship was apparent between the academic achievement of students and their clinical performance at Indiana University. The correlation coefficients obtained between the clinical performance and preprofessional GPA (r = .29) and total academic achievement GPA (r = .39) were not high. The high level of significance (P < .001), however, was sufficient evidence to indicate that a student whose classwork was poor did not tend to do well in the clinic and a student who excelled academically did well clinically.

In answer to the second concern in this study, some aspects of the didactic courses seemed to correlate more positively with the clinical performance of the students. As might have been expected, the data showed that the best indicator of clinical ratings, before completion of the program, was achievement in physical therapy courses (r = .43). Next in rank was preprofessional academic performance (r = .29), followed by performance in biological and physical sciences (r = .28). Achievement in the behavioral sciences, although statistically significant (P < .001), appeared to be less related to clinical ratings (r = .23).

Beyond the stated purposes of the study, other observations could be made regarding the various interrelationships in the GPAs. High correlation values were noted between total academic and preprofessional grades (r = .88). Biological-physical science grades also appeared to be good indicators of success in the total program (r = .84), in the preprofessional curriculum (r = .83), and in physical therapy courses (r = .67).

TABLE 3
*Intercorrelation of GPAs in the Various
Performance Areas (P < .001)*

Performance Areas	1	2	3	4	5	6
1. Clinical performance	...	.39	.29	.28	.23	.43
2. Academic achievement		...	.88	.84	.72	.73
3. Preprofessional achievement			...	.83	.80	.55
4. Achievement in biological and physical sciences				...	.67	.67
5. Achievement in behavioral sciences					...	.49
6. Achievement in physical therapy courses						...

DISCUSSION

The results of this investigation were consistent with those of previous studies in physical therapy, confirming that academic grades are positively related to performance in the clinic. Coefficients of correlation reported by others had ranged from .05 to .01 levels of statistical significance. On the basis of the Indiana findings, one can be more confident ($P < .001$) that "better students do perform better in the clinic" as measured by their clinical grades. The difference in the levels of significance between this and previous studies may have resulted from the method of quantification of letter grades and reduction of possible sources of error related to heterogeneity of the subject's background, education level, work experience, and age.

One of the most important goals of selection of students in a physical therapy curriculum is academic success, although on-the-job performance after leaving college is of equal importance. The findings of this study show that a significant relationship exists between success in the biological sciences and achievement in the preprofessional ($r = .84$) and professional ($r = .83$) years of study. Those persons involved with the selection of criteria for admission of students into physical therapy programs should note that of all nonintellective[1,4-6] and intellective predictors[13,15,16] studied by various investigators, academic achievement appears to be the strongest criterion identified thus far, and that GPAs in the biological and physical sciences may be the best indicators of academic success.

The necessary balance and the types of courses to be included in a curriculum are of particular interest to program planners. The present basic national curriculum requirements in physical therapy emphasize biophysical sciences but also require the behavioral sciences, although to a lesser extent. The data from this study help validate the relationship of these subjects to physical therapy education and their relative measurable importance.

No attempt was made in the Indiana study to relate academic grades to actual employment ratings of the graduates; therefore, the results should be interpreted with caution and only as partial cues to performance on the job. Another limitation of this study pertains to the problems associated with measurements of achievement in courses and in the clinic. Reliable and valid evaluation tools are lacking and grades, therefore, are fallible. In physical therapy education, an acute need exists for the exploration and development of measurement tools and further analysis of academic predictors of job success.

SUMMARY AND CONCLUSIONS

In 1972, a study was designed at Indiana University to investigate the relationship of academic achievement and clinical performance of students in physical therapy. Previous research had shown that a positive relationship exists between the two variables as measured by grades. Five null hypotheses were stated and tested at the .05 level of significance, comparing students' grades in preprofessional courses, total academic programs, biological sciences, behavioral sciences, physical therapy courses, and the clinical practicums. The analysis of data pertaining to 285 graduates yielded correlation coefficients between clinical grades and the other GPAs ranging from .23 to .43, $P < .001$. High relationships were observed between preprofessional and total academic grades ($r = .88$), between achievement in biophysical sciences and total academic achievement ($r = .84$), and achievement in physical therapy courses and total academic achievement ($r = .73$).

In conclusion, academically better students generally tend to perform better in the clinic. The preprofessional GPA of a student can be a strong indicator of his success in the professional studies, but the best indicator of success may be the student's grades in the biological sciences which correlate highly with the preprofessional, professional, and physical therapy GPAs. For the Indiana graduates, the balance and types of courses required in physical therapy are apparently sound as judged by their relationship with clinical ratings of students. Reliable and valid measurement tools need to be developed to better assess academic and clinical performance. Further investigation of the relationship of academic achievement with actual on-the-job ratings of physical therapists is recommended.

REFERENCES

1. Pinkston D, Margolis B: Student selection for physical therapy education: A project in progress. Phys Ther 50:1710-1714, 1970
2. Council on Medical Education and Hospitals of the American Medical Association: Essentials of an Acceptable School of Physical Therapy, Chicago, 1955
3. Gobetz W: Physical therapy school admission test batteries: Report on the student selection test research program. Phys Ther Rev 34:429-437, 1954
4. James A: A Study of Relationship Between the A-Z Temperament Traits and the Clinical Practice Grade of Physical Therapy Students. Unpublished master's thesis. Boston, Massachusetts, Boston University, 1960
5. Duntman G, Anderson H, Barry J: Characteristics of Students in the Health Related Professions. Gainesville, Florida, University of Florida, 1966
6. Graham W, McIntyre F, Johnson G, et al: Selection of Students for Physical Therapy Educational Program—Part III: Use of Biographical Information Data to Predict Job Performance. Cleveland, Ohio, Case Western Reserve University, 1971
7. Taylor C: Measurement and Prediction of Nursing Performance. Unpublished report. Salt Lake City, Utah, University of Utah, 1964
8. Taylor C, Nahm H, Quinn M, et al: Report on Measurement and Prediction of Nursing Performance—Part I. Salt Lake City, Utah, University of Utah, 1965
9. Taylor C, Nahm H, Loy L, et al: Selection and Recruitment of Nurses and Nursing Students: A Review of Research Studies and Practices. Salt Lake City, Utah, University of Utah Press, 1966
10. Weiss I: Prediction of academic success in dental school. J Appl Psychol 36:11-14, 1952
11. Gough H, Hall W, Harris R: Admissions procedures as forecasters of performance in medical training. J Med Educ 38:989-998, 1963
12. Gaier E: The criterion problem in the prediction of medical school success. J Appl Psychol 36:316-322, 1952
13. Anderson H, Jantzen A: A prediction of clinical performance. Am J Occup Ther 19:76-78, 1965
14. Englehart H: An investigation of the relationship between college grades and the on-the-job performance during clinical training of occupational therapy students. Am J Occup Ther 11:97-101, 1957
15. Stockmeyer S: The Relationship of Clinical and Academic Grades in Physical Therapy. Unpublished master's thesis. Palo Alto, California, Stanford University, 1959
16. Everett M: The Relationship of Preliminary Academic Achievement to Performance in Physical Therapy Education. Unpublished master's thesis. Palo Alto, California, Stanford University, 1962
17. Kelly T: Educational Guidance. New York, Teachers College, Columbia University, 1914

THE AUTHORS

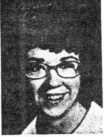

Gretchen S. Tidd received a bachelor's degree in physical therapy from The Ohio State University and a master's degree from Indiana University. She has been an area supervisor at the Institute of Physical Medicine and Rehabilitation in Peoria, Illinois, a supervisor of clinical education at the Convalescent Hospital for Children in Cincinnati, Ohio, and a consultant to the Wayne Township Schools in Indianapolis, Indiana. She is currently employed as an assistant professor at Indiana University and as a staff therapist for the Home Care Agency of Greater Indianapolis.

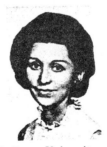

Tali A. Conine received a bachelor's and a master's degree in physical therapy from New York University, and a health science degree from Indiana University. She has served with the World Health Organization. Dr. Conine is currently professor of education and physical therapy and is chairman of Graduate Allied Health Sciences Education at Indiana University, Schools of Education and Medicine, Indianapolis, Indiana.

Teaching
and Clinical
Education

Teaching Physical Therapy Students to Reflect:
A Suggestion for Clinical Education

G Jensen, PhD, PT
B Denton, MA, PT

ABSTRACT: *The ability of practitioners to think about what is done and why and to assess past actions, current situations, and possible outcomes is vital to professional practice that is reflective and not routine. Twenty-three graduate students enrolled in a first professional degree program in physical therapy used a structured journal-writing activity during their first clinical experience as a method of reflective inquiry. Students were asked to keep a journal throughout their clinical experience according to a set of guidelines. Student journals and feedback surveys were coded and analyzed using qualitative data analysis techniques. Results demonstrated that students had a consistent focus on self-concerns and self-growth. The journal served as an outlet for student feelings and as a structured method for cognitive reflection. It provided students with a method of tracking their development throughout the clinical experience. Structured journal writing provided students with a framework for reconstructing events and thinking more critically about their actions. Recommendations for development of further activities for encouraging reflective practice are offered.*

INTRODUCTION

Many practitioners, locked into a view of themselves as technical experts, find little in the world of practice to occasion reflection. For them, uncertainty is a threat; its admission, a sign of weakness. They have become proficient at techniques of selective inattention. ... Yet reflection-in-action is not a rare event. There are teachers, managers, engineers,

Dr Jensen is Associate Professor, Division of Physical Therapy, School of Health Related Professions, The University of Alabama at Birmingham, Birmingham, AL 35294. Ms Denton is Associate Professor and Academic Coordinator of Clinical Education, Division of Physical Therapy, School of Health Related Professions, The University of Alabama at Birmingham. This article was adapted from a presentation at the Annual Conference of the American Physical Therapy Association, Nashville, TN, June 11–15, 1989.

and artists for whom reflection-in-action is the "prose" they speak as they display and develop the ordinary artistry of their everyday lives. Such individuals are willing to embrace error, accept confusion, and reflect critically on their previously examined assumptions.[1(pp251–252)]

Schon, in his model of professional practice, argued that professional practice could be improved if practitioners were encouraged to reflect more on their actions rather than simply to rely on their acquired technical knowledge.[2] His model, based on studies of professionals such as architects, town planners, scientists, and psychotherapists,[2,3] has stimulated a great deal of interest and research among educators in other professions.[4–8] We believe that physical therapists, like other professionals, practice in an environment where clinical problems often defy technical solutions. Creating opportunities for physical therapy students to learn the skills and attitudes required for reflective practice may be one way of better preparing students to handle the complexity of practice; that is, to consider the consequences of their work as well as to apply their technical expertise. The purpose of this article is to describe one education program's experience with the implementation and evaluation of a method of reflective inquiry used during physical therapy students' first clinical experience.

What is reflection and reflective practice? John Dewey first characterized *reflection* as a specialized form of thinking critical for effective teaching.[9] He maintained that reflection stems from doubt or perplexity in a directly experienced situation, which, in turn, leads to purposeful inquiry and problem resolution. According to Dewey, "The function of reflective thought is, therefore, to transform a situation in which there is experienced obscurity, doubt, conflict, disturbance of some sort, into a situation that is clear, coherent, settled and harmonious."[9(p99)] Reflection does not merely grow out of a direct experience, but it refers back to it as well, so that the aim

and outcome arise out of the direct experience. Key components of reflection are the presence of a *directly experienced situation* and the *process of thinking about what to do, when, and why*. Dewey also asserted that reflective thinking frees us from using routine thinking and action. He described *routine action* as being guided primarily by tradition and external authority, whereas *reflective action* requires active and careful consideration of beliefs and knowledge.[9]

Schon[2,3] and others[4,5,10] viewed Dewey's concept of reflective thinking and action as critical not only for teachers, but for practice in many professions. Furthermore, Schon argued that it is the capacity of successful practitioners to "reflect-in-action" that enables them to deal with the complexity and uncertainty of practice.[2]

Teaching, medicine, and occupational therapy are among the professions that are implementing programs to promote reflective thinking.[4,7,8] A growing body of research in teacher education reveals that many teachers are not reflective practitioners and that reflection will not occur in teaching unless it is facilitated as teachers learn to teach.[4,11] Structured programs have been successful in providing opportunities for students to learn the knowledge and skills of reflective practice.[4–6] In occupational therapy, Parham[7] argued that the reflective occupational therapist uses theory as a key element in problem setting and problem solving in clinical practice. She believes that the development of sound reasoning in the professional therapist is dependent on providing experiences that promote reflection. In medicine, Hewson et al[8] advocate that reflection is part of a cognitive apprenticeship; that is, the development of a practical knowledge base, thinking skills, and motor skills in patient care activities.

Although there are programs in other professions constructed to promote reflective thinking among students, little has been written about implementation of such activities in physical therapy. At the American Physical Therapy Association clinical education conference in Rock Eagle, Ga, in 1985,

Reprinted with permission from the Section for Education, APTA

Carol Davis urged educators to recognize the value of reflective thinking and to teach for it:

> We must, as Schon suggests, recognize the demand for reflection-in-action and *teach for it.*[12(p64)]

At the University of Alabama at Birmingham, we implemented a structured journal-writing activity as a method of reflective inquiry during physical therapy students' first full-time clinical experience. The idea of journal writing during a clinical experience is not new in physical therapy. Others have used student diaries during clinical experiences in physical therapy to facilitate student recognition of the affective domain.[13,14] Previous research in teacher education, however, demonstrated that structured journal writing can be a vehicle for reflective thinking.[4-6]

Facilitating reflection also requires creating conditions that allow for reenactment or reconstruction of events to occur.[6] The conditions we created for the journal writing were guidelines adapted from Schwab's four *commonplaces* of teaching.[15] Schwab[15] suggested that in order for teaching to occur, someone (a teacher) must be teaching someone (a student) about something (a curriculum) at some place (a milieu). Several researchers in teacher education[4,6,16] have used Schwab's four categories as a structural foundation for reflective activities. The four commonplaces we posed for physical therapy were patient, student physical therapist, curriculum, and context.

METHOD

The participants in this field experience were 23 students enrolled in a graduate-level first professional degree program in physical therapy. Students were asked to keep a journal throughout their first full-time clinical affiliation, a 3½-week assignment following the first three terms of course work. They were assigned to a variety of settings where they could gain experience in beginning-level evaluation and treatment skills. Prior to the clinical experience, a 1-hour class session was spent introducing the students to the concept of reflection by defining the process, sharing examples of reflective activities implemented in other professions, and discussing the journal guidelines and ground rules. These journal guidelines and ground rules provided students with a framework for systematic reflection on their development as physical therapists and their actions in the clinic (Tab. 1).

At the end of the clinical experience, journals were returned to us for coding and analysis. Journals were required but were not graded to encourage students to write

Table 1

Examples of Journal Guidelines and Journal-Writing Ground Rules Provided for Students

Guidelines	Ground Rules
1. Student therapist: How do you feel about your role as a therapist?	1. Write at least two journal entries per week. Write more if you wish.
2. Patient: What are your thoughts about a particular patient?	2. Respond to the four areas at least once each week. If the areas are not conducive to writing, write whatever you want.
3. Curriculum: What are your needs now that you are immersed in the clinical environment?	3. Keep entries in a small notebook. Date the entries. Indicate the major category and return the journal to us after your clinical experience.
4. Context: What strikes you about how the department runs, the organization, and the health care system?	

Figure 1

Initial coding scheme based on Schwab[15] and other coding categories that emerged from data.

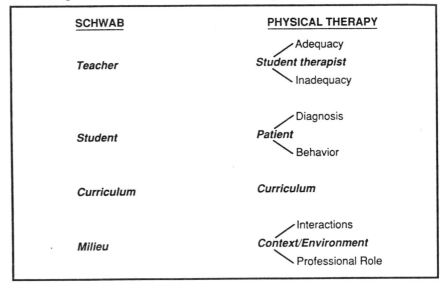

freely without the pressure of a grade. Two weeks after completion of their clinical assignment, students were given a short questionnaire with four open-ended questions asking students what they had learned from the journal-writing activity, what they found most and least enjoyable about journal writing, and how they felt about keeping a journal again if it was not required. The student questionnaire responses also were analyzed.

Data Analysis

The coding scheme for all data emerged during the analysis of data.[17] Both authors initially read one half of the journals and coded them using the four commonplaces as initial coding categories. We then met and discussed the need for further expan-

sion of the coding categories and revised them to include a total of six coding categories. These six categories were expansions or subcategories of the commonplaces we identified for physical therapy (Fig. 1). Two categories were from the student physical therapist commonplace (self-adequacy and self-inadequacy), two were from the commonplace of patient (patient diagnosis and behavior), and two categories were from the environmental context (personnel interactions and professional role). The commonplace of curriculum did not appear as a separate category because we found that references to curriculum frequently were part of student expressions of self-adequacy or self-inadequacy. These six final categories were defined and then used for rereading and coding of all journals (Tab. 2). Codes were

Table 2

Definitions of the Six Finalized Coding Categories for Journals

Coding Category	Definition
Patient:	
1. Patient diagnosis	References made to medical diagnosis and medical record information.
2. Patient behavior	References made to how the patient reacts to surroundings. Patient cooperation with treatment.
Student therapist/curriculum:	
3. Self-adequacy	Expressions of self-satisfaction and self-confidence.
4. Self-inadequacy	Expressions of frustration and insecurity in lack of knowledge or skills or perceived gaps in current knowledge.
Context/environment:	
5. Personnel interaction	References made to staff interactions or observations about the organization.
6. Professional role	References made to students' expectations of physical therapy and their future role as a therapist.

Figure 2

Percentages of frequency counts (N=462 coded passages) for each of the six journal categories.

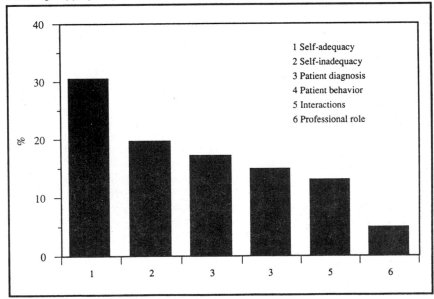

1 Self-adequacy
2 Self-inadequacy
3 Patient diagnosis
4 Patient behavior
5 Interactions
6 Professional role

assigned to a series of sentences or to a journal passage that represented one of the six identified categories. A sample of journals was coded by both authors to check the reliability of the coding scheme ($\bar{X}$=92% agreement; Kappa=.80).

Student questionnaire data were first sorted by listing all student responses for each of the four questions (eg, what students learned, what they enjoyed most and least). An inductive content analysis process then was used to look across all student responses and identify common themes.[18]

RESULTS

The purpose of this project was to gain further insight into the effect of structured journal writing as a tool for facilitating reflection among physical therapy students, from the students' perspective. The findings reported are drawn from the students' journals and students' self-report data on their assessment of the experience.

Journal Data: Focus on Self

In coding the journals according to the six coding categories, we identified 462 coded passages. The coding categories of student self-adequacy (31%) and self-inadequacy (20%) received the greatest number of entries (Fig. 2). Of the 23 journals, three journals were more documentary in nature. These three journals contained a majority of statements related to patient diagnoses and behaviors. The coding categories of personnel interactions (13%) and students' professional role (5%) had the fewest entries.

Student self-adequacy. The largest number of coding references were in the category of self-adequacy and satisfaction. Many of the journal entries here represent increased student confidence and independence as well as students' recognition of their application of classroom knowledge to clinical practice. The following journal entries of two students are typical:

> I have been amazed what is in my brain from last year, ready to be put together and I have the answers. I think this is one reason my clinical has gone so well. I finally have the confidence. I realize that what I learned last year is in there and I have so much to be learned, so I don't worry when I'm faced with those things I don't know yet.

> It feels good to become more independent and to be trusted by patients and other therapists. I really appreciated that (discussion with clinical instructor before and after an evaluation) and felt good as a student physical therapist.

Student self-inadequacy. The second-largest coding category was student self-inadequacy and frustration. Here the journal appeared to be an outlet for expressions of frustration about the knowledge gap between where students were in the educational process and where they perceived they needed to be. This knowledge gap included psychomotor skills and cognitive decision-making skills.

> It is very stressful to be totally disoriented physically as well as feeling painfully conspicuous as the "new kid on the block" who doesn't know how to do anything.

> Sometimes I get frustrated because I feel I have all this book knowledge but I have trouble recalling and putting it together. I have to remind myself this is what clinical is for and these things come with experience.

> A skill that has given me trouble (it occurred with this patient and two or three others) is simple goniometry. I'm fidgety and I never get the same measurement as the PT! That makes me feel inadequate and dumb, so I guess I need to practice.

Patient diagnosis and patient behavior. The percentage of codes for these two categories were similar: 17% for patient diagnosis and 15% for patient behavior (Fig. 2.). The journal entries pertaining to the patient diagnostic category frequently reported the medical background of the patient.

We have a 26-year-old pt who had a AK amputation of the left LE and lost the lateral aspect of the R lower leg as a result of a concrete wall falling on him.

One of my patients is a woman in her forties with low back pain caused by a motor vehicle accident in March 1988.

Journal entries that addressed the behavioral aspects of the patient often demonstrated student insights into the complexity of patient care:

Anyway, we got this patient up and he takes a few steps, stands straight and walks 10 feet quite well. It brought home to me you can't prejudge a patient's ability.

Today we had a CVA patient. He was a very frustrated man with aphasia and hemiplegia. . . . He had the hardest time putting on his socks and every time my CI went to help, the patient would swat at him. It was so sad. We could've helped him so much if he had just let us. He would've been a great candidate for rehabilitation but he wouldn't give in. It made me realize that we only do for the patient what the patient will let us do; we can't make a patient do what we want no matter how good we think it would be for the patient.

We found that a small number of students had a more documentary than reflective approach to journal writing. These student journal entries gave the patient data, both diagnostic and behavioral, without any discussion or reflection on their experience.

2 CVAs, L, AKA, fx pelvis, arthritic, postop hip replacement with leg length discrepancy. Helped with discharge eval on AKA with COPD.

Case I, 60 year old white female with a THR, revealed apprehension to having treatment by SPT; after communication gap was crossed, no problems; she enjoyed setting goals and achieving them.

Personnel interaction/professional role. These categories were the least-used categories in our coding scheme (Fig. 2). The journal entries again represented an emphasis on self. Students remarked on interaction among the staff, but more frequently, remarked on how the staff related to them:

Staff is really friendly—everyone seems to enjoy each other's company.

The people in this department continue to get along great. They're a close-knit group of people and do a lot of things outside the hospital. Relationships between the PT and technicians seem good, even though I don't see much interaction and they all seem to like me.

Examples of references to their professional role as a physical therapist were less frequent but often represented student's concerns for their future responsibilities as therapists:

Case I is an 89-year-old male with a right CVA, became comatose after 48 hours and soon after past (sic) away with the PT and me in the room. This was a big moment in my life. It is amazing what true death can do to you. At the moment of death one wonders many questions: 1) How important is PT in times like these? 2) Should PT really be applied to a patient who is assumed dying? 3) Does this patient really care, concerning PT?

Yesterday I shared in a patient's joy and triumph, but today I experienced a patient's defeat. . . . Her wound is not healing, and next week the doctor will amputate. . . . It's not easy to work with someone and admit defeat. It's made me think about the fact that not all patients will be helped with PT. Being idealistic, I would like to think this is not true; however, reality tells me differently.

Most journals contained numerous entries at or near the beginning (during the first few days) that expressed students' feelings of inadequacy, frustration, and insecurity. As the experience progressed, these types of comments became fewer. Comments related to self-adequacy increased in frequency as students commented on their feelings of self-satisfaction and confidence. The following examples compare student comments from week one to week three.

(Week 1): I don't feel like I'm making as much of a difference with the patients. . . . (Week 3): I have gained a good deal of experience in evaluating and assessing patients. I am really enjoying this now.

(Week 1): At times I felt and still feel awkward, and it seems I'm in the way. I feel like a little puppy dog at times, following my CI around. (Week 3): I

feel so much more comfortable in my position. I feel more confident in what I do and feel more accepted by the staff and patients.

(Week 1): I don't like seeing needles and big open wounds. (Week 3): I really enjoyed returning to the burn unit today. I'm glad I was exposed to it and am very interested in the area.

Student Feedback: Multipurpose Role of the Journal

We identified three themes in the student questionnaire data regarding the role of the journal: 1) the journal served as a vehicle for expressions of their feelings about the clinical experience; 2) the journal allowed for cognitive reflection; that is, students thought about what they did and why, and how they were applying and integrating their knowledge; and 3) the journal provided an opportunity for them to look back on their growth and development throughout the clinical experience.

Outlet for feelings. For many students, the focus again was on the affective domain and their own self-adequacy. The journal was an outlet for expression of their feelings and provided them the opportunity to express frustrations and triumphs. Here are some examples of student responses:

Helped me reflect and keep in touch with myself . . . a way of expressing feelings rather than holding them in.

Helped me verbalize in times of stress or change to objectify my feelings and reactions to the situation. Alice in Wonderland said, "How can I know what I think until I see what I say?"

The fact that I could write about bad experiences and get them off my chest.

Cognitive reflection. Another element highlighted by students was how the journals gave them a framework for looking more critically at their knowledge base. The journals were a structured way of looking back on the day and thinking about what they did and why and how they integrated information.

Helped me remember cases I'd seen during the day and enabled me to think twice about my actions.

Helped me take time to review my day and assimilate the new information I had learned. Helped me think through aspects of my clinical experience that I found helpful or unhelpful in an organized manner.

Helped me bring my thoughts together and really pinpoint what I was learning, thinking, and experiencing.

Learning to bring ideas together to see how clinical experiences brought book learning to reality.

Development. Finally, the journal experience was a vehicle for students to track their own growth and development throughout the clinical experience. Once again, students' focus was on their own self-adequacy and self-inadequacy.

Reading the journal and seeing the progress from being a scared, incompetent PT student to a student who felt she had the knowledge to approach some patients and work with them.

To look back and see the difference from the first to the end.

It was fun to see on paper how many things I was learning.

For most students (60%), the journal writing was a positive experience that they would do again. Limitations for some students had to do with not liking to write and preferring to discuss their experience with their clinical instructor or classmates; a few students felt constrained by the structure of the categories and the lack of privacy.

DISCUSSION

This project was implemented in the context of a graduate-level first professional degree program in physical therapy, and our sample may not represent the larger population of physical therapy students. We believe, however, that our findings are useful in providing us with a better understanding of the phenomenon of reflection in a physical therapy education program.

Our findings demonstrate that for these beginning physical therapy students, structured journal writing did document and promote student reflection. Over one half (51%) of the coded journal passages related to student expressions about self, self-adequacy, or self-inadequacy. We also observed a shift in the journals from concerns about self-inadequacy in the early part of the clinical experience toward expressions of self-adequacy and confidence by the middle and later stages of the experience. Recognition of this shift in their feelings was a positive aspect of the reflective journal writing for the students.

Student focus on self and self-concerns is not inconsistent with what others have found in looking at the development of student teachers.[19,20] Fuller[19] and Goodman[20] both reported that experienced teachers are more concerned about student progress, while novice teachers usually are

more concerned with self-adequacy and survival. Researchers have noted in other professional programs that providing students with structured opportunities to respond to the emotional aspect of their development results not only in expression and validation of feelings, but often in a critical analysis of the basis for their feelings.[4,7] Opportunity for expression and validation of feelings also has been cited as an important component of clinical education in physical therapy.[13,14] Although feelings dominated student reflections in our study, it was not to the exclusion of reflections on experiences with patients, staff, and the students' future professional role.

Schon argued that professional students must be taught a process of reenactment, in a clinical setting, to encourage the development of critical judgment and clinical decision making.[2,3] If we want to enhance the development of critical thinking skills and clinical judgment in future therapists, then we may want to consider the benefits of educating a "reflective practitioner."[3] To do this, we will need to provide opportunities for students to reflect and to learn the knowledge and skills of reflective practice.

Designing programs that help students develop the skills of reflection is not without difficulty. The barriers to reflection identified in the teaching profession include the complexity of the classroom and the isolation of teachers.[4,5,16] Beginning physical therapy students frequently are overwhelmed with the demands of clinical practice and with a fear of failure in a clinical experience. In a fast-paced clinic, it may appear to students that practice is more routine than reflective. Students may focus on their own survival needs and be unable to move to a level of analysis that requires skills they have not yet developed. It may, therefore, be easier to function reflexively to survive. Reflection requires time and an understanding of the knowledge and skills that promote reflection.[4-6] A framework that facilitates reflective practice may help students develop a better understanding of the processes they are experiencing.

This structured journal-writing activity is but one beginning method of encouraging development of reflective skills in students. We could consider designing opportunities for reflection that would include different conditions such as discussion with colleagues, thorough critique of materials, and structured opportunities to debrief with clinical instructors.[5,6] Looking at students' experiences over time and throughout their entire educational experience could provide

information on how one develops clinical judgment. Educators may gain insight into how to facilitate the development of clinical decision making in students through knowing more about ways students process their experiences. Opportunities for reflection may also be beneficial in the development of clinical instructors as they struggle with the complexity and spontaneity of clinical teaching. Continued research that examines prospective therapists' reflections and the conditions that promote reflection should be conducted.

CONCLUSION

As educators, we have the challenge of preparing students to practice in a complex and uncertain environment. Developing opportunities for students to learn the knowledge and skills of reflective practice is one suggestion for meeting this challenge. Evidence from other professions demonstrates that reflection affects how one develops as a professional by influencing how successfully one is able to learn from her or his experience.[2-4,6] Our findings suggest that a structured journal-writing activity served as a vehicle for students to reconstruct events or to reflect on events that they had experienced during their clinical experience. This structured opportunity for reflection is an example of the kind of activity that could be integrated into current educational experiences.

ACKNOWLEDGMENTS

We are indebted to the physical therapy students from the Division of Physical Therapy, The University of Alabama at Birmingham, for sharing their experiences with us. We also are grateful to Dr. Anna Richert, Assistant Professor, Mills College, whose enthusiasm and commitment to teaching others about the reflection process knows no limits.

REFERENCES

1. Schon D: The crisis of professional knowledge and the pursuit of an epistemology of practice. In Christensen C (ed): Teaching and the Case Method. Boston, MA, Harvard Business School, 1987, pp 241–253
2. Schon D: The Reflective Practitioner: How Professionals Think in Action. New York, NY, Basic Books, Inc, 1983
3. Schon D: Educating the Reflective Practitioner. San Francisco, CA, Jossey-Bass, Inc, Publishers, 1987
4. Zeichner KM, Liston D: Teaching student teachers to reflect. Harvard Educational Review 57(1):23–48, 1987
5. Grimmett P, Erickson G (eds): Reflection in Teacher Education. New York, NY, Teachers College Press, 1988
6. Richert A: Reflex to reflection: Facilitating Reflection in Novice Teachers. Doctoral Dissertation. Stanford, CA, Stanford University School of Education, 1988

7. Parham LD: Applying theory to practice. In: Proceedings of the Occupational Therapy Association's Conference on Education, Target 2000. Rockville, MD, June 22–26, 1986, pp 119–122

8. Hewson M, Hewson P, Jensen N: The Role of Reflection in Professional Medical Education: A Conceptual Change Interpretation. Read at the Annual Meeting of the American Educational Research Association. San Francisco, CA, March 27–31, 1989

9. Dewey J: How We Think: A Restatement of the Relation of Reflective Thinking to the Educative Process. Chicago, IL, Henry Regnery Co, 1933

10. Van Manen M: Linking ways of knowing with ways of being practical. Curriculum Inquiry 6:205–228, 1977

11. Lortie D: Schoolteacher: A Sociological Study. Chicago, IL, University of Chicago Press, 1975

12. Davis C: Professional socialization: Process that empowers. In: Leadership for Change in Physical Therapy Clinical Education. Alexandria, VA, Department of Education, American Physical Therapy Association, 1986, pp 53–70

13. Senter J, Black T: Teaching and monitoring the affective domain through use of a clinical education diary. Physical Therapy Education: Section for Education, Winter 1980

14. Davis C: Evaluating student clinical performance in the affective domain. Journal of Physical Therapy Education 1(1):19–20, 1987

15. Schwab J: The practical 3: Translation into curriculum. School Review 81:501–522, 1973

16. Posner G: Field Experience. Methods of Reflective Teaching, ed 2. New York, NY, Longman Inc, 1989

17. Merriam S: Case Study Research in Education: A Qualitative Approach. San Francisco, CA, Jossey-Bass Inc, Publishers, 1988, pp 123–146

18. Berg B: Qualitative Research Methods for the Social Sciences. Boston, MA, Allyn and Bacon, 1989, pp 105–129

19. Fuller F: Concerns of teachers: A developmental conceptualization. American Education Research Journal 6:207–226, 1975

20. Goodman J: What students learn from early field experiences: A case study and critical analysis. Journal of Teacher Education (Nov–Dec): 42–48, 1985

Preparation of Entry-level Students for Future Roles as Clinical Instructors

Patricia A Halcarz, MS, PT, NCS
Donna K Marzouk, PT
Elaine Avila, MS, PT
Mary S Bowser, MS, PT
Linda Hurm, MS, PT

ABSTRACT: In the clinical rotation sites affiliated with Indiana University, physical therapists commonly assume the position of clinical instructor within a year of entry into the profession. Most entry-level curricula do not incorporate instruction in the skills necessary to become an effective clinical instructor. This article discusses the 5-year evolution of an entry-level course designed to provide knowledge on the development of a clinical education program and the roles and responsibilities of clinical educators. The format and resources utilized to develop this body of knowledge regarding clinical instruction are presented so that other programs can adopt such a segment into their own curriculum.

INTRODUCTION

The importance of the clinical instructor (CI) in providing quality clinical education of the entry-level physical therapist is being addressed at the national level.[1-3] The American Physical Therapy Association has held two conferences—Rock Eagle (1985) and Split Rock (1987)—to discuss future clinical education models. The development of clinical faculty was one of four main themes at the conference on Pivotal Issues at Split Rock. Faculty development from a clinical perspective was addressed by speakers such as Jacqueline Montgomery at this conference. She stated that CIs should be prepared for "their teaching role."[1]

Ms Halcarz is Physical Therapy Consultant, Nova Care, 9292 N Meridian St, Indianapolis, IN 46260 . Ms Marzouk is Assistant Professor, Texas Woman's University, Houston, TX 77030, and a doctoral candidate, Physical Therapy Program, Department of Allied Health Sciences, School of Medicine, Indiana University, Indianapolis, IN 46202. Ms Avila is Academic Coordinator of Clinical Education and Assistant Professor, Physical Therapy Program, Department of Allied Health Sciences, School of Medicine, Indiana University. Ms Bowser is Director of Surgical (Administrator) Service, St. Vincent's Hospital and Health Care Center, 2001 86th St, Indianapolis, IN 46260. Ms Hurm is Manager of Rehabilitation Services, St. Vincent's Hospital and Health Care Center.

The need for CIs to be knowledgeable about and have experiences related to teaching, learning, educational methodology, and the climate of the environment, along with adult learning theories and principles, was further defined by Montgomery.[1] Scully and Shepard reported that CIs perceive a lack of preparation for their role in education.[4] In 1976, Moore and Perry identified this problem with data from a survey of CIs, demonstrating that only 25% had attended teachers' training.[5] Because no standard criteria for preparation of the CI currently exist, clinical facilities and academic institutions continue to develop their individual programs.[6]

The CI is defined as a person who is responsible for the direct instruction and supervision of the physical therapy student in the clinical education setting. Preparation for the role of CI is primarily accomplished through informal methods within the clinical setting. The potential for formalized development exists in methods such as facility in-service seminars and workshops conducted by educational institutions and consortia. According to Montgomery, in addition to the lack of formal training as a CI, new clinicians also lack the "experience, maturity and wisdom" to serve as mentors to the student physical therapist.[1] Examination of the curriculum vitaes of our clinical faculty suggests that many CIs assume this role within 1 to 2 years of entry into the profession.

Review of the literature revealed few published reports on methods of teaching therapists to be CIs included in entry-level physical therapy curriculum. Perry reported that "a few" advanced academic programs are including skills necessary for the role of a CI.[5] To better prepare students for their eventual role as a CI, the faculty at Indiana University have incorporated a clinical instruction component into the academic portion of the physical therapy curriculum.

This article presents our innovative course for development of potential CIs in an effort to stimulate discussion of alternative models to educate CIs within entry-level physical therapy programs.

DEVELOPMENT OF CLINICAL EDUCATION COMPONENT

Since the fall semester of 1986, a component of our administration course, Administration and Management Skills for Physical Therapists, has been devoted to clinical education and the role of the clinical instructor. This component is taught by the academic coordinator of clinical education (ACCE) and a faculty member who formerly was a center coordinator of clinical education (CCCE). Both faculty members also are involved in the local clinical education interest group.

Format of Clinical Education Component

As a requirement in the administration course, small groups of students (seven groups of four students each) develop a hypothetical physical therapy service that includes a budget, personnel requirements, equipment, and space requirements in the chosen setting. Using this chosen service as a basis, the students are asked to develop a corresponding clinical education program that is the terminal objective of this component.

Information essential for developing the clinical education program is presented within this course. The following topics are covered in a series of 6 hours of lecture and discussion:

1. Criteria for establishing a clinical education program both from the clinical and the academic perspective.[7-9]

2. The roles and responsibilities of the ACCE, CCCE, CI, and student in clinical education.[7]

3. Methods of communication, feedback guidelines, and learning styles.[10]

4. Methods of evaluation including the use of logs and the critical incident method

Reprinted with permission from the Section for Education, APTA

(positive and negative observations) of documentation for evaluation.[11]

5. Current issues in clinical education, including year-long clinical rotations and certification of CIs.[12]

6. Methods of developing a philosophy statement of clinical education.[7]

CLINICAL EDUCATION PROJECT AND OPEN FORUM

Each group is required to develop a clinical education program designed for the selected hypothetical physical therapy service.

The clinical education program includes

1. A written philosophy statement of clinical education for the hypothetical department.

2. The table of contents for the proposed "Student Handbook for Clinical Education."

3. The roles and responsibilities of the CI, CCCE, ACCE, and student.

4. A student evaluation form and justification for its selection. (Blue MACS* and other established evaluation tools are made available for review and inclusion.)

5. A list of references that includes interviews with CCCEs and course instructors.

To assist in developing the clinical education program, students are required to read *Developing a Clinical Education Program from the Clinician's Perspective*,[7] and *Establishing a Clinical Education Program at Your Facility: What You Need to Consider and Why*.[8]

In addition to the above, students are also required to utilize two outside references. Related articles, texts, and existing student handbooks are available in a program file.

To promote interaction, students are required to contact CCCEs from a list of individuals who have given their approval to be contacted. Interviews with these CCCEs are utilized not only to assist with development of the model clinical education program but also are used as a basis for information shared during an open forum. Topic areas for questions to CCCEs include instruction provided by CCCEs to new CIs, individual facility's self-evaluation of their clinical education program, facility rewards and areas of concern in providing clinical education, views on development of professional socialization, evaluation tools, and future trends in clinical education. The Table is a sample of questions provided to help students plan their interviews.

The open forum is designed to discuss controversial topics involved in clinical edu-

*Texas Consortium for Physical Therapy Clinical Education Inc, 1989.

cation, including certification of CIs and rewards and drawbacks to instituting a clinical education program as well as those topics on the list of questions (Table). The format of this discussion is an informal setting in which a topic is introduced by a student from one of the groups. Each group then has the opportunity to present supporting or opposing views to the stated opinion.

Information gained through the interviews with local CIs and CCEs is utilized in the open forum. The discussion is held in a 3-hour block of time. The purpose of this discussion is not to come to a uniform opinion but to expose students to the varying opinions of CIs on these topics. Each project is graded, with specific points assigned for each of the five areas previously listed as required components of the model clinical education program. This score comprised 15% of the total course grade.

DISCUSSION

The evolution of this institutional component has been a multistep process. Many of the changes implemented have been based on suggestions from the students, although most of the input from course evaluations was positive. The overall impact on the students has not been evaluated because our students do not return to campus after completing senior clinical rotations. Future surveys of these graduates are planned to assess the effectiveness of this instruction.

The first time this component was included in the administration course, it was presented separately from the rest of the course. The development of a hypothetical clinical education program was a separate project from the group's hypothetical physical therapy service. The next step in the process will be to integrate information regarding clinical instruction into the lecture series from the beginning of the administration course and to incorporate the clinical education program directly into the hypothetical physical therapy service. A proposed future step is projected to include information on methods of conducting research in the area of clinical education into the lectures and project.

Table

Sample Clinical Education Questionnaire for Clinical Instructor Interviews

Preparation for New Clinical Instructors:

1. What criteria do your facility use to determine readiness of staff to become clinical instructors?

2. What type of education or training is provided to prepare staff who will become clinical instructors?

3. What do you feel is lacking in development of new clinical instructors? At your facility or service? On a national level?

4. How much experience is required for a physical therapist to become a clinical instructor at your facility?

Rewards and Areas of Concern in Clinical Education for Clinical Instructors and Administrators in Clinical Education Site:

1. What are the benefits in having your staff and facility involved in clinical education?

2. What are the disadvantages of having your staff or facility involved in clinical education?

Professionalism:

1. What effect did the participation of the staff have on your clinical education program? What effect will it have next year?

2. What professional groups does your staff participate in (American Physical Therapy Association, Orthopaedic Study Group, Neurology Group/Section, Pediatrics Section)? What benefits does the participation of staff have on your clinical education program?

Student Handbook Entries:

1. Does your facility or service have a student handbook? If not, is your facility in the process of developing a handbook?

2. If your facility or service has a student handbook, what information do you include in the handbook? How often do you update the handbook? Do you give the handbook to the student prior to the clinical education experience?

Evaluation Tools:

1. What type of evaluation does your facility utilize to evaluate the student performance, clinical instructor performance, quality of the clinical education experience, and academic institution participation?

Opinion of the Interviewer:

1. What do you feel are the minimum criteria that a physical therapist or facility should meet to be considered a viable clinical education site?

2. What factors do you consider to assess whether you or your staff can provide a quality clinical education experience in the year ahead?

3. What do you see as issues that will need to be addressed in clinical education in the next few years?

4. What do you feel is the optimal length of time and number of clinical education experiences for all entry-level physical therapy students?

Physical therapy curricula routinely include instruction for teaching peers, patients, and family members but rarely include instruction in skills necessary to teach student therapists in the clinical setting. By receiving information on clinical education, it is hoped that students can integrate these previously learned teaching skills into the framework of clinical education. No research is available to substantiate that the ability to teach patients and peers automatically transfers to the ability necessary to teach students in the clinic.

STRENGTHS AND WEAKNESSES

The major strength of this instructional component is the formalization of issues in clinical education that usually is otherwise left to chance. In addition, it is proposed that the students will gain the following:

1. An increased sensitivity to the dynamics that may be present in a clinical situation.

2. A heightened awareness of the need for effective communication skill in a clinical practice.

3. The ability to be an objective consumer of clinical education.

4. Improved self-assessment skills.

5. Increased knowledge of responsibilities of the CI, CCCE, ACCE, and student in the clinic.

The above benefits may affect the student as a potential CI but also as a student physical therapist on clinical rotation.

A weakness of this instructional component is that, although information on clinical education is presented, a mechanism for practicing these skills is not available. This component also does not address the fact that new clinicians may lack the wisdom and experience necessary to become a competent mentor. Our goal is to bridge the gap partially with knowledge of the clinical education process until the clinician gains the "wisdom and experience" necessary to become a CI.

FUTURE CONSIDERATIONS

A future consideration will be to promote increased involvement of area CCCEs and CIs in the development and execution of this project to promote collaboration of students (potential CIs) and CIs in various settings. This collaboration can be accomplished by increasing the number of CIs willing to be interviewed as well as by identifying mentors from local clinics to assist students in this project. Feedback also will be solicited from CCCEs regarding the impact of the student interviews on potential benefits to the clinic and perceived inconveniences.

A follow-up study is planned to survey graduates who have participated in this course to determine the impact of the course on their clinical rotations and on their role as a CI. Suggestions for future inclusions or exclusions also will be solicited. In addition to graduates, employers will be polled regarding the impact of this information on clinical education programs.

By sharing this information with the physical therapy community, it is hoped that discussion and disclosure of other methods of education specifically aimed at clinical instruction would be encouraged. We believe that the inclusion of a formal education component of clinical instruction in the physical therapy curriculum is a vital aspect of our students' education and should not be left to chance.

REFERENCES

1. Montgomery J. Clinical faculty: revitalization for 2001. In: *Pivotal Issues in Clinical Education.* Alexandria, VA: American Physical Therapy Association, Section for Education; 1988.

2. Perry JF. Who is responsible for preparing clinical educators? In: *Pivotal Issues in Clinical Education.* Alexandria, VA: American Physical Therapy Association, Section on Education; 1988.

3. Clendenin MA: Clinical faculty development: panel summation and discussion. In: *Pivotal Issues in Clinical Education.* Alexandria, VA: American Physical Therapy Association, Section on Education; 1988.

4. Scully RM, Shepard KF. Clinical teaching in physical therapy education. *Phys Ther.* 1983;63(3):349–358.

5. Moore ML, Perry JF. *Clinical Education in Physical Therapy: Present Status/Future Needs.* Washington, DC; American Physical Therapy Association, Section for Education; 1976;4.45.

6. Perry JF: Who is responsible for preparing clinical educators? In: *Pivotal Issues in Clinical Education.* Alexandria, VA: American Physical Therapy Association, Section on Education; 1988.

7. Windom P: Developing a clinical education program from the clinician's perspective. *Phys Ther.* 1982; 62(11):1604–1609.

8. Haskins AR: Establishing a clinical education program at your facility: What you need to consider and why. In: *Physical Therapy Education.* Alexandria, VA: American Physical Therapy Association, Section for Education; 1984.

9. *Project on Clinical Education in Physical Therapy.* Contract No. 1-AH-44112. Alexandria, VA: American Physical Therapy Association, Section for Education; 1976.

10. Kolb DA, Rubin IM, McIntyre JM. *Organizational Psychology: An Experienced Approach.* Englewood, NJ: Prentice Hall; 1971.

11. McDaniel LV. The critical incident method in evaluation. *Phys Ther.* 1964;44(4):235–242.

12. Echternach JL, Sanders BS, Towne LL. *Physical Therapy: Considerations for Alternative Models.* Alexandria, VA: American Physical Therapy Association; September 1985.

special communication

Rapping with a Chaplain

JAMES T. WAGNER, M Div, EdS

Group discussions for senior physical therapy students, led by the hospital chaplain, were held at the University of Florida Medical Center. The idea for these "rap sessions" originated with the Department of Physical Therapy at Shands Teaching Hospital. The content of the discussions grew out of the students' experiences during their clinical assignments. The experience was deemed beneficial to the learning process by students, clinic staff, and faculty and helped to create a more relaxed atmosphere for learning in the clinic.

Group discussions, led by the hospital chaplain, were made available to senior physical therapy students in the College of Health Related Professions at the University of Florida. The suggestion for such meetings originated with the physical therapy clinic staff at Shands Teaching Hospital who provide supervision for students during their clinical affiliation. Staff interest in such discussions emerged from reflection on their own educational backgrounds, where formal opportunities for discussions were lacking, and from frequent inquiries, questions, and comments from the students. The decision was made, therefore, to schedule time for senior students if they wished an opportunity to meet weekly throughout the academic quarter. The students were free to establish both structure and format of these meetings. Two conditions were imposed on the student discussions. First, group therapy was not the intended purpose. The expectation was that topics, information, or issues not covered in the classroom, as well as concerns emerging from clinical work, would become the focus of the group discussions. Second, unless the students indicated otherwise, I, as Health Center Chaplain, would serve as facilitator for the

discussions. Other participants in the group would be decided upon by the students.

Topics of discussion chosen and explored by the groups ranged widely. The following subjects were common to all the groups:

1. Graduation and the approaching role shift from student to health professional; coping with feelings of inadequacy; and establishing support systems in a new community.
2. The problem of causing the patient pain during treatment and the need to redefine pain in clinical situations as giving care.
3. Difficulties in interprofessional relationships such as learning territorial rights in the hospital setting, being able to articulate one's skills and insights to other health care roles, and the feeling of being intimidated by physicians.
4. The issue of continuing to feel useful and purposeful as a therapist while facing limited goals in working with either the patient with permanent functional loss or the patient with catastrophic illness.
5. Various ethical issues in health care such as abortion, the use of extraordinary means of life support with terminal patients, and the complexities in separating personal from professional values.
6. Problems posed in treating patients who manifest or raise the following issues: seductive behavior, depression, psychosomatic disorders, denial, peers in age, those

Chaplain Wagner is Director, Department of Pastoral Care, J. Hillis Miller Health Center, and Assistant Professor, College of Health Related Professions, University of Florida, Gainesville, FL 32610.

unable or unwilling to follow home care plans, dependency, manipulation, and communicating with the child-patient.

7. The problem of the therapist coping when identifying with and becoming overly involved with a particular patient to the extent that professional and personal aspects of the relationship become confused.

To date, four groups of senior students have elected to participate in the discussions. The size of the groups ranged from seven to nine members, including both men and women. The weekly lunch meetings followed a morning in which the students worked with patients in the clinic setting. Three groups decided upon an open agenda for each meeting, whereas one group used the first session to establish topics for the entire quarter. Having done this, however, the group abandoned their own schedule and essentially followed an open format. Each group invited specific clinic staff members to attend, usually an individual with whom they felt comfortable. Ambivalence was expressed by each group with regard to inviting faculty to participate. Without a clear invitation extended, no faculty attended. Both students and faculty expressed concern that candid conversation might be inhibited if they were to meet together in this type of setting. Whether the presence of faculty would or would not inhibit open discussion is not discernible. It is notable that confidentiality was an issue in only one group.

Evaluation of the groups took place in several ways. The last meeting of each group was used to review the experience. In a separate meeting, the clinic staff who had participated discussed their own assessment of the effort. Among the students, three of the groups expressed very positive feelings about the discussions. They suggested that such group meetings would be effective during the spring quarter of the junior year, a time when the students are first exposed to the clinical setting and treatment of patients. One group expressed ambivalent feelings on the value of their time invested, citing a busy schedule and the lack of group cohesiveness. The affirmative feedback focused on the opportunity not only to continue subjects touched upon in the classroom, but also to discuss formally issues raised in the clinical experiences. From this perspective, representatives from the clinical staff who participated in each group were of invaluable assistance.

Clinic staff members indicated several positive reactions from having participated in the groups. Some of the issues discussed were of current interest to them and gave them the opportunity to share personal feelings and arrive at more adequate positions. Further, and perhaps of greatest significance, was the fact that the informal and relaxed atmosphere during the group discussions enhanced the supervisory relationship between the clinic staff and the students which resulted in improved work while students were in the clinic setting. The students seemed less anxious about learning and a more effective colleague relationship between clinic staff and students emerged. Although the correlation is uncertain, the faculty reported that, for the first time, student evaluations of the curriculum did not include negative comments about opportunities to explore emotional issues in health care. The use of group discussions for physical therapy students was deemed valuable and the wish was expressed that they be continued.

SELECTED READINGS

1. Bergmann T: Children in the Hospital. New York, International Universities Press, 1965
2. Cramond WA: Psychotherapy of the dying patient. Br Med J 3:389-393, 1970
3. Duff R, Hollingshead A: Sickness and Society. New York, Harper & Row, Publishers, 1968
4. Hamburg DA, Adams JE: A perspective on coping behavior. Arch Gen Psychiatry 17:277-284, 1967
5. Holder AR: The right to refuse necessary treatment. JAMA 221:335-336, 1972
6. Howe LW, Howe MM: Personalizing Education. New York, Hart Publishing Co, Inc, 1975
7. Kinnick BC: Group discussion and group counseling applied to student problem solving. In Dierich RC, Dye HA (eds): Group Procedures: Purposes, Processes, and Outcomes. Atlanta, Houghton Mifflin Co, 1972, pp 29-38
8. Lindemann E: Symptomatology and management of acute grief. Arch Gen Psychiatry 17:141-148, 1944
9. Robinson L: Psychological Aspects of the Care of Hospitalized Patients. Philadelphia, F. A. Davis Co, 1968
10. Simon SB, Howe LW, Kirshenbaum H: Values Clarification. New York, Hart Publishing Co, Inc, 1972
11. Skipper J, Leonard R: Social Interaction and Patient Care. Philadelphia, J. B. Lippincott Co, 1965
12. Smith HL: Ethics and the New Medicine. Nashville, Abingdon Press, 1970
13. Taylor C: In Horizontal Orbit: Hospitals and the Cult of Efficiency. Atlanta, Holt, Rinehart and Winston, 1970

Legal Status of Students in Clinical Education

Legal Status of Students of Health Sciences in Clinical Education

MARGARET L. MOORE, M.S.

▶ *The legal status of students in the health sciences should be well-understood by students, by administrators and faculty of the university which enrolled them, and by supervisors of the affiliated institutions to which they are assigned for the clinical part of their educational program. Three of the areas that need special attention and understanding are liability insurance, workman's compensation insurance, and contracts.* ◀

COLLEGES AND UNIVERSITIES offer many professional curricula which require students to gain educational experience in a realistic setting. The student teacher usually acquires this experience in the classroom of the public school; the student in the health sciences acquires it in a variety of facilities, agencies, and hospitals dealing with health and welfare programs. Each year there is an increase in the number of health-professions students assigned to a variety of clinical settings as a necessary part of their educational program.

The legal status of the student in any of these situations concerns not only the responsible university and faculty, but also the supervisors and the institution with which the college or university is affiliated. The entire issue is especially relevant today, because ours is a legalistic, claims-conscious society. The proficiency and integrity or persons in the health professions are being closely scrutinized by the public, the consumers of their health care. A review of the literature in the area of health and hospitals indicates the rapidly increasing number of court actions in all health-related areas. Since the student is frequently involved in these situations, the problem is compounded.

Because there is not enough information to focus on any one discipline, an attempt is made to study a variety of court cases involving students in the health sciences and thus to identify principles and policies which relate to and can be applied to the physical therapy student.

THE PROBLEM

More than three-fourths of the forty-eight curricula in physical therapy in this country are at the baccalaureate level; therefore, we are concerned primarily with the junior and senior college student. Approximately 20 percent of the group are men and 80 percent are women.

In order to obtain accreditation from the American Medical Association and the American Physical Therapy Association, the physical

Miss Moore is on leave of absence for 1968–1969 from her position as Associate Professor of Physical Therapy and Director of the Division of Physical Therapy, School of Medicine, University of North Carolina. She is currently a trainee of the American Physical Therapy Association and the Social Rehabilitation Services of the U.S. Department of Health, Education, and Welfare at the Graduate School of Arts and Sciences, Duke University, Durham, North Carolina 27706.

therapy curriculum must include clinical education. A minimum of 650 hours is stated as a requirement in the AMA publication *Essentials of a School of Physical Therapy*,[1] but most schools offer the student a greater number of hours. When students of the health professions perform in a clinical setting, they do not hold any form of certification. Rather, they are completing a required part of the educational program, prerequisite to graduation and licensure or state or national registration.

The centers to which students are assigned include institutional programs such as the teaching hospital of the university which offers the curriculum, community hospitals sponsored by local governments, private hospitals, voluntary agency facilities, public health programs in local health departments, public health programs associated with the state board of health, and visiting nurse programs. The student frequently rotates through four to six clinical assignments which may represent governmental, charitable, or private and proprietary institutions. Because students from one school may be placed in institutions in more than one state, the laws of the several states should be considered.

In some of these affiliated institutions, members of the faculty from the parent school are employed for the basic supervision of students; in most placements, however, the student is under the guidance of a chief clinical supervisor, and may be reassigned to a staff physical therapist employed in the facility or agency. (The term "facility" is used in this paper to refer to any type of clinical assignment.)

There is no fixed pattern of time, length, or place for the clinical experience, particularly for the undergraduate physical therapy student working for the baccalaureate degree. These variables have significant bearing on the legal status of the student in clinical education. A similar statement could be made for students in other health disciplines.

THE UNIVERSITY'S ROLE

Although in North Carolina there is state authority for hospitals to have educational activities, there does not appear to be a state statute allowing a university to establish curricula in the health sciences which require clinical education and, therefore, to place students in clinical facilities. Whether these provisions exist in other states was not investigated.

Provisions which allow for construction and operation of public hospitals and provide for training schools for nurses are found in General Statutes 131–19 and 131–23 of the State of North Carolina. Article Twelve of the Hospital Authority's Law, Powers of Authority, implies that hospitals have the authority to offer education benefits to students other than those specifically identified in the foregoing paragraph. Hospitals for the mentally ill are covered under North Carolina General Statutes 122–1.2 and 122–69.1, and include provisions for training.[2]

These seem to be the only state statutes specifically applicable to the authority of the university to place, and the hospitals of the state to accept, students in the health sciences for clinical education.

Further involvement of the university is identified in court cases. In Nickley v. Skemp, the participants in the case were interns and undergraduate student nurses who were judged to be employed by the hospital.[3]

In Christiensen v. Des Moines Still College, an often-quoted case, the suit related to an injury sustained by a patient who had been treated only by a senior student in osteopathy

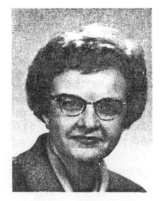

the author _____

Margaret L. Moore has been director of physical therapy at the Medical Center of the University of North Carolina in Chapel Hill for seventeen years, and is also an associate professor of physical therapy. She is currently on a twelve-month leave of absence while enrolled as a full-time student in the Graduate School of Arts and Sciences at Duke University as a trainee of the Social Rehabilitation Services and the American Physical Therapy Association.

Miss Moore is the author of several articles in PHYSICAL THERAPY, including "The Fallacy of Peaceful Change," "Paralysis of the Trapezius Muscle," "The Personnel Shortage: Its Effects on the Qualified Physical Therapist," "A Guide for the Chief Physical Therapist: Organizational Responsibilities," and "There are Challenges in Electrotherapy."

at Still College of Osteopathy and Surgery. A suit was brought for negligence and won by the plaintiff. The court ruled:

> . . . in performing adminstrative or semi-professional tasks assigned to them by authorities at clinic operated by a college, students and interns not yet licensed to practice osteopathy were servants or employees of the college.[4]

In this instance the college was, therefore, held liable for the actions of the employee who was its student. The college was also held responsible for the student, and this responsibility was not referred to the physician who was in charge of the patient. The physician never appeared in the student's treatment area and was not a party to the suit.

Three other cases involved the university's or college's responsibility for their students in the area of clinical education. In Otten v. State in 1949, a student nurse enrolled at the University of Minnesota under the Cadet Nurse Training Act was declared employed by the university and not by Minneapolis General Hospital, to which she was assigned. When she contracted clinical tuberculosis, the university was responsible for her workmen's compensation coverage under the terms of her "employment" at the university. The fact that the university maintained a faculty member to supervise students at the hospital was also a factor in the case.[5]

In Cook v. Buffalo General Hospital, a student nurse enrolled at the Children's Hospital, School of Nursing, was assigned to Buffalo General Hospital for special work. She contracted tuberculosis during her clinical education. She received acute care by her "primary employer," which was her school of nursing, and then workmen's compensation was granted against the "special employer," which was Buffalo General Hospital. The court ruled that it was not inconsistent to have two employers.[6, 8]

The case of Judd v. Sanatorium Commission of Hennepin County (1948) involved the University of Minnesota and a student dietitian who injured her hand during her internship year. In this case, however, the student had completed degree requirements and, to fulfill requirements for certification as a dietitian, she was assigned to the sanatorium, with approval of the university, for her year of directed experience. No faculty member from the university was present in the sanatorium, and the university exercised no control over the student in this assignment. Because her education required the internship,

the court ruled that she was an apprentice dietitian; therefore, she was covered by workmen's compensation insurance. She was declared an employee and an apprentice dietitian in this category since she did receive board, room, and laundry.[7, 8]

Lesnick presents the university's or school's role, stating that the student's application for enrollment, and the university's acceptance, is in the nature of a contract between the student and the institution. In the case of the student nurses and the university, Lesnick states: "The contract of employment is deemed to exist whether or not the student receives monetary payment."[9] When the university maintains full control of the student in clinical education, the university remains responsible.

AFFILIATED INSTITUTIONS

An important aspect of the student's legal status is the place where he gains experience in the application of his professional knowledge and skills. If the institution is immune from suit, the chances are that little action could be

---

66 *It is generally agreed that the physician is liable (1) when the assistant is on salary and employed by him; (2) when the assistant is under his immediate control and supervision; and (3) when his own negligence occurs in the directions given in the performance of a task which results in court action.*99

---

brought against a student except in extreme situations. At one time, both federal and state government hospitals were immune from suit. There also was a time when all charitable institutions were immune. The most vulnerable institution was the private hospital which was not charitable in nature. Many changes have occurred, and continue to occur, in the area of the immunity of hospitals and related agenices. Despite the fact that several courts have declared that they had no right to remove immunity and that only the legislature could do so, many courts have made changes in case interpretations which have had a great effect on liability.

In 1951, the North Carolina General Assembly passed the State Torts Claims Act. By following the procedures set forth in this act, claimants can now seek redress for injuries allegedly suffered at the hands of employees of state hospitals. The act set a limit of $10,-000 for damages in any one case, and followed by a few years the 1946 enactment by Congress of the Federal Torts Claims Act, which waived the sovereign immunity of the federal government for its employees, provided that the employee was acting within the scope of his employment.[2]

The doctrine of sovereign immunity is still maintained by more than half the states, although that number decreases each year. Such immunity is usually extended to the counties

---

66 *The legal status of the student concerns not only the responsible university and faculty but also the supervisors and the institution with which the university is affiliated.* 99

---

and municipalities because they are governmental subdivisions of the state. It should be remembered, however, that

> . . . the cloak of immunity does not extend to the negligent employee's liability as an individual, unless the legislation specifically so provides.[10]

Who would pay for the insurance that would be involved in suits against governmental units? The courts in several instances have stated:

> . . . there is no justification or reason for absolute immunity if the public funds are protected . . . liability insurance, to the extent that it protects the public funds, removes the reason for, and thus immunity to, suit.[11]

At the same time, the charitable hospital,

which is either public or private, has been facing the removal of its immunity status. One of the classic, oft-repeated statements in court cases dealing with immunity comes from the case of Hungerford v. Benevolent Association:

> Negligence law is common law . . . the fact that a rule has been followed for fifty years is not convincing reason why it must be followed for another fifty years if the reason for the law has ceased to exist . . . when courts have recognized the need for remedies for new injuries, the remedies have been found.[12]

Another frequently quoted case involved a community hospital in North Carolina. The court maintained that the doctrine of charitable immunity no longer applies to hospitals; the doctrine applies only to "beneficiaries of the charity." The case involved a nurse, who, in giving a penicillin injection, damaged a radial nerve and caused the patient to become paralyzed. The question was not whether the nurse was negligent, but whether the hospital could be sued for her acts. The case went through two lower courts before reaching the North Carolina Supreme Court. At the Supreme Court hearing, Judge Sharpe wrote the majority opinion, stating that:

> . . . liability for tortious conduct is a general rule; immunity is the exception, and charity is no common law defense to tort . . . there can be little doubt that immunity fosters neglect and breeds irresponsibility while liability promotes care and caution.[13]

At the time of these hearings, thirty states had fully removed immunity from charitable hospitals; other states had partially removed it. Seven who still maintained full immunity were Arkansas, Maine, Maryland, Massachusetts, Missouri, Rhode Island, and South Carolina.

THE STUDENT

Relationship with Clinical Facility

A key question in any possible suit is, Will the student be declared an employee of the facility, a visitor to the facility, or an agent of the facility? Expressing the dilemma which faces hospital administrators and educators, Ligon commented: "The possible negligent acts of the hospital employees are as numerous and varied in nature as to defy classification."[2]

An employee is generally classified as one who is working for wages or salary; his relationship is essentially contractual in nature and is to be determined by the rules governing the establishment of contracts expressed or implied.

The American Physical Therapy Association has studied only briefly the legal status of the student, usually through the Subcommittee on Insurance of its Board of Directors. The minutes of the 1964 meeting of the board contain this statement:

> A legal interpretation has been obtained indicating that unless there is a written statement from the institution or clinical facility to the contrary, it is very possible that the supervising physical therapist could be named in a legal action arising out of the student's negligence. . . . That MacGinnis and Associates (insurance agents) be required to express an opinion as to the value of the supervisors of affiliating students, securing from the institution a statement to be given to the student that he classifies as an employee with or without stipend for the period of his affiliation, so there could be clear determination that his acts would be covered in the sense of the supervisors being covered in the event of such an act by the student.[14]

In October 1965, the subcommittee reported to the Board of Directors:

> The supervisors of hospitals, rehabilitation centers (institutions) where students have affiliations, request that their respective administrators (directors, executive boards, and so forth) let these students understand that while they are there as affiliate students, they are considered as employees of that institution and that there should be a statement relating to the legal responsibility of both the student and the institution . . . the intent here is that the affiliating hospital make some statement to these students which would clarify their particular position in regard to their protection or nonprotection from a legal point of view.[14]

The 1968 publication *Problems in Hospital Law* contains the following statement:

> Hospitals are ordinarily liable for the negligence of all nonprofessional employees, such as orderlies, elevator operators, and student assistants, under respondeat superior.[10]

A more extensive statement appears in the same volume in the section on student nurses. Lesnick and Anderson concur in these opinions.[9]

However, there is disagreement or lack of clarity at the University of North Carolina in Chapel Hill regarding the Attorney General's opinions associated with dental, nursing, and medical students. In 1960, a dental student injured a patient in the public dental clinic. No suit was brought, but the incident raised ques-

66 *Ours is a legalistic, claims-conscious society. The proficiency and integrity of persons in the health professions are being closely scrutinized by the public, the consumers of their health care.* 99

tions, and an opinion was requested from the Attorney General. He stated only that the dental student is not an employee of the university, a statement which was not entirely satisfactory and comforting to the School of Dentistry faculty. Subsequent correspondence in 1961 repeated this opinion but reminded the institution that a student was liable for his own acts of negligence.[15]

In reply to a subsequent request for guidance on student nurses, the university's assistant business manager advised the administrator of the North Carolina Memorial Hospital that student nurses and physicians could not be considered employees but might be called "agents," and that the hospital probably would not be held liable for their acts anyway. In the same letter, however, he did recommend that nurses carry personal liability insurance.[15] In previous correspondence between the School of Dentistry and the university, permission was granted to purchase liability insurance for dental students from funds collected for dental care, as long as the insurance was not paid for from out-of-state funds.

Many cases in the literature deal with the treatment of a patient by a student without the patient's consent. One of the most frequently quoted is Inderbitzen v. Lane Hospital, in which the hospital was found liable because a patient was frequently examined by medical students against her wishes, and in spite of her protests.[16]

In a 1941 case in Georgia, a student nurse was found to be improperly trained and inexperienced in applying an electric pad to the patient. The court ruled that the employee was incompetent, incapable, and careless. Although the hospital maintained that the physician was responsible for the prescribed treatment, the courts found the hospital liable for the acts of the student nurse.[17]

In 1959, in Memorial Hospital v. Oakes, an

accident resulted in the death of a patient who had been in an oxygen tent. Although the suit was brought against the hospital, a student nurse who had been involved in his care was mentioned frequently in the case. The plaintiff claimed that the hospital had been negligent in the selection and retention of its employees, and classified the student nurse as an employee. The hospital was classified as a charitable institution and had to show to the courts that it selected its employees wisely. The court reviewed the instructions the patient had received on the dangers of the oxygen tent. The hospital was found not liable for the patient's death, but the question of the student's place as a negligent employee was a major aspect of the case.[18]

The case of Bakal v. University Heights Sanatorium involved a student nurse working under the direction of a physician in applying equipment needed for electrocautery. The patient brought suit against the hospital, and the courts found that the nurse in this instance was not employed by the hospital, but was, in fact, employed and working under the direction of the physician; therefore, the hospital was not liable for her acts. Had the suit been brought against the physician, the case might have had a different ending.[19]

In 1956, a medical technologist with only six weeks of training was involved in a laboratory error which resulted in harm to the patient.[20] The court pointed out that the technologist was an employee of the hospital and not, as the institution attempted to maintain, an independent practitioner. The court called attention to the brief length of her training and questioned her adequacy for performance. Although this case did not involve a student, the technologist's level of education and training should lead to thoughtful consideration of the liability of students who have had little experience and training before they are assigned to a clinical situation.

Relationship with Supervisors

The following quotation comes from the report of the Subcommittee on Insurance of the APTA Board of Directors and appears in the minutes of the board of July 1964:

A legal interpretation has been obtained indicating that unless there is a written statement from the institution or clinical facility to the contrary, it is very possible that the supervising physical therapist could be named in a legal action arising out of the student's negligence. This subcommittee considers this a hazy area which should be clarified.[14]

66The patient has the right to expect the same level of care on an individual task performed by a student as he would receive from a professional person in the same locale.99

Ligon points out that a negligent employee is always personally liable for his own negligence without regard to the type of hospital which employs him.[2]

Problems in Hospital Law goes into some explanation of the role of the student, the supervisor, and the institution:

The supervisor is liable only for her own negligence in carrying out her supervisory duties. If she assigns a task to an individual who is incompetent to perform it, or if her instructions are inadequate or her supervision insufficient for the circumstances, she may be found liable.[10]

Hershey states:

No state extends freedom from responsibility to someone who is in his late teens and mentally competent and would not effect his liability. A student must be afforded reasonable supervision and guidance by his instructors.[21]

Relationship with Referring Physician

It is generally agreed that the physician is liable (1) when the assistant is on salary and employed by him; (2) when the assistant is under his immediate control and supervision; and (3) when his own negligence occurs in the directions given in the performance of a task to which court action results. Garber and Tyree state:

When the intern has been loaned to a surgeon, and works under his direction, the hospital will not be held liable. This means that the employee is functioning as an agent of the physician and not as an employee of the hospital in this situation, and the physician is then the responsible respondeat superior.[11]

It was for the reason in that statement that the decision in Rath v. Beth El Hospital in 1952 was dismissed by the court. The court held that the intern in this case was working for the physician rather than the hospital and, therefore, the hospital was not found liable for his actions.[22]

In a 1965 case, suit was brought by a family against the physicians responsible for the direction of the blood bank at the local hospital. As a result of incorrectly matched blood, a patient died from reaction to transfusion. The suit alleged that the pathologists were responsible for the death of the patient because of inadequately trained and supervised medical technologists. In this instance the court ruled that the medical technologists were provided by the hospital and employed by it, but only assigned to the laboratory, and that the pathologists did not intimately and personally supervise all activities of duly qualified personnel.[23]

New Academic Arrangements

Opinions differ as to the impact of the new collegiate nursing programs, and perhaps of other health science areas, on the status of the student as an employee. In Lesnick's 1955 publication, the opinion is that programs at the junior college and university level will rule out the student as an employee of the hospital.[9] However, the 1968 publication *Problems in Hospital Law* maintains that hospitals under the doctrine of respondeat supervisor will remain liable for the student assistants.[10] All agree that the student's basic responsibility for his conduct is to himself. As an individual, unless he has a proper defense, he is liable for the payment of damages to anyone he injures through his own negligent conduct. It has been stated frequently that the student's vulnerability for suit for his own negligence exists regardless of the type of institution to which he is assigned.

The patient has the right to expect the same level of care on an individual task performed by a student as he would expect to receive from a professional person in the same locale. The standard of practice to which the student would be held is well stated by Hershey: "A student nurse's conduct would also be measured against that of the professional nurse in a state that has a mandatory licensing act." [21] Or, as it is wisely put in *Problems in Hospital Law:*

> Although it may seem a harsh rule at first, a student is held to the standard of a competent professional nurse in the performance of nursing duties. The courts have indicated in several judicial decisions that anyone who acts as a nurse in performing duties customarily performed by professional nurses is held to the standard of the professional nurse. The patient

has the right to expect the competent performance of nursing services, even if the care is provided by students as part of their clinical experience. From the patient's point of view it would be unfair to deprive him of the opportunity to recover from the injury because the hospital has undertaken to utilize students to provide nursing care to him.[10]

INSURANCE

Liability Insurance

What about the wisdom and availability of liability insurance for the institution, the supervisor, and the student in the clinical setting? What effect does the existence of liability insurance have on court action?

In 1965, at the request of the American Physical Therapy Association, the Council of Physical Therapy School Directors conducted a sur-

---

"All health sciences students, clinical and academic faculty, and professional staff should possess personal liability insurance, regardless of whether the policy is purchased by the individual or by the college, university, or facility."

---

vey on personal liability insurance coverage for school faculty, supervisors, and students when treating patients. Twenty-eight schools of physical therapy participated. Nineteen of them indicated that their students were not covered by personal liability insurance, while eight schools reported that their students were covered. Seven of those eight had coverage which had been secured by the facilities and not by the individuals. Few facilities had anything in writing between the parent institution and the clinical center relative to the student's liability status. The facilities were divided on whether the institution's insurance indirectly covered the student, but thought that the supervisor's liability was covered. Only three institutions indicated that the coverage of the faculty member also covered the student. Seven facilities indicated there was no coverage, and twelve indicated that coverage was variable.

The basic conclusion of the study was that very little liability coverage of students exists, and that even physical therapy educators are not clear about their current status in relation to their students in other facilities and to the supervisors of their students who are in a clinical setting.[24]

Some have claimed that the existence of liability insurance increases susceptibility to suit and increases the possibility of the court's judgment in behalf of the plaintiff, but the courts in several instances have ruled otherwise.[8, 10, 25]

Workmen's Compensation

As long as the student is classified as an employee or beneficiary of the charity, he is eligible for insurance coverage from the institution he is serving in an employed status. This principle is agreed to by Lesnick and Anderson,[9] Judd v. Sanatorium,[7] and Cook v. Buffalo General Hospital.[27] An important aspect which bears repeating is that Cook was a student nurse assigned to a second hospital for part of her education and was ruled by the courts to be an employee of *both* institutions. She could, in fact, have been eligible for workmen's compensation insurance from both institutions at the same time. In the Judd case, the student dietitian was fully assigned to the sanatorium for a year of internship, and was classified as an employee. Workmen's compensation insurance was payable to her for an injury she sustained in a kitchen accident. The level of compensation as ruled in Smith v. St. Mary's Hospital was on the basis of board, lodging, other benefits, and a graduate nurse's salary.

CONTRACTS

In its 1965 session, the Board of Directors of the American Physical Therapy Association and the Council of Physical Therapy School Directors made reference to the desirability of formal contracts between parent college and clinical facility.[14, 24] Few such contracts are currently in effect. The contracts and the legality of such arrangements need further study.

SUMMARY

The health sciences student faces, and should be aware of, a variety of situations with legal implications in the course of his clinical education. The health sciences educator should be aware of the legal situations which the student may encounter in his clinical education. Administrative authorities in universities and colleges should be aware of the legal situations faced by their health sciences students in regard to the clinical part of their education. The professional and administrative staffs of the clinical affiliation centers should clarify for themselves, and for the students involved, the legal status of the assigned student.

The best protection against any tort liability action is the quality of the total educational process—from wise selection and retention of highly qualified students to soundness in education offered and to wise selection and development of clinical affiliation centers and of associated professional staffs.

The health-care facilities with which universities and colleges are affiliated for educational purposes will be increasingly liable for suit as legislative action and court decisions diminish both governmental and charitable immunity.

The health science student may well be classified as an employee by the affiliating center, even though he may receive no award of monetary value, and as such is the beneficiary of the institution's insurance coverage.

The assignment of a student to a clinical center does not relieve the parent university or school of its responsibility for the student.

The clinical supervisor, faculty member, or referring physician is responsible only for his direct supervisory actions in relation to the health sciences student. Also, each individual student, staff, or faculty member is ultimately responsible for his own negligent action.

The health sciences student is held to the standard of the competent professional in the specialty in the performance of his duties.

There may be a need to develop well-structured contracts between the parent school or university and each affiliating facility. All health sciences students, clinical and academic faculty, and professional staff should possess personal liability insurance, regardless of whether the policy is purchased by the individual or by the college, university, or facility.

REFERENCES

1. Council on Medical Education of the American Medical Association. Essentials of a School of Physical Therapy. Chicago: American Medical Association, 1955.

2. Ligon, Roddy M., Jr. Law and Government: North Carolina Hospital Law. Chapel Hill: Institute of Government, 1964.
3. Nickley v. Skemp, 239 N.W. 426 (1931).
4. Christiensen v. Des Moines Still College, 82 N.W. (2d) 741 (1957).
5. Otten v. State, 40 N.W. (2d) 81 (1949).
6. Cook v. Buffalo General Hospital, 308 N.Y. 480, 127 N.E. (2d) 66 (1955).
7. Judd v. Sanatorium Commission of Hennepin County, 227 Minn. 303, 35 N.W. (2d) 430 (1948).
8. Hayt, Emanuel, Lillian Hayt, August Groeschel, and Dorothy McMillan. Law of Hospital and Nurse. New York: Hospital Textbook Co., 1958.
9. Lesnick, Milton Jack, and Bernice E. Anderson. Nursing Practice and the Law, 2d Ed. Philadelphia: J. B. Lippincott Co., 1955.
10. Health Law Center. Problems in Hospital Law. Pittsburgh: The Aspen Corporation, 1968.
11. Garber, Lee O., ed. Law and the School Business Manager. Danville, Illinois: The Interstate Printers & Publishers, Inc., 1957.
12. Hungerford v. Benevolent Association, 235 Ore. 412, 584 P. (2d) 1009 (1963).
13. Rabon v. Hospital, 26 N.C. 1 (1966).
14. American Physical Therapy Association. Correspondence, Beth Phillips to Margaret L. Moore, June 19, 1968.
15. University of North Carolina. Correspondence, Attorney General to J. A. Williams, December 20, 1960; J. A. Williams to Attorney General, March 17, 1961; Attorney General to J. A. Williams, May 8, 1961; J. A. Williams to E. B. Crawford, Jr., October 6, 1965.
16. Inderbitzen v. Lane Hospital, 12 P. (2d) 744 (1932).
17. Piedmont Hospital v. Anderson, 16 S.E. (2d) 90 (1941).
18. Memorial Hospital v. Oakes, 108 S.E. (2d) 388 (1959).
19. Bakal v. University Heights Sanatorium, 101 N.Y.S. (2d) 385 (1950).
20. Berg v. New York Society, 154 N.Y.S. (2d) 455 (1956).
21. Hershey, Nathan. Student, instructor, and liability. Amer. J. Nurs., 65:122–123, March 1965.
22. Rath v. Beth El Hospital, 110 N.Y.S. (2d) 583 (1952).
23. Davis v. Wilson, 265 N.C. 139, 143 S.E. (2d) 107 (1965).
24. Council of Physical Therapy School Directors. Survey Regarding Liability Insurance Coverage, June 1965. (Mimeographed.)
25. Herndon v. Massey, 217 N.C. 610, 8 S.E. (2d) 914 (1940).
26. Bernstein v. Beth Israel Hospital, 104 N.E. 694 (1923), 236 N.Y. 268.
27. Smith v. St. Mary's Hospital, 259 N.Y.S. (2d) 373 (1965).

Methods of Student/Clinical Site Placement

Computer-Assisted Student Clinical Placements

Jancis K Dennis, MAppSci, PT
Bella J May, EdD, PT

ABSTRACT: *Student clinical placement is a time-consuming process that can be enhanced by computerization. A computer-assisted allocation process using optical scanning device scoring forms for gathering of student data and SmartWare® data bases for hospital information has been effective in reducing faculty time in assigning students to clinics. A statistical analysis software program has been adapted for developing data displays depicting student demographic information and student requests for clinical placement by clinical education course and facility. The printout of a facility data base depicts available slots of placement, and students are placed through the application of an algorithm based on decision rules identified by the academic coordinators of clinical education. The development of the process is described in some detail, and its advantages and limitations are briefly discussed.*

INTRODUCTION

Academic coordinators of clinical education (ACCEs) spend considerable time on administrative tasks such as determining available clinical sites and allocating students. Many ACCEs have expressed dissatisfaction with their work load and with the administrative efficiency of their specific role.[1] Van Swearingen[2] suggested that such administrative tasks do not demand the professional skills of an ACCE.

As ACCEs in the Department of Physical Therapy at the Medical College of Georgia (MCG), we are responsible for student placement in an entry-level physical therapy program, a physical therapist assistant program, and a small graduate program. Greater numbers of students, proposed increases in student clinical hours, as well as placement emergencies created by staff shortages have increased our administrative work load. As-

Ms Dennis is Assistant Professor and Academic Coordinator of Clinical Education, Department of Physical Therapy, Medical College of Georgia, 1120 15th St, Augusta, GA 30912. Dr May is Professor and Academic Coordinator of Clinical Education, Department of Physical Therapy, Medical College of Georgia.

signing students to clinical facilities is one of the time-consuming administrative tasks that is also duplicative when facilities, faced with sudden and critical staff shortages, cancel assignments.

There are few reports of methods designed to improve the placement process, although the problem has been discussed by ACCEs.[3–6] Carey and associates[3] discussed the use of a computer program to assign students for patient evaluations in one academic course; the authors did not present the specific algorithm but suggested that computers could be used for a broad range of administrative activities. Van Swearingen[2] most recently described a sorting system and the use of an algorithm based on reading student records from 1 through n to improve the efficiency of clinical placement and student placement match. The manually applied algorithm was designed for eventual computer use.

To reduce our administrative work load, we are developing a fully computerized information management system that will maintain both facility and student data bases for use in the ongoing administration of the clinical education program. One component of the final system is a computerized clinical placement program that will compare information in the student and facility data bases to assign students to facilities. We began by clarifying our decision rules and stipulating the algorithm that guides our decision making. To be effective, a fully computerized program must be based on the decision rules used by humans to achieve the same task.[7]

Clinical assignment is an interactive process between student and ACCE. The experienced ACCE has a highly structured knowledge base about clinical facilities, center coordinators of clinical education (CCCEs), clinical instructors (CIs), and the students; students have their own criteria that affect their requests for placement. The manual allocation process, although slow and awkward, does utilize the ACCE's experience and considers special student needs. We value retaining the individualized approach but recognize the need for greater efficiency. Therefore, to streamline the current assignment process and to prepare for the final

program, we decided on an interim step of computer-assisted assignment using Opscan* optical scanner scoring forms and a small computer program that presents us with ordered data for our consideration. The steps we followed were as follows:
1. Identification of our decision process.
2. Identification of the data needed to facilitate the decision process.
3. Collection and display of the data.
4. Implementation of the procedure.
5. Evaluation and revision of the procedures.
6. Computerization.

THE DECISION PROCESS
Background

Clinical placement at MCG involves three full-time periods of clinical education (a one-week, a four-week, and a six-week) for the physical therapist assistant program and six full-time periods (three one-week, a four-week, and two six-week) for the entry-level physical therapy program. Graduate students are placed individually. Clinical education is integrated throughout the curriculum.

Placement Criteria

We developed a list of the criteria we believe affected our placement decisions and asked students to rank the factors they considered important. We also gave them an opportunity to add other items. The list that evolved is presented without concern for priority:
- the student's preference;
- the student's concerns for housing and other costs;
- facility accessibility (eg, does the student have a car?);
- the student's other clinical experiences and need for a balanced experience (eg, a student should go out of Augusta for at least one long-term clinical course; a student should have at least one inpatient experience);
- the student's interest in a specialty area;
- the student's stated preferred supervisory style;

*National Computer Systems, 1100 Prairie Lakes Dr, Minneapolis, MN 55440.

- the student's preferred method of obtaining feedback;
- the student's previous experiences in the particular clinic, either through work or volunteer time;
- the facility requirements for student type (eg, "please do not send us students who are not self-reliant");
- the availability of the right type of experience at the facility at the time it was needed (eg, was the rehabilitation section open when students needed rehabilitation experiences? Were physical therapist assistants employed in the clinic to serve as a role model for physical therapist assistant students?);
- the "quality" of the educational program of the facility as determined by the ACCE (to date, we have made no attempt to quantify our quality ratings).

Table 1

Excerpt from Student Profile Matrix: Prior Experience[a]

Student Number	Facility Number								
	11	12	13	14	15	16	17	18	19
std 1	1	-	-	-	2	-	-	-	-
std 2	-	-	-	-	-	-	-	-	-
std 3	-	-	-	-	-	-	-	-	-
std 4	-	-	-	-	-	-	-	-	-
std 5	-	-	-	-	-	-	-	-	2
std 6	-	2	-	-	-	-	-	-	-
std 7	-	-	-	-	-	1	-	-	-
std 8	-	-	-	-	-	1	-	-	-
std 9	-	-	-	-	-	-	-	-	-
std 10	-	-	-	1	-	-	1	-	-
std 11	-	-	-	-	-	-	-	1	-
std 12	-	-	1	-	-	-	-	-	-

[a] 1 = I have observed at this clinic for at least five days; 2 = I have been employed at this clinic. This table indicates, for example, that Student 1 has observed at facility 11 and has worked at facility 15.

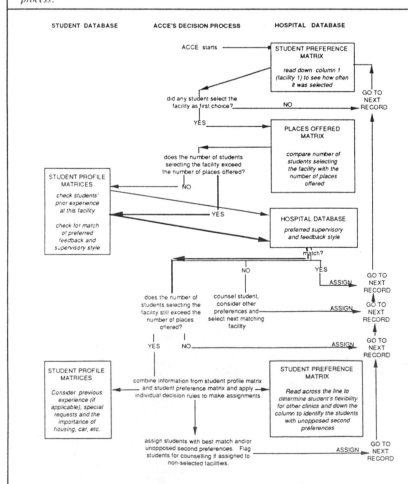

Figure

Decision algorithm showing the decision process and the data displays used to facilitate the process.

The Algorithm

As we started to write our actual decision process, we realized that some rules were constant and immutable (eg, each student must have a neurological rehabilitation experience) while others were multifaceted and interdependent (eg, Jane has limited her listings because of financial considerations; she would have a good experience at facility X, which is the first choice of Betty, who has school-aged children and can only go out of town in the summer). We decided that we had a two-part decision process: 1) a systematic routine that we followed to assign students in the absence of conflict, and 2) a set of complex decision rules applied under conditions of conflict. The complex rules are almost individual because of their multivariate nature. For a computer-assisted decision process, we needed to separate the complex individual tasks from the routine tasks and obtain data displays that would assist with the routine tasks. The complex tasks we would continue to do on an as-needed basis until a computer system utilizing these rules was fully developed.

DATA NEEDED FOR THE DECISION PROCESS

When we wrote the algorithm we realized that specific data displays would facilitate our allocation task. We identified three categories of data: 1) hospital data, 2) student data, and 3) a selection matrix showing student preferences for each hospital. We could access the hospital data from our own information system stored in SmartWare®

data bases[†], but the student data (choices, past experiences, and factors important in their choices) were only available as individual student records. It was at this point that we decided students would enter their data on Opscan sheets and the Division of Research Computing, using the SPSS X2™ program[‡], could generate reports in the desired format.

Our basic decision algorithm is shown in the Figure. We appreciate that each educational program may have different decision criteria and processes, and have included our algorithm as illustrative, not necessarily as a tested protocol for universal adoption. The factors that enter into the complex decision rules discussed above are shown in italics.

Facsimilies of the three displays we receive are presented in the Tables as described below:

1. A student-by-hospital matrix indicating students' prior experience at the facility (Tab. 1).
2. A student profile indicating the importance of different factors in placement selection, supervisory and feedback style preferences, and availability of a car (Tab. 2). We refer to these two tables as Student Profile Matrices 1 and 2, respectively.
3. A student-by-hospital matrix indicating student ranking for each facility (Tab. 3). We refer to this as the Student Preference Matrix.

[†]Innovative Software Inc, PO Box 15998, Lenexa, KS 66215.

[‡]SPSSX™ Inc, 444 N Michigan Ave, Chicago, IL 60611.

Table 2
Excerpt from Student Profile Matrix: Preferred Modes of Supervision and Feedback and Importance of Different Factors in Selection of Facility

Student Number	Student Data[a]										
	Car	F/B	Sup 1	Sup 2	Chal	AGS ngt	AGS w/e	Hme	ACC	Meals	Drive
std 1	0	2	2	2	2	4	5	3	5	5	5
std 2	0	3	3	1	1	0	0	2	5	5	5
std 3	0	1	3	2	1	0	0	0	3	2	0
std 4	0	3	3	3	2	0	0	0	3	3	0
std 5	0	2	3	2	1	1	2	0	4	3	5
std 6	0	2	2	2	1	1	3	4	5	5	4
std 7	0	1	2	2	2	0	1	5	3	2	4
std 34	0	2	3	2	1	0	0	5	5	5	5
std 35	0	2	2	2	1	3	5	3	4	4	4
std 36	0	3	3	1	1	2	1	5	3	0	4
std 37	0	0	1	1	1	0	0	5	2	0	5
std 38	0	3	4	4	1	0	0	5	5	5	5
std 39	0	3	3	2	1	2	1	5	3	0	4
std 40	0	3	2	2	1	4	0	5	3	0	0

[a]For Key, see appropriate sections of Appendix—Form for the Selection of Clinical Affiliation Sites—Student Information: Car = IIA; F/B = IIB; Sup 1 = IIC; Sup 2 = IID; Chal = IIE; AGS ngt = IIF; AGS w/e = IIG; Hme = IIH; ACC = IIi; Meals = IIJ; Drive = IIK.

Our SmartWare® data bases provide us with a list of available places for each clinical facility by each clinical education period and a profile of each facility indicating the experiences offered and the supervisory and feedback policies.

COLLECTION AND DISPLAY OF DATA
Data Collection

The Appendix depicts the form we use to collect data from the students. Subtest 1 requests information on the student's past experiences with a particular clinic because we prefer to assign students to facilities that are new to them. However, with growing student numbers and an increasing number of multifaceted clinical sites, we may well assign a student to the same facility for a one-week and a six-week period.

Initially we requested information on students' financial and special needs as well as interest in specialty placements. Checking each student's listing prior to assignment was cumbersome and time consuming. We believe that students share in the responsibility for their education and that clinical placements are most effective if they can be a joint rather than a one-sided decision. We therefore instructed students to include housing, costs, and specialty interests in determining their preferences for clinical sites. We continue to gather information on the importance of location as well as supervisory and feedback preferences but use it only to assist in complex situations.

In Subtest II, students list their first and second choices for each period of clinical education and select other clinics they are willing to attend (Appendix). This gives us a large repository of options for use if too many students want the same facility. Compliance is encouraged by stating (and building into the computer program) that incorrectly completed forms are rejected by the computer and are not considered until all other students have been placed.

Depending on the number of clinics available for the sequence of affiliations, it may

Table 3
Excerpt from Student Preference Matrix[a,b]

Student Number	Facility Number									
	65	66	67	68	69	70	71	72	73	74
std 1	-	-	-	4	7	9	2	-	-	-
std 2	9	9	9	9	9	9	9	9	9	9
std 3	-	-	-	-	-	-	-	-	-	-
std 4	-	-	-	2	-	-	-	-	-	-
std 5	-	-	-	-	-	-	-	-	-	-
std 6	9	9	9	1	9	9	3	9	9	9
std 35	-	-	-	-	-	-	9	-	-	9
std 36	-	-	-	-	-	-	8	-	-	-
std 37	-	-	-	-	-	-	-	-	-	-
std 38	-	-	-	-	-	-	-	8	-	-
std 39	-	-	-	-	-	-	6	-	-	-
std 40	-	-	1	-	-	3	-	-	4	-

[a]Key: 1 = This is my first choice for a one-week; 2 = This is my second choice for a one-week; 3 = This is my third choice for a one-week; 4 = This is my fourth choice for a one-week; 5 = This is my fifth choice for a one-week; 6 = This is my sixth choice for a one-week; 7 = This is my first choice for the four-week; 8 = This is my second choice for the four-week; 9 = I would be prepared to affiliate with this facility.
[b]Note the relative ease in scanning each column for the number of first preference. For example, facilities 67 and 68 each have one unopposed choice.

take one or two 10-item Opscan forms to gather all the information. One form is used for demographic and past experience information and the other for actual clinic preference statements. Each clinic is numbered, and each question on the answer sheet refers to a particular clinic. A numbered list of clinics with available places for each period is posted for the students. A book of information about each clinic is developed and made available to the classes. Each clinic is listed with general information, staff and patient population, available amenities, and the clinic's preferred supervisory and feedback style depicted by statements similar to those on the student's information sheets (Appendix).

Approximately two weeks before the Opscan sheets are due, we meet with the students to review the allocation process and their clinical education manuals. The manuals contain the objectives for each clinical period, the sequence of clinical experiences, the total program calendar, and the evaluation forms used to determine achievement of the objectives. Students are encouraged to clarify the goals of any education period before making selections. We also share some of our basic decision rules (eg, each student must go out of town for at least one full-time rotation) and encourage students to consider them in their selection.

Data Displays

The Subtest I data, prior experience at the facility, is displayed in Student Profile Matrix 1 (Tab. 1). These data are used primarily to check that students have not worked at a facility that we chose for them if they have not been assigned to their first or second choices.

The Student Profile Matrix 2 (Tab. 2) indicates the importance of different factors in their placement selection, their supervisory and feedback style preferences, and whether they have a car. These data are used to ensure a match between the student and the facility and/or to determine selection for students whose first and second preferences are not available.

The Student Preference Matrix (Subtest II data) (Tab. 3) was our primary allocation guide. Beginning with facility 1, we scanned down the column looking for the number 1, which indicated how many students wanted this facility as their first choice and compared the number of requests with the number of places offered by the facility for the particular clinical education course.

IMPLEMENTING THE PROCEDURE

We begin with the Student Preference Matrix, processing each facility to see how

Appendix
Form for the Selection of Clinical Affiliation Sites

Department of Physical Therapy
Medical College of Georgia

This form will be used to assign you to three 1-week and one 4-week clinical affiliations. All clinics have been listed by number and appear on the set of papers posted on the bulletin board. Availability for either a 1-week block or the 4-week block are indicated by the number under the clinical period. The number refers to the number of students that can be accommodated during that period.

Your task is to select six facilities for possible 1-week assignments and two facilities for possible 4-week assignment. Keep the objectives of these affiliations in mind and try to select a variety of inpatient and outpatient general facilities. Duplicating selection will not necessarily increase the likelihood of being assigned to that facility. In allocating you to a place, we will determine the time of the affiliation, depending obviously on availability but also on demand. To the extent possible, we will try to assign you to a facility of your choice but may need to assign you to another facility depending on your educational needs, availability, and demand. This increases the importance of your ranking each facility in Subtest I.

Please complete the Opscan sheets as indicated. Part of the allocation task will be done by computer and part by hand, so it is important that the Opscan form be completed accurately. Mistakes on the Opscan sheet will lead the computer to "throw out" your answer sheet, and you will be manually assigned to available places after all other assignments have been completed.

The first set of questions and Subtest I are to be answered on the first Opscan sheet; mark this sheet with an "M" under the sex code.

STUDENT INFORMATION

I.   Enter your full name (last name first) as you would for any test.

II. Key in your answers to the following questions beginning in slot A under Identification Number:

A.   I have access to a car.   0 (yes)
     1 (no)

B.   I prefer feedback to be:
- given when I ask or if there are problems   0
- somewhere between 1 and 3   1
- negotiated with the CI   2
- somewhere between 3 and 5   3
- daily written feedback with logs and charts   4

C.   In the early clinics, I prefer supervision to be:
- very loose, direct supervision only when asked or when there is a problem   0
- fairly loose, direct supervision when the CI thinks best   1
- negotiated with the CI at the beginning   2
- fairly direct, with the CI in the same general area   3
- direct, with the CI with me most of the time   4

D.   In the 4-week clinic, I prefer supervision to be:
- very loose, direct supervision only when asked or when there is a problem   0
- fairly loose, direct supervision when the CI thinks best   1
- negotiated with the CI at the beginning   2
- fairly direct, with the CI in the same general area   3
- direct, with the CI with me most of the time   4

E.   In the 4-week affiliation, I hope to be:
- really challenged from the beginning   0
- eased in gently and then challenged   1
- allowed to proceed at my own pace   2
- asked for challenge as I feel ready   3

Rank the following items in terms of their importance to your clinical assignment (5 = very important; 0 = does not matter):

F.   I can come back to Augusta every night.
G.   I can come back to Augusta every weekend.
H.   I can live at home.
I.   There are free accommodations available to me.
J.   There are free or inexpensive meals.
K.   I can drive to the facility.

(continued next page)

Appendix
Form for the Selection of Clinical Affiliation Sites
(continued from previous page)

SUBTEST I

Now refer to the facility list. The number against each facility is to be considered as one question. That is, the next question (question 1 on the Opscan), is facility 1 on the sheet.

Answer **Experience in This Clinic** individually for each facility using the following code (eg, if you have affiliated at Hospital "X" for one week you will mark (B) on the Opscan sheet opposite the number for Hospital "X," and if you have never been to Facility "Y," you will leave the item blank).

Experience in this Clinic

A. I have observed at this clinic for at least five days but have not worked as a volunteer, aide, or assistant.

B. I have been employed at this clinic either as an aide or an assistant.

SUBTEST II

Use second Opscan sheet. Enter SEX = F

You are now asked to go back through all the facilities and classify the facility according to its level of appeal to you. We are assuming that you will compute appeal on the basis of the type of experience offered and financial, housing, and other personal considerations. You will not be asked about your housing or finances directly in this questionnaire. **Use the following key to indicate your choices for affiliation. Do not make more than one mark for each facility.**

A. I would be delighted to affiliate with this facility, and it is my first choice for a one-week period.

B. I would be delighted to affiliate with this facility, and it is my second choice for a one-week period.

C. I would be delighted to affiliate with this facility, and it is my third choice for a one-week period.

D. I would be delighted to affiliate with this facility, and it is my fourth choice for a one-week period.

E. I would be delighted to affiliate with this facility, and it is my fifth choice for a one-week period.

F. I would be delighted to affiliate with this facility, and it is my sixth choice for a one-week period.

G. I would be delighted to affiliate with this facility, and it is my first choice for my four-week general.

H. I would be delighted to affiliate with this facility, and it is my second choice for my four-week general.

I. I would be prepared to affiliate with this facility.

J. I would be delighted to go to this facility for a one-week and my four-week affiliation.

If the facility is out of the question for you, leave it blank.

---

many students designated that clinic as first preference. If no student selected a facility as first preference, we move on to the next facility. If the number of students selecting a facility does not exceed the number of places offered, assignment is made once we have checked the student profile for a reasonable match. Here we apply complex and individual decision criteria. If there is a mismatch, we may assign temporarily and counsel the student, or assign the student to the next highest available and matching preference.

Generally we expect to assign about 75% of the class based on first choices. In the remaining 25% of cases, the conflict is resolved in one of the following ways:

1. Enough of the students' second preferences may be available to resolve the conflict easily.

2. Students have indicated second preferences in already highly contended facilities but have indicated enough options to allow us to be flexible in our assignment.

3. The conflict is irresolute because the second preferences are highly contended and none of the students has indicated a willingness to be assigned to an appropriate facility.

Regardless of the problem, we use the same decision rules to make assignments. We choose to allocate first or second preferences on the basis of perceived "sameness" of the experience to the students involved. We compare the student's second preferences and "willing to affiliate" selections with the availability list and then match data seeking what we perceive to be the fairest decision.

As we proceed with the assignment process, we develop a list of hospitals that we consider offer high-quality clinical experiences but that have not been selected as first or second preference by any student. Students indicating a willingness are assigned to one of those facilities using the match criteria described above.

In the case of irresolute conflict, we generally counsel the student(s) involved, suggesting alternatives from our list, but this problem arises in a very small percentage of cases.

If the placement task involves multiple clinical placements (eg, three 1-week assignments plus one long-term assignment or two long-term assignments), we work sequentially, handling only one clinical education course at a time. Students who are not assigned their first preference in one period are "flagged" for assignment to their first choices in the next period.

PROCEDURE EVALUATION AND REVISION

We tested the algorithm by comparing the placements with similar placements done manually and with a self-allocation completed by the students using the same algorithm. We also compared student satisfaction with the Opscan placements, the manual placements, and the self-select placements. Under the self-select system, we placed a list of all available clinical sites on the bulletin board and had the students sign up for the site they wanted for each clinical education course. Students were told they could only sign up for the number of available places and had to resolve conflicts between themselves. That is, if more students wanted one facility than the facility had available space, the students had to decide who would get the spots. We asked for a finished list with all students placed. Some students were unable to negotiate a compromise and came to us seeking assistance. We suggested ways of compromising but left the final decisions to the students.

The major difference between the manual and Opscan allocation system was time. The manual system took approximately 35 hours, and the Opscan system took about 15 hours of faculty time including discussion with individual students. Students reported about equal satisfaction with the results of the two systems.

The self-select system took no more than about 6 hours of faculty time; however, students expressed considerable dissatisfaction with the system, and the results were not always desirable from an educational point of view. Students had difficulty resolving conflicts and did not always find their classmates as willing to compromise as desired. In some instances students did not give themselves a balanced series of clinical experiences, selecting all outpatient orthopedic facilities or all small inpatient centers.

DISCUSSION

The Opscan system of student placement seems to be an effective bridge between manual allocation and a completely computerized system. While we are still working on the development of a completely computerized match system, we are using the Opscan system with greater efficiency and effectiveness. Students are satisfied with the system because it allows their input but leaves the conflict resolution to the faculty. Once complete, assignments are posted and students are given one week to request any change. After that, clinics are notified of the placement and no further changes can be made except by the clinic or for emergency rea-

sons. The Opscan system allows for faculty input to ensure that students have balance in their clinical assignments. The system is relatively easy and inexpensive to use and is readily available to all universities and colleges. The major limitations are that it is more cumbersome than a fully computerized system and uses a variety of paper records.

We have used the system now for three different periods of allocation and have more clearly identified the routine as compared with the complex situation. Although the Figure depicts the algorithm as it would be followed by a computer, we are aware that we deviate from the sequence in certain situations where our knowledge of the facility and the student may lead us to suggest other placements than were initially selected. There will always be a need for some personal input into the process. Until the full computer program is developed, however, we have found

that the use of the Opscan system for data displays saves us considerable time while making routine decisions automatic and more complex decisions easier.

REFERENCES

1. Harris MJ, Fogel M, Biacconiere M: Job satisfaction among academic co-ordinators of clinical education. Phys Ther 67:958–963, 1987
2. Van Swearingen JM: Systematic placement of physical therapy students. Phys Ther 67:394–398, 1987
3. Carey JR, Ellingham C, Chen Y: Computer-based solution to a clinical education problem in a physical therapy course. Phys Ther 66:1725–1729, 1986
4. Leadership for Change in Physical Therapy Clinical Education. Alexandria, VA, American Physical Therapy Association, 1986
5. Pivotal Issues in Clinical Education: Present Status/Future Needs. Alexandria, VA, American Physical Therapy Association, 1988
6. Renner JB, Block FE, Craig JW: A scheduling algorithm for medical student clerkships. J Med Ed 63:657–658, 1988
7. Williamson M: Artificial Intelligence for Microcomputers. New York, NY, Brady Communications Co Inc, 1986

Computer-based Solution to a Clinical Education Problem in a Physical Therapy Course

JAMES R. CAREY,
CORINNE ELLINGHAM,
and YIGANG CHEN

This article describes the solution to a logistical problem involving the assignment of multiple clinical experiences to students in an undergraduate physical therapy course. Physical therapy faculty members collaborated with a computer programmer to formulate a computer program that would satisfy the organizational needs imposed by this problem. We suggest that the skills of the physical therapist combined with those of a computer programmer can be used to generate effective, computer-based solutions to many other problems related to the organization of data and to decision making in physical therapy.

Key Words: Computers; Education, physical therapist; Organization and administration; Physical therapy.

Use of computer technology rapidly has become common practice in solving the complicated problems in many professions. Physical therapy education is no exception: Educators have used the computer to provide alternative methods for individualized instruction of students[1,2] as well as to summarize the various clinical experiences of students during full-time clinical practicums.[3] The purpose of this article is to illustrate how a personal computer, in conjunction with a specially constructed program, can be applied to solve a decision-making problem involving the weekly assignment of students to clinics as part of an academic course. We propose that, by gaining a familiarity with the following problem and the corresponding computer-based solution, individuals may become inspired to conceive novel, computer-assisted solutions to their own unique problems. Furthermore, we emphasize that a sound understanding of the operations of a computer, although obviously helpful, is not a prerequisite for creating a satisfying computer-based solution. Individuals, however, should be able to 1) define the overall problem; 2) recruit the appropriate resources, including a computer and programmer; and 3) imaginatively express to the programmer whatever convenience features may be desired to simplify the problem.

PROBLEM

Physical Medicine 5289–Patient Assessment is a course taken by senior physical therapy students at the University of Minnesota in final preparation for their subsequent full-time clinical affiliations. The course is designed to integrate the classroom and the clinic, and the weekly course structure is divided into three parts. The first part of the course involves model evaluations whereby a clinical or academic instructor reviews and demonstrates the proper evaluation procedure for a patient with a particular diagnosis. In the second part, students are assigned a one-hour clinical rotation in one of the area clinics to perform an evaluation of a patient with a known diagnosis. After this examination, students submit a written report of their findings and their proposed treatment plan to the faculty for critiquing. The third part entails a case-study presentation to the class by one or more of the students.

Of these three components, assignment of the students to appropriate clinics is the most important in arranging an optimal learning experience for every student each week. This clinical assignment task proved to be the most difficult, however, because of numerous factors that required consideration in making the weekly decisions. Each individual from the class of 30 students is assigned 10 different clinical rotations over a 10-week academic quarter. The first 8 patient evaluations are performed in pairs with 2 students examining 1 patient; the last 2 evaluations are performed individually. To maximize the learning experience for all individuals, we desired to expose each student to a different diagnosis, clinical site, and student partner in each of their 10 clinical rotations. Therefore, the problem to be solved was to assign a total of 300 clinical rotations to the 30 students over the 10-week period without duplicating the diagnosis, site, or partner for any student.

In previous years, this organizational task was accomplished through painstaking efforts with pencil and paper that were extremely time-consuming. Errors of duplication in the assignments were inevitable and, as the data accumulated in the latter weeks of the quarter, the organizational chart became confusing and unmanageable.

SOLUTION

The solution to this problem was simple given the following resources that were available: 1) an Apple IIe com-

Mr. Carey is Instructor, Program of Physical Therapy, University of Minnesota, PO Box 388 Mayo, 420 Delaware St SE, Minneapolis, MN 55455 (USA).

Ms. Ellingham is Assistant Professor and Academic Coordinator of Clinical Education, Program of Physical Therapy, University of Minnesota.

Mr. Chen is Research Assistant, Department of Physical Medicine and Rehabilitation, University of Minnesota.

This project was supported in part by contributions to the University of Minnesota Foundation–Physical Therapy Program.

This article was submitted August 19, 1985; was with the authors for revision 10 weeks, and was accepted March 3, 1986. Potential Conflict of Interest: 4.

puter* with an 80-column card. 2) a printer interfaced with the computer. and 3) a modest budget with which to contract the services of a computer programmer. The programmer was a research assistant who was enrolled in the University of Minnesota Graduate School with a major in computer sciences. His previous experience afforded him skill in the operation of Apple computers and knowledge of the programming language of BASIC.

The solution process commenced with the course instructors imagining and describing an idealistic filing system to the programmer. The desired model called for a weekly tabulation of the various categories of clinical rotation information for each student. Figure 1 shows an example of such data tabulation for student #1 for the first six weeks of the course. The selected categories of pertinent information were the week number. date. appointed time. clinical site. patient diagnosis. student partner. and whether the student had been assigned to present a case study.

The assignment of clinical rotations to students for a given week was preceded by determining which clinical sites with the desired patient diagnoses were available. At the beginning of each week. area clinics were contacted to identify one or two patients with a specified diagnosis. After obtaining permission from the patients and their physicians. the clinics would respond within one or two days indicating the available patients for that week.

The computer greatly facilitated the subsequent matching of students with the most appropriate clinics by displaying the "individual file" of each student. which conveniently summarized the previous assignments for that individual (Fig. 1). By scanning such a display. we could assess rapidly the remaining needs of the student and eliminate duplication errors as the next assignment was typed into the succeeding line of the file.

In addition to this clear and concise organizational display. we also used the computer to record two clinical rotation assignments for each entry of data. For example. as we typed the clinical rotation for week #7 into the individual file for student #1 (Fig. 2. top diagram). the computer automatically entered the same information into the designated

* Apple Computer. Inc. 20525 Mariani Ave. Cupertino. CA 95014.

```
NAME: JULIE A.              S#: 1
W#  DATE    TIME    SITE            DIAGNOSIS            WITH              P
------------------------------------------------------------------------------
1   1/10    2;00    BETHESDA H      HIP FX              30 DONNA W.
2   1/17    2;00    FAIRVIEW H      LOW BACK PAIN        5 ANNE B.
3   1/24    2;30    U OF MINN H     ARTHRITIS/KNEE      12 DAVID F.          Y
4   1/31    2;00    SISTER KENNY    CVA                 23 DAWN P.
5   2/7     1;30    COURAGE CENTER  SCI                 19 MICHAEL M.
6   2/14    2;00    COMO SCHOOL     PEDS                16 ROBIN K.
7                                                        0
8                                                        0
9                                                        0
10                                                       0
```

Fig. 1. Individual file for student #1 showing categories of clinical rotation information and a summary of the student's clinical assignments through the first six weeks of the course. "With" indicates column for partner's name, and "P" indicates column for yes (Y) for case-study presentation.

```
NAME: JULIE A.              S#: 1
W#  DATE    TIME    SITE            DIAGNOSIS            WITH              P
------------------------------------------------------------------------------
1   1/10    2;00    BETHESDA H      HIP FX              30 DONNA W.
2   1/17    2;00    FAIRVIEW H      LOW BACK PAIN        5 ANNE B.
3   1/24    2;30    U OF MINN H     ARTHRITIS/KNEE      12 DAVID F.          Y
4   1/31    2;00    SISTER KENNY    CVA                 23 DAWN P.
5   2/7     1;30    COURAGE CENTER  SCI                 19 MICHAEL M.
6   2/14    2;00    COMO SCHOOL     PEDS                16 ROBIN K.
7   2/21    2;00    VETERANS H      AMPUTEE             11 JANICE D.
8                                                        0
9                                                        0
10                                                       0
```

```
NAME: JANICE D.             S#: 11
W#  DATE    TIME    SITE            DIAGNOSIS            WITH              P
------------------------------------------------------------------------------
1   1/10    2;00    FAIRVIEW H      NECK PAIN           25 TANYA R.
2   1/17    2;00    U OF MINN H     SHOULDER PAIN       16 ROBIN K.          Y
3   1/24    1;30    CAROLINE CTR    CHI                 27 PETER S.
4   1/31    2;00    HENN MED CTR    PNI                 17 SUSAN M.
5   2/7     2;00    SISTER KENNY    MS                  29 JOSEPH W.
6   2/14    2;00    SHRINERS H      PEDS                18 LINDA M.
7   2/21    2;00    VETERANS H      AMPUTEE              1 JULIE A.
8                                                        0
9                                                        0
10                                                       0
```

Fig. 2. Individual file: (Top) for student #1 after the clinical rotation for week #7 was assigned; (bottom) for student #11 showing the automatic recording of the same week #7 assignment after "11" was typed into the "With" column of student #1's individual file.

partner's (student #11) individual file (Fig. 2. bottom diagram). thus expediting the assignment process considerably. The information for both students also was entered automatically into a "class file." which displayed a composite of the clinical rotation assignments for all students during the specified week. Figure 3 (top diagram) shows the class file after we typed the clinical rotation information for student #1 into week #7.

This process of assigning a clinical rotation to an individual. and concurrently to the corresponding partner. continued until the class list for that particular week was complete. Thus.

only 15 entries were needed to complete the 30 assignments during the weeks when partners were used. Figure 3 (bottom diagram) shows the completed class file for week #7. A printed copy of this list then was posted to inform the students of their assignments.

This simultaneous entry of data into two student files initially presented a problem with the proper selection of a partner. In the assignment of student #1 during week #7, for example. we easily could assign her next clinical site and patient with her previous clinical history displayed. The selection of a partner for student #1. who had not been assigned the same clinical site or diagnosis previously, however, was impossible without checking the proposed partner's individual file for possible duplication. Such verification required frequent alternation between individual files, which was prohibitively confusing and time-consuming.

We resolved this initial difficulty with partner selection by describing the problem to the programmer and suggesting an alert system that would indicate a duplication between the current rotation assignment and a previous assignment of the proposed partner without actually displaying the proposed partner's file. The programmer accomplished this task by programming the computer to search the individual file of the proposed partner automatically when that student's number was entered into the partner category. The computer then would instantaneously identify any matches between the current and former rotation assignments for that proposed partner. In Figure 2 (top diagram), for example, if student #1 had been assigned to evaluate a patient with multiple sclerosis instead of an amputee during week #7, then as soon as student #11 was entered as the proposed partner the computer would sound a "beep," and the cursor would shift to the diagnosis column of student #1's file, indicating that student #11 previously had evaluated such a patient (Fig. 2, bottom diagram). Pressing the "Return" key would move the cursor back to the partner column, and either a different partner could be substituted or the proposed partner could be retained despite the match. Such duplications were permitted occasionally when a student needed additional experience evaluating a certain type of patient.

The computer also was programmed to perform several additional functions that made the entire process of clinical rotation assignment and record keeping organized and efficient. These optional functions were listed as various menu items available for selection at will. One such choice allowed for the inclusion of descriptive comments in a student's individual file (Fig. 4).

The most convenient optional function was the "Help" function, which could search the individual files of all students for a specified diagnosis and indicate those students who had not evaluated a patient with that particular diagnosis. For example, if a patient with

```
FMED 5289 PATIENT ASSESSMENT-WINTER 1985 - CLINICAL ROTATIONS
Week# 7
```

S#	NAME	DATE	TIME	SITE	DIAGNOSIS	WITH P
1	JULIE A.	2/21	2:00	VETERANS H	AMPUTEE	11
2	MARK A.					0
3	KAREN B.					0
4	MARY B.					0
5	ANNE B.					0
6	JESSICA C.					0
7	KRISTA C.					0
8	SUSAN C.					0
9	TASHA D.					0
10	BARBARA D.					0
11	JANICE D.	2/21	2:00	VETERANS H	AMPUTEE	1
12	DAVID F.					0
13	SCOTT H.					0
14	MARGARET H.					0
15	SONYA J.					0
16	ROBIN K.					0
17	SUSAN M.					0
18	LINDA M.					0
19	MICHAEL M.					0
20	MICHELLE N.					0
21	ANN N.					0
22	LORI O.					0
23	DAWN P.					0
24	JOHN P.					0
25	TANYA R.					0
26	MARY S.					0
27	PETER S.					0
28	LAURIE T.					0
29	JOSEPH W.					0
30	DONNA W.					0

```
FMED 5289 PATIENT ASSESSMENT-WINTER 1985 - CLINICAL ROTATIONS
Week# 7
```

S#	NAME	DATE	TIME	SITE	DIAGNOSIS	WITH P	
1	JULIE A.	2/21	2:00	VETERANS H	AMPUTEE	11	
2	MARK A.	2/21	2:00	SISTER KENNY	SCI	25	
3	KAREN B.	2/21	2:00	COURAGE CENTER	PEDS	17	
4	MARY B.	2/21	2:00	METRO MED CTR	CVA	14	
5	ANNE B.	2/21	2:00	VETERANS H	AMPUTEE	29	
6	JESSICA C.	2/21	1:30	UNITED H	CVA	27	
7	KRISTA C.	2/21	1:30	ST JOSEPHS H	CVA	18	
8	SUSAN C.	2/21	2:30	U OF MINN H	ALS	21	Y
9	TASHA D.	2/21	2:00	METHODIST H	PARKINSONS	23	
10	BARBARA D.	2/21	2:00	FAIRVIEW H	MS	20	
11	JANICE D.	2/21	2:00	VETERANS H	AMPUTEE	1	
12	DAVID F.	2/21	2:00	EBENEZER	CVA	19	
13	SCOTT H.	2/21	2:00	COURAGE CENTER	CHI	16	
14	MARGARET H.	2/21	2:00	METRO MED CTR	CVA	4	
15	SONYA J.	2/21	2:00	U OF MINN H	AMPUTEE/CVA	30	
16	ROBIN K.	2/21	2:00	COURAGE CENTER	CHI	13	
17	SUSAN M.	2/21	2:00	COURAGE CENTER	PEDS	3	
18	LINDA M.	2/21	1:30	ST JOSEPHS H	CVA	7	
19	MICHAEL M.	2/21	2:00	EBENEZER	CVA	12	
20	MICHELLE N.	2/21	2:00	FAIRVIEW H	MS	10	
21	ANN N.	2/21	2:30	U OF MINN H	ALS	8	Y
22	LORI O.	2/21	2:00	MIDWAY H	MULTIPLE FX	28	
23	DAWN P.	2/21	2:00	METHODIST H	PARKINSONS	9	
24	JOHN P.	2/21	1:30	GILLETTE H	PEDS/CHI	26	
25	TANYA R.	2/21	2:00	SISTER KENNY	SCI	2	
26	MARY S.	2/21	1:30	GILLETTE H	PEDS/CHI	24	
27	PETER S.	2/21	1:30	UNITED H	CVA	6	
28	LAURIE T.	2/21	2:00	MIDWAY H	MULTIPLE FX	22	
29	JOSEPH W.	2/21	2:00	VETERANS H	AMPUTEE	5	
30	DONNA W.	2/21	2:00	U OF MINN H	AMPUTEE/CVA	15	

Fig. 3. (Top) Class file for week #7 showing the automatic recording of paired clinical rotation assignments after student #1's clinical rotation information was entered; (bottom) completed class file for week #7 after clinical rotations were assigned to the remaining 14 pairs of students.

a spinal cord injury was available for evaluation during a particular week, but the majority of the class already had completed such an evaluation, then the Help function could be activated to screen rapidly the diagnosis category in all individual files for the term "SCI." Those students lacking this term in their file then would be listed as the remaining candidates appropriate for this assignment. The time required for completion of this task was less than two seconds.

We also could use this service to help select the pool of available diagnoses to be assigned during the last weeks of the quarter. For example, we desired that each student complete one pediatric evaluation, but not all of the students could be accommodated by the pediatric clinics during the same week. Therefore, to identify those students remaining to perform such an evaluation and, correspondingly, the number of patients needed to accomplish this objective, a diagnosis search for "PEDS" could be executed.

Similarly, the computer also could identify in one or two seconds which students had not been to a particular clinical site or which students had not participated in a case-study presentation. Such search capability greatly simplified the clinical rotation assignments during the closing, more complicated, weeks of the quarter.

Another optional function listed in the main menu was the search of the clinical site category in all individual files and the subsequent tabulation of the frequency with which each site was visited (Fig. 5). Such documentation was valuable for each school's records and for the records maintained at each clinical site.

```
NAME: MICHELLE N.        50: 20
NO  DATE    TIME    SITE            DIAGNOSIS

1   1/10    2:00    METHODIST H     MULTIPLE FX        6 'TH              P
2   1/17    2:00    GALLERY PT      LOW BACK PAIN     27 PE-----------
3   1/29    4:15    COPLIN PT       HAND INJURY        5 ANNE C.
4   1/31    2:00    U OF MINN H     SCI                9 TASHA A.
5   2/7     1:30    SISTER KENNY    CHI               12 DAVID F.         Y
6   2/14    2:00    COURAGE CENTER  PEDS               4 MARY B.
7   2/21    2:00    FAIRVIEW H      MS                10 BARBARA D.
8   2/28    2:00    EBENEZER        CVA               13 SCOTT H.
9   3/7     1:30    HOOVER SCHOOL   PEDS               0
10                                                     0

* PATIENT CANCELLED APPOINTMENT ON 1/24 - WILL RESCHEDULE EVALUATION FOR 1/29.
* HAD DIFFICULTY WITH PEDIATRIC EVALUATION ON 2/14 - SHOULD REPEAT EVAL.
```

Fig. 4. Individual file for student #20 through the ninth week, showing pertinent comments.

SITE	# OF STUDENTS UP TO DATE	SITE	# OF STUDENTS UP TO DATE
BETHESDA H	9	U OF MINN H	33
CENTER PT	9	UNITED H	12
COURAGE CENTER	16	FAIRVIEW H	14
MULTICARE ASSOC	6	ST ANTH ORTHO	6
GALLERY PT	5	GILLETTE H	4
ST MARYS H	4	COMO SCHOOL	3
ST JOHNS H	6	EBENEZER	6
PARK NICOLLET	8	HOOVER SCHOOL	4
SISTER KENNY	24	COPLIN PT	11
METHODIST H	16	VETERANS H	23
RAMSEY H	8	METRO MED CTR	16
CAROLINE CTR	6	ST JOSEPHS H	10
MIDWAY H	10	HENN MED CTR	8
ST MARYS REHAB	4	SHRINERS H	3
BRIDGEVIEW	5	LAKE RIDGE HC	8
DOWLING SCHOOL	3		

Fig. 5. Clinical sites that were visited during the 10-week period and the total number of students who visited each site.

Limitations

Certain limitations are imposed on the application of personal computers to such organizational tasks. Although speed of operation was not crucial to the solution of our clinical education problem, it could prove to be a deterring factor in a more complicated problem involving multiple calculations.

A more common problem is the available memory space. The basic Apple IIe computer can accommodate a maximum of 64 kilobytes (K) of information where 1 K is equal to 1,024 bytes or typewritten characters. About 22K of the total memory space, however, are designated to the Read Only Memory that executes the basic functions of the computer, such as the disk-operating system, monitor routines, and language interpreter. The remaining 42K of memory space, known as the Random Access Memory, are accessible to the user for special programming and data entry.

The custom-made program for this project and the space reserved for 10 weeks of clinical rotation data for 30 students consumed about 40K of memory space. Thus, only 1K or 2K of memory space are available for further use. If, in the future, additional weeks of clinical rotations are added, the present system must be modified to accommodate the additional data. Such modification would involve purchasing a memory expansion card.

Another limitation to the use of personal computers to solve such organizational tasks is the structuring of files so that all pertinent data can be displayed on the screen without alternating among different sections of the same file. The computer monitor used in this project had a vertical dimension that allowed 24 rows of data to be displayed on the screen. This dimension posed no restriction for individual files that used 10 rows for rotation assignments, 4 rows for comments, and several rows for labeling, spacing, and menu listing. The full class file, however, could not be displayed on one screen because the number of students exceeded the vertical dimension limit. This complication was reduced by programming the computer to scroll upward or downward along the class file by pressing the "U" or "D" key, respectively.

The width dimension of the monitor was expanded from the basic capacity of 40 columns by adding an 80-column card. Despite the addition, the restriction of 80 characters to a line necessitated abbreviation under the site and diagnosis categories so that all categories of an individual file could be viewed simultaneously. Any characters typed into a given category that exceeded the allotted number for that category would be truncated.

Commercial Options

A wide selection of database software packages is available commercially. The advantages of these commercial programs are their immediate availability and their adaptability for solving a variety of fundamental organizational problems. Their disadvantage, however, is their limited capability to execute the specialized functions required for the solutions to more unique problems. For example, the capability to search a proposed partner's file automatically and to identify immediately a rotation duplication, as described earlier, was not available in the commercial database programs.

Cost and Benefits

The cost of developing a computer-based program to meet a department's specific needs depends on the difficulty of the problem and the familiarity of the programmer with the computer. The solution of our logistical problem required a total of 42 hours of the programmer's time and 10 hours for the course instructors to finalize the program. The time required to complete the weekly assignments using the computer-assisted approach was reduced by an average of 40%, compared with the manual method. We project that, because of the savings in faculty time, the cost of developing this program will be

recovered fully during the second academic period of use. In addition to the improved efficiency, the implementation of computer-based problem solving resulted in an improved, professional appearance of the weekly documents and the elimination of duplication errors.

SUMMARY

A computer-based solution to a complicated problem in a physical therapy academic course has been described. Construction of the computer program was achieved by collaboration between the physical therapy faculty, with only minimal knowledge of computers, and a computer programmer, having only minimal knowledge of the problem.

Although this particular solution is directed to one highly specific clinical education problem, we propose that a multitude of unique physical therapy problems exists in education, administration, and clinical practice that can be solved more efficiently and economically through custom-made computer programs than by conventional methods. Such problems might include the assignment of students to affiliation

sites, inspection of voluminous admissions committee data, identification of trends in diagnoses and in modality usage, or the scheduling of patients in a large clinic. The computer possesses numerous capabilities for the development of innovative and effective solutions to such problems. Actualization of this dormant potential can be accomplished readily by uniting the problem-recognition and imaginative skills of the physical therapist with the technical skills of the computer programmer.

Acknowledgments. Grateful appreciation is extended to Mr. John Allison and Mr. Glenn Scudder for their kind assistance in the development of this manuscript.

REFERENCES

1. Williams CS, Chalmers RJ, Salter PM: Microcomputers in physical therapy education. Physiotherapy 68:318–319, 1982
2. Lee EC, Watson DR, Argo JK, et al: A model for competency-based, computer-managed instruction in allied health. J Allied Health 11:106–114, 1982
3. Abdelhak M, Green VL: A quantitative computerized recording method in clinical education: A pilot project. J Allied Health 8:237–246, 1979

Systematic Clinical Placement of Physical Therapy Students

JESSIE M. VAN SWEARINGEN

The focus of this article is a description of a management information system (MIS) designed to handle the task of matching physical therapy students with clinical education facilities in fulfillment of clinical requirements of the physical therapy curriculum. The use of a specialized MIS for the assignment of physical therapy students to clinical sites has resulted in a high degree of suitable placements, pairing students' needs with the resources of clinical sites. Multiple applications of the system to the placement task also have resulted in successful matching. The clinical placement system was designed to facilitate adaptation to an automated system in the future. Applications of the proposed computer-assisted placement system and the advantages of such a system in terms of administration and research in clinical education also are presented.

Key Words: *Computers, Education, Physical therapy.*

Each year, and often several times a year, Academic Coordinators of Clinical Education spend excess amounts of valuable research and teaching time manually solving the puzzle of matching physical therapy students with suitable clinical education facilities in fulfillment of the clinical requirements of the physical therapy education program. The long hours ACCEs spend matching students with clinical sites do not require the physical therapy educational and clinical background or talents the ACCEs may possess in the areas of teaching, research, service, or administration. The matching task primarily requires time and patience.[1]

Management information systems (MISs) handle large volumes of information, store information in an organized manner, allow ready access to the information, permit sorting and recombining of information, and provide a mechanism for easily adding to or correcting the stored information. With the increasing number of physical therapy students and the number and diversity of clinical education facilities currently used by physical therapy programs, an MIS designed to handle the clinical placement task and the storage of clinical site information may provide a tremendous benefit in terms of time and human resource savings. An MIS for clinical placement was developed and subsequently tested by the Program in Physical Therapy at the University of Pittsburgh in coordination with the School of Library and Information Sciences.

The purpose of this article is to describe the algorithm (a set of step-by-step instructions describing how to accomplish a task[2]) developed initially to manage the task of placing physical therapy students in clinical education facilities. I also shall discuss recent adaptations of the manual algorithm for future implementation of the clinical placement MIS with an IBM personal computer.*

BACKGROUND

Currently, the task of matching physical therapy students to suitable placements for the clinical education component of the Program in Physical Therapy at the University of Pittsburgh occurs at least twice a year and involves placing a minimum of 70 students, each in three different clinical sites, for full-time affiliations. Students participate in a four-week, full-time affiliation at the completion of their first year in the program and in two consecutive six-week affiliations in the final term of their second year. The major goal of designing an MIS was placement of students for the full-time affiliations only. Assignments of students for the two part-time affiliations that also occur during the two-year program were not a concern of the original MIS project.

System Components

The MIS design that matches physical therapy students with clinical affiliations involves four basic components: 1) the student record, 2) the clinical site (agency) record, 3) the sorting mechanism, and 4) the matching process.

Student record. The student record includes relevant criteria, generated by each physical therapy student, on which to base the clinical site assignment. After reviewing past student request forms, we found the following criteria to be the most significant in making assignments that were satisfactory for the student: 1) specialty (eg, pediatrics, rehabilitation, sports, general or acute care); 2) geographic location of the site (ie, city or region); 3) car access (ie, availability of transportation); 4) session preference (ie, first or second session in the final full-time affiliations); 5) priority criterion (ie, the criterion

Ms. Van Swearingen is Assistant Professor, Program in Physical Therapy, University of Pittsburgh, 109B Pennsylvania Hall, Pittsburgh, PA 15261 (USA).

This paper was presented at the Sixty-First Annual Conference of the American Physical Therapy Association, New Orleans, LA, June 16–20, 1985.

This article was submitted October 18, 1985; was with the author for revision 19 weeks; and was accepted June 18, 1986. Potential Conflict of Interest: 4.

* International Business Machines Corp, Old Orchard Rd, Armonk, NY 10504.

that must be satisfied: choice of specialty or geographic location); and 6) priority rating, determined by the ACCE based on information provided by students and not represented by the other criteria (ie, individual circumstances).

The priority rating may include such things as dependent children, job commitments, or the involvement of the student in graduate courses. A priority rating also may include current limitations of the clinical education program, such as the available number of sites of a certain specialty and the number of students interested in that type of specialty for the term for which the assignments are being made.

Clinical site (agency) record. This component is complementary to the student record and includes 1) name of the site, 2) geographic location of the site (ie, address or city or region), 3) specialty or specialties offered, 4) car needed or not needed, 5) room and board availability, and 6) number of affiliations available each session. All information for this record can be obtained from the clinical site information requested on the forms of the American Physical Therapy Association's accreditation self-study material (originally forms B, C, and Ca).[3]

Sorting mechanism. The aim of the sorting mechanism is to enhance the "best-fit" concept, that is, matching the greatest number of students with their chosen affiliations without extensive reprocessing of requests. The sorting mechanism is a "decision tree" designed to approach methodically what was originally a trial-and-error process. The sorting mechanism depends on a concept called *ordered processing*. Ordered processing involves processing student requests with the most restrictive criteria combinations first. The criteria combinations are derived from combinations of the first five criteria of the student record. In addition, ordered processing means that students with special needs should be processed early using a priority rating determined by the ACCE.

To illustrate ordered processing, consider the situation of the Physical Therapy Program at the University of Pittsburgh during the academic year 1984–1985. Pediatric requests were the most difficult to satisfy because many physical therapy students were interested in pediatric affiliations, and few clinical pediatric affiliations were available for the winter term of the final full-time affiliations. The second most difficult student request to satisfy was one for a particular geographic location because of the proportionally large number of students requesting affiliations at that location. The sorting mechanism, therefore, resulted in ordered processing with student requests for pediatric affiliations first and specific area requests second.

The sorting mechanism allows 96 possible student requests to be considered through the use of a decision table (Table). The decision table, like decision trees, provides the user with a systematic approach to sorting student requests based on selected criteria of the student request and the current clinical site environment.[4,5] Such decision analysis encourages the user to identify present options and to specify important future factors in the decision scheme.[4] The decision table, therefore, illustrates a systematic, sequential approach to ordering student requests, or ordered processing, for the matching process.

The decision table is used by sorting from left to right across the field such that student requests are sorted initially from the least restrictive criteria and subsequently from progressively more restrictive criteria. The result of sorting in this fashion brings those student requests that are most difficult

TABLE
Sorting Mechanism Decision Table[a]

Car	Area	Session	Priority	Specialty
No	Pgh[b]	yes	yes	peds[c]
Yes	Pgh	yes	yes	peds
No	Pgh, out of Pgh	yes	yes	peds
Yes	Pgh, out of Pgh	yes	yes	peds
No	out of Pgh	yes	yes	peds
Yes	out of Pgh	yes	yes	peds
No	Pgh	no	yes	peds
.	.	.	.	.
.	.	.	.	.
.	.	.	.	.
No	Pgh	yes	no	peds
.	.	.	.	.
No	Pgh	no	no	peds
.	.	.	.	.
.	.	.	.	.
.	.	.	.	.
No	Pgh	yes	yes	sports/ortho[d]
.	.	.	.	.
No	Pgh	yes	yes	rehab[e]
.	.	.	.	.
No	Pgh	yes	yes	gen/acute[f]

[a] Used by Program in Physical Therapy, University of Pittsburgh, winter term, academic year 1984–1985.
[b] Pgh = Pittsburgh.
[c] peds = pediatrics.
[d] sports/ortho = sports medicine and orthopedics.
[e] rehab = rehabilitation.
[f] gen/acute = general-acute care.

to satisfy to the top in the ordered processing. The order of the combinations of criteria illustrated is the template for priority ordering resulting from application of the sort mechanism. Student records sorted this way ensure that the most difficult requests to satisfy are "in line" to be processed first, based on the particular set of conditions directing the ordered processing, such as those described for the winter term.

Matching process. This process involves matching the requests of physical therapy students with a clinical site satisfying the stipulated criteria. The design of this process represents an adaptation of an algorithm derived by Wolfe[6] for scheduling rooms for courses in a university setting. Three aspects of the algorithm are important—the report, the rules, and the handling of unresolved conflicts.

The report portion of the algorithm yields a listing of clinical site affiliations with students assigned in each session. Three basic rules governing the matching process are included in the rules portion of the algorithm. The first rule is that data are ordered for processing. The second rule is that criteria without priority, as indicated by the student, may be relaxed to resolve conflicts. Rule three directs that problems should be referred to the system manager for a solution when no acceptable match between student request and available clinical sites is achieved. Management of unresolved conflicts is

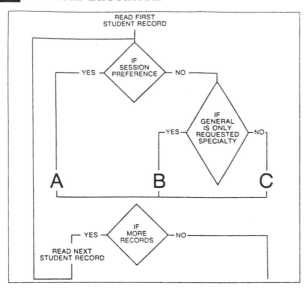

Fig. 1. Processing algorithm: matching process overview. A, B, C refer to routines represented in Figures 2, 3, and 6.

the third aspect of the adapted algorithm. Unresolved conflicts result in the system printing a note acknowledging the conflicts. After such conflicts have been resolved, the process continues.

The most difficult matching task to manage occurs during the term in which the students participate in two consecutive affiliations at two different clinical sites (ie, their final full-time affiliations). Three major types of student requests illustrate this process. Each type requires that a different series of steps of the general matching process should be used. An overview of the matching procedures is presented in Figure 1.

The first procedure involves requests for two general-acute care specialty affiliations and is the simplest request to match. In this type of student request, both affiliations requested are for general-acute care specialty settings. The student lists six site choices, which are checked sequentially until two sites have been assigned (Fig. 2).

Requests with two specialties and no session preference represent the most difficult type of requests to satisfy. The flexibility of being able to match the specialty in either session requires an involved process to check both sessions for the choices, then for the criteria, then with the criteria relaxed, if necessary, to obtain a suitable match. After finding a suitable match for the first affiliation, the second specialty is assigned in the remaining session (Figs. 3–5).

The third type of request involves session preference criteria. Although seemingly a more restrictive routine, the matching process is simpler than the previous routines. Each specialty is processed only once in the requested session (Fig. 6).

DISCUSSION

Implementing the MIS consisted of placing 60 physical therapy students in two consecutive affiliations each. The results were that 88% of the students received two of their six choices for clinical sites and that all placements satisfied a minimum of 80% of each student's criteria for site selection. The process was conducted by a person who was unfamiliar

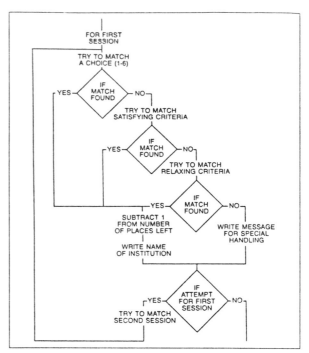

Fig. 2. Routine B: Procedure for managing a student request for two general-acute care specialty affiliations.

with either the students or the clinical sites. Processing time was reduced from 80 hours using the traditional trial-and-error method to 3 hours for both the sorting and matching procedures of the designed algorithm. Similar results have been achieved in three subsequent applications of the manual MIS to the clinical placement task.

Adaptation to the Computer

The manual algorithm is being adapted for use with an IBM personal computer. The advantages of computer-assisted placement over the manual system do not include a large savings of processing time. Modest operator time still will be required to enter student and clinical site data, which must precede the sorting mechanism and matching process. Computer-assisted placement, however, will offer the following advantages:

1. Savings in ACCE time, because the system operator may be a secretary or administrative assistant.

2. A means of recording and storing student and clinical site information with easy access to the data for updating. (This capability is ideal because of the constantly changing nature of clinical site information.)

3. Increased likelihood of ensuring a best-fit match of the student with the clinical assignment requested. (The computer-assisted system is better able to check all possible student-site matches with the maximum number of requested criteria satisfied.)

4. Potential for compiling several types of reports quickly, such as a list of sites with the students assigned or a list of sites without the students assigned. (The list of unused sites can be organized by specialty, by geographic locations, or by sessions the site is available for student affiliates.)

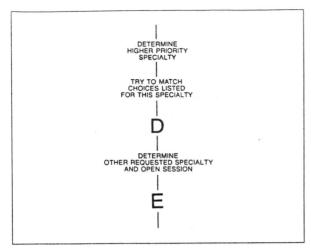

Fig. 3. Routine C: Procedure for managing a student request for two specialty affiliations and no session preference.

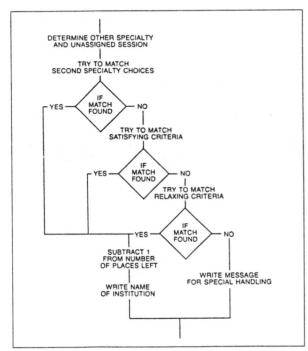

Fig. 4. Routine D: Procedure for matching the priority specialty affiliation.

5. Compilation of a record of information on clinical site usage for future reference. (This information may be useful in recognizing trends in clinical education such as types of affiliations most often requested and yearly alterations in the availability of sites geographically or by specialty.)

CONCLUSION

The application of an MIS to the task of clinical placement of physical therapy students yielded a manual algorithm for matching the students with clinical sites. The MIS has been shown to be valid (ie, the MIS manages the task with a high degree of acceptable placements) and reliable (ie, similar

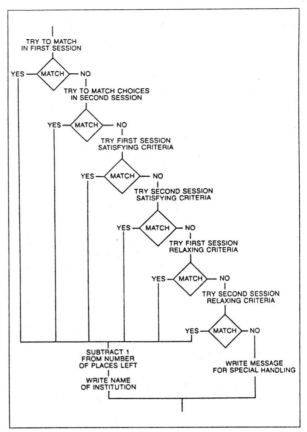

Fig. 5. Routine E: Procedure for matching the second specialty affiliation.

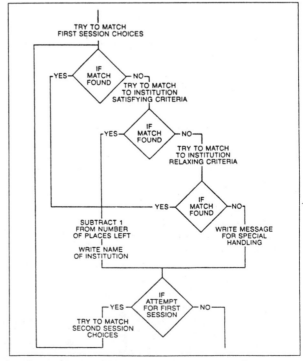

Fig. 6. Routine A: Procedure for managing a student request with session preference criteria.

results were obtained in four separate applications of the system).

The MIS we have designed currently is undergoing adaptations to be compatible with a computer that not only will handle the matching task but also will provide an efficient and useful means of storing, recalling, and updating the vast amount of clinical site data that physical therapy education programs collect.

Acknowledgment. I acknowledge the assistance of Catherine S. Kletterer in the development and design of the MIS.

REFERENCES

1. Moore ML, Perry JF: Clinical Education in Physical Therapy: Present Status/Future Needs. Washington, DC, Section for Education, American Physical Therapy Association, 1976, pp 2–17—2–18, 3–39
2. Reggia JA, Tuhrim S (eds): Computer-Assisted Decision Making. New York, NY, Springer-Verlag New York Inc, 1985, vol 1, pp 264–267
3. Accreditation Handbook. Washington, DC, American Physical Therapy Association, 1979
4. Ford RC, Heaton CP: Principles of Management: A Decision-Making Approach. Reston, VA, Reston Publishing Co Inc, 1980, pp 97–103
5. Patrick EA: Decision Analysis in Medicine. Boca Raton, FL, CRC Press Inc, 1979, pp 40–41
6. Wolfe TE: A Course-Scheduling Algorithm for Mini-computer Systems. Master's Thesis. Pittsburgh, PA, University of Pittsburgh, 1972

Survey of Center Clinical Coordinators: Format of Clinical Education and Preferred Methods of Communication

Nancy Peatman   Ruth Hall

Richard Albro   H Mary Owens

Marilyn DeMont   Jeanne Previty

Meredith Drench   Pamela Roberts

Michael Emery   Neil Schuster

ABSTRACT: The purpose of this study was to identify current clinical education formats and preferred methods of communication between physical therapy education programs and clinical education centers (CECs). Three-hundred seventy-seven questionnaires were analyzed in this study. The majority of center coordinators of clinical education (CCCEs) (78%) would prefer to receive requests for student placements from all academic programs at one time and confirmation of student placements two to three months in advance (63%). Most CCCEs (87%) would be comfortable having academic coordinators of clinical education (ACCEs) share information about the availability of an unfilled student spot at their facility. Fifty-six percent of CCCEs would consider allocating a spot to a program with which they were not currently contracted. On-site visits by ACCEs were considered to be essential when requested (66%), with problem students only (49%), or with changes in the ACCE or CCCE (42%). The results of this study will be useful in planning for change in clinical education (ACCEs) and in guiding cooperative efforts between academic institutions and CECs.

Ms Peatman is ACCE, Department of Physical Therapy, University of Lowell, Lowell, MA 01854. Mr Albro is Assistant Professor, Department of Physical Therapy, Quinnipiac College, Hamden, CT. He was ACCE, Department of Physical Therapy, Quinnipiac College, when this study was conducted. Ms DeMont is Assistant Professor and ACCE, Department of Physical Therapy, Boston University, Boston, MA. Ms Drench is Lecturer, Department of Physical Therapy, Northeastern University, Boston, MA. She was Clinical Assistant Professor and ACCE, Department of Physical Therapy, Northeastern University, when this study was conducted. Mr Emery is Assistant Professor and ACCE, Department of Physical Therapy, University of Vermont, Burlington, VT. Ms Hall is retired after 29 years as a physical therapy educator. She was Associate Professor and ACCE, Department of Physical Therapy, North-

eastern University, Boston, MA, when this study was conducted. Ms Owens is Director of Professional Development, Rehabilitation Associates of Cape Cod, Chatham, MA. She was Assistant Professor and ACCE, Simmons College, Boston, MA, when this study was conducted. Ms Previty is Assistant Professor and Chairperson, Department of Physical Therapy, Springfield College, Springfield, MA. She was ACCE, Department of Physical Therapy, Springfield College, when this study was conducted. Ms Roberts is Associate Professor and Associate Director, Physical Therapy Program, School of Allied Health Professions, University of Connecticut, Storrs, CT. She was ACCE, School of Allied Health Professions, University of Connecticut, when this study was conducted. Mr Schuster is Assistant Professor and ACCE, Division of Physical Therapy, University of New England, Biddeford, ME.

INTRODUCTION

Planning for the future of physical therapy clinical education has received considerable attention in the past few years.[1-6] It has been the focus of task forces,[7,8] national meetings, special-interest groups, and a landmark conference in 1985 entitled "Leadership for Change in Physical Therapy Clinical Education."[9]

All of this attention is warranted. Changes in the health care needs of society and in the health care delivery system have resulted in changes in the practice of physical therapy. Changes in practice and practice environments have influenced physical therapy didactic education and may significantly affect the clinical education process. For this reason, those involved in the preparation of future physical therapists have been forced to reexamine current practices and trends related to clinical education. Clinical education centers (CECs) share this responsibility with academic institutions. In keeping with this premise, changes in policy should not be made unilaterally by the academic institution. Rather, these decisions should be made only after careful consideration of the recommendations, views, and preferences of the CECs. Where possible, the development of regional clinical education consortia would further ensure the spirit of cooperation in effecting change.

Recognizing the need for cooperative efforts, the New England Consortium of Academic Coordinators of Clinical Education (NEC-ACCE) was developed in 1984. It is comprised of the academic coordinators of clinical education (ACCEs) from nine New England entry-level physical therapy programs. In addition to promoting clinical faculty development and developing research efforts in clinical education, one of the primary goals of the consortium is to promote cooperative efforts in the planning and administration of clinical education.

To identify areas in which cooperative efforts could be most effective, the consortium polled all affiliated CECs that were contracted with one or more of the nine New England programs. Of particular interest was feedback on current formats of clinical education, how the center coordinators of clinical education (CCCEs) allot student slots when several academic programs are involved, the preferred methods of communication with the academic institutions, and the perceived need for a common evaluation tool. The results of this survey are described here, followed by a discussion of the implications of these results in planning for clinical education of the future.

METHOD

A master list of CECs was compiled. Each academic institution in the consortium was assigned a number from 1 to 9 for identification purposes. These numbers were used to indicate the use of a CEC by a particular school. School 1 began the process by mailing its CEC list to School 2. School 2 added their ID number to any facility on School 1's list with which they were also contracted. School 2 then attached a list of facilities that were unique to them and mailed the combined list to School 3. ID 3 was added beside any facility also used by School 3. Additional facilities used only by School 3 were listed separately. This expanding working document was then sent to School 4, where the process continued. This process was completed when School 9 mailed the entire package back to School 1 for alphabetization and the final draft. This process took approximately three months by mail. At the time of this study, 520 CECs that had signed contractual agreements with one or more consortium schools were included on the master list.

The master list was subdivided into nine responsibility lists, one for each New England program. Care was taken to ensure that each academic program was "responsible" for CECs with whom they had a contract. Logically, any CEC under contractual agreement to only one institution would appear on that school's responsibility list. Further division of CECs was done equitably and with consideration for geographic location. The purpose of the responsibility list was one of efficiency. That is, it prevented duplicate mailing of consortium-related information by nine different academic programs.

Portions of two day-long meetings were devoted to identifying questions to be included on a survey. This survey would be mailed to all CECs on the master list to gather input from the center coordinators on selected issues. Feedback would be used to guide future consortium activity as well as to assist individual ACCEs in developing clinical education policies. The following primary content areas were determined to be of common interest to members of the consortium.

Sharing Clinical Spots

Consortium members had long been concerned with the ever-present need for more CECs. The availability of sites never seemed to be adequate to meet the needs of the current student population. Last-minute cancellations of guaranteed spots were the rule rather than the exception. Members had informally discussed the possibility of sharing clinical sites, especially in last-minute crisis situations. Input from clinical educators regarding their degree of comfort with this type of policy was desired. In addition, it was important to know whether CCCEs would prefer to be notified by the ACCE who no longer needed the spot. Finally, and of some significance in terms of future planning, it was critical to establish whether CCCEs would consider accepting a student from a school with whom they were not formally affiliated by contract.

Clinical Visitations

Each consortium school had a different policy related to visiting clinical facilities. Some visited each student on each rotation, others visited each facility one time per year, and others visited on request only. Determining when a CCCE found a visit to be essential would be helpful to all programs in terms of future planning, budgeting, and policy changes.

Communication

Members were interested in identifying changes in communication patterns between the academic institutions and the CECs that would or could have some immediate impact. Of specific interest was how far in advance CCCEs needed confirmation of student placement and whether and when they preferred requests for student placements from all academic institutions at one time.

Some members believed it was necessary to revise their current evaluation tools. This need, combined with recent discussion at the national, regional, and local levels related to a common evaluation tool, suggested the final question related to communication: Is a common evaluation tool a priority?

Current Patterns of Clinical Education

Planning for change in clinical education warranted a review of current patterns. Of particular interest were the number of physical therapists eligible to be clinical instructors and the type of facility responding. Information was requested relative to current levels of students educated at a particular facility, the ratio of clinical instructors to students, and how many students could be accommodated in any one month. It was also important to solicit the CCCEs' opinions on perceived "ideal" length of clinical affiliations for each level of student.

Priorities in Allocating Slots

The consortium was interested in identifying which factors were most important in influencing a CCCE's decision to allocate a slot to a particular academic program. Members speculated that academic preparation, duration of contract, format of a curriculum, level of student, geographic location, time of affiliation, length of affiliation, relationship with the ACCE, and recruitment potential might be considered in this decision. Relationship with the ACCE was interpreted to mean a form of loyalty to the individual as opposed to the academic institution. Members of the consortium believed that loyalty could develop as a result of longstanding clinical education associations between the

ACCE and the CCCE or through knowledge of the ACCE through professional meetings or committee work. Relationship could also be defined as a loyalty that developed as a result of friendship with the ACCE.

After the identification of the above-mentioned key areas, a 17-item questionnaire was developed to address these issues. The final draft was a combination of closed- and open-ended questions and included one rank-order item. A cover letter was drafted to explain the purpose of the survey and to encourage a high response rate from the CCCEs.

The questionnaire was mailed by consortium members to each CEC on their responsibility list. Completed documents were returned to the originating institutions, where each questionnaire was coded and entered onto a Fortran coding sheet. Fortran sheets were mailed with the original surveys to the University of Connecticut for data entry and frequency analysis using the Statistical Package for the Social Sciences (SPSS-X).

RESULTS

Of the 520 mailed questionnaires, 377 (75%) were returned and analyzed in this study. The majority of the respondents (54%) were from acute care facilities, followed by rehabilitation centers (19%). Home health, private practice, and nursing home therapists combined accounted for 12% of the responses. The category "other" accounted for 15% of the responses and included pediatric and outpatient facilities.

Senior-year students were the most commonly accepted students by CCCEs (89%). Junior-year students were the next-most favored (70%). When asked what the ideal length of a clinical experience was for each level of student, the most frequent response was 6 weeks for a physical therapist assistant, sophomore-year, junior-year, basic master's I, or doctoral-level student; 8 weeks for a senior-year, basic master's II, or advanced master's student; and 24 weeks for a student on a cooperative (co-op) experience. (The co-op experience is integral to Northeastern University's five-year undergraduate physical therapy curriculum. This program incorporates 12 to 18 months of work experience [co-op] interspersed with academic preparation. Students who are on co-op work as physical therapy aides using skills learned thus far in school. The clinical education component of the curriculum is separate from the co-op experience.) Table 1 lists the three most frequently identified ideal lengths of affiliation for each level of student and also includes the range of responses received for this item.

Table 1
Levels of Students Accepted by 377 Clinical Education Centers and "Ideal" Durations of Affiliation

Level	Number of Centers (%)	Ideal Length of Affiliation		
		Most Common Responses (wk)	Frequency	Range (wk)
PTA[a]	128 (46)	6	74	1–40
		7	23	
		4	23	
Sophomore	78 (21)	6	21	1–11
		4	12	
		1	11	
Junior	265 (70)	6	116	1–10
		4	37	
		7	33	
Senior	336 (89)	8	111	1–60
		6	104	
		7	84	
Co-op[b]	65 (17)	24	17	2–50
		12	14	
		18	4	
Basic Masters I	107 (28)	6	43	1–60
		7	24	
		8	23	
Basic Masters II	109 (29)	8	44	1–12
		6	30	
		7	21	
Advanced Masters	16 (4)	8	4	2–80
		2,6,12	2	
		5,7,80	1	
Doctoral	3 (1)	6	2	6–8
		8	1	

[a] Physical therapist assistant.
[b] Student on a cooperative experience program.

The mean number of staff eligible to be clinical instructors was 4.8. The mean number of students educated in a facility in a typical year was 9.6. The most frequent response (mode), however, was 4. In addition, 374 (94%) of the CCCEs indicated that the ratio of clinical instructors to students was one to one.

The most frequent response (mode) to how many students are in a CEC during any one month was one. The range of responses to this item, however, was from 0 to 12. Clinical coordinators were least able or least willing to accommodate students during July, August, and December. This was reflected by the increased percentage of facilities accepting zero students during these months. Table 2 summarizes the above information and indicates how many of the responding facilities accommodate only one student at a time.

Five items on the questionnaire related specifically to communication and the mechanics of placing students in clinical facilities. The majority of respondents (78%) preferred to receive requests for student placement from all affiliated academic programs at one time. Our data indicate that June and September were the best months for these requests to be received. Clinical coordinators also preferred to receive confirmation of student placement at least two months in advance of the students' arrival. In the event that an academic institution would not be using a slot originally reserved for them, the majority of the respondents (87%) stated they would be either very comfortable or comfortable in allocating that slot to another academic program. They would prefer, however, to be notified that the slot was no longer needed before being approached by another institution. In addition, 56% of the clinical educators stated they would consider allocating the slot to another institution, even if there was no previously existing contract. A summary of these results is shown in Table 3.

There has been considerable regional and national discussion in the past few years about the need for a common evaluation tool. Among the clinical educators surveyed in this study, the responses were evenly divided on this issue. When asked whether a common evaluation tool was a priority, 181 respondents (48%) answered "yes," while 186 respondents (49%) answered "no."

Table 4 describes various factors considered by the clinical coordinators when allocating available slots to academic institutions. The time of the affiliation, level and academic preparation of the student, length of the affiliation, and duration of the contract were ranked first, second, or third by the majority of the respondents. Not as essential were the format of the curriculum, recruitment possibilities, geographic location of the program, and relationship with the ACCE.

Finally, the majority of the respondents considered an on-site visit by the ACCE essential under the following circumstances: 1) when requested (66%); 2) with a change in the ACCE or CCCE (42%); 3) with problem students only (49%); 4) once per year during student placement (33%); 5) at the time of major curriculum change (33%); 6) with each student (31%); and 7) never (.5%).

Table 2
Patterns of Student Acceptance in 377 Clinical Education Centers (CECs)

Month	Mode	Number of Students Accepted Per Month		
		Number of CECs	Range of Responses	No Students Accepted (%)
January	1	182	0–12	13
February	1	186	0–12	12
March	1	181	0–12	13
April	1	189	0–12	13
May	1	194	0–12	10
June	1	163	0–12	24
July	1	139	0–12	35
August	1	130	0–12	40
September	1	174	0–12	21
October	1	185	0–12	18
November	1	182	0–10	18
December	1	158	0–10	31

Table 3

Respondents' Communication Preferences Regarding Clinical Placement

	Frequency of Response	Percentage
All placement requests received at one time?		
Yes	295	78
No	10	3
Do not care	62	16
Sharing a clinical spot acceptable?		
Very comfortable	141	37
Comfortable	187	50
Uncomfortable	45	12
No response	4	1
Prior approval necessary?		
Yes	278	74
No	92	24
Do not care	7	2
Non-contracted school accepted?		
Yes	212	56
No	162	43
No response	3	.8
Confirmation in advance required?		
1 month	57	15
2 months	123	33
3 months	113	30
4 months	52	14
4 months	23	6

DISCUSSION

Sharing Clinical Spots

The results of this study as they relate to the sharing of clinical spots are very encouraging. Most CCCEs are willing to participate in a networking system among the academic institutions provided that the spot is "released" by the assigned institution before being "shared." Even more encouraging to ACCEs is the fact that many CCCEs would be willing to reallocate the slot to a school with which they are not currently contracted. The latter implies willingness to negotiate and sign a clinical agreement on short notice.

The incumbent realities and problems faced in clinical placement may hamper the development of widespread networking. Cutbacks in staffing patterns, budgets, and the effects of diagnosis-related groups continue to decrease the number of slots allocated to any one academic institution. Fewer available slots per facility and variations in the lengths and dates of affiliations among academic institutions further restrict the planned use of networking. In crisis situations, such as the inevitable last-minute cancellation of a student assignment, ACCEs can be somewhat comfortable in contacting one another

for possible solutions. Knowledge of the affiliation dates and durations of other entry-level programs is helpful in determining the direction in which to proceed. Ongoing documentation of unfilled clinical spots would provide additional information as to the feasibility of networking on other than an emergency basis.

Clinical Visitations

Among the nine entry-level programs in New England, considerable variation exists in CEC site visitation policy. For example, some ACCEs visit each student on each rotation, while others visit once per year and not necessarily at the time of student placement. Financial constraints restrict long-distance, out-of-state visits for some ACCEs, while others incorporate these costs directly into their budgets.

To date, no plan exists to standardize visitation policies among the New England institutions. The information gained from this portion of the study may help to support changes in existing policy on a school-by-school basis.

The majority of respondents (66%) indicated that they found a visit to be essential when requested. The next-most frequently

checked response was with problem students only (49%). It was not possible to determine whether either of these responses were exclusive of all others. Theoretically, the latter could be included in a positive response to the former. Further study would be needed to extract the single-most important factor in determining the need for a site visit.

Communication

Before the results of this study were tabulated, the NEC-ACCE established a common mailing date for student request forms. Each of the nine programs mails its requests for the next calendar year on June 1, with a suggested return date of June 30. It was hoped that this strategy would simplify the assignment process for CCCEs whose deal with more than one academic institution. The word-of-mouth response to this policy change has been overwhelmingly positive. The results of this study indicate that 78% of the respondents prefer this approach. The data also reflect that June and September are the preferred months for CCCEs to receive these requests.

CCCEs prefer to receive confirmation of student placement two to three months before the actual starting date. The ACCEs should bear this in mind when establishing deadlines and budgeting time to match students to facilities. Extra time should be allowed for the juggling of placements that inevitably occurs.

It was surprising to note, in the midst of so much discussion about the need for a common evaluation tool, that the respondents were evenly divided on this issue. The questionnaires were returned just before the Leadership for Change conference in Rock Eagle, GA, in 1985.[9] Since that time, the proceedings from the conference have been shared at individual clinical education workshops and clinical faculty institutes. If this question were repeated, the response might now be quite different.

Current Patterns of Clinical Education

The results of this study corroborate the well-known fact that the majority of physical therapy clinical education occurs on a one-to-one basis. Although Emery experimented with a three-to-one student-to-supervisor ratio,[10] no other published data exist on the feasibility of alternative supervisory ratios in physical therapy. In light of the recommendations from the Leadership for Change conference[9] and the emphasis given to clinical education in the new *Proposed Standards for Accreditation of Physical Therapy Programs*,[11] further exploration of alternative models is necessary. This

Table 4

Factors Considered by Clinical Coordinators when Allocating Clinical Spots

Factor	Rank Order	Frequence of Response	Combined Frequency
Academic preparation of	1	111	212
students from a particular	2	53	
program	3	48	
Duration of contract	1	51	151
or loyalty with a	2	46	
particular program	3	54	
Format of a particular	1	9	73
academic program	2	30	
	3	34	
Geographic location	1	11	39
	2	14	
	3	14	
Length of affiliation	1	9	136
	2	47	
	3	80	
Academic level of student	1	63	208
	2	84	
	3	61	
Recruitment	1	4	21
	2	4	
	3	13	
Relationship with ACCE[a]	1	2	24
	2	10	
	3	12	
Time of affiliation	1	100	223
	2	73	
	3	53	
Other	1	20	37
	2	11	
	3	6	

[a] Academic coordinator of clinical education.

Priorities in Allocating Slots

The timing of the affiliation is one of the primary considerations of CCCEs when assigning available slots to the academic institutions. Physical therapy programs planning to move to a post-baccalaureate degree program may want to survey the existing CECs in their respective areas to use facilities in a low-demand time. July and August, however, should be avoided. This is probably because short staffing occurs during summer vacation. The academic preparation and level of the student are also considered essential, followed by the duration of the contract or the facility's loyalty to a particular institution. Over time, the clinical facility's expectations of students at various levels and from various schools become more well defined. It is not surprising, then, that the above-mentioned factors are weighted more heavily when assigning available clinical slots.

The actual format of the physical therapy curriculum was not considered an essential criterion. It may be that this item was interpreted as being the same as "level of student."

Geographic location, relationship with the ACCE, and recruitment potential do not influence the CCCE's decision very strongly. It would be interesting to determine, however, whether recruitment is a strong motivator for accepting students in general. In New England, even with nine entry-level programs, demand for physical therapists exceeds supply. Recruitment of previous students would clearly shorten the orientation time to the facility, staff, and client populations.

CONCLUSION

Cooperative efforts between academic and clinical faculty are paramount in achieving an effective clinical education program. Input from CCCEs and clinical instructors provide valuable data for academic institutions when planning for change in a rapidly growing field. In this time of increased emphasis on education in physical therapy, further investigation is still warranted. Topics requiring continued inquiry include but are not limited to the need and feasibility of a common evaluation tool and alternative methods of clinical education. Adequate investigation and experimentation in both areas is necessary before a decision-making process begins.

REFERENCES

1. Physical Therapy Education and Societal Needs: Guidelines for Physical Therapy Education (Final Report). Alexandria, VA, Department of Education, American Physical Therapy Association, 1984

exploration should not be restricted to reviewing the overall format of clinical education. Rather, it should also incorporate the need for creativity on a smaller scale (ie, within individual clinical facilities). Future research on the cost-effectiveness of various student-to-supervisor ratios is warranted. In addition, clinical-instructor workshops should include topics such as planning learning experiences for more than one student at a time.

The majority of CECs provide experiences considered appropriate for senior-level students. Many of these same facilities also provide junior-level experiences. It is not clear from the data how many facilities restrict their acceptances to one particular level of student. Many CECs are reserving available spots for seniors only; some further restrict their student population to last-affiliation seniors. The reasons may include the perceived increased cost of taking a

junior student,[12] specialization within the field of physical therapy, and the increased need for consultation skills in the general acute care setting. Whatever the cause, the effects are experienced by programs trying to provide adequate early exposure to juniors and, in some instances, to sophomores. This situation strengthens the argument for the development of more creative approaches to clinical education.

The range of perceived ideal lengths of clinical experiences for different levels of students is very broad but includes only scattered responses at the extremes. The data from this survey support the existing clinical education models within New England (ie, most clinical blocks last six to eight weeks). Because of the similarity between these responses and the existing format of clinical education, the data may be more reflective of current practice than the ideal.

2. Planning for Clinical Education in 1990. Alexandria, VA, Department of Education, American Physical Therapy Association, 1984

3. Issues affecting the financing of clinical education. In: Survey of Joint Commission on Nursing and the Joint Commission on Medicine. Washington, DC, Health Care Financing Administration, Bureau of Health Professions, United States Department of Health and Human Services, December 1984

4. Current Patterns for Providing Clinical Education in Physical Therapy Education. Alexandria, VA, Department of Education, American Physical Therapy Association, August 1985

5. Clinical Education in Physical Therapy: Considerations for Alternative Models. Alexandria, VA, Department of Education, American Physical Therapy Association, 1985

6. Report on Clinical Education for the Entry-level Physical Therapist: Consortia, Clinical Education Conferences and Students Early Patient Contacts. Alexandria, VA, Department of Education, American Physical Therapy Association, January 1987

7. Alternative Models for Clinical Education in Physical Therapy. Alexandria, VA, Task Force on Clinical Education, Department of Education, American Physical Therapy Association, 1985

8. Selected Issues Regarding Alternative Models for Clinical Education in Physical Therapy. Alexandria, VA, Task Force on Clinical Education, Department of Education, American Physical Therapy Association, 1985

9. Leadership for Change in Physical Therapy Education: Rock Eagle, Georgia. Alexandria, VA, Department of Education, American Physical Therapy Association, March 1986

10. Emery M, Nalette E: Student-staffed clinics: Creative clinical education during times of constraint. Clinical Management 6(2):6-10, 1986

11. Accreditation of Education Programs of the Physical Therapist: Proposed Standards for Accreditation of Education Programs for the Physical Therapist. Alexandria, VA, Task Force on Revision of the Accreditation Standards and Criteria, American Physical Therapy Association, November 1986

12. Lopopolo RB: Financial model to determine the effect of clinical education programs on physical therapy departments. Phys Ther 64:1396-1402, 1984

Survey of Student Clinical Practice

Implications for Educational Programs

PATRICIA A. WELLS
and EVA LESSARD

The purpose of this survey was to analyze the content of physical therapy students' clinical education programs. We developed and used patient and student record forms that elicited information on the age and sex of the patient groups, the types of pathological conditions, the number and types of treatments administered, the levels of assessments, the levels of supervision of students by clinical instructors, the time spent with patients, and the specialized educational activities at each facility. One hundred seventy-six students participated in the three-year survey; each student completed 600 hours of study for a total of 105,600 hours. The results of this study revealed that musculoskeletal disorders (47.26%) were reported most frequently; fractures of the lower extremities constituted 10.5% of those disorders. Therapeutic exercise was the most frequently used treatment procedure (57.3%). The data obtained through this survey may be useful for evaluating curricula and developing improved practice-specific education programs.

Key Words: *Education; Physical therapy; Students, health occupations.*

Clinical education is an intricate, but essential, process in the physical therapy education program. Although this educational process is beset by many problems, such as the lack of scientific proof of its efficacy, there really is no viable alternative.[1] Clinical education is a shared responsibility that requires a cooperative effort between the academic faculty and the clinical staff.[2] The academic faculty has the task of preparing students during classroom hours with the pertinent theoretical framework required to provide direct patient care. The clinical instructors have the responsibility of ensuring that students can observe, participate, and eventually treat patients effectively and compassionately with entry-level competence.

Physical therapy journals contain many articles that relate to clinical education. Some articles analyze competencies and trends in clinical practice, teaching skills in clinical practice, or clinical teaching in physical therapy ed-

Ms. Wells is Assistant Professor and Coordinator, Clinical Education Program, Division of Physical Therapy, School of Physical and Occupational Therapy, McGill University. 3654 Drummond St. Montreal, Quebec, Canada H3G 1Y5.

Mrs. Lessard is Assistant Clinical Coordinator, Division of Physical Therapy, School of Physical and Occupational Therapy, McGill University.

This study was supported by a grant from the Centre for Teaching and Learning, McGill University.

Address all correspondence to Ms. Wells.

This article was submitted March 1, 1985, was with the authors for revision three weeks, and was accepted October 3, 1985.

ucation.[3-6] With the exception of a report of a pilot study,[7] however, a review of the literature did not reveal any studies that systematically investigated either the disorders treated or the therapeutic approaches used by physical therapy students. A review of the literature of the last five years associated with the disciplines of medicine, nursing, and dentistry revealed only one article[8] detailing the clinical experiences of nursing students. That author reported on a computer-based information system that can be used by the academic faculty to select appropriate clinical placements for students and by students to identify their own learning needs, but did not refer specifically to the students' experiences or the therapeutic procedures used.

According to Scully, clinical education has many overlapping components.[9] Because of their interdependence, both the academic and the clinical faculties must be fully aware of developments in each other's domains. Specific data on students' clinical experiences would enable the academic faculty to develop professional courses that are practice specific, thus freeing the clinical faculty to focus attention on patient-specific teaching. To provide specific information on students' clinical experiences and to analyze the clinical education curricula, we conducted a three-year survey at the clinical institutions associated with McGill University.

METHOD

We compiled a coding list enumerating 55 diagnostic categories for use in the survey (Appendix). Additionally, we developed a coding list of 78 treatment procedures used (available on request from authors). The diagnostic and treatment procedure lists were compiled using information derived from an American Physical Therapy Association publication,[10] from a published survey of clinical education programs at the hospitals and centers affiliated with McGill University,[7] and from a survey of the clinical education program of a Canadian hospital's outpatient department (P. Girard, Hôpital St-Jean-du-Haut-Richelieu, St-Jean, Québec, 1978). A patient record form was used to elicit information concerning the students' clinical rotations (first, second, and final year). This information included each patient's age, sex, primary diagnosis, and surgical factor (if applicable); the students' level of participation in patient assessments; and the treatment procedures used. The student's level of participation in the patient's treatments, the treatment time factor, and the type of facility also were recorded. A student record form also was used to elicit information regarding student participation in the in-service educational activities at each institution. The coding lists, the two record forms, and the instructional guidelines for students and supervising therapists were

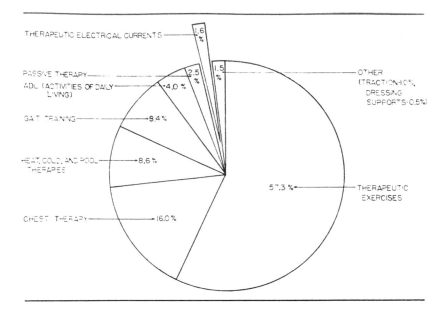

Figure. Frequency distribution of treatment procedure categories. Passive therapy includes connective tissue massage, soft-tissue mobilization, classic massage, and acupressure.

TABLE 1
Frequency Distribution of Diagnostic Categories

Category	% Total Cases
Musculoskeletal	47.26
Medicine	25.99
Neurology	14.90
Arthritides	7.43
Other	4.33
Miscoded	0.09
TOTAL	100.00

TABLE 2
Frequency Distribution of Procedure Use—Therapeutic Exercise Category

Category	% Total Use
Active	13.7
Home programs	9.0
Progressive resistive	7.2
Active assistive	7.0
Presurgical and postsurgical	4.3
Passive	3.8
Neuromuscular (eg, PNF, Rood)	3.1
Balance	3.0
Stretching	2.5
Postural	1.7
Relaxation	1.0
Other (eg, Postnatal)	1.0
TOTAL	57.3

incorporated into a book format. The books were distributed to students before their initial rotation during the first academic year, who retained them for the three-year period. Verbal instruction in the use of the forms was given by the academic clinical coordinator. Each student was requested to complete one precoded data form for every patient seen during a clinical rotation. Only one student record form for each rotation was completed.

Data recorded on these forms were verified by supervising therapists. At the end of each rotation, the completed forms were returned to the academic clinical coordinator, reviewed, and sent to McGill University's computing center for analysis.

The survey provided data for three full years relative to the clinical experiences of 176 students. In the areas of musculoskeletal disorders, acute neurology, medicine, pediatrics, surgery, and rehabilitation, 105,600 hours of clinical practice were completed at 28 teaching facilities. The data were analyzed using frequency distributions of each item in the patient and student record forms. Cross-tabulation of data provided additional information concerning variations in approach to treatments, procedures used, levels of assessment and treatment, and time spent with the patients. Data concerning individual students' clinical experiences also were computed and recorded in each student's university clinical file. These data were made available to the academic faculties and to the hospital and center coordinators of clinical education programs.

RESULTS

Although considerable data were collected and analyzed, we will report in this article only the diagnostic categories and treatment procedures. The frequency distribution of the diagnostic categories is shown in Table 1. Soft-tissue injuries accounted for 24.7% of the disorders in the musculoskeletal category and fractures accounted for 16%. In the medicine category, respiratory disorders represented 6.02% of the total number of cases; digestive, endocrine, and metabolic system disorders, including surgical factors (eg, cholecystectomy), represented 5.14%; and cardiac disorders accounted for 2.78%. In the neurology category, cerebrovascular accidents accounted for 6.37% of the total and disorders of the central nervous system accounted for 5.11%. All other neu-

TABLE 3
Frequency Distribution of Procedure Use—Chest Therapy Category

Category	% Total Use
Breathing exercises	4.7
Bronchial drainage	3.5
Presurgical and postsurgical cardiac	2.4
Intensive care unit	1.5
Exercise tolerance	1.9
Home program	1.0
Suctioning	0.6
Other	0.4
TOTAL	16.0

TABLE 4
Frequency Distribution of Procedure Use—Heat, Cold, and Pool Therapies Category

Category	% Total Use
Hot packs	2.80
Ultrasound	1.90
Cryotherapy	1.50
Whirlpool baths	1.10
Pool	0.40
Shortwave diathermy	0.30
Infrared	0.20
Wax baths	0.20
Hubbard tank	0.10
Microwave	0.04
Ultraviolet	0.03
Contrast baths	0.03
TOTAL	8.60

rological disorders constituted 3.42% of the total number of cases. In the arthritides category, osteoarthritis of the extremities and the spine together represented 4.6% of the total and rheumatoid arthritis constituted 1.74%.

The frequency distribution of the students' use of specific physical therapeutic procedures is shown in the Figure. Chest therapy and therapeutic exercises constituted 73.3% of all treatment provided. The specific frequency distributions by major categories (ie, therapeutic exercise; chest therapy; and heat, cold, and pool therapies) are shown in Tables 2, 3, and 4, respectively.

DISCUSSION

The goal of professional physical therapy programs is to educate and graduate a generalist.[11] This therapist must be capable of assessing patients and executing treatment programs for patient groups referred for physical therapy.

Currently, and in the future, the academic faculty in physical therapy programs must fulfill the university's criteria for excellence in teaching, research, and administration. In accomplishing their teaching and research objectives, academic faculty members often must become specialized. Nonclinical research may result in alienating the academic faculty from the clinical environment, which may cause a disparity between academic and clinical curricula. Documentation of students' clinical experiences may be one way to maintain integration of the two groups because it identifies the critical knowledge base necessary for entry-level physical therapists. The results of the pilot survey of this study,[7] for example, were used to make some appropriate curriculum changes at McGill University. The finding of a high frequency of use of therapeutic exercises has resulted in an increase in the number of theoretical hours devoted to the areas of kinesiology, exercise physiology, and biomechanics. Theoretical hours in the use of therapeutic electrical currents and passive therapy (eg, connective tissue massage, soft-tissue mobilization, classic massage, and acupressure) were reduced. The findings of our three-year survey provide further justification for such changes.

Our three-year survey revealed that therapeutic exercise is still the most prevalent procedure used by student therapists under the supervision of clinical therapists. Its frequency of use has increased in comparison with the pilot study.[7] The significant increase in home exercise programs may reflect decreased health care funding and may indicate a greater reliance on community-based programs and decreased institutionalization. Do current therapeutic exercise courses reflect this trend? Are students being educated to prepare patients for an essentially unsupervised home program and to instruct family members regarding therapeutic exercise goals and procedures? Are methods of obtaining patient compliance, timing, and examination procedures during follow-up visits being taught? Educators and clinicians should consider these questions when they evaluate their educational programs.

Another value of surveys of this nature is that they objectify the longstand-

---

APPENDIX
Coding List of Diagnostic Categories

Arthritides and Musculoskeletal Disorders

Osteoarthritis of spine
Osteoarthritis of extremities
Rheumatoid arthritis and allied conditions
Back pain (nonspecific diagnosis)
    Cervical
    Cervical with radiation
    Thoracic
    Lumbar
Congenital anomalies and epiphyseal disorders
Contusion, lacerations
Crushing injuries
Degenerative disk disease, herniated disks, and other mechanical derangements
Dislocations—upper and lower extremities
Fracture and fracture dislocation—upper limb
Fracture and fracture dislocation—lower limb
Fractures—spine, ribs, pelvis
Meniscectomies
Multiple injuries, including motor vehicle accidents
Musculoskeletal disorders—miscellaneous diagnoses
Osteomyelitis and other bone diseases
Periarthritis—frozen shoulder
Sprains, strains—joints, ligaments adjacent to muscles in the neck and thoracic region
Sprains, strains—joints, ligaments adjacent to muscles in the lumbosacral region
Tears—muscles, ligaments
Tendonitis, bursitis, capsulitis, synovitis—upper limb
Tendonitis, bursitis, capsulitis, synovitis—lower limb

Medicine

Blood diseases and diseases of blood-forming organs
Burns
Cardiac disorders
Central circulatory disorders (great vessels)
Digestive, endocrine, metabolic system disorders (eg, cholecystitis, gout, diabetes)
Diseases of the eye and ear
Diseases of the genitourinary system
Diseases of skin and subcutaneous tissue
Psychiatry
Neoplasms, growths, tumors—malignant and benign
Peripheral vascular disease
Pregnancy
Infectious diseases
Respiratory disease—acute and chronic
Other (eg, genetic disorders, hyperlipidemia)

Neurology

Cerebrovascular accidents
Diseases of the central nervous system
Disorders of spinal and peripheral nerves, peripheral ganglia, neuromuscular junction, and autonomic nervous system
Head injuries and skull fractures
Myopathies
Neuropathies (eg, alcoholic, Guillain-Barré)
Peripheral nerve and plexus injuries
Spinal cord and root injuries

---

ing assumption that certain pathologies are seen more frequently than others. Voss, for example, postulated that musculoskeletal disorders constitute a large proportion of the pathologies seen in physical therapy.[12] Our survey not only substantiated Voss's assumption, but also specifically identified orthopedic conditions of high incidence, such as fractures of the upper and lower extremities, and those of low incidence, such as thoracic injuries. Such information on the actual frequency of disorders may enable educators to devote adequate time to teaching the latest approaches, including medical and surgical management and physical therapeutic treatments that are consonant with total patient management.

Our pilot survey demonstrated a low incidence of modality use in the therapeutic electrical currents and passive therapy.[7] The three-year survey confirmed that clinical usage of these modalities continues to decrease. Such concrete evidence should not be ignored by curriculum committees in the ongoing review and development of professional courses.

After an initial survey has been conducted, and academic faculty, clinicians, and researchers have been made aware of the discernible trends, a periodic review at three- to five-year intervals may reveal changing patterns in pathologies and treatment procedures. The results obtained from the analyzed data may facilitate revisions in the professional curriculum. At McGill University, the exercise therapy courses are being revised and a new pathology-specific exercise program will be implemented. The survey provides clinicians with a heightened awareness of current treatment procedures and trends in pathologies. The results also will provide a source of information to develop continuing education courses.

The information from the survey gives the academic clinical coordinator insight to the quality of the clinical program in each affiliated institution, such as in-service educational experiences and types of treatments administered. This information may be used by clinical coordinators to prepare clinical education seminars. Such surveys also may help to identify areas in which clinical research is lacking, such as validation of chest therapeutic procedures, hip replacement, and home exercise protocols.

CONCLUSION

The establishment of an objective data base on students' clinical experiences benefits educators, clinicians, and students. It provides data for educators when changes in curricula are being considered. Improvements in academic preparation enable clinicians to provide as much "hands on" experience as possible. Students, through the process of identifying personal clinical experiences, are made more discerning of their needs and expectations in clinical affiliations. As physical therapy continues to develop as a profession, the demand for the accountability of professional knowledge and therapeutic approaches will increase. The establishment of an objective clinical education knowledge base may provide a viable reference in the accounting process.

Acknowledgment. We thank the clinical educators and the physical therapy undergraduate students for their support during the survey.

REFERENCES

1. Deusinger S: Implications for the academic institution. In: Planning for Clinical Education in 1990: A Forum Presented June 16, 1983, Kansas City, Missouri. Alexandria, VA, American Physical Therapy Association, Department of Education, May, 1984
2. Windom PA: Developing a clinical education program from the clinician's perspective. Phys Ther 62:1604–1609, 1982
3. Aston-McCrimmon E: Trends in clinical practice: An analysis of competencies. Physiotherapy Canada 36:184–188, 1984
4. Davis CM, Anderson MJ, Jagger D: Competency: The what, why, and how of it. Phys Ther 59:1088–1094, 1979
5. May BJ: Teaching: A skill in clinical practice. Phys Ther 63:1627–1633, 1983
6. Olsen SL: Teaching treatment planning: A problem-solving model. Phys Ther 63:526–529, 1983
7. Wells PA, Lessard E: Analysis of clinical experiences of physical therapy students in a Canadian university. Physiotherapy Canada 35:92–99, 1983
8. Ellis PH: Matching students with clinical experiences by computer. Nurs Outlook 30:29–30, 1982
9. Scully R: Purpose and perception of clinical education. In: Planning for Clinical Education in 1990: A Forum Presented June 16, 1983, Kansas City, Missouri. Alexandria, VA, American Physical Therapy Association, Department of Education, May, 1984
10. American Physical Therapy Association: Competencies in Physical Therapy: An Analysis of Practice, ed 2. San Diego, CA, Courseware Inc, 1979
11. Gwyer J: Introduction. In: Planning for Clinical Education in 1990: A Forum Presented June 16, 1983, Kansas City, Missouri. Alexandria, VA, American Physical Therapy Association, Department of Education, May, 1984
12. Voss DE: Seventeenth Mary McMillan lecture: "Everything is there before you discover it." Phys Ther 62:1617–1624, 1982

Plan to Provide Specialty Training in Rehabilitation

Carolyn K Rozier
Andrea Morgenthaler
Lisa Protsman

ABSTRACT: *The purpose of the project was to provide specialty training in rehabilitation of multi-handicapped adults in order to improve the quality of preparation and to increase the number of students seeking this area for employment after graduation. The approach taken was to develop a plan to increase the integration of the teaching of rehabilitation skills between the academic and the clinical setting. A clinical facility was selected as a primary site for clinical experiences and a clinician was hired to assist the faculty in developing and planning the clinical experiences. All students participated in the program, which integrated academic and clinical work, and specific students were selected as trainees to be given additional training in rehabilitation of multi-handicapped adults. All students were able to observe the immediate results of various rehabilitation treatment methods and to discuss these methods with the faculty. New skill statements developed for the "Blue MACS" for use with the trainees have now been included as optional skills for all students. After graduation, of 15 students who accepted the specialty training in rehabilitation, 10 began working immediately in a primary rehabilitation facility and 3 are working in a rehabilitation unit at a hospital.*

In an effort to determine the best way to integrate long-term neurological rehabilitation training into the curriculum, patterns of clinical education were investigated. In many curricula, students do not apply theory to clinical practice until the end of the academic curriculum. To enhance a student's ability to apply theory, many teaching methods have been designed and many patterns of clinical education have been developed.[14] Some require

Dr Rozier is Dean, School of Physical Therapy, Texas Woman's University, Denton, TX 76204. Ms Morgenthaler is Instructor, School of Physical Therapy, Texas Woman's University, Houston, TX 77030. Ms Protsman was RSA Grant Coordinator, School of Physical Therapy, Texas Woman's University, and is now at Providence Hospital, El Paso, TX.

students to attend the clinic one day or half a day per week for a semester, several weeks during a semester, or several weeks between semesters. Students often do not integrate material from their academic courses into their clinical experience regardless of when the experience is offered.[5,6] Closer integration of the didactic material on long-term rehabilitation with the learning in the clinical setting could reinforce the interest of the student in this particular specialty and increase the number of students who accept initial employment in a long-term rehabilitation setting.[7]

Integration of didactic and clinical learning poses many problems. For example, course instructors often do not control what the student sees or does in the clinic. Lack of control in the clinical setting makes it more difficult for the instructor to facilitate the student's integration of material. One strategy for integrating this material has been to use patient-centered problem solving. Patient-centered cases seem to facilitate the transmission and application of theory to clinical practice because the student takes an active part in studying representative cases, rather than merely observing a large number of cases in a clinic.[8] The student does not, however, immediately develop the psychomotor skills needed for clinical practice.

In an attempt to integrate clinical material with theory, some health professions have indicated that the persons supervising the students in the clinic should be the academic faculty.[9] In this manner the academic faculty become role models for the students. This method is not always practical, but in any method for integration, a close relationship between the clinical and academic work is desired. The faculty should be clearly aware of the goals and objectives of their courses and how these objectives are related to the clinical experience of the student.

The faculty of the School of Physical Therapy, Texas Woman's University, Hous-

ton Campus, developed a method to integrate academic classroom theory on rehabilitation with simultaneous clinical experiences. There are approximately 80 upper-level undergraduate students and 52 entry-level master's students on the campus. A physical therapy clinician was employed with grant funds to work half-time for Texas Woman's University and half-time for the clinical facility. The faculty chose course objectives relating to long-term rehabilitation that they would like to correlate and enhance with clinical experiences.

The project was funded by an RSA grant and was developed by the part-time clinician, the faculty, and an advisory committee. The advisory committee included representatives from community agencies for the handicapped and other health professions. The faculty involved in courses that had rehabilitation content indicated the type of experiences that they felt were appropriate in the clinical setting to reinforce didactic material. The clinician then arranged for these experiences.

The choice of the clinical facility was made carefully; it had to meet the needs of the students and have a philosophy congruent with those of the curriculum and the rehabilitation emphasis.[10] The center chosen was Medical Center del Oro Hospital in Houston, Texas, a rehabilitation center of 70 beds with a staff of 20 physical therapists, 8 physical therapist assistants, 2 aides, and a secretary. Six support services in addition to physical therapy are occupational therapy, cognitive training, recreation therapy, speech pathology, neuropsychology, and social services. The Center also offers biofeedback, vocational counseling, driver's education, and a specialized unit for rehabilitation of the brain-impaired adult. A contract was developed with Medical Center del Oro, similar to many clinical affiliation agreements, that delineated the responsibility for patient care, the responsibility of the students in the facility, the protection of civil

Figure
Additional "Blue MACS" Skills

Skill #55: Participates in the rehabilitation process through active involvement with the entire treatment plan.
Skill #56: Evaluates the neurological and functional status of patient with closed-head injury.
Skill #57: Plans and implements a treatment program for patient with closed-head injury.
Skill #58: Evaluates the neurological and functional status of a stroke patient.
Skill #59: Plans and implements a treatment program for the stroke patient.
Skill #60: Selects and performs techniques indicated to evaluate and modify transitional movements, eg, rolling, coming to sit, sit to stand.
Skill #61: Uses appropriate techniques in evaluation of patient with spinal cord injury.
Skill #62: Uses appropriate techniques in treatment of patient with spinal cord injury.
Skill #63: Utilizes appropriate techniques in the evaluation and treatment of the multiply injured adult.
Skill #64: Assesses indication for, fit of, and proper care of serial or inhibitive cast or tone-inhibiting orthosis.
Skill #65: Participates in the vocational rehabilitation process through active involvement with vocational rehabilitation (VR) personnel.

rights, and the provision for contract modifications. The contract also specified that the grant clinician would be employed half-time by the facility and half-time by the University. Faculty would be allowed to accompany students to the facility and to perform patient treatment and evaluations.

Two groups of students were included in this project. All junior and senior physical therapy students and entry-level graduate students received the integrated clinical experiences for many of the rehabilitation objectives in the curriculum. Fifteen students were selected by an application process to receive additional training in rehabilitation, and were known as "rehabilitation trainees." These trainees received a stipend of grant funds.

Courses with rehabilitation objectives were involved in this integrated plan. The clinician arranged for the experiences at Medical Center del Oro. Some of the beginning courses for the juniors or first-year graduate students required a much different type of experience than did courses that were offered when the students were seniors or second-year graduate students. The academic faculty and/or the clinician accompanied groups of students to Medical Center del Oro.

The clinical activities performed were gait assessments, stroke evaluations, and neuro-developmental treatment for patients with stroke or closed-head injury. The students observed treatment techniques performed by the facility's therapists and by the academic faculty. Patient evaluations by students were done in groups as well as individually. The students went into the community with the rehabilitation patients to assess architectural barriers. In addition,

three students elected to work on research projects at Medical Center del Oro. The focus of these projects was to assess characteristics of gait in brain-injured patients.

Integration of didactic coursework with the clinical experience was accomplished by having the students go to the clinic as soon as possible after receiving the information in the didactic class. The faculty member teaching the selected rehabilitation activity in the didactic class went to the facility with groups of 6 to 12 students. Students went to the facility only during weeks when specific activities were introduced in class; they spent an average of two hours per month at del Oro. The time spent at the facility was considered part of the laboratory for the course. The faculty members served as role models for the students and were able to point out pertinent information related to the class when reviewing a patient.

Other objectives of the facility experience were to enable the student to plan a comprehensive program for the severely disabled in cooperation with other disciplines and agencies, to assess architectural barriers in the environment, and to develop skill in adapting environments for accessibility to the handicapped. Students reviewed the rights of the handicapped and observed the role of advisory groups. The students took an active role in educating the handicapped about their rights and assessing physical needs for vocational placement.

Integration also was needed to proceed in a reverse direction from the clinical experience back into the classroom. The faculty member would have a class discussion following the experience at Medical Center del Oro. The students were tested on the practical application of the theory in laboratories

after they had been to the Center. The students presented case studies of patients they had seen in the clinic, which allowed the faculty member and the other students to share information. Patients seen at the Center were used as models for treatment planning programs presented or discussed in class. The students also were given case studies on their examinations in which they had to design program plans that required integration of the didactic and clinical material.

Supplemental activities for the rehabilitation trainees included a special rehabilitation course designed to complement established rehabilitation coursework and augment specific skills in rehabilitation. Trainees were then assigned to selected clinical affiliations with rehabilitation specialties for their long-term internships. The "Blue MACS" was used as the clinical evaluation tool for all of the students, and new evaluation and treatment skills were added for the trainees (Figure). One skill, casting for inhibition of muscle tone, was not available at all facilities. Clinical and rehabilitation settings accepted the new skills and several facilities have adopted them as requirements for all students at their facilities.

After using this plan for three years, a number of limiting factors were identified. Planning the integrated clinical experiences was difficult because the types and numbers of patients were not always available at the exact time that the students were ready for a particular skill. It was also difficult to arrange for a particular patient with a specific diagnosis to be treated at a time when the students were available and not required to be in another class. There was limited space in the physical therapy department, and patients also had busy schedules with various other services.

Other than prompt integration of clinic and class material, benefits to the students were varied, and not all were related to rehabilitation objectives. The beginning student was able to have time to adjust to being in a clinic with multi-handicapped patients. Students who had progressed further in their coursework were able to practice skills in a clinical environment and were able to see a variety of patient types. Students were introduced to rehabilitation treatment of the total patient, and they participated in the team approach to treatment with the other services at the Center. Students learned to deal with other medical problems that they might not have been studying at the time; because they were treating patients who had various problems, they learned how to deal with these medical complications. The students were exposed to a variety of treatment approaches other than what they had learned in class. Not only were the students able to practice a treatment, but they were able to identify issues relating to community health and professional behavior.

The del Oro experience provided benefits to the academic faculty and clinical physical therapists. Faculty members, who could refer to the patients that both the faculty and students had seen in the clinic, were given a new tool to assist them in classroom teaching. The experiences allowed the faculty to maintain and practice their own therapeutic skills. The agreement with Medical Center del Oro also gave easier access to a patient population for research on behalf of faculty and students. Interaction between faculty and clinical physical therapists led to a sharing of new treatment techniques. The faculty and clinicians were able to consult with one another on difficult cases. Faculty members gave in-service programs for the facility and served as mentors to the clinical staff who were interested in pursuing research projects. Staff members at Medical Center del Oro were given priority in attending continuing education courses given by the University.

An employee evaluation form was sent to employers of graduates who had been trainees in the special program. Ten are now working in a rehabilitation facility and three are working in a rehabilitation unit of a facility. The employers indicated that the trainees were above average for new graduates, that it took less time than usual for orientation to the facility, and that the amount of supervision required in the first few months was less than usual.

The integration of classroom theory in rehabilitation and clinical application in the plan developed by the Texas Woman's University faculty has been successful and will be expanded in the future. Faculty and students have been enthusiastic about the introduction of certain didactic course material which is followed by a clinical experience with a patient who exemplifies that classroom material. These experiences assist not only with integration in rehabilitation classes, but in other classes that are occurring in the same semester. The special rehabilitation course and internships have proven successful as methods to encourage students to become employed in a rehabilitation facility. In the future, different curricular objectives will be added to this plan and an additional clinical facility will be selected for the simultaneous integration of academic and clinical work.

ACKNOWLEDGMENTS

The authors acknowledge the assistance provided by the United States Department of Education under grant number G068400007 in partial support of the activities reported here.

REFERENCES

1. French RM: Clinical laboratory education. In Hamburg J (ed): Review of Allied Health Education, No. 1. Lexington, KY, The University Press of Kentucky, 1974, pp 120–135
2. Hein JW: The dilemma in dental education. In Hamburg J (ed): Review of Allied Health Education, No. 1. Lexington, KY, The University Press of Kentucky, 1974, pp 93–119
3. Howard DR, Lewis DE: Evolution of the physician's assistant. In Hamburg J (ed): Review of Allied Health Education, No. 1. Lexington, KY, The University Press of Kentucky, 1974, pp 181–200
4. Soule AB: Radiologic technology. In Hamburg J (ed): Review of Allied Health Education, No. 1. Lexington, KY, The University Press of Kentucky, 1974, pp 136–180
5. Walish JF, Olson RE, Schuit D: Effects of a concurrent clinical education assignment on student concerns. Phys Ther 66:233–236, 1986
6. Smillie C, Wong J, Arklie M: A proposed framework for evaluation of support courses in a nursing curriculum. J Adv Nurs 9:487–492, 1984
7. Scanlan CL: Integrating didactic and clinical education: High patient contact. In Ford CW (ed): Clinical Education for the Allied Health Professions. St. Louis, MO, C V Mosby Co, 1978, pp 113–114
8. Myers C, Shannon P, Sundstrom C: Strategies in clinical teaching. Am J Occup Ther 23:30–34, 1969
9. Rodgers JM: An examination of research priorities in nurse education. J Adv Nurs 10:233–236, 1985
10. Gwyer J, Barr JS, Talmor Z: Selection of clinical education centers in physical therapy. J Allied Health 11:272–281, 1982

Impact of Previous Nursing Home Work Experience on Student Physical Therapists' Employment Interests

Rita A Wong, MS, PT

ABSTRACT: Physical therapy students' interest in future employment in chronic care settings was studied, particularly as it relates to previous nursing home work experience. Using a 7-point Likert scale, 127 students indicated their interest in future employment in nine work settings (three chronic care settings and six non-chronic care settings). The results revealed significantly less student interest in chronic care versus non-chronic care settings (P<.001). Forty-seven students had had nursing home work experience, and 60% of those students stated that their nursing home experience made them less interested in working with elderly patients. Students who had enjoyed the nursing home work experience demonstrated significantly more interest in future employment in chronic care settings than did students without nursing home experience (P<.008). Students who had disliked their nursing home work experience demonstrated no significant difference in interest from students without nursing home experience.

INTRODUCTION

The number of individuals aged 65 years or older is rapidly increasing,[1] as is the demand for physical therapists in the field of geriatrics. Although physical therapy for geriatric patients spans most practice settings, the segment highlighted in this study is chronic care. This aspect of geriatrics is particularly vulnerable to the current shortage of physical therapists.[2] The combined effect of ageism and chronicityism (negativism toward the care of chronically ill patients) impedes geriatrically focused chronic care settings from attracting and retaining qualified practitioners.[3]

Although the majority of elderly adults are healthy and functionally independent, a significant minority of that population has chronic, disabling conditions. Seventeen per-

Ms Wong is Assistant Professor, Physical Therapy Program, School of Allied Health Professions, University of Connecticut, U-101, Storrs, CT 06269-2101.

cent of individuals between 65 and 74 years of age are dependent in at least one personal care activity. This percentage jumps to 49% in individuals over 85 years of age, with 22% requiring nursing home care.[1] Interventions to minimize the effects of these long-term illnesses and impairments will require an increasing physical therapy emphasis.

Despite the increasing demand, student interest in the elderly population is low. One recent study concluded that 76% of a sample of 326 physical therapy students did not intend to work with older patients after graduation.[4] Both chronicityism and ageism were reflected in student responses. Factors such as "depressing environment" and "low desire to work with chronic illness" as well as a belief that older people are "less motivated" and "more frustrating to work with" than younger people were common reasons given by students for their low interest.

Many strategies for increasing student interest in geriatrics have been suggested.[5,6-10] One strategy is based on the hypothesis that negative attitudes toward elderly people stem from a lack of familiarity with this age group. If an individual's exposure to older people increases, the stereotypical negative biases will decrease.[8,10,11]

Care must be taken, however, in applying this hypothesis. If students' initial introduction to elderly people is limited to patients who are debilitated and frail, negative stereotypes may be reinforced, not dispelled.[8] Students may need to confront one set of biases at a time; ageism or chronicityism. Few studies exist, however, that objectively evaluate this premise.

I became acutely aware of a potential problem with early student exposure to nursing home elderly patients through my role as an academic educator. I coordinate a junior-year clinical arts course that assigns students to one of about 25 different clinical settings for a one-day-per-week clinical experience. Frequently students come to me pleading not to be assigned to a nursing home: "I've worked in a nursing home before and hated

it," "I want to get 'real' physical therapy experience." Never, however, in six years, has a student pleaded with me not to be assigned to an outpatient or sports therapy setting, although many entering students also have experience in these areas.

This study attempted to quantify the level of student interest in chronic care work settings and to document students' perceptions of the effect of previous nursing home work experience on their future practice plans.

Two hypotheses were examined: 1) Physical therapy students are less interested in working in chronic care settings than in non-chronic care settings, and 2) Interest in working in chronic care settings will differ among students based on the students' positive, negative, or lack of nursing home work experience.

METHOD
Subjects

During the spring 1988 semester, a questionnaire was completed by 127 physical therapy students in the entry-level bachelor of science program at the University of Connecticut. The subjects were upper division students who had not yet begun their final full-time clinical rotations. The average age of the respondents was 22.5 years (range= 19–37 years); 89% were women; 8% were non-Caucasian.

Procedure

The project was approved by the institution's Committee for the Use of Human Subjects in Research. The questionnaire was pretested with 25 physical therapy students and was reviewed by two faculty members. Suggested changes to increase the clarity and representativeness of the questions were incorporated into the final instrument.

Students completed the three-item questionnaire during regular class time. In question one, students indicated their interest in future employment in nine work settings using a 7-point Likert scale (1=extremely uninterested; 7=extremely interested). In questions two and three, students reported whether they had nursing home work experience and, if they did, how this experience affected them. Specifically, did the experience increase or decrease their interest in future work with elderly patients? Students were asked to complete a sentence explaining why the nursing home experience affected them in the manner they reported.

Based on the results of the questionnaire, the subjects were placed into one of three categories: 1) those for whom the nursing home experience increased their interest in geriatrics (positive experience), 2) those for whom the experience decreased their interest in geriatrics (negative experience), and 3) those without any nursing home experience (no experience).

On a separate form, subjects gave their opinion as to whether each of the nine settings identified in the questionnaire represented chronic or non-chronic care. Any setting with at least an 85% agreement as chronic care was categorized as chronic care for the purposes of data analysis. Through this process, the settings of long-term care, hospice, and nursing home were categorized as chronic care.

Data Analysis

The mean interest score for each of the nine work settings was calculated as well as the average interest score for the three chronic care settings and the average interest score for the six non-chronic care settings.

An analysis of variance (ANOVA) was used to evaluate overall differences among the three categories of subjects for the chronic care interest variable. Student t tests were used *post hoc* to determine significant differences between the scores of the "no-experience" group and each of the two "experience" groups. As discussed and summarized by Gardner, parametric statistics are appropriate for this type of summated scale data that hold an intermediate position between ordinal and interval scales of measurement.[12]

Responses to the sentence-completion question were organized according to recurring statements and themes.

RESULTS

One of the 127 subjects did not complete all of the questions, and these data were eliminated. The figure identifies the mean interest scores for all 126 subjects for each work setting.

Student Interest

The scores for the three settings that students identified as chronic care (long-term care, hospice, and nursing home) were averaged to form the chronic care interest score. The chronic care interest score was 3.2 on the 7-point Likert scale. The scores for the remaining six settings were averaged to form the non-chronic care interest score. The non-chronic care score was 5.1 on the same 7-point Likert scale. A student t test for correlated samples demonstrated significantly less student interest in chronic care work settings than non-chronic care settings ($t=18.1$; $df=125$; $P<.001$).

Nursing Home Experience

Forty-seven (37%) of the 126 subjects had previous nursing home work experience. Twenty-eight students categorized their nursing home experience as negative; the remaining 19 categorized it as positive.

The mean scores and standard deviations for student interest in chronic care employment for subjects in the three categories of nursing home experience are summarized in the Table. Using the Statistical Package for the Social Sciences (SPSSx),[13] an ANOVA was used to compare these scores. This analysis yielded significant differences among the three groups ($F=6.03$; $df=2, 123$; $P<.003$).

Two *post hoc* student t tests were performed to evaluate how each of the two groups with nursing home experience individually compared with the group with no experience.

The 19 students who categorized their nursing home work experience as positive demonstrated more interest in future work in the chronic care environment than students with no nursing home experience ($t=2.72$; $df=96$; $P<.008$). The interest scores of the 28 students who found the nursing home experience to be negative did not differ significantly from the scores of subjects with no nursing home experience.

In the sentence-completion question, one or both of the following themes were mentioned by 60% of the subjects who had had a positive nursing home experience: 1) I enjoyed the interactions with or personalities of my elderly patients, and 2) I felt needed and appreciated by my elderly patients. Twenty-nine percent of the subjects credited the high quality of care as a major influence, and 18% stated that the experience had decreased their stereotypical view of elderly individuals and had left them more open to future work with this population.

Seventy percent of the subjects with a negative nursing home experience included at least one of the following three related themes in their sentence-completion answer: 1) The care given was mostly maintenance, 2) The work was not challenging, or 3) I could not help the patient improve. Three subjects stated that they found the atmosphere depressing. Another three subjects commented only that they "were not interested in geriatrics."

DISCUSSION

The results of this study demonstrate that physical therapy students have low interest in chronic care work settings. Even the group

Figure
Student interest in working in each of nine different settings.

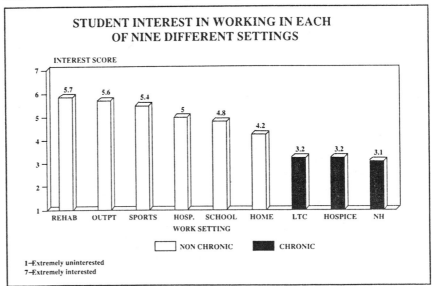

Table

Student Interest in Future Employment in Chronic Care Settings for Three Categories of Previous Nursing Home Work Experience[a]

Type of Experience	Mean Interest Score[b]	SD
Positive[c]	4.0	1.4
None[d]	3.1	1.3
Negative[e]	2.8	1.2

[a] $P<.001$.

[b] 7-point Likert scale (1=extremely uninterested, 2=extremely interested).

[c] A nursing home work experience that increased subjects' interest in future work in geriatrics.

[d] No nursing home work experience.

[e] A nursing home work experience that decreased subjects' interest in future work in geriatrics.

that expressed the greatest interest in chronic care employment—those who had had a positive nursing home experience—barely reached the neutral score of 4 on the 7-point scale. In comparison, subjects expressed much more interest in non-chronic care employment, scoring 5.1 on the same 7-point scale.

Thirty-seven percent of the total sample had worked in a nursing home. The majority (60%) stated that the nursing home experience had decreased their interest in future work in geriatrics. When these same subjects were asked to indicate their interest in future employment in chronic care settings, their interest scores were not significantly different from subjects with no nursing home experience. In contrast, the subjects who believed that the nursing home experience had increased their interest in geriatrics scored significantly higher than subjects with no nursing home experience.

The *ex-post facto* nature of the study precludes definitive interpretation of these findings. It is not known whether students' interest levels prior to the nursing home experience were similar to those reported later. Perhaps students who choose a nursing home environment to obtain early health care experience have different interests and expectations than students who choose other environments. A study is needed to evaluate this point.

The sentence-completion question provided some insights into different reactions to a nursing home experience. The reasons given for a positive experience usually related to the emotional rewards received from helping the elderly patient and to the enjoyment of interpersonal linkages with patients. These students enjoyed working with the nursing home elderly patients on a personal level. They felt good about helping people, they felt that the elderly patients appreciated their efforts, and they believed that their interventions made a difference in the comfort and quality of life of their patients. Very few students credited activities that provided intellectual challenge as a basis for their future interest in chronic care employment.

Students who perceived the experience as negative frequently referred to activities that limited the intellectual challenge of the situation as key factors in their disinterest. These students cited the maintenance nature of the care as a major disincentive. They felt frustrated by their inability to help patients improve. They perceived maintenance care as the primary objective of nursing home intervention—a type of care they found uninteresting and nonchallenging. "All I did was walk patients" was a typical response. They did not believe that they could use the professional skills taught in school in the chronic care setting with geriatric patients. They believed that the setting did not provide "real" physical therapy.

The emphasis of our health care system fosters the bias that the chronic care setting is unchallenging and unrewarding. Most of the external rewards and prestige for health care practitioners are entwined in "curing" the patient, not in caring for him.[3,5,6] Students working in the chronic care setting often try to apply treatment concepts based on the acute care model of intervention: diagnose and cure. When these techniques fail, frustration and a sense of personal failure result. Disinterest in the population soon follows.[14]

The physical therapy profession needs to utilize the resources of practitioners from chronic care settings to develop supportive environments in which to introduce students to the chronically ill geriatric patient. If students enter their professional training with a low value for chronic care settings, they will be more likely to neglect this aspect of their academic preparation than areas of practice for which they have a high value.[15] The problem is compounded if clinical and academic faculty have a low value for the chronic care setting and give low priority to teaching students the principles and importance of chronic care interventions.

Committed, insightful clinicians and educators are needed who can help students adapt their problem-solving strategies to patients with predominantly chronic health problems. Intellectual rigor and compassion are needed to work effectively in the chronic care setting.

Further research should be conducted on such questions as: What specific experiences will have a significant impact (positive or negative) on student interest in chronic care interventions? Does the presence of both ageism and chronicityism have a greater impact on student attitudes than the presence of only one of these variables? Can academic and clinical faculty reverse negative student attitudes about chronically ill elderly patients? Is there an ideal age at which to focus on attitude change toward the chronically ill elderly patient? Can nursing home personnel develop an effective program to enhance students' attitudes toward chronically ill elderly patients? How do students' full-time clinical rotations affect their attitudes toward chronic care geriatrics? Will student attitudes toward chronically ill elderly patients change significantly with greater work experience?

CONCLUSION

The field of physical therapy for geriatric patients is expanding rapidly. The area of chronic care geriatrics also is expanding. Currently students are disinterested in this area of practice. With the shortage of physical therapists evident in many parts of the country, it is unreasonable to assume that students will gravitate toward settings for which they have a low interest when there are numerous employment opportunities in settings for which they have a high interest level.[2]

As physical therapy educators, we should examine closely student (and faculty) attitudes, stereotypical beliefs, and knowledge bases in the area of chronic care geriatrics and develop strategies to heighten interest and knowledge.

REFERENCES

1. *Aging America: Trends and Projections.* 1987–1988 edition. United States Senate Special Committee on Aging. Washington, DC: Department of Health and Human Services.

2. Russell T. The PT personnel shortage. *Clinical Management.* 1990;10(2):15.

3. Wong R. Negative attitudes toward chronic-care intervention: an overview of a growing challenge. *Geritopics.* 1990;13(2):11–14.

4. Coren A, Andressi M, Blood H, et al. Factors related to physical therapy students' decisions to work with elderly patients. *Phys Ther.* 1987;67:60–65.

5. Kutner NG. Medical students' orientation toward the chronically ill. *J Med Educ.* 1978;53:111–118.

6. Halstead L, Halstead M. Chronic illness and humanism: rehabilitation as a model for teaching humanistic and scientific health care. *Arch Phys Med Rehabil.* 1978;59:53–57.

7. Strasburg DM. Gerontological content in entry-level physical therapy education. *Gerontology and Geriatrics Education.* 1984;4(4):65–73.

8. Gordan SK, Hallauer DS. Impact of a friendly visiting

program on attitudes of college students toward the aged: a pedagogical note. *Gerontologist*. 1976;16:371–376.

9. Wilson JF, Hafferty FW. Long-term effects of a seminar on aging and health for first-year medical students. *Gerontologist* 1983:23:319–324.

10. Heller B, Walsh FJ. Changing nursing students' attitudes toward the aged: an experimental study. *J Nursing Educ*. 1976;15(5):9–17.

11. McTavish D. Perceptions of old people: a review of research methodologies and findings. *Gerontologist*. 1971; Winter; 90–108.

12. Gardner PL. Scales and statistics. *Rev Educ Research*. 1975;45:43–57.

13. Norusis M. *Statistical Package for the Social Sciences (SPSS/PC)*. Chicago, IL: SPSS, Inc; 1984.

14. Perkins DN. *Knowledge as Design*. Hillsdale, NJ; Lawrence Erlbaum Assoc, Publishers; 1986.

15. Brody S. Rehabilitation and the nursing home. In: Schneider E, ed. *The Teaching Nursing Home*. New York, NY: Raven Press; 1985:147–156.

Clinical Education in the Nursing Home Setting

Preliminary Report

CARL T. ANDERSON, M.A.,
and KATHRYN A. SAWNER, B.S.

Methods for evaluation of students' attitudes toward types of patients and types of employment settings are of critical concern to physical therapy educators and clinical practitioners. The following is a preliminary report of a study in progress and presents a method being utilized for evaluation of student attitudes toward a specific physical therapy clinical employment setting and the effect of undergraduate clinical education experiences on these attitudes. The authors recommend similar study in evaluation of these attitudes toward other types of physical therapy clinical education settings. The word attitude, as used in this paper, may be defined as a mental position or feeling with regard to a fact or state.

Inherent in the physical therapy educator's philosophy of preparing the student to assume his ultimate professional role is acquainting the student with as many different types of clinical settings for physical therapy practice as are educationally meaningful to and structurally feasible for the student.

Acquainting the student with nursing home physical therapy is seen as highly desirable both

Mr. Anderson was Assistant Professor of Physical Therapy, State University of New York at Buffalo, at the time this paper was originally submitted. He is currently Coordinator, Rural Health Manpower Project, Regional Medical Program for Western New York, 2929 Main Street, Buffalo, New York 14214, and Clinical Assistant Professor, Department of Physical Therapy, State University of New York at Buffalo.

Miss Sawner is Assistant Professor of Physical Therapy and Director of Clinical Education, State University of New York at Buffalo, 264 Winspear Avenue, Buffalo, New York 14215.

The study was supported in part by grant 44-P-10095/2-07,08 from the Rehabilitation Services Administration, Social and Rehabilitation Service, Department of Health, Education, and Welfare.

from the standpoint of the student's overall preparedness for clinical practice and from the standpoint of the expanding emphasis on comprehensive geriatric care. The work of Tuckman and Lorge showed "attitudes toward aging have shown that individuals differing in age, education, and life experience subscribe substantially to the misconceptions and stereotypes about old people."[1] Further, from his work on professional perspectives on the aged, Coe stated, "It does not appear that a therapist could meet any expectations of the aged patient if . . . stereotypes were strongly held. The practitioner would, so to speak, have developed a negative 'set' about older patients even before actually seeing a particular aged patient."[2]

A part of the physical therapy educator's responsibility is recognized as helping to meet the manpower demands of the field. Acquainting the student with geriatric care during his undergraduate preparation is seen as an ideal way of increasing the potential number of physical therapists employed in nursing home settings. Finding a nursing home in this area suitable as a site for full-time clinical education for students was possible in only one nursing home because of only part-time physical therapy coverage in most facilities, problems inherent in scheduling, and legal constraints. Part-time affiliation, i.e., half a day, has been and continues to be available in a second nursing home. The authors, therefore, determined to develop additional clinical affiliations in nursing home settings in which the student would be provided an environment appropriate to enriching his appreciation of and involvement in geriatric rehabilitation. In so doing, an attempt is being made to determine the extent to which the undergraduate student's attitudes toward geriatric patients are influenced by his clinical education experiences.

This project was not designed to show a change in student skill in managing a geriatric caseload; rather, the project was designed to show attitudinal change toward a specific type of clinical setting because of the student's preprofessional involvement in that setting.

METHOD

To implement this project, a nursing home facility agreed to participate in the establishment of a nursing home physical therapy clinical instruction unit. Funds to initiate the project were provided through a Department of Health, Education, and Welfare, Social and Rehabilitation Service, Rehabilitation Services Administration (RSA) training grant awarded in June 1970 for the 1970-1971 academic year. Additional funds have been appropriated to continue the work of this project during the 1971-1972 academic year.

RSA grant funds have provided for a full-time physical therapist to give clinical instruction in the nursing home for junior and senior physical therapy students, and to give comprehensive rehabilitative services, upon physician referral, to patients of the nursing home. The physical therapist selected for the project has had several years experience with geriatric patients through her employment in public health agencies and with clinical education of physical therapy students.

The many specific subobjectives of the overall project, both patient-service related and

student-instruction related, will not be delineated here. The focus of this report will be on one subobjective: to ascertain if, by exposure to and involvement in geriatric care in a nursing home setting, a change in the student's attitudes occurs toward working with geriatric patients or working in a nursing home setting.

Evaluation of this project necessitated development of a specific evaluation protocol. Since "objectives form the basis of any evaluation effort,"[3] the objectives as stated in the original grant application served as a baseline for evaluation. The following tools are being utilized to evaluate the student's attitudinal change: attitude scale, log diary, forced selection schema, and longitudinal employment study. Since not all students will be receiving clinical education within the nursing home, those who do not will serve as a control group. These tools will provide for a measure of changes in attitudes of the control group as a result of overall preparation, and a change in attitude of the experimental group, whose overall preparation is essentially the same as the control group, but who will have been exposed to clinical education in the nursing home.*

Evaluation Tools

Attitude Scale. The purpose of this scale, developed and validated specifically for this study, is to measure the student's attitudes toward nursing homes, the role of physical therapy within the nursing home, and the resident patients themselves. Search of literature that might have been useful to determine physical therapy students' attitudes toward nursing homes and geriatric patients was unsuccessful. The developed attitude scale will be administered to each student at the beginning of his professional preparation and three times additionally during his professional preparation, regardless of whether he receives clinical experience in a nursing home during that time. By thus subjecting all students, the investigators will have a means of assessing the change in

---

* Unless unusual circumstances prevail, both the experimental and the control groups will be derived by assignment during the junior year and electively by the student during the senior year.

attitude of those students who do receive nursing home clinical education experience with those who do not. (An assumption is made that all students will be involved in the physical therapy management of geriatric patients in other than the nursing home setting.)

Forced Selection Schema. This evaluation instrument will be used to show the effect of the project on the student's choice of employment site. The device consists of nine specific physical therapy work specialties randomized into multiple sets of four specialties. Within each set, the student is forced to arrange, in order from most preferable to least preferable, the areas in which he desires to work following graduation. The forced selection schema will be presented to all students at the inception of their physical therapy program and four times during the two years of professional education, terminating with their final day as undergraduate students, and will be illustrative of the students' change in choice of work site.

Log Diary. Each student in the experimental group will maintain a daily record of his observations and activities in the nursing home setting. The record of daily activity will be analyzed for statements showing the student's direct involvement in the problems of geriatric care, planning effective—or ineffective—methods of treatment, and other such activities. From such a record, inferences may also be drawn regarding the student's level of appreciation for the problems involved in management of geriatric patients.

Longitudinal Employment Study. During the length of the project and for five years following project completion, records on employment of persons who take part in the project will be kept. Any change in employment patterns toward nursing home settings could be noted in contrast to the control group. Although no inferences can be drawn at this time, two of the eight project participants from the spring 1971 graduating class have chosen nursing home employment following graduation.

PRELIMINARY REPORT

Although the direct patient-services related aspects of the project have been in effect since October 1970, clinical education in the project site for full-time physical therapy interns was not initiated until January 1971. To date, eight senior students participated in the project for two- to three-week periods during the internship semester (January through May 1971). The only previously described project evaluation tool which was available for these students was the log diary; however, immediately prior to his internship semester and immediately after his nursing home experience, each student was asked to submit ten statements descriptive of "how you feel about working with geriatric patients or about working in a nursing home." The investigators hoped that this would provide some rough measure of attitudinal change. Final project evaluation will be based on data gathered throughout the project's five-year duration. This preliminary report includes the preaffiliation and postaffiliation attitudinal statements written by two students during the first complete year of the project. They are representative of materials prepared by the eight project participants and are intended to serve only as a positive indication of the quality of the attitudinal changes which have occurred following a nursing home internship.

Student One

1. Preaffiliation attitudes
   a. I think it is difficult to relate to the older patient.
   b. I really don't feel confident with the older patient.
   c. It is hard to motivate geriatric patients.
   d. I don't know how to interact with the patient in terms of the problems that he may be subjected to.
   e. Working with geriatric patients is discouraging because of the limited goals.
   f. I am afraid I would get into a routine with the patients.
   g. Aides in this type of situation are familiar with the routine and may be hard to work with.
   h. The routine of seeing the same type of patient may not be stimulating.
   i. I'm not too excited about going.
2. Postaffiliation attitudes
   a. The patients are very challenging.
   b. Geriatric patients are very enjoyable to

work with.

c. Patients in a nursing home need a great deal of stimulation.

d. Geriatric patients must be treated in terms of their individual needs.

e. They do not linger on their personal problems.

f. Working in a nursing home can be very stimulating.

g. The patients can improve and markedly.

h. Geriatric patients can be very inspiring.

i. You need an inventive mind for treatments because of patients' other complications.

j. Patients in a nursing home are similar, if not exactly the same, as patients found in a general hospital.

Student Two

1. Preaffiliation attitudes

   a. Right now, the last place I would care to work in is a nursing home.

   b. Seeing mostly old people every day would tend to get me down.

   c. I don't think I have the type of patience needed to work with geriatric patients.

   d. Most of the experiences I have had with old people have been less than pleasant; these experiences have turned me off to working with old people.

   e. Whenever I have visited a nursing home, I have come away depressed. There always seems to be so much sadness and loneliness that I don't think I could take it every day.

   f. Geriatric patients often present other medical and psychological problems than just their major complaint. I'm not sure I can effectively cope with all these aspects of these patients.

   g. I feel such an age difference between me and geriatric patients that I often find it difficult to communicate with them.

   h. A nursing home does not generally have a rapid turnover of patients; I think I might get tired of the same patient all the time.

   i. I just don't feel geared to working with old people. I guess they're just not my thing.

   j. I guess I never considered a nursing home as a stimulating atmosphere in which to work.

2. Postaffiliation attitudes

   a. I did not look forward to this affiliation but now that it's over I can say that I really enjoyed myself.

   b. Before my affiliation here, I felt that physical therapy was almost wasted on old people. Now I see that it does have definite value in this situation.

   c. Physical therapy for geriatric patients can help these people to become more independent and less of a "problem" to the nursing staff.

   d. I would now seriously consider working in a nursing home some day. Before my affiliation here, I would never have considered this.

   e. I went into this affiliation with a definitely negative and apprehensive attitude and I came out with a decidedly positive attitude toward geriatric work.

   f. So many of these patients were such hard workers—they even requested more physical therapy than they were already getting.

   g. Geriatric work is very rewarding, as much for the emotional gains one makes as the physical gains.

   h. I felt that physical therapy, especially the group therapy sessions, was a good socializing factor as well as physical help.

   i. I think geriatric patients are probably generally the most appreciative and hard working patients around.

   j. I would not trade my nursing home experience for the world. It really changed my attitude about elderly people.

SUMMARY

In response to a need to develop a geriatric clinical educational experience for undergraduate physical therapy students, the Department of Physical Therapy was awarded a Rehabilitation Services Administration training grant to establish a clinical instruction unit in a nursing home. With the development of criteria, an attempt is being made to evaluate the effect of clinical education in a nursing home on the attitudes of undergraduate physical therapy students toward geriatric patients and toward being employed in a nursing home after graduation. Four evaluation tools have been presented which will be utilized throughout the project's five-year duration: attitude scale, log diary, forced selection schema, and longitudinal employment study.

Developing a model for evaluation of student attitude change toward a specific patient sample in a specific clinical setting has generated implications for further study. Stated in general terms, what influence does exposure of students to any type of clinical educational facility have on choice of future employment setting? Is there a recency-primacy effect, such that the student's first (primacy) or final affiliation (recency) is more influential in his decision-making toward desired site of employment?

Acknowledgment. Frank L. Husted, Ed.D., Dean, School of Allied Health Professions, Temple University, Philadelphia, Pennsylvania, is the evaluation consultant for this project.

REFERENCES

1. Tuckman J, Lorge I: The projection of personal symptom into stereotype about aging. J Gerontol 13:70-73, 1958
2. Coe RM: Professional perspectives in the aged. Gerontologist 7:114-119, 1967
3. Husted FL: The Application of Educational Principles of Evaluation of Industrial Supervisory Training. Unpublished doctoral dissertation. Buffalo, University of Buffalo, 1961

THE AUTHORS

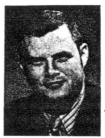

Carl T. Anderson received a B.S. degree in physical education from Augustana College, and a certificate and master's degree in physical therapy from the University of Iowa. Currently he is Coordinator, Rural Health Manpower Project, Regional Medical Program for Western New York, and Clinical Assistant Professor, Department of Physical Therapy, State University of New York at Buffalo.

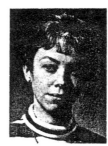

Kathryn A. Sawner received her B.S. in physical therapy from the State University of New York at Buffalo. She was a staff physical therapist at the New York State Rehabilitation Hospital, West Haverstraw, New York, before joining the faculty of the Department of Physical Therapy, State University of New York at Buffalo. She is currently director of clinical education and assistant professor in physical therapy, State University of New York at Buffalo, with major interests in clinical education of physical therapy students and training of the hemiplegic patient.

Career Profile of and Feedback from Graduates of a Midwest Curriculum

PATRICIA A. HAGEMAN

The purpose of this survey study was to create a career-activity profile of all physical therapy graduates from the University of Nebraska Medical Center (1972–1985) and to gather evaluative information for the planning of a postbaccalaureate entry-level degree program for physical therapy. A majority of the survey respondents (91%) were employed in physical therapy when the survey was made and were satisfied with their undergraduate program. A majority of the respondents resided in Nebraska or surrounding states and identified similar changes within the physical therapy profession. The results supported the hypothesis that a negative correlation would exist between the salaries of full-time physical therapists and the size of the population they serve. Graduates' recommendations to increase clinical education and student exposure to specialties were included in the University of Nebraska's postbaccalaureate physical therapy degree proposal. This graduate feedback system was helpful with physical therapy program planning to meet the identified needs of this regional area.

Key Words: *Education, graduate; Education: physical therapist, general.*

Physical therapy educators continually are reassessing and updating their curricula to meet the changing needs of the profession. Educators currently are directing their efforts toward reevaluating, changing, and reconstructing physical therapy academic programs to meet the expanded didactic and clinical education requirements identified in the proposed *Standards for Accreditation* of entry-level physical therapy programs.[1] Educators also are responding to the strong nationwide support of postbaccalaureate entry-level education that was reflected in a unanimous vote of support by the 1986 House of Delegates.[2]

Educational programs must meet updated professional standards and should reflect and react to the needs of the regional area they serve. The primary goal of the University of Nebraska's physical therapy curriculum is to remedy the physical therapist shortages in the Midwest, especially in Nebraska and in rural areas of the surrounding states. Several studies indicate that graduates' assessment of their educational preparation for physical therapy practice is a valuable tool for evaluating a physical therapy curriculum.[3–7]

Previous formal follow-up studies of physical therapy graduates provided information about their employment and professional activities,[3–7] satisfaction with education,[3–7] and perception of change in physical therapy practice and prestige.[6] With the numerous changes occurring in physical therapy education, another assessment of a physical therapy program by the graduates is timely.

The specific purposes of this questionnaire follow-up study of the physical therapy graduates from the University of Nebraska were 1) to create a descriptive employment and career-activity profile of the University of Nebraska Medical Center's physical therapy graduates and 2) to gather evaluative information regarding their educational experience, recommendations for planning of a postbaccalaureate degree program, and perceived changes within the profession.

Relative to the need for physical therapists in rural areas, I hypothesized that an inverse relationship would be observed between the salaries of full-time therapists and the population density of the area the therapists served. Specifically, the more rural the area, the higher the salary.

METHOD

Procedure

The sample consisted of 218 graduates from the University of Nebraska Medical Center from 1972, the first graduating class, to 1985. A two-page questionnaire with an open- and closed-question format was used to collect the graduates' 1) personal data, 2) employment data, 3) professional activities, 4) evaluation of educational experience, 5) recommendations for future planning of a postbaccalaureate degree program, and 6) perception of changes within the profession in the last five years (Appendix). A cover letter explaining the questionnaire and a preaddressed stamped envelope were sent with the questionnaire. To ensure anonymity, the graduates were not asked to identify themselves by name and nonrespondents received no follow-up mailing. Only questionnaires returned within 60 days of mailing were analyzed.

Data Analysis

I calculated the survey's frequency of response, means, and percentages and computed a Spearman rank order correlation coefficient to test for a significant relationship between the salary of full-time therapists and the population of the region that they serve. A chi-square analysis was used to check the

P. Hageman, MS, is Assistant Professor, Division of Physical Therapy Education, University of Nebraska Medical Center, 42nd and Dewey Ave, Omaha, NE 68105 (USA).

This article was submitted August 28, 1986; was with the author for revision six weeks; and was accepted April 6, 1987. Potential Conflict of Interest: 4.

significance of the graduates' responses about perceived changes within the profession.

RESULTS

The rate of return for the questionnaire was 65%, with 141 graduates responding. Men represented 31% of the respondents and 32% of the total number of graduates.

Eighty-six (61%) of the respondents lived in Nebraska at the time of the survey, and 24 (17%) of the respondents resided in surrounding states. The remainder of the respondents lived in 17 other states.

Employment

One hundred twenty-eight (91%) of the respondents currently were employed in the field of physical therapy, 104 (81%) full time and 24 (19%) part time. The most frequently cited reasons for not being employed in physical therapy were related to raising a family or to changing careers.

Of the 128 respondents employed full time or part time in physical therapy who specified their job position, 47% were staff therapists, 21% were chiefs or directors of physical therapy, and 20% were self-employed.

The most common employment setting of the full-time physical therapists was reported as acute care hospitals (37%). Multiple settings was the second most common type of employment setting of the full-time therapists (24%). Numerous combinations of various settings were reported. One respondent, for example, practiced in acute care, extended care, and nursing home settings. Private practice settings ranked next, with 18% of the respondents employed full time.

Overall, 97% of the men and 88% of the women who responded to this survey were employed in physical therapy. Thirty percent of the men compared with 16% of the women were department chiefs or directors (Tab. 1). Twenty-six percent of the men and 16% of the women were self-employed. Full-time female therapists in this study earned less than full-time male physical therapists (Tab. 2). Sixty percent of the men employed full time reported annual earnings over $27,000, compared with 36% of the women employed full time.

Fifty-two percent of the respondents employed in physical therapy either full time or part time indicated that they practiced in areas with a population of 100,000 people or less. Fourteen percent worked in areas with 1,001 to 10,000 people, and 26% practiced in areas with a population of 10,001 to 50,000 people.

Professional Activities

This survey revealed that 84% of all respondents were members of the American Physical Therapy Association. Over 90% of the respondents perceived an increased need in the past five years for participation in continuing education. Eight-eight percent of the respondents attended the continuing education courses yearly, and 51% of these respondents attended more than 20 hours of continuing education a year.

Rating of Educational Experience

The survey asked graduates to describe specific aspects of their undergraduate physical therapy education using a five-point semantic scale (5 = outstanding, 4 = very satisfactory, 3 = satisfactory, 2 = marginal, and 1 = unsatisfactory). Over 95% of the respondents rated their overall educational experience at the University of Nebraska Medical Center as satisfactory or better, with 75% of these responses in the very satisfactory or outstanding categories.

The highest-rated curriculum content area was anatomy and basic science background, with 100% of the responses being very satisfactory or outstanding; 64% of these responses were in the outstanding category. The lowest-ranked curriculum content area was principles of administration, which 72% of the respondents rated satisfactory or outstanding. Although this was the lowest-ranked area, the majority of responses in this category were satisfactory or better.

Transition Recommendations

The most frequent response listed by graduates as the area that the faculty should emphasize when changing from a baccalaureate to a postbaccalaureate degree program was exposure to physical therapy specialties (31% of responses). Clinical experience was ranked second, with 28% of the responses. The remaining responses were divided among seven other areas (Tab. 3).

Perceived Changes

Chi-square analysis of graduates' responses to perceived changes within the practice of physical therapy over the past five years revealed that a significant number of respondents perceived changes in the following areas: 1) increased caseloads, 2) increased need for documentation, 3) increased prestige of physical therapists among physicians and other health care workers and in communities, 4) increased acceptance by physical therapists of autonomous

TABLE 1

Positions Held by Male and Female Physical Therapists Employed Full Time or Part Time (N = 128)

Position	Male		Female	
	n	%	n	%
Staff physical therapist	16	37.2	45	52.9
Chief-director	13	30.2	14	16.5
Senior physical therapist	1	2.3	8	9.4
Self-employed	11	25.6	14	16.5
Other	1	4.7	4	4.7
TOTAL	43	100.0	85	100.0

TABLE 2

Annual Income (Before Deductions) for Physical Therapists Employed Full Time

Annual Income Before Deductions	Total Number of Physical Therapists Employed Full Time	Men		Women	
		n	%	n	%
$18,001–$21,000	12	4	9.5	8	12.9
$21,001–$24,000	24	5	11.9	19	30.6
$24,001–$27,000	20	8	19.1	12	19.4
Over $27,000	47	25	59.5	22	35.5
No response	1			1	1.6
TOTAL	104	42	100.0	62	100.0

practice by a physical therapist, 5) increased numbers of open physical therapy referrals from physicians, and 6) increased need for continuing education (Tab. 4). A significant number of respondents perceived a decrease in the acceptance of physician-owned physical therapy services (POPTS) by physical therapists.

The graduates were asked to identify the greatest problem or challenge facing the physical therapy profession today. The three most frequently listed answers in a total of 27 different responses were: 1) the development of physical therapy as a profession (21%), 2) increasing public awareness of physical therapy (13%), and 3) practice without physician referral (11%). Other responses included

quality of care versus a large patient caseload (6%), research to justify the profession (5%), and justification of the physical therapist's status within the health care environment (4%). The remaining 40% of the responses were divided among 21 different answers.

DISCUSSION

The questionnaire response rate of 65% is good, because this study covered 14 years of graduates and no follow-up reminder was mailed. This response rate is similar to that of a study of Marquette University physical therapy graduates from 1956 to 1980 conducted by Morrison et al.[6] Data from therapists who did not respond to this study, however, could alter the results of this study.

Employment

This survey indicated that only 9% of the respondents were no longer employed as physical therapists. This dropout rate is similar to a 12% dropout rate reported by Morrison et al[6] and a 4.7% dropout rate published by Blood[7] of graduates from Stanford University (1970–1980). Morrison et al[6] suggested that the reduction in dropouts from physical therapy practice could be attributed to the trend in the 1970s and 1980s of increasing numbers of working women and two-salary households. Earlier studies by Worthingham of 1961 graduates[3] and by Conine of 1960 to 1970 graduates[5] showed much higher dropout rates of 32% and 23%, respectively.

The reported employment settings of physical therapists from the University of Nebraska are presented differently than in other studies because many of these graduates worked in multiple settings instead of in one type of employment facility. They described their employment as either separate practice settings or as multiple settings under the direction of one facility or corporation. Employment in multiple settings may be a reflection of the changing health care system, which often incorporates several settings (eg, nursing homes and extended care facilities) into one corporation. Many physical therapy departments are expanding their services to include nursing homes, home health

TABLE 3
Graduate Recommendations for Areas to Emphasize in a Postbaccalaureate Degree Physical Therapy Program

Area	Responses	
	n	%
Exposure to specialties	44	31.2
Clinical experience	39	27.7
Research	17	12.0
Classroom laboratory practice	11	7.8
Legal-ethical	9	6.4
Anatomy-basic science	8	5.7
Introduction to teaching skills	7	5.0
Other	4	2.8
No opinion	2	1.4
TOTAL	141	100.0

TABLE 4
Graduates' Perception of Changes in the Practice of Physical Therapy over the Past Five Years

Practice Area	Responses						χ^2
	Increase		No Change		Decrease		
	n	%	n	%	n	%	
Caseload (n = 141)	102	72.3	21	14.9	18	12.8	94.95*
Need for documentation (n = 140)	133	95.0	7	5.0	0	0.0	240.00*
Prestige of physical therapists among other health care workers (n = 140)	107	76.4	33	23.6	0	0.0	128.67*
Prestige of physical therapists among physicians (n = 138)	98	71.1	38	27.5	2	1.4	102.26*
Prestige of physical therapists among the community (n = 137)	101	73.8	34	24.8	2	1.4	111.78*
Number of open physician referrals for physical therapy (n = 136)	121	89.0	15	11.0	0	0.0	191.92*
Need for continuing education (n = 141)	129	91.5	11	7.8	1	0.7	215.66*
Acceptance by physical therapists of autonomous practice by physical therapists (n = 133)	98	73.7	32	24.1	3	2.2	106.93*
Acceptance by physicians of autonomous practice by physical therapists (n = 140)	33	23.6	87	62.1	20	14.2	54.10*
Acceptance by physical therapists of physician-owned physical therapy services (n = 133)	17	12.8	38	28.6	78	58.6	43.32*

*$df = 2$; $p < .001$.

TABLE 5

Relationship[a] Between Salaries of Physical Therapists Employed Full Time[b] and the Population of the Areas They Serve

Population of Area Served	Salary Ranges			
	$18,000–$21,000	$21,001–$24,000	$24,001–$27,000	Over $27,000
	Number of Therapists	Number of Therapists	Number of Therapists	Number of Therapists
1,001–10,000	0	0	1	7
10,001–20,000	2	0	1	5
20,001–50,000	0	8	5	7
50,001–100,000	2	3	1	7
100,001–300,000	1	6	3	8
Over 300,000	8	6	9	13

[a] $n = 103$, $r = -.20$, $p < .05$.
[b] 103 out of 104 full-time therapists responding.

agencies, school systems, and extended care facilities. Physical therapists in small communities may be more likely than those in larger communities to contract their services or to be employed in multiple settings.

The percentage of practicing physical therapists in acute care general hospitals traditionally is high. This percentage ranges from 30.5% reported by Blood[7] in 1984 to 56% reported by Conine[5] in 1972. The 37% of University of Nebraska graduates employed full time in an acute care setting is within this range. This percentage, however, may not reflect the total number of University of Nebraska graduates practicing in acute care settings, because those who practice in multiple settings may spend part of their time in an acute care setting.

The 18% of the respondents who work full time in private practice settings is much higher than the 7% reported in a 1982 study of Marquette University graduates[6] and the 3% from a 1972 study of Indiana University graduates.[5] The increased number of graduates who work in private practice settings may be the result of physical therapy promotion by the Private Practice Section of the APTA and greater acceptance of private practitioners within the medical community.

A primary concern of the University of Nebraska Board of Regents (the governing body for the University), is to meet the staffing needs for physical therapy in the state of Nebraska. The results of this study indicate that the majority of University of Nebraska physical therapy graduates remain in Nebraska or move to surrounding states, including states without a physical therapy education program such as South Dakota and Wyoming.

The majority of respondents lived in Nebraska (61%) or surrounding states (17%) with few densely populated areas. The survey results suggest that the University of Nebraska program is meeting its goal to fill physical therapy positions in the state and in less-densely populated areas.

A significant negative correlation was determined between the salary of full-time physical therapists and the size of population they serve using a Spearman rank order correlation ($r = -.20$, $p < .05$) (Tab. 5). Analysis of the data revealed that in smaller populations a greater percentage of physical therapists had a higher salary. This finding may be due to greater numbers of therapists in private practice in the rural areas or smaller communities paying professionals more to attract them to the area.

Strong overall differences in salary and employment status were observed between male and female graduates practicing physical therapy full time. This study did not attempt to identify or analyze confounding factors that could have influenced these differences. Kemp et al[8] studied therapists with similar employment profiles and found significant differences in salary and employment status between sexes. The Kemp et al study showed that male graduates were more likely than female graduates to earn a higher salary and to be self-employed or hold supervisory positions.[8] Kemp et al suggested that these trends may be due to men demonstrating a greater initiative in pursuing leadership positions and higher salaries. Women also may be more likely to interrupt their careers because of family responsibilities, which may affect their salary and status within the field.[8]

Perceived Changes in Physical Therapy

The University of Nebraska graduates perceived many changes in the practice of physical therapy over the past five years. Similar to 1982 Marquette University graduates,[6] University of Nebraska graduates perceived larger caseloads and an increased need for documentation and continuing education. Morrison et al[6] attributed such responses to the rising demand for accountability within the health care system by consumers.

In contrast with the Marquette University graduates,[6] University of Nebraska graduates perceived an increase in the prestige of physical therapy among physicians and other health care workers and in the community. This perception may have resulted from major regional marketing efforts by the Nebraska chapter of the APTA.[9] Perceived increases in open referrals from physicians may be a direct reflection of increased competencies demonstrated by physical therapists and improved relations between physicians and therapists.

Curriculum Planning Implications

The survey results about professional education and perceived changes within the profession were helpful in the evaluation and development of course offerings and instructional methods, especially during the development of the University of Nebraska Medical Center's postbaccalaureate degree proposal. The survey respondents highlighted strengths and weaknesses of the baccalaureate physical therapy program and gave suggestions for the postbaccalaureate program.

The anatomy and basic science courses required of the University of Nebraska physical therapy students appear, on the basis of this survey, to be an asset and will continue as part of the professional program. Administrative skills was identified as the weakest curriculum content area, similar to the findings of another program.[5] This component of the curriculum will be restructured and sequenced differently in the future. Graduates indicated that emphasizing administrative skills during the educational program would assist future graduates to meet the increased need for documentation of services, public relation activity, and cost accountability.

Although the goal of the professional entry-level degree of the University of

Nebraska program is to educate a qualified general practitioner, graduates of this program recommended that a postbaccalaureate degree program include greater exposure to physical therapy specialties and additional time for clinical education. The University of Nebraska's postbaccalaureate degree proposal included these recommendations in an effort to improve the patient care skills of new graduates. The new graduate may be better qualified to practice in rural areas if these recommendations are considered and implemented.

Care must be taken when applying the results of this study to other programs or regions of the country. Ongoing assessment of physical therapy programs by graduates helps the faculty improve the professional skills of their graduates through curriculum changes. Future studies should focus on responsibilities and difficulties encountered by graduates during their first professional position. Graduates' perceptions of changes in the physical therapy practice as the profession advances to a postbaccalaureate entry-level degree also should be noted.

CONCLUSIONS

The results of a questionnaire follow-up study of the graduates from the University of Nebraska Medical Center from 1972 to 1985 demonstrate that

1. University of Nebraska physical therapy graduates had a low dropout rate from the profession.
2. The majority of the graduates practiced in Nebraska or surrounding states, and these graduates accepted positions in rural areas.
3. A significant negative correlation existed between the salaries of full-time physical therapists and the size of the population they serve.
4. Male-female differences existed in employment characteristics including salary.
5. The graduates were satisfied with their professional educational experience and provided valuable feedback for evaluating this curriculum.
6. The graduates' perceptions of changes occurring within the profession were similar.

REFERENCES

1. Proposed standards for accreditation of education programs for the physical therapist: A preliminary report. Task Force on Revision of the Accreditation Standards and Criteria, Commission on Accreditation in Education of the American Physical Therapy Association, January 1986

2. Morton T: Board, House take actions on wide spectrum of issues: Full House supports raised entry level. Progress Report of the American Physical Therapy Association 15(7):1, 8, 1986

3. Worthingham CA: The 1961 and 1965 graduates of the physical therapy schools. Phys Ther 49:476–499, 1969

4. Nelson C: Evaluation of a physical therapy curriculum: A method. Phys Ther 51:1307–1311, 1971

5. Conine TA: A survey of the graduates of a professional physical therapy program. Phys Ther 52:855–861, 1972

6. Morrison MA, Linder MT, Aubert EJ: Follow-up of the graduates of one curriculum: 1956–1980. Phys Ther 62:1307–1312, 1982

7. Blood H: Entry-level master's degree: A decade of experience. Phys Ther 64:208–212, 1984

8. Kemp NI, Scholz CA, Sanford TL, et al: Salary and status differences between male and female physical therapists. Phys Ther 59:1095–1101, 1979

9. Morton T: Nebraska chapter wins four awards in APTA public relations contest. Progress Report of the American Physical Therapy Association 15(7):4, 6, 1986

APPENDIX
Examples of Questions Used in the Survey

Example: *EVALUATION OF YOUR PHYSICAL THERAPY EDUCATION PROGRAM*

Directions: Please circle the appropriate value that corresponds to your evaluation of each area.

```
5 = outstanding
4 = very satisfactory
3 = satisfactory
2 = marginal
1 = unsatisfactory
```

SPECIFIC AREA	RANK
1. Overall educational experience	5 4 3 2 1
2. Anatomy-basic science background	5 4 3 2 1

Example: *TRANSITION TO THE POSTBACCALAUREATE ENTRY-LEVEL PROGRAM*

Directions: In planning the curriculum for the transition to the postbaccalaureate degree program for physical therapists, the faculty especially needs to emphasize which area? (Check one only.)

_____ Anatomy-basic science background   _____ Teaching

_____ Classroom laboratory practice   _____ Research

_____ Clinical experience   _____ Legal-ethical issues

_____ Exposure to specialties   _____ Other (specify)
_____

Example: *PERCEPTION OF CHANGES IN THE PRACTICE OF PHYSICAL THERAPY OVER THE PAST FIVE YEARS*

Directions: Please circle the appropriate value to evaluate each area.

```
3 = increase
2 = no change
1 = decrease
```

AREA	RANK
1. Caseload	3 2 1
2. Need for documentation	3 2 1

Personality Characteristics and Expressed Career Choice of Graduating Physical Therapy Students

SUSAN ROVEZZI-CARROLL
and RONNIE LEAVITT

We examined the personality characteristics of physical therapy students (N = 45) who had different career goals. We used the Myers-Briggs Type Indicator and a brief demographic information sheet to collect data at the conclusion of the 1982 spring semester. Analyses of variance indicated statistically significant differences ($p < .01$) between those who desired careers as generalist clinicians versus specialist clinicians. The specialist group represented adaptive, curious problem solvers; the generalists demonstrated characteristics of precision, order, and preferences for routine procedure. The findings have implications for the job satisfaction of physical therapists and have ramifications for curriculum planning.

Key words: *Education, Personality assessment, Physical therapy.*

Stereotypical personality characteristics are frequently used to portray members of different occupational groups. Business persons are considered entrepreneurial; artists, creative and spontaneous; and lawyers, logical and convincing. Health-care professionals have also been subjects of such stereotyping. People generally consider the nurse as a caring helper; a physician, as bright and knowledgeable; and the physical therapist, as the enthusiastic muscle mover.

Both theoretical support and empirical documentation for stereotyping occupational groups by personality characteristics exist. One of the oldest approaches to career choice is the trait-factor theory that assumes a straightforward linking between a person's abilities and interests and the work world.[1] A modern version of the trait-factor theory is Davis's "birds of a feather" theory, which proposes that occupational groups exhibit increasingly homogeneous personality traits over time.[2]

A frequently used method of testing the trait-factor theory of career choice has been to extend it to groups of college students in the same curriculum. Here, researchers empirically relate personality traits to different major fields of study, and assume that these college students will ultimately represent an occupational membership in terms of specific personality traits.

Lehmann and Ikenberry,[3] Elton,[4] and Osipow et al[5] conducted classic studies of this nature by using traditional major fields of study. More recent inquiries comparing health-related major fields of study have been undertaken, and results have shown personality differences of practitioners exist also in the health fields.[6-13] Additionally, some researchers have examined personality differences within a health field to document subgroup personality differences. Medical students in specialty fields have been shown to possess differing personality characteristics.[14, 15] Studies of nursing students in specialty areas have produced similar findings.[16, 17]

The concept of specialization in physical therapy is not new. Official recognition of a trend toward specialization came in 1975, however, when the first special interest sections were approved by the American Physical Therapy Association. Specialization emerged as a response to new and meaningful needs of patients. In 1978, a task force report on specialization described the identification of specialty areas of advanced clinical competence as forging ahead into "new territories" and "trailblazing."[18] In the area of pediatrics, the petition to the APTA Board of Directors for the establishment of the specialty area in pediatrics claimed that entry-level physical therapists were not equipped to address maximally the needs of the expanding pediatric population who were often located in nontraditional health-care settings.[19]

Currently, the Board for the Certification of Advanced Clinical Competence formally recognizes six specialty areas in physical therapy. A meaningful research question is whether personality differences within subgroups of the physical therapy profession itself exist. The literature has substantively documented that physical therapists and students in training are highly "people-oriented" and empathic.[9, 12, 13] The specialization trend raises the possibility that physical therapists who choose specialty careers are different from those who select careers as generalist clinicians.

The purpose of the current study was to determine if statistically significant differences exist between graduating physical therapy students who expressed the career goal of generalist clinicians and those who expressed the career goal of specialist clinicians. Because the nature of the research was exploratory, the nondirectional, null hypothesis was no personality differences exist between graduating physical therapy students who desire generalist clinical careers and those who desire specialist clinical careers.

Dr. Rovezzi-Carroll is Assistant Professor, Graduate Program, School of Allied Health Professions, University of Connecticut, U-101, Storrs. CT 06268 (USA). When this article was written, she was Assistant Professor, Department of Physical Therapy, School of Allied Health Professions, University of Connecticut.

Ms. Leavitt is Assistant Professor, Department of Physical Therapy, School of Allied Health Professions, University of Connecticut.

This paper was presented at the Fifty-ninth Annual Conference of the American Physical Therapy Association, Kansas City, MO, June 14–18, 1983.

This article was submitted September 23, 1983; was with the authors for revision 19 weeks; and was accepted May 2, 1984.

TABLE 1
Comparison of Personality Characteristics on Myers-Briggs Type Indicator

Continuous Scores on Myers-Briggs Type Indicator	Generalist		Specialist	
	$\overline{X}$	s	$\overline{X}$	s
Extroversion and Introversion	85	28	93	26
Sensing and Intuition	82	26	99	18
Thinking and Feeling	110	31	116	18
Judging and Perceiving	79	28	104	26

METHOD

The sample was from the class of 1982 who were graduating with physical therapy degrees at the University of Connecticut School of Allied Health Professions (N = 45). The program of study in this postsecondary program included didactic, clinical, and interdisciplinary experiences with the awarding of a Bachelor of Science degree. Ninety-two percent of the sample were women; the mean chronological age was 22 years old.

We collected data by administering two instruments. The first instrument was the Myers-Briggs Type Indicator (MBTI). The MBTI is a personality test with a forced-choice, self-report inventory and it consists of 126 items with bipolar, nonthreatening responses. Four scales are used to measure personal preferences.

Extroversion and Introversion (E/I). A person who attends to the outer world of people and objects is an E. A person who prefers to focus on the inner world of ideas and reflects before engaging in action is an I.

Sensing and Intuition (S/N). A person who is realistic, observes by way of the senses, and works well with facts is an S. A person who is imaginative, idea-oriented, and good at problem solving is an N.

Thinking and Feeling (T/F). A person who is analytical and values impersonal, objective logic is a T. A person who weighs personal values, sympathizes, and believes that human dislikes and likes are important is an F.

Judging and Perceiving (J/P). A person who lives in an orderly and decided fashion is a J. A person who is flexible, adaptive, and spontaneous is a P.

Reliability data for the MBTI were reported by the split-half procedure and reflected coefficients mostly above .80. Validity data of both a congruent and concurrent nature were reported to be satisfactory, correlating with other personality measures and nonstandardized data.[20,21] The test has been used often to measure personality characteristics of health professionals.[10,12]

The second instrument was a brief, demographic information sheet that elicited career choice information. The key item asked respondents to select a career goal that they desired for themselves. Responses included the following: 1) generalist clinician, 2) specialist clinician (eg, pediatrics, orthopedics, or sports medicine), 3) researcher, 4) manager or administrator, 5) educator or faculty member, or 6) other. Most respondents chose the specialist clinician career goal (n = 28) and the generalist clinician career goal (n = 17). Five subjects selected other responses including research (n = 2), manager or administrator (n = 2), and educator or faculty member (n = 1). These subgroups were eliminated from the current study because of the small number of subjects in each subgroup.

We administered the two instruments to subjects during a two-hour testing session at the conclusion of the spring semester of the senior year. We explained to the subjects the purposes of the research and use of the data to ensure informed consent and voluntary participation. Anonymity was assured.

Data Analysis

We selected a one-way analysis of variance (ANOVA) for the statistical analysis. The independent variable was physical therapy career goal with two categories, generalist clinician (n = 17) and specialist clinician (n = 28). We used four separate dependent variables corresponding to the four scales of MBTI—Extroversion and Introversion, Sensing and Intuition, Thinking and Feeling, and Judging and Perceiving. The four ANOVAS were calculated by using the Statistical Package for the Social Sciences (SPSS) computer program.[22] We selected a probability level of $p < .01$ to determine statistical significance.

RESULTS

The results from the sample data indicated statistically significant differences between the two physical therapy groups on selected personality characteristics. Table 1 reports means and standard deviations. Specifically, we found statistically significant differences on the Sensing and Intuition scale ($F = 6.85$; $df = 1, 43$; $p < .01$) and the Judging and Perceiving scale ($F = 8.92$; $df = 1, 43$; $p < .01$). We found no statistically significant differences on the Extroversion and Introversion scale ($F = 1.05$; $df = 1, 43$; $p = NS$) or the Thinking and Feeling scale ($F = .61$; $df = 1, 43$; $p = NS$). Table 2 gives the ANOVA results.

The results demonstrated that significant personality differences ($p < .01$) existed between the physical therapy students who desired careers as generalist clinicians and who scored higher on the Sensing and Judging scale and those who desired to be specialist clinicians and who scored higher on the Intuitive and Perceiving scale. We rejected the null hypothesis. Both groups were homogeneous in their preferences for the categories of Extroversion and Feeling, a finding that corroborated previous research.[9,12,13]

TABLE 2
Analysis of Variance for Groups: Personality Characteristics

Source of Variation	df	SS	MS	F
Extroversion and Introversion	1	757	757	1.05
Error	43	31046	722	
Sensing and Intuition	1	3170	3170	6.85*
Error	43	19866	462	
Thinking and Feeling	1	328	328	0.61
Error	43	23177	539	
Judging and Perceiving	1	6406	6406	8.92*
Error	43	30874	718	

* Significant at $p < .01$.

DISCUSSION

According to the MBTI Manual, people who prefer the Sensing and Judging dimensions can be characterized as individuals who like to follow-through on plans and projects without interruption. These persons like routine and dislike new problems unless they have a standard way to solve them. Additionally, people who score high on the Sensing and Judging scale enjoy practicing old skills rather than learning new ones and become impatient with complicated details. They are precise individuals and make few errors based on their adherence to facts.[20]

On the other hand, people who score high on the Intuitive and Perceiving scale are very proficient at adapting to new situations, tend to be curious, and enjoy problem solving. They often work in bursts of energy, dislike routine, and sometimes make errors because of neglected precision. They have a propensity to work in less familiar situations, are patient when complications arise, and welcome new innovative solutions to problems.[20]

Specialist Clinician

The findings suggest a meaningful link between personality characteristics and expressed career choice. The specialist clinician group scored as curious, adaptive problem solvers; the generalist scored as precise, routine-oriented, and procedural. Although the literature is limited with regard to the topic of specialization in physical therapy, the specialists will clearly be called on to pioneer into new theoretical territories, pursue research inquiry, and develop clinical knowledge and practice in their designated specialty.[18] Possessing problem-solving characteristics appears congruent with the specialists' role responsibilities.

Specialists will probably be employed in nontraditional settings. The mandate of PL 94-142 in its clause of "least restrictive settings" indicates that physical therapists, as specialists, will be employed more regularly in public schools. Other sites include business and industrial settings, community agencies, and athletic training facilities. In these nontraditional settings, physical therapists with specialized knowledge will be required to deal with complex patient problems. Furthermore, the physical therapist will interact with a diversified collection of professionals and lay persons. In an educational setting alone, Mullins describes the physical therapist as part of a transdisciplinary team working with educators, administrators, parents, private agency personnel, union officials, and school staff.[23] Nontraditional health-care settings, diversified and complex patient problems, and the transdisciplinary team concept necessitate that the physical therapist specialist be adaptive, flexible, innovative, and comfortable with ambiguity.

Generalist Clinician

The generalist clinician group from this study appeared to prefer routine tasks, precision, and certainty. These characteristics are congruent with the generalist clinicians' role responsibilities. The generalist clinicians will most likely practice their skills in a more traditional physical therapy setting. This may take the form of a general hospital or rehabilitation center, well-equipped with human and technological resources for physical therapy.[19] Such a setting may follow a daily routine of scheduling patients, record keeping, staff meetings, and other time delineations. Because the patients will represent the more typical and traditional physical therapy problems, the generalist can also adhere to established protocol. Interaction will rest predominantly with members of health-related professions, providing more peer contact, and allowing the generalists to practice skills on their own "turf." Traditional health-care settings, adherence to daily routines, typical patient problems, and the predominance of health-professional service delivery appear to be compatible with the personality characteristics of the generalist clinician who prefers to function in an ordered and certain environment, practice traditional skills, and apply well-known and familiar solutions to problems.

Practical Implications

This study has practical implications for both physical therapy faculty and their students. Faculty advisors may find the additional information regarding personality characteristics and career choices helpful in counseling high school students and transfer students applying to the physical therapy program. Also, the same information would be useful to graduates of the program, as they leave postsecondary education and enter the world of work. Selecting employment sites that are congruent with personality preferences may contribute to job satisfaction and job stability.

The results of the current study have ramifications for curriculum planning. Students in the two groups studied may have different learning style preferences. Students who desire a generalist experience may grow and respond cognitively to concrete, task-oriented learning experiences. Students who desire a specialist experience, however, may demand a flexible, nonstructured approach to learning. Faculty members should be responsive to such preferences. Additionally, faculty members may determine that both sets of students need to nurture the preferences of their counterpart peer group. Specialist-oriented students may need to emphasize development of organizational skills; generalist-oriented students might benefit from more problem-solving tasks. Both sets of personality characteristics appear imperative for physical therapists to function optimally in the complex health-care system.

CONCLUSION

We found statistically significant differences between graduating physical therapy students who desired generalist clinician experience and those who desired specialist clinician experience. The specialists were more adaptive problem solvers. The generalists were routine-oriented and comfortable with procedure and stability.

These findings necessitate further research. As specialists in the field of physical therapy increase, research might compare personality characteristics of actual specialists with generalist clinicians. Classifications might be extended among the specialty areas, for instance, to compare sports physical therapy with pediatrics or with cardiopulmonary or with other specialties. Such investigations will enrich the understanding of the current and future professional membership at a critical time when roles of physical therapists in the health-care arena are becoming more complex, diversified, and dynamic.

REFERENCES

1. Parsons F: Choosing a Vocation. Boston, MA, Houghton Mifflin Co, 1967 (Reprinted from 1909 edition)
2. Davis JA: Great Aspirations: Career Decisions and Educational Plans During College. Chicago, IL, National Opinions Research Center, 1965, vol 1, no. 90
3. Lehmann IJ, Ikenberry SO: Critical Thinking, Attitudes and Values in Higher Education. East Lansing, MI, Michigan State University Press, 1967
4. Elton CT: Male career role and vocational choice: The prediction with personality variables. Journal of Counseling Psychology 14:99–105, 1967
5. Osipow S, Ashby J, Wall H: Personality types and vocational choice: A test of Holland's theory. Personnel and Guidance Journal 45:37–42, 1966
6. Rovezzi-Carroll S, Fitz P: Predicting major fields of study in allied health education with selected personality characteristics. College Student Journal (18)1:43–51, 1984
7. Dunteman GH: Characteristics of Students in Health Related Professions. Gainesville, FL, University Presses of Florida, 1966
8. Bergman JS: A Comparative Study of Certain Personality Characteristics of Students Enrolled in Selected Health Programs at the University of Alabama. Doctoral dissertation. Birmingham, AL, University of Alabama, 1974
9. Holstrom EL: Changing characteristics of students in health fields. J Allied Health 4:9–13, 1975
10. Rezler AG, Buckley JM: A comparison of personality types among female student health professionals. J Med Educ 52:475–477, 1977
11. Rezler AG, French RM: Personality types and learning preferences of six allied health professions. J Allied Health 4:20–26, 1975
12. McCaully MH: Application of the MBTI to Medicine and Other Health Professions. Monograph 1. Washington, DC, US Dept of Health, Education, and Welfare, 1978
13. Wellock LM: Comparison of opinions, attitudes, and interests of physical therapy students with other students at the University of Michigan. Phys Ther 55:371–375, 1975
14. Otis GD, Weiss JR: Patterns of medical career preference. J Med Educ 48:116–123, 1973
15. Schoenfield J, Donner L: The effect of serving as a psychotherapist on students with different specialty preferences. J Med Educ 47:203–209, 1972
16. Reavley W, Wilson LJ: Personality structure of general and psychiatric nurses: A comparison. Int J Nurs Stud 9:225–234, 1972
17. Tronnes HF: A Comparative Study of Personality Characteristics Among Selected Nursing Specialties in a Voluntary Nonprofit General Acute Hospital. Thesis. Minneapolis, MN, University of Minnesota, 1966
18. Task force report: Certification of advanced clinical competence may come before 1978 House. Progress Report of the American Physical Therapy Association 7(1):10–11, 1978
19. Petition to Board of Directors. Washington, DC, Pediatrics Section of the American Physical Therapy Association, 1980
20. Myers IB: The Myers-Briggs Type Indicators Manual. Princeton, NJ, Educational Testing Service, 1962
21. Stricker LJ, Ross J: Intercorrelations and reliability of the MBTI scales. Psychol Rep 12:287–293, 1963
22. Nie NH, Hull CH, Jenkins JG, et al: Statistical Package for the Social Sciences. New York, NY, McGraw-Hill Inc, 1970
23. Mullins J: New challenges for physical therapy practitioners in educational settings. Phys Ther 61:496–502, 1981

Clinical
Education
Consortia

Texas Consortium for Physical Therapy Clinical Education

A Model for Interinstitutional Consortium Arrangements

SANDRA RADTKA,
NANCY DRAGOTTA,
SUZANNE NEEDHAM,
SUSAN S. SMITH,
and JUNE TUCKER

This article describes the Texas Consortium for Physical Therapy Clinical Education, which exemplifies one type of collaborative arrangement among universities. Coordination of physical therapy clinical education among five Texas universities is the major function of the Texas Consortium. Although originally developed from a federally funded project (1977–1980), it currently functions with sole financial support from the participating universities. The collaborative efforts of the Texas Consortium have resulted in 1) developing and implementing a common evaluation tool for students' clinical performance; 2) coordinating development of new clinical education centers, development of clinical instructors, and visits to students at clinical education centers; and 3) developing and using a shared computer program for data on clinical education centers. The successful functioning of the Texas Consortium with a resultant decrease in duplication of time, effort, and costs of clinical education demonstrates that this type of arrangement is feasible and beneficial.

Key Words: *Academic medical centers; Education, clinical; Physical therapy; University consortia.*

Development of educational alliances among various universities or between departments within a university was cited as an important recommendation for allied health fields by the National Commission on Allied Health Education.[1] Collaborative arrangements among academic physical therapy programs for coordination of clinical education exemplify one type of educational alliance. The results of the Project on Clinical Education in Physical Therapy by the Section for Education of the American Physical Therapy Association included a recommendation for the formation of these regional planning committees or consortium arrangements for physical therapy clinical education.[2] It was suggested that the goals of these committees include improved use of current clinical education centers, development of new clinical education centers in underutilized areas, and expansion of learning opportunities within clinical education centers.

The Texas Consortium for Physical Therapy Clinical Education is one of several consortium arrangements for physical therapy clinical education programs that have developed during the past five years.[3] The successful functioning of the Texas Consortium demonstrates that this type of cooperative effort is feasible and beneficial. It can serve as a model for other physical therapy programs interested in developing similar alliances.

ORGANIZATION OF THE TEXAS CONSORTIUM

The academic coordinators of clinical education (ACCEs) from the Texas physical therapy programs

Ms. Radtka was Academic Coordinator of Clinical Education, Texas Woman's University, School of Physical Therapy, Denton, TX. She is currently a doctoral student at the University of California at Berkeley.

Mrs. Dragotta is Academic Coordinator of Clinical Education, Program in Physical Therapy, University of Texas at San Antonio, University of Texas Health Science Center, San Antonio, TX 78285.

Major Needham was Academic Coordinator of Clinical Education, Program in Physical Therapy, US Army-Baylor University, Fort Sam Houston, TX 78234.

Mrs. Smith was Academic Coordinator of Clinical Education and currently is an Instructor, Department of Physical Therapy, University of Texas Health Science Center at Dallas, Dallas, TX 75235.

Ms. Tucker was Project Coordinator for the Texas Consortium for Physical Therapy Clinical Education, Texas Woman's University, Houston, TX 77030.

Address correspondence to Ms. Radkta, 3597 Somerset, Castro Valley, CA 94546 (USA).

This article was submitted August 31, 1981; was with the author for revision 24 weeks; and was accepted for publication December 1, 1982.

collaborated on the initial development of a grant proposal for the Physical Therapy Consortium for Clinical Education in Texas.[4] The proposal was awarded an Allied Health Special Improvement Project Grant with funding from 1977 to 1980 at Texas Woman's University in Houston. The participants in the consortium were a project coordinator, an administrative secretary, and the ACCEs from the five Texas physical therapy programs at Texas Woman's University at Denton, Dallas, and Houston, University of Texas Health Science Center at Dallas, University of Texas Medical Branch at Galveston, University of Texas Health Science Center at San Antonio, and U.S. Army-Baylor University at Fort Sam Houston. Additional consultants for part of the project included education and evaluation experts and eight physical therapy clinicians representing various clinical settings and geographical areas.

The original purposes of the project were 1) to develop statewide planning among the physical therapy programs; 2) to facilitate assessment and development of new and current clinical education centers; 3) to improve patterns of utilizing clinical education centers; 4) to improve coordination among the physical therapy programs in Texas and between the academic and the clinical portions of their curricula; and 5) to enhance the quality of learning experiences in clinical education.

After federal funding for the project was terminated, the participating physical therapy programs assumed sole financial responsibility for continuing the cooperative arrangement. The current committee for the Texas Consortium consists of the five ACCEs, with one member appointed chairman on an annual basis. The consortium functions through a system of individually delegated and shared responsibilities and develops new projects as well as continues the original goals of the grant.

PRODUCTS OF THE TEXAS CONSORTIUM

Major products resulted from the original project, and many products have been expanded by the current Texas Consortium. These include Mastery and Assessment of Clinical Skills (Blue MACS), workshops for clinical instructors, computerized data on clinical education centers, development of new clinical education centers, shared visits to students at clinical education centers, student evaluation of clinical education, and a master clinical affiliation schedule.

Blue MACS

One of the most significant accomplishments of the Texas Consortium was the development and implementation of a common evaluation tool for assessing physical therapy students' clinical performance. The Blue MACS is a competency-based and criterion-referenced evaluation tool.[5] Developing the instrument was a coordinated effort involving consortium members, consultants, and numerous physical therapy clinicians at various centers. After pilot tests, the first edition was implemented in 1979 by all five Texas physical therapy programs. The instrument has been revised twice based on feedback from physical therapy students and clinical instructors. It is anticipated that the instrument will continue to require periodic updating to reflect changes in the practice of physical therapy.

Several physical therapy programs outside of Texas are currently using the Blue MACS. The Texas Consortium continues to present workshops on the development, purposes, and use of the Blue MACS to those in programs who are interested. In addition, communication is maintained with those programs using the Blue MACS in order to promote mutual sharing of information on its implementation and suggestions for future revisions.

Workshops for Clinical Instructors

The presentation of combined workshops for all clinical instructors participating in the Texas Consortium is another important product. The workshops are planned and conducted by the consortium. Various aspects of clinical teaching, training sessions on using the Blue MACS, and separate business meetings for each of the program's clinical instructors are included in these workshops. Initially, two consortium members had federal funds for clinical education workshops. These funds were used to financially support the combined workshops. Currently, the federal funds are not available, and the workshops are being sponsored by each consortium member on a rotating basis.

Computerized Data on Clinical Education Centers

Another important achievement is the development of a computer program to store data on the clinical education centers used by Texas Consortium members. The staff members from each clinical education center complete a revised version of a document, "Self-Assessment of the Clinical Education Site in Physical Therapy," that was originally developed by the Project on Clinical Education in Physical Therapy.[2] This document enables those in both the clinical education center and the academic program to evaluate whether the center meets the Standards for Clinical Education Centers in Physical Therapy.[6]

Data collected from these forms are entered into the computer and retrieved on computer print-outs available to any consortium member. Print-outs include a mailing list of clinical centers, a cross-referenced directory of clinical centers, and all pertinent clinical center information required for accreditation reports. All consortium members share computer storage costs and also have individual costs computed for entering, editing, and printing the data. The information is updated annually so that current accreditation reports may be obtained.

Development of New Clinical Education Centers

Members also cooperate in the development of new clinical education centers. On-site evaluation visits to potential clinical education centers are made by one member. A common form, "Summary Evaluation of a Clinical Education Site in Physical Therapy," that was originally developed by the Project on Clinical Education in Physical Therapy[2] is completed by the ACCE visiting the center. This information is shared with other Texas Consortium members interested in initiating affiliations with the center.

Shared Visits to Students at Clinical Education Centers

Many clinical education centers affiliate with more than one of the Texas physical therapy programs. This results in simultaneous placement of students from these different programs at one center for clinical education. Members of the Texas Consortium save time by visiting one another's students during periods of maximal use of the clinical education centers. The ACCE conducting a visit is provided with information from the other ACCEs about the various students before the visit. A common report form, "Record of Student Supervision During Affiliations," is completed after the visit and sent to the appropriate ACCE.

Student Evaluation of Clinical Education

Another cooperative project of the Texas Consortium is the implementation of common forms for student evaluation of clinical education. One form that was originally developed by the Project on Clinical Education in Physical Therapy,[2] "Evaluation of the Individual Assignment," is used by students to evaluate the affiliation at the individual clinical education center. Another form that also originated from the Project on Clinical Education in Physical Therapy,[2] "Overview of Total Experience," is used by students to evaluate their total clinical education program. Both forms were revised to be used with a computer and to reflect changes suggested by Texas Consortium members.

Master Clinical Affiliation Schedule

A master clinical affiliation schedule of the dates of affiliations for the five physical therapy programs and the four physical therapist assistant programs in Texas is developed annually. The ACCEs can determine peak and low times for clinical affiliations in this geographical area by reviewing the master schedule. This information enables them to plan for clinical center availability and to project future changes in affiliation scheduling. Also, the staffs of clinical education centers can review the affiliation dates and plan more effectively for the utilization of their center.

COSTS OF THE TEXAS CONSORTIUM

Costs of initial development of consortium arrangements are dependent on the extent of proposed goals and activities for cooperative efforts. Because of the broad scope of the intended projects, the initial cost of developing the Texas consortium averaged $52,000 annually for three years and was provided by federal grant funds. Sixty-six percent of this figure represented personnel costs for the project director and secretary. Approximately 8 percent represented consultant services, 12 percent travel expenses, 4 percent equipment and supplies, and 10 percent other costs including computer programing and printing.

Since termination of the federal grant project, each consortium member provides travel monies of approximately $350 a year for their ACCE to attend three or four consortium meetings and one annual combined clinical instructors' workshop. This figure reflects the large geographical area included in this consortium. Travel costs can be reduced if phone communication and written correspondence are substituted for meetings.

Computer costs range from $200 to $300 annually for each consortium member, depending on the number of clinical education centers used by the program. Other costs absorbed by each university participating in the consortium include secretarial support, supplies, postage, printing, phone, and time for the ACCE to continue implementing and developing consortium goals. The annual combined clinical instructors' workshop represents another major expense. The workshop is sponsored and funded by one of the consortium members on a rotating basis.

ADVANTAGES AND DISADVANTAGES OF COOPERATIVE ARRANGEMENTS

Many benefits have been derived from the collaborative efforts of the Texas Consortium, including a decrease in the duplication of time, effort, and costs of clinical education for the clinical education centers and more effective use of the financial resources and personnel of the academic programs. In addition, increased communication between the clinical education centers and academic programs has resulted in better integration of the clinical and the academic portions of the curricula.

Clinical instructors have expressed satisfaction in using a uniform clinical education evaluation tool.

Consistent use of the Blue MACS has decreased training time for new clinical instructors. Workshops for clinical instructors using the Blue MACS have resulted in more uniform, objective clinical evaluation of students. In addition, combined workshops involving all Texas programs have meant less clinical instructor time away from their facilities.

Those in clinical education centers have realized a decrease in the duplication of paperwork as a result of computerizing clinical center information and sharing it among consortium members. Shared visits to students at clinical centers by ACCEs have decreased clinical instructor time spent in scheduling and meeting with visiting ACCEs. Cooperative development of new clinical education centers by consortium members has decreased duplication of paperwork for those in both the academic programs and the clinical centers. In addition, the staff members in academic programs have realized a reduction in time and travel expense for clinical center visits.

A consortium is not developed without difficulties, however. Considerable time is spent by ACCEs on consortium projects. Because of the high attrition rate among ACCEs, significant initial training time is required to orient new ACCEs to consortium procedures. Also, there is concern about the equitable distribution and prompt execution of individual and shared consortium responsibilities. Obtaining interinstitutional cooperation on joint financial arrangements, scheduling clinical affiliations, and coordinating academic calendars is a continual challenge. Limited travel, maintenance, and operation budgets for universities and clinical centers may restrict some collaborative efforts. Many of these problems, however, can be partially alleviated by administrative support and commitment from individuals in universities and clinical centers.

FUTURE GOALS AND POTENTIAL APPLICATION

The Texas Consortium has identified several potential projects for future development. With implementation of the third edition of the Blue MACS, the Texas Consortium plans to conduct interrater reliability and concurrent validity studies on the instrument. Other long-range plans include the development of additional computer programs using the current data on clinical education centers. One potential program would identify available clinical learning experiences to ensure students of a well-rounded exposure to all competencies necessary for entry into the profession. Another possibility includes developing computerized scheduling of students for clinical affiliations. Analysis of students' evaluation of the individual clinical education center would also be a useful computer program.

Cooperative planning for clinical education could expand to other programs in the region, resulting in a regional planning committee for clinical education. Such expanded collaborative efforts could result in increased shared visits of students at clinical education centers, more combined workshops for clinical instructors, and better utilization of existing and new clinical education centers. With decreasing resources available to academic programs and clinical education centers, regional coordination would be cost-effective.

CONCLUSIONS

A consortium for the coordination of clinical education among five Texas physical therapy programs has resulted in decreased duplication of time, effort, and costs associated with clinical education. The successful functioning of the Texas Consortium demonstrates that this type of cooperative association is feasible and beneficial. The Texas Consortium can serve as a model for staff in other programs interested in developing similar arrangements. It may also serve as the beginning framework for an expanded regional approach to cooperative clinical education planning.

Acknowledgments. The assistance of the following is gratefully acknowledged: Ann Langley, Don Woerz, Mary Lucas, and June Tucker, who served as ACCEs for Texas Woman's University, University of Texas Health Science Center at Dallas, U.S. Army-Baylor University, and University of Texas Medical Branch at Galveston, respectively, and participated in the initial development of the project; Nancy Watts, PhD, and Martyn Hotvedt, PhD, consultants to the project; Linda Herson, secretary for the project; all ACCEs serving on the advisory board of the project; physical therapy clinical consultants to the project; and clinical instructors in the Texas Consortium.

REFERENCES

1. National Commission on Allied Health Education: The Future of Allied Health Education. San Francisco, CA, Jossey-Bass Inc, Publishers, 1980, pp 201–203
2. Moore ML, Perry JF: Clinical Education in Physical Therapy: Present Status/Future Needs. Washington, DC, Section for Education, American Physical Therapy Association, 1976, pp 2.11–2.12
3. Newman J, Pittenger M: Education for the 1980s: Student Performance Evaluation Through Consortium Efforts. Read at the American Physical Therapy Association Combined Sections Meeting, Reno, NV, 1981
4. Final Report on the Physical Therapy Consortium for Clinical Education in Texas. Allied Health Special Improvement Project, Grant #5-D12-AH80206-03, Department of Health, Education and Welfare. Houston, TX, Texas Woman's University, 1980
5. Texas Consortium for Physical Therapy Education: Blue MACS or Mastery and Assessment of Clinical Skills. Galveston, TX, University of Texas Medical Branch, 1981
6. Barr JS, Gwyer J, Talmore Z: Standards for Clinical Education in Physical Therapy: A Manual for Evaluation and Selection of Clinical Education Centers. Washington, DC, American Physical Therapy Association, 1980

Experience with a Consortium for Exploring and Arranging Clinical Education Programs

PAULETTE M. KONDELA, MS,
and TERRY HATMAKER, MPH

The Clinical Allied Health Education Center, a prototypic agency, was established to assist in addressing clinical education issues of various allied health professions within the western half of lower Michigan. The agency aids in coordinating the clinical phase of the education of students in the educational programs. In the process of establishing new clinical education sites, the individuals involved in the physical therapy educational program and at the potential site address issues related to the exploration, evaluation, development, and implementation of the clinical education program. The experience and process in establishing the relationship between the Curriculum in Physical Therapy at the University of Michigan and the Clinical Allied Health Education Center are described.

EXPLORATION, EVALUATION, DEVELOPMENT, AND IMPLEMENTATION

The exploration of potential clinical education sites by individuals involved in physical therapy educational programs presupposes a need. This need could be influenced by many factors including: 1) an increased number of students to be placed, 2) a decrease in the number of ongoing commitments from clinical education sites, 3) a desire to expand the educational program in order to meet a variety of objectives, or 4) a desire to expand the educational program geographically in order to provide students with variations in experiences based upon urban-rural factors or upon ethnic considerations. Once a need is clearly established, the individuals involved in the educational program survey the availability of potential clinical education sites either by directly contacting persons at the site or indirectly acquiring information from individuals who have knowledge about the site. At this time, the persons involved in the educational program begin to evaluate the potential site according to estab-

lished criteria. Standards to be considered in this exploration and evaluation have been clearly described by Moore and Perry.[1]

Following the initial exploration, evaluation, and subsequent interest expressed in further negotiation by persons at the facility, a representative or representatives from the educational program conduct an on-site visit to further evaluate the site, to respond to questions, and to describe the procedures to be implemented. Steps to formulate a mutually acceptable agreement for affiliation are initiated once a decision to establish a clinical education program is made by individuals involved in the educational program and persons at the new facility.

The clinical education program is implemented according to the terms of the formal agreement. Students are assigned to the facility and progress through their clinical experience. Procedures which are mutually acceptable to individuals at the clinical education site and at the educational program are followed.

Although the steps previously described appear to be simple, the process of establishing several new clinical education sites at the same time can be time-consuming and complicated. Attempts to coordinate the exploration and development of multiple sites concurrently require careful planning in order to utilize time and manpower most efficiently.

Ms. Kondela is Instructor in Physical Therapy and Coordinator of Clinical Education, Department of Physical Medicine and Rehabilitation, University of Michigan, Ann Arbor, MI 48109.

Mr. Hatmaker, at the time this article was written, was Assistant to the Director, Clinical Allied Health Education Center, Grand Rapids, MI 49503.

TABLE 1

*Services Provided by Clinical Allied Health
Education Center*

Administrative Services:

Central scheduling—Scheduling of all clinical experiences for allied health students from member institutions. This includes exploration of new clinical sites and scheduling of interinstitutional rotations whenever possible.

Formal agreements development—Developing contractual agreements with member institutions for specific services and financial support.

Financial management—Developing a cost-accounting mechanism to analyze clinical education costs.

Staffing—Developing the mechanisms for joint appointments of clinical faculty, including fiscal arrangements, and articulation of responsibilities and lines of authority.

Instructional Development Services:

Faculty development—Pre-service and in-service programs in teacher education.

Continuing education—Formal and informal courses and workshops in allied health disciplines.

Evaluation—Providing consultation for both academic and clinical areas including the accreditation process.

Informational Services:

Community education—Developing materials depicting allied health clinical education.

Communications system—Developing a feedback system for students, faculty, and administration.

Resource center—Establishing an area center to provide information and counseling in various allied health disciplines.

Publications—Preparing and disseminating newsletters, journal articles, and monographs when appropriate.

CLINICAL ALLIED HEALTH EDUCATION CENTER

The Clinical Allied Health Education Center in Grand Rapids, Michigan, is a consortium of educational and health care institutions which is designed to function as a national prototype for the systemization and coordination of the clinical phase of the education of allied health students. The Center was funded through 1977 by a contract agreement with the Division of Associated Health Professions of the Department of Health, Education, and Welfare. More than 20 allied health professions are served by the Center. Among them are physical therapy, medical records, respiratory therapy, medical technology, and nuclear medicine. The Center negotiates with approximately 20 health care institutions and some 80 to 100 individual practitioners' offices in order to render its services. The services provided to both the allied health programs and the health care institutions are listed in Table 1.

EXPERIENCE WITH THE CENTER

For the clinical education period during 1976, the physical therapy faculty at the University of Michigan needed to explore potential clinical education sites because of a temporary increase in enrollment and a decrease in ongoing commitments from several facilities which had undergone significant staff changes. The University of Michigan Medical School, in which the Curriculum in Physical Therapy is a part of the Department of Physical Medicine and Rehabilitation, had already established a relationship with the Clinical Allied Health Education Center in which there was no financial commitment involved. Late in 1975, the Coordinator of Clinical Education for the Curriculum in Physical Therapy contacted the Center and described the need for additional clinical education sites. Staff of the Center requested and reviewed the objectives of the clinical education program as well as various other critical documents and procedures; for example, the criteria for selection of clinical education sites, the agreement for affiliation, and the student evaluation forms and procedures. The Assistant to the Director of the Center was identified as the contact person and liaison between the faculty and persons at the potential sites. The Coordinator of Clinical Education supplied the Center representative with a list of areas to be considered in the initial exploration of potential sites (Tab. 2). The instructions given to the Center representative were highly detailed and essential to all that he was to accomplish. The Center representative explored seven potential sites via telephone contact with the chief physical therapists and submitted written recommendations to the Co-

TABLE 2

*Considerations in Early Exploration of Potential Clinical
Education Sites*

   I. Bed capacity or agency capacity
  II. Types of patients seen in physical therapy
 III. Ratio of inpatient to outpatient load
 IV. Special learning experiences available
  V. Staff
     A. Physical therapists
       1. Educational background
       2. Years and types of experience
       3. Supervisory experience
     B. Physical therapist assistants
       1. Educational background
       2. Years of experience
     C. Supportive staff
     D. Related allied health professionals
 VI. General comments
VII. Placement possibility

ordinator of Clinical Education based on the specific criteria provided by the educational program. The Coordinator studied the information, considered the recommendations, and requested further exploration and evaluation through personal on-site visits. The Center representative coordinated the on-site visits and accompanied the Coordinator of Clinical Education in order to facilitate planning, development, and communication as well as to evaluate the site further in terms of the criteria for selection. A mutual decision was subsequently reached to establish a clinical education relationship with two of three facilities visited and to renew the relationship with a third facility which had affiliated previously with the program. The Center representative proceeded with all negotiations in establishing an agreement for affiliation with each of the facilities. He counseled the departmental representatives regarding the mechanical aspects of the clinical education program as defined by the curriculum. In addition, he sought answers and clarified information regarding financial and liability questions. Although the Center was capable of scheduling the rotations, this service was not requested by the faculty. During the implementation of the clinical education program, the Center representative provided student housing information and acted as a local contact person for students and supervisors if problems arose. He was capable of counseling students, although this service was not used. After the rotations, the Center representative contacted the chief physical therapists for feedback regarding the desirability of continuing the affiliation and subsequently coordinated the re-evaluation prior to renewing the agreements for affiliation for the following year. Evaluation of supervisor and student performance were not within the scope of the service provided by the Center representative. He was, however, an active representative of both the facility and the educational program in handling administrative and procedural matters.

The relationship with the Center has continued since 1975 with its primary yearly role of re-evaluating the facilities' continued participation in the clinical education program, re-negotiation of the annual agreement for affiliation, and implementation of the on-going programs.

ADVANTAGES OF RELATIONSHIP

Among the specific advantages of this kind of relationship are the following:
1. The Center provides the service of individuals who are knowledgeable in clinical education methods and skills.

2. The Center representative is
   - well known and accepted by administrators of health care institutions and educational programs involved.
   - knowledgeable about the objectives, policies, and procedures of the health care institutions and their educational programs.
   - knowledgeable of all allied health commitments of the institution and thereby more sensitive to demands placed on the institution.
   - readily available and a competent resource for investigating procedural and administrative questions.
   - aware of supply and demand of potential student housing sites and can advise students accordingly.
   - available to counsel students with problems which might arise during the internship.
3. Communication is facilitated because the Center representative is the sole contact person for several allied health programs (asset to institution) or for an entire geographic area (asset to educational program).

DISADVANTAGES OF RELATIONSHIP

No clear disadvantages were noted in this relationship. Potential weaknesses which are inherent but which did not negatively affect the relationship described could include 1) lack of financial commitment assuring continued service, 2) problems associated with a temporarily funded federal project, and 3) dependency by an educational program on an individual not professionally trained as a physical therapist.

CONCLUSION

The relationship between the staff of the Clinical Allied Health Education Center and the faculty of the Curriculum in Physical Therapy at the University of Michigan appears to be highly successful. No disadvantages or apparent problems have been noted. From our perspective this prototypic agency has proved to be effective and efficient. Through this relationship the faculty's efforts to explore, evaluate, develop, and implement clinical education in one geographic area have been optimized.

REFERENCE

1. Moore ML, Perry JF: Clinical Education in Physical Therapy: Present Status/Future Needs. Washington, DC, American Physical Therapy Association, 1976, Appendix B-12-22